Traumatic Brain Injury Rehabilitation

Children and Adolescents

Traumatic Brain Injury Rehabilitation

Children and Adolescents

Second Edition

Mark Ylvisaker, Ph.D.

Assistant Professor of Communication Disorders,
College of Saint Rose, Albany, New York

with 29 contributors

Butterworth–Heinemann
Boston   Oxford   Johannesburg   Melbourne   New Delhi   Singapore

Butterworth–Heinemann supports the efforts of American Forests and the Global ReLeaf program in its campaign for the betterment of trees, forests, and our environment.

Library of Congress Cataloging-in-Publication Data

Traumatic brain injury rehabilitation : children and adolescents /
  [edited by] Mark Ylvisaker. -- 2nd ed.
    p.   cm.
  Rev. ed. of: Head injury rehabilitation. c1985.
  Includes bibliographical references and index.
  ISBN 0-7506-9972-8
  1. Brain--Wounds and injuries--Complications. 2. Brain-damaged children--Rehabilitation.   I. Ylvisaker, Mark, 1944- . II. Head injury rehabilitation.
   [DNLM: 1. Brain Injuries--in infancy & childhood. 2. Brain Injuries--rehabilitation.   WS 340 T7775 1997]
  RJ496.B7T726   1997
  617.4'81044'083--dc21
  DNLM/DLC
  for Library of Congress   97-26005
                                              CIP

British Library Cataloguing-in-Publication Data
A catalogue record for this book is available from the British Library.

The publisher offers special discounts on bulk orders of this book.
For information, please contact:

Manager of Special Sales
Butterworth–Heinemann
313 Washington Street
Newton, MA 02158-1626
Tel: 617-928-2500
Fax: 617-928-2620

For information on all Butterworth–Heinemann publications available,
contact our World Wide Web home page at: http://www.bh.com.

10 9 8 7 6 5 4 3 2 1

Printed in the United States of America

This book is dedicated to Kathy, Jess, and Ben,
the best wife, daughter, and son in the history of the world!

Contents

Contributing Authors

Colleen Connolly Chester, M.S., CCC-SLP
Senior Speech-Language Therapist, The Rehabilitation Institute, Pittsburgh

Anna J.L. Chorazy, M.D.
Medical Director, The Rehabilitation Institute, Pittsburgh; Clinical Associate Professor of Pediatrics, Children's Hospital of Pittsburgh, University of Pittsburgh School of Medicine

Patricia K. Crumrine, M.D.
Associate Professor of Pediatrics, University of Pittsburgh School of Medicine; Director of Pediatric Epilepsy and EEG, Department of Child Neurology, Children's Hospital of Pittsburgh

Larry Edelman, M.S.
Senior Instructor in Pediatrics, University of Colorado Health Sciences Center, Denver

Linda Ewing-Cobbs, Ph.D.
Associate Professor of Pediatrics, University of Texas Health Science Center, Houston

Timothy J. Feeney, Ph.D.
Assistant Professor of Education, The Sage Colleges, Troy, New York

Jack M. Fletcher, Ph.D.
Professor of Pediatrics and Neurosurgery, University of Texas Houston Medical School; Neuropsychologist, Department of Pediatrics, Hermann Children's Hospital, Houston

Robert T. Fraser, Ph.D.
Director of Vocational Services, Harborview Medical Center, Seattle; Professor of Neurology, University of Washington School of Medicine, Seattle

Gerard A. Gioia, Ph.D.
Assistant Professor of Psychiatry, Johns Hopkins University School of Medicine, Baltimore; Director of Pediatric Psychology and Neuropsychology, Mt. Washington Pediatric Hospital, Baltimore

Julie Haarbauer-Krupa, M.A., CCC
Speech Pathologist, Rehabilitation Specialists of Georgia, Marietta; Clinical Instructor, Department of Special Education, Georgia State University, Atlanta

Jeanne M. Hanchett, M.D.
Clinical Associate Professor of Pediatrics, Children's Hospital of Pittsburgh, University of Pittsburgh School of Medicine; Staff Pediatrician, The Rehabilitation Institute, Pittsburgh

Kim Henry, B.S., B.S.E.E.
Rehabilitation Technology Specialist, Technical Support and Training, Sentient Systems Technology, Inc., Pittsburgh; Clinical Adjunct Instructor of Rehabilitation Science and Technology, School of Health Rehabilitation Sciences, University of Pittsburgh

Susan I. Krouse, P.T.
Brain Injury Clinical Supervisor and Physical Therapist, The Rehabilitation Institute, Pittsburgh

Amy Karas Lane, O.T.R./L.
Occupational Therapy Clinical Supervisor, The Rehabilitation Institute, Pittsburgh

Daniel Leger, R.N.
Pediatric Program Case Manager, The Rehabilitation Institute, Pittsburgh

Harvey S. Levin, Ph.D.
Professor and Director of Research, Department of Physical Medicine and Rehabilitation, Baylor College of Medicine, Houston

Jeri A. Logemann, Ph.D., CCC-SLP
Ralph and Jean Sundin Professor of Communication Sciences and Disorders, Northwestern University, Evanston, Illinois; Professor of Otolaryngology and Maxillofacial Surgery and Neurology, Northwestern University Medical School, Chicago; Professor, Cleft Palate, Northwestern University Dental School, Chicago

Phyllis-Ann Mandella, R.D.
Director of Nutritional Services, The Rehabilitation Institute, Pittsburgh

June Marshall, M.S., R.N.
Clinical Nurse Specialist, Perioperative Services, Children's Medical Center of Dallas; Clinical Assistant Professor of Nursing, Texas Woman's University, Dallas

Nancy F. Meserve, M.Ed.
Special Education Supervisor, Monroe 2–Orleans BOCES, Spencerport, New York

Gregory J. O'Shanick, M.D.
Medical Director, Brain Injury Association, Inc., Washington, D.C.;
Medical Director, Center for Neurorehabilitation Services, Richmond, Virginia

Carol Ann Robson, M.A., CCC-SLP
Supervisor of Brain Injury and Neurological Programs and Department
Co-Manager, Speech-Language Therapy, The Rehabilitation Institute, Pittsburgh

Mary Louise Russell, M.D.
Director, Children's Rehabilitation Services, Children's Hospital of Pittsburgh;
Pediatric Physiatrist, Pediatric Medical Services, The Rehabilitation Institute, Pittsburgh

Carol Wedel Sellars, Ph.D., CCC
Supervisor of Speech Pathology, Department of Rehabilitation, Gillette
Children's Specialty Healthcare, St. Paul, Minnesota

Elisabeth D. Sherwin, Ph.D.
Assistant Professor of Psychology, Georgia Southern University, Statesboro

Cynthia L. Smith, M.D.
Attending Pediatric Physiatrist, Department of Physical Medicine, Children's
Hospital of Pittsburgh; Pediatric Physiatrist, Pediatric Medical Services, The Rehabilitation Institute, Pittsburgh

Shirley F. Szekeres, Ph.D.
Associate Professor and Chair of Speech-Language Pathology, Nazareth
College of Rochester, Rochester, New York

Terri Tarquinio, O.T.R./L.
Occupational Therapist and Specialist in Rehabilitation Technology,
The Rehabilitation Institute, Pittsburgh

Pamela K. Waaland, Ph.D.
Clinical Faculty, Virginia Commonwealth University Medical College of Virginia
School of Medicine, Richmond; Affiliated Staff, St. Mary's Hospital, Richmond

Mark Ylvisaker, Ph.D.
Assistant Professor of Communication Disorders, College of Saint
Rose, Albany, New York

Preface

The real introduction to this book is provided in Chapter 1, much of which was written by young people with a history of traumatic brain injury (TBI) and their parents. They paint a picture of the real world of injury and disability, a picture that is different for each child and for each family member—and a picture that is forever incomplete. Rehabilitation and education professionals have the opportunity and responsibility to positively influence the ongoing painting of these pictures. Their work will be increasingly effective as they listen to the people they serve and embrace a collaborative orientation to their service.

This is a revised edition of *Head Injury Rehabilitation: Children and Adolescents*, published in 1985. Although that book was only a first, fledgling attempt to organize a comprehensive approach to pediatric TBI rehabilitation, it was found to be useful by many practitioners and family members. This positive reception was due in large part to the fact that the book was written by practicing clinicians, most of whom had worked together for several years, fashioning creative interventions for children and adolescents with TBI.

Much has happened since 1985. There has been substantial growth in the clinical and research literatures, along with a proliferation of providers delivering rehabilitation programs specifically designed for this population. In addition, changes in special education law have included the addition of TBI as an official educational disability, which has motivated a sharp growth in the literature dealing with the educational needs of these students. Taken together, these developments have resulted in increasing numbers of children with TBI being served by professionals sensitive to the needs of this group, which are in many cases unique.

At the same time, economic forces have dramatically reduced lengths of stay in children's hospitals and rehabilitation programs. These ongoing changes in the health care delivery system combine with the recognition of chronic and often growing disability after severe TBI in children to demonstrate the importance of seeing rehabilitation not as a brief service delivered in a medical setting, but rather as an ongoing effort to help the child and family achieve real-world goals in real-world settings. This shift in perspective from the early 1980s to the late 1990s can be detected in most of the chapters of this book.

In the late 1970s and early 1980s, those of us who were active in the field of pediatric TBI rehabilitation worked hard to understand the critical themes that defined this disability group and the ways in which these themes might be importantly different from those central to the experience of children and adolescents with other, better understood disabilities. We struggled to create and validate rehabilitation procedures and systems of care that would best serve the population. In the late 1980s, people with whom I worked became increasingly alert to the need to integrate important lessons learned by clinicians and investigators working in related fields (e.g., developmental disabilities, learning disabilities) while retaining a sensitivity to possibly unique features of TBI as a disability category. This healthy broadening of the professional horizon in TBI rehabilitation is evident in many chapters of this book.

As I write the preface to this revised edition, four critical concepts dominate my thinking as we anticipate the next century in pediatric rehabilitation. First, the only reasonable approach to pediatric TBI is prevention. Severe brain injury creates chronic disability. Those of us who work in this field of rehabilitation are justifiably enthusiastic about intervention procedures, systems of care, and laws that offer potential for improving the outcome and quality of life of children and adolescents with disability after TBI. However, there is no cure; disability persists. The future may hold breakthroughs in neuropharmacology and neurosurgery that will challenge this sober assessment. As this book goes to press, however, prevention of injuries is the only satisfactory answer to the extraordinary problem of TBI in children.

Similarly, the best approach to intervention after TBI is prevention of growing disability. When appropriate supports and services are in place and alert professionals act in a proactive manner to prevent the medical, academic, social, behavioral, and other complications frequently associated with TBI, children with severe injuries often enjoy a long-term outcome that far exceeds early expectations. In contrast, when a passive wait-and-see approach is taken, the frequent result is academic and social failure, which in turn creates developmental problems that typically require more effort and resources than would have been required by early preventive efforts.

Third, with decreasing lengths of stay in rehabilitation centers and shrinking resources for rehabilitation, professionals must redouble their efforts to collaborate with everyday people in the child's world. For most children with chronic disability after TBI, the most critical deliverers of rehabilitation services are everyday people in the child's life, including family members, school staff, paraprofessionals, and others. These everyday people can be expected to do their jobs well only if well-informed rehabilitation specialists create effective alliances with them and work to ensure that they are as informed, competent, and supported as possible.

Finally, related to this commitment to collaborating with everyday people in the child's life is a frank recognition that good rehabilitation must include a focus on real-world issues and provision of services and supports in real-world settings. This focus is necessitated both by the ongoing reduction in resources for medical rehabilitation and, more positively, by the growing body of evidence that learning occurs more efficiently in the contexts in which that learning must be applied.

This book is long and may seem intimidating to active clinicians who have little time for study in their busy lives and who, therefore, seek to improve their practice without investing large quantities of precious time. I hope that the book offers readers a handsome return on their investment and that they will find an appropriate balance of principles and rationale, on the one hand, with practical assessment and intervention procedures on the other. The authors have sought to present principles and procedures that are practical and applicable to a wide range of ages, disabilities, and domains of professional practice. They have also maintained a commitment to scholarship essential to a book that is intended to be more than a "how-to" manual. My hope is that their work will offer direction to those charged with helping children with TBI and their families create successful and satisfying lives.

Mark Ylvisaker

Acknowledgments

Many acknowledgments and thanks are in order after completing a project of this magnitude. My wife, Kathy, has provided me with many wonderful ideas for serving children and adolescents with special needs. In addition, she has put up with all too many long days of work and tired recitations of "I'd really like to do that, but unfortunately I have to get this chapter done." She is an incredible wife. My daughter, Jessica, did much of the artwork for the book. Her talent knows no bounds. My son, Ben, has been my computer consultant for some time and is entirely responsible for my current state of helplessness in that area. I thank him for that contribution, sort of.

The contributors to this book are a dedicated group of clinicians and investigators whose wisdom derives largely from their work in the trenches, where the best lessons in rehabilitation are learned. I thank them for the many early mornings and late nights they added to their real-world schedules to complete their contribution to this book.

Mainly I want to thank the hundreds of children and adolescents with traumatic brain injury I have known over the years, as well as their families. I thank them for sharing intense times in their lives with me, for giving me a real-world education in the realities of brain injury in young people, and for being a constant source of inspiration in my life.

Chapter 1

Traumatic Brain Injury in Children and Adolescents: Introduction

Mark Ylvisaker

This book is about people, young people whose lives have been changed in dramatic ways by an event that resulted in injury to their brain. Associated with the changes in these individual lives are changes in countless other lives, including those of family members and friends. Rehabilitation professionals have the honor and the responsibility of working with these people as they recreate meaning, hope, success, and satisfaction in their lives. We do our jobs well only if we listen to the people we serve. Because this book is ultimately about people and the meaning that they create for themselves in their lives after a life-altering injury, it is appropriate that these people be permitted to introduce the subject of this text.

Kelly: Injured at Age 16

Poignant Stains

Mutely I wonder
what would have happened
had I been two minutes earlier
my mind is now covered in grime
thinking, who did this—
who decided it was going to be us?
And all the doctors,
lifeless eyes, and
condescending attitudes
would never have been ours
to deal with
so much has been taken away
and I can't help but feel
guilty for not being
content with these changes

could have been worse, but
we'll never feel the same again
we aren't the same
Added negativity, the positive just drowns
all these feelings create the
emptiness
because no one knows except
us and we never talk to each other
am I alone?
"Alive She Cried,"*
I wonder mutely
Why.

Ryan: Injured at Age 16

My head injury was a turning point in my life that directed me onto a new path. Since the injury, I've learned the importance of such wonderful things as learning and living. In the beginning of my recovery, I remember not accepting the reality or the consequences of this new term I never stopped hearing— *head injury*. I told myself I would abolish the memory of this traumatic event. So I began to do just that. In me there grew a quiet aggressiveness that let me persevere tirelessly toward a triumph within my soul. I do not know if I have reached this peak yet, but if I was told that I have, I would believe it.

My head injury has done something to me that nothing else will ever do to me. It was terribly traumatic, but, most importantly, it taught me that nothing is impossible and that makes me very happy. The long hours of therapy were not positive for me, but they paid off beautifully. Ironically, professionals helped with their upsetting prognoses. Of course, it

---

*Jim Morrison, The Doors.

was probably hard for them to present bad news to me and my parents. But I wasn't going to accept their predictions. I worked to prove them wrong and now, almost 2 years after my injury, I am attending college, studying until the lights go out—and on my face glows a smile of triumph.

This is what they need: Kids must know that they still have a power—a power they may not have known existed. If they discover this strength and use it, they will learn what it is to succeed. They will be proud. I learned this as I reflected on all of the work and doctor appointments and therapy sessions. I reflected and pieced things together in one train of thought. These sessions of recollective, ponderous thought gave me the fuel to accelerate toward the light that shone in the distance of the one-lane road to recovery. In dealing with difficulty, I abandoned feelings of difficulty. I have worked the hardest I have ever worked in my life. In return, I have received great pleasure in knowing that I have succeeded.

Karin: Injured at Age 14

What kind of character am I writing into my life for myself?? I hope that my character will play the role of hero! I know about being a hero. I was a starter on my fourth-grade softball team and hit a home run (well, with the help of some errors). In sixth grade, I played clarinet in the all-star band; so I must have been good? Mainly I know about being a hero because I survived an accident that should have killed me. And when I was discharged from rehab, they told me that I would probably not graduate from high school. Because of that, high school graduation was very special to me. They said that college was a definite no, which made college graduation even more special to me. Eight years ago, I never even expected to go to college, let alone to graduate only 1 year after my freshman class. So I'm a hero, right?

But despite all of this, I think mainly I feel like a victim. Many people would not think I should say that; but that's the way I feel. My two best friends before the accident abandoned me. Before the accident I was an excellent roller skater, but now I've gotten out of the habit of roller skating. I have been told that I was always smiling before the accident, and I was always surrounded by my friends. In college, I couldn't keep a roommate for more than one semester. They all moved out. Before the accident, I always had something to do, especially on my birthday. I was very active. Now, for my birthday, I don't do much. My mom takes me out to dinner, usually, which is not good for my figure. Since I have stopped doing my exercises, I have gained a great deal of weight.

I guess this is me, the victim. I get angry now when things don't go my way. My mom says that I have always been like that, but it seems to be worse now. I flip out about the littlest and stupidest things you could ever imagine. Mom says I need to grow up. But my childhood was stolen from me, so I don't want to grow up.

Sometimes I forget just how fortunate I have been since the accident. And I really want to be a hero. If I could just get a job that actually lasts longer than 3 weeks, I think that I will most definitely play the role of hero. I will be a hero because I will be able to support myself and maybe even help Mom out a little. I want to work for an attorney; just like my last job—but one where I'll actually get paid. Maybe God has a job for me and I just haven't found it yet? Also, I'd like to play the role of wife. Maybe not the mother role, but definitely wife. I will be a hero, maybe.

Kathy, Mother of Ryan, Injured at Age 16

I'm not sure I understand the meaning in Ryan's accident. There is no answer to why it happened. However, the meaningful change in me is that I will never again take anyone I love for granted, assuming that they will be here tomorrow.

Hardest for me was getting used to the new Ryan. I would watch every move, listen to every word, and compare the old Ryan with the new. Two years later, I am only just discovering that this "new" Ryan is a great kid whom I admire and love. I envy his love of life and the peace that I see in him. He will never be what he was, but he is becoming someone he never could have been.

Prayer was most helpful to me, followed by my wonderful friends who listened without judgment and advice—the ones who didn't try to "fix" what couldn't be fixed. Professionals could take a lesson from some of my friends, a lesson in compassion, a lesson in understanding. It is much easier to hear bad news from a person you feel truly cares.

And the news doesn't all have to be bad. Families need hope; they need to know about children who have defied the odds and have done well after the worst injuries. Without hope, people give in and give up. With hope, it is possible to work hard, remain determined, bounce back. Ryan now attends college on an academic scholarship; and he has good friends, some old ones and some new ones. If we had believed the professional who told us he would lose his friends and not finish high school, we might have given up.

But Ryan didn't give up. We are thrilled for him. Prayer, hope, and determination!

Beth, Mother of John, Injured at Age 14

"I'm not complaining too much . . . The reality is not exactly what the song started out to be, but it's not a bad song" (Robert James Waller, *The Bridges of Madison County*). There have been many good things that have grown in our lives since John's accident, 14 years ago. The seeds were sown early in his rehabilitation when professionals took the time to listen to me, gave me opportunities to learn, and supported me in all of my efforts. They helped me believe that I could manage apparently impossible situations and that there would always be support when it was needed. They helped me to be a "whatever it takes" person—and I have succeeded.

In counseling, I learned skills that I still practice: analytical problem solving, caregiver care, network building, humor, and self-talk. Self-talk has been the easiest for me. My head is filled with wisdom, passed down through others, wisdom that creates perspective, calm, resilience, and power: This too shall pass; it takes a village to raise a child; there is nothing new under the sun; one day at a time; don't make a mountain out of a molehill; Rome wasn't built in a day; save your ammunition for the big fight. . . .

I was wisely cautioned early on to take good care of myself. I am a single parent: Who would be there for John if I failed? In the beginning, caring for myself meant occasionally staying in bed all day, sleeping, and reading. But it worked; I am still here, healthy and happy. And I still allow time in the day for exercise, quiet time, hobbies, and real time off occasionally.

Professionals also stressed the importance of building networks of support. During the crisis weeks in the acute-care hospital, I learned from family and friends what caring and support mean. And over the years, I have cast my net widely, yielding many friends, a world of learning and sharing, and a wealth of information. We must watch that we do not become isolated. We may need help creating our networks of support.

In our family, we have always used humor to survive tough times and, since the accident, I have laughed through many crises that may otherwise have been unbearable. But it was only recently that John and I both decided to take humor seriously. We became clowns. We both graduated from clown school and our education continues through monthly classes, charity events, conferences, and practice. Think about it—clowns get laughs for acting inappropriately!!!

Professionals encouraged me to learn everything I could learn about brain injury. For me, knowledge is therapeutic. Mysteries are more frightening than events and conditions that I understand. I would not have succeeded in my role as John's case manager over the years without a solid base of knowledge. I was also urged to be an active participant, not just a passive receiver of information. So I became active in the Brain Injury Association; I began to help other families; I went to meetings and made contacts. It was in this way that I regained control and the strength that a sense of control creates.

A physician once looked at me—after I had asked a critical question in her area of expertise— and said, "I don't know." I was dumbfounded to hear these words from a medical person. But the honesty in the statement not only created admiration for the physician; it also gave me permission to learn and to explore creatively. I was no longer intimidated by experts. I felt an invitation to join a community of honest people searching for answers.

And there certainly are questions for which we have no good answers. John was injured as he was entering his teen years and therefore beginning to explore sexuality. Over the years, programs have addressed his "inappropriate" sexual acting out with behavior modification, educational classes, psychosocial group discussions on relationships, private counseling, and medication. Fine. But what John really needed was a girlfriend. It has been our experience that most providers of rehabilitation are afraid to allow their residents to make friends. This subject continues to be mainly taboo. No professional ever willingly discussed with me, John's main advocate and caregiver, how to answer his questions, how to help him meet his needs. I have had to be the one to explore the real world of handicapped dating, masturbation, surrogates. This has been an adventure I could never have anticipated. Visualize a gray-haired mother (grandmother!!) reading through soft-porn ads, scanning the yellow pages, asking the hotel concierges in Las Vegas for information about how to get John to the Chicken Ranch (brothel) so that he could assure himself that his performance abilities were normal and so that his self-esteem could be restored. Then I had to explain brain injury to a delightful madam at the Chicken Ranch. Finally, I had found somebody willing and able to talk about the real world!

Why can't rehabilitation address life in the real world—and all of life in the whole real world? Why can't sexuality be part of rehabilitation? Why does a mother need to take responsibility for helping her young adult son find ways to become a man and feel complete?

In retrospect, I look at the last question and answer it myself: Why not the mother? I am the caregiver. But I did not do it alone. John helped. Other people helped. It was a problem. We solved it. There will be other problems and we will solve them together.

Judy, Mother of Karin, Injured at Age 14

Prayer was the most important and powerful of all meanings for me. When I got to the hospital, the chaplain was there to comfort me. He was strength at that most important time when I needed to be calm. My son was driving and he had some injuries, but not as serious as my daughter's, so I needed to be there for him as well as for her. I had to be careful not to judge him or blame him in any way. The chaplain stayed with me until my daughter was stabilized; then he made arrangements for my son to be taken home and cared for by neighbors so I could stay with my daughter. Family and neighbors were very caring and helpful, and continue to be so—watching our house when we are away, giving us a ride when we need one, sending us food from their gardens, sitting with us and talking.

Staff at the rehabilitation hospital treated Karin—and me—with love, respect, and kindness. That is what helped the most. For 7½ months they were there for us, explaining everything they did and making me part of Karin's routines—even making use of my knowledge and expertise. Their truthfulness and integrity meant a great deal, never condescending, never too busy to talk and offer encouragement. And they encouraged me to be hopeful. They are still excited to see us when we visit. Some have become personal friends, and they keep in touch since they have left and gone on to other jobs. They are very pleased with Karin's progress.

Most difficult for me is watching Karin struggle to become whole again. She was intelligent and self-sufficient before the accident, and so mature at the age of 14. Now she is childlike in some ways and gets very frustrated. She lacks self-confidence. She feels her friends have abandoned her. She has no patience with herself or anyone else. The medical problems are taken care of, but she still has a long way to go with the social and emotional problems. It frustrates me that I can't make it right for her. I keep thinking if I can help her get the confidence to be self-sufficient, she will be able to be her own person. It gets harder and harder. My life is to get her to be able to care for herself, have self-confidence to function on her own, and to be whole again. Karin was spared for a purpose, and I thank God each and every day that I can watch her grow again. Because that is what it's like—watching your child grow again.

Kathleen, Mother of Megan, Injured at Age 5

"When in the course of human events it becomes necessary for one people to dissolve the political bonds which have connected them to another. . . ." With the exception of the word *political*, the beginning of the Declaration of Independence sounds like a description of what happens after a brain injury and a new battle for independence begins. Who's involved?

A defining of fundamental issues and relationships occurs after brain injury for more than the survivor. Parents, siblings, and all those who support the child in this struggle are involved. I can think of no more polarizing injury. It produces sets of extremes. After an often breathtaking journey through basic physical survival, the struggle immediately begins to chart new ground where strengths and abilities can flourish—all in the face of staggering losses, losses that ricochet throughout the lives of everyone connected to the child. Despite watching it happen repeatedly, I remain amazed at the resilience and creativity—or paralysis and destruction—that result from this adversity.

I have never survived a brain injury but have watched the struggles of my 5-year-old daughter, alternating among holding my breath, sighing in relief, struggling in silence, and bursting with pride and joy. I have experienced and watched the process of healing in some family members, despite the fact that there was no "cure." And I have been enriched beyond imagination by the resolute friendship and steadfast love I've encountered in this 17-year journey. I've repeatedly seen the persistent bravery and fighting spirit that searches for independence evident in many injured children. I've seen it matched by an equally insistent need for dependence on others. Some people insist someone else negotiate their decisions, thus avoiding risks. All deal with overwhelming loss and fear. One fights for independence, overcoming the terrible predictions—you will never walk, live on your own, talk, think clearly, finish school. . . . Another is seemingly paralyzed in spirit, unable to set goals and grow. I have watched people with eyes flashing while they struggle to whisper an answer or type out a comment or question. One child reaches out to another to coach or cajole him through the same struggle. Other children complain how hard their life is. We all have moments in our lives when we may do these things. I do know that we can encourage either response in others. We all play a part in supporting chronic winning or chronic whining. I have done both. Winning is better!

An important guide for my thinking now is knowing that individuals do their own work. I haven't done it for my daughter. I have applauded it, encouraged it, coached it, assisted it; but she does it or doesn't do it. It's her work. Children who are injured need to learn or relearn how to set and accomplish their goals. I think that initially we all hope for a "cure." However, what we do when there are still things that just don't "get better" is the more persistent challenge. Creating the opportunity for healing the wounds that aren't cured—that's the role of a good rehabilitation team. I believe that some survivors are a decision away from beginning the process of healing, and with the right support— maybe mixed with confrontation—they can begin. I know that support from my relationships with God, family, friends, neighbors, and church helps me when I wrestle with a complex problem. I want to be understood in my pain and struggle. Then I can have patience with myself as I work out my solution.

I believe that understanding means having someone "stand under" and support me while I totter tenuously, until my own feet and legs can carry me again. I believe that one of the main things we can do for survivors of brain injury is to understand them—that is, "stand under" them while they do their work. It is often exhausting. At times, it is scary. We sometimes need to take a break and laugh at our mistakes. We sometimes need to be uncooperative. It is a long journey. The victories are exhilarating. It is a privilege to watch them; it is an even greater privilege to participate.

I have seen the power of "standing under" by a whole group of people committed to the task of rehabilitation. Everyone is richer for sharing and respecting each other's competencies and discovering solutions together. Everyone needs support in the process, even professionals. This ensures that we avoid forcing our opinions and agendas on the survivors, families, or professionals. We avoid helping survivors do what we want them to do so that we can feel good about ourselves. We avoid promoting a need for us to the point that survivors compromise or fear their independence. We are more able to respect their choices to "get better" or not. We do it best when we are simultaneously working on our own goals and solutions. How can we teach what we don't know? Can we know something if we don't do it? It's the only way to trust ourselves and survivors in this process. It's the secret to avoid taking a seeming "failure" personally. We are participating in the formation of someone's life in her most vulnerable moments. It is a constant challenge to learn how best to coach kids through this process. But that's the job. It's called loving people, and it's worthy of our best efforts.

So how do we practice standing under those who are experiencing the extreme circumstances of brain injury? Who makes up the team? I am a mom, and I'm on the team. I am not supposed to be my child's therapist. I tried it. It didn't work, and I jeopardized my relationship with my daughter. In the beginning, I was frantic to do anything that would help her "get better." I was encouraged to be her therapist, and I was a very cooperative mom. For a time, my daughter lost herself

and her mom. Her older sister lost her best friend and saw her mom turn into a quasi-therapist—another loss. When you're 8 years old, your imagination runs free. If you simultaneously see your sister, mom, and dad all acting weird—well, *terror* is the closest word I can think of. Sadness, frustration, and anger. I want things the way they were. Doesn't everyone? But they're not. What's next? Can I be safe?

Providing parents and siblings access to information on a continuing basis, explaining and allowing mourning—that is, standing under each family member in the journey through this pain—are critical components if the family is actively to promote rehabilitation. The alternative jeopardizes the process. Children need to know that they can still be buddies but that things will be different and sometimes really hard. Talking about these things is crucial but is more effective if parents aren't always involved. We can find help through community resources, churches, and possibly professional counselors. Parents and children want to talk to people who feel that *their* agendas are important. Children have felt isolated and frightened because they were ignored or talked to as if they couldn't understand. It does not have to be formal counseling or a support group. Siblings are a particularly powerful influence at home and in the community. They can understand that different is okay. They make a difference. We must recognize and use their strengths.

Brain injury combines staggering loss with enormous opportunities for new life. I grieve the loss of the old familiar life and its relationships. It was imperfect but comfortable; now it's gone. In one instant. Little things repeatedly remind me of it . . . and I grieve again. At the same time, I learn to focus on the possibilities for a new life. I can do better by working with others and remembering what I may have forgotten. And I embrace the privilege of participating in my daughter's creation of her life, by standing under her until she moves forward, declaring her independence.

Central Themes of Rehabilitation After TBI in Children and Adolescents

These statements from young people and their parents, John's Rules at the end of this chapter, and the experience of professionals who have been actively engaged in pediatric rehabilitation combine to yield important themes that are elaborated throughout this book.

Variety

Kelly, Ryan, Karin, and John are very different from one another, as are their parents. They all had different lives before their injury, and the injuries created even more profound differences among these interesting people. The same can be said of the thousands of children and adolescents who have a severe brain injury in the United States every year. Traumatic brain injury (TBI) is unlike other disability categories, in that there is nothing common to all members of this group other than the medical event labeled TBI. Differences are a consequence of the child's age, ability and achievement levels, culture, and personality before the injury; the nature and severity of the injury or injuries; the quality of early medical intervention; the quality of ongoing rehabilitation and educational services; the response of family and friends, including their ability to provide ongoing support for the child; available resources and opportunities; and the young person's own resilience and evolving response to life with disability.

Frank acknowledgment of this extreme variety in the population has implications for the clinical and educational practices of rehabilitation and education professionals. On the negative side, extreme variety implies that the development of specific test batteries and intervention programs and curricula for this disability group is unwise. In many cases, assessment and intervention materials and strategies developed for other disability populations are equally useful for children and adolescents with TBI. In *every* case, decisions about assessment, intervention, and support must be based on highly individualized considerations, not simply on the diagnosis of TBI.

Commonalities

Having acknowledged the extreme variability within this group of people, it is equally important to understand the central tendencies—the themes—that make TBI a useful disability category and justify books on the subject. The fact that the injury and subsequent disability are acquired after a period of normal development creates important themes that may distinguish this group from those children and adolescents whose disabilities have existed since birth. For example, children and adolescents with TBI often experience unspeakable losses, including the loss of abilities, anticipated levels of accomplishment, cherished activities, and friends. It is difficult for anybody— particularly young people just beginning to understand themselves and to choose their life's path—to acknowledge extreme losses, mourn those losses, and move on with a life defined by new limits, modified goals, and different circles of people. In Chapter 16, Sherwin and O'Shanick describe some of the supports that may be helpful for children and adolescents struggling with these losses as they build their new lives.

Family members also mourn the loss of the child they knew and loved, while also learning to know and love the child who emerges over time after the injury. This mourning is complicated by the reality that, in one important

sense, there was no loss—the child lived. It may also be complicated by the ill-conceived counsel of unwise professionals that family members *accept* the reality of fundamental change in their child—a reality that they know in their hearts is *unacceptable*. In Chapter 16, Waaland describes ways that rehabilitation professionals can be helpful to family members as they attempt to adjust to a life that is often punctuated by ongoing crises.

Other commonalities within the population of children and adolescents with TBI are created by known vulnerabilities within the brain during and after the injury. For example, it has long been known that the frontal lobes, associated with general executive or self-control functions, and the limbic system, associated with memory and a variety of behavioral and emotional functions, are particularly vulnerable in closed head injury as well as other types of brain injury. In Chapter 2, Ewing-Cobbs and colleagues describe the many cognitive, social, behavioral, and academic consequences of injury to these areas of the developing brain. To be sure, specific types of injury do not necessarily predict specific types and severity of deficit. Functional outcome is the result of a complex interaction between the child's preinjury functioning, injury, and postinjury supports and challenges. Furthermore, multiple areas of impairment interact in complex ways. Nevertheless, the particular vulnerabilities associated with TBI in children necessitate a disproportionate focus on cognitive, social, behavioral, and academic domains of intervention in their rehabilitation, thereby explaining the relative weights assigned to these domains in this book.

A final group of commonalities is due to the epidemiologic fact that TBI is not evenly distributed in the population. There are groups of children and adolescents at risk for TBI, including children who had behavior or learning problems before the injury, adolescents who were extreme risk takers before the injury, and children whose disadvantaged families had difficulty managing their lives before the injury. Certainly, many children and adolescents with TBI do not come from these high-risk groups. However, the challenges associated with the risk factors must be acknowledged, because they influence the types of services and supports that may be necessary after the injury.

Developmental Themes

Children are not short adults. Their lives are dominated by quite different abilities, needs, interests, activities, limitations, relationships, and biological vulnerabilities at different ages. Young children are also much more integrally connected within their family and dependent on their family than are adults.

Child and Family

Brain injuries in children are also injuries in families. Although it may make sense to consider adults, distinct from their families, as isolated targets of rehabilitation efforts, the target of pediatric rehabilitation must be the child in the context of the family. Parents are not only the primary support for their children, ultimately they are also the primary deliverers of long-term rehabilitation services. This extraordinary responsibility is placed on them at a time when they are most vulnerable because of their own need to mourn their losses. Therefore, pediatric rehabilitation programs must make every effort to serve and support family members, including siblings and possibly extended family members as well as parents, in their attempts to positively influence the child's outcome. In Chapter 16, Waaland describes many of these services and supports.

The importance of supporting families in pediatric rehabilitation is underscored by the repeated finding that the child's long-term outcome is profoundly influenced by the quality of life at home after the injury. That is, children who are well understood by their families and effectively managed at home tend to have a better outcome, particularly in behavioral and psychosocial domains, than comparably injured children who do not enjoy this advantage.

Age at Injury

The needs of children injured in infancy differ in important ways from those of older preschoolers, which in turn differ from those of young school-age children, which in turn differ from those of adolescents. For example, school is the primary context for ongoing rehabilitation for school-age children, but not for very young children or adults. Furthermore, within the group of school-age children, the academic demands and the school context differ dramatically from early grade school to high school. Because of their importance in pediatric rehabilitation, school themes are specifically addressed in Chapters 17 and 18. In many of the other chapters of this book, the authors explicitly address the differences in the needs of children at different developmental stages. The cognitive, psychosocial, and family needs of preschoolers are specifically addressed in Chapter 14.

Age and Brain Plasticity

It has long been assumed that youth confers an advantage in outcome after brain injury, an assumption that may partially explain the slow development of programs for children with TBI. In Chapter 2, Ewing-Cobbs and colleagues cite several sources of evidence that call this traditional principle into question, particularly in relation to functions associated with the vulnerable prefrontal and limbic areas of the brain. Investigators and clinicians have increasingly highlighted the possibility of delayed consequences of brain injury in young people. That is, a specific injury may not manifest itself functionally until later in development when the function associated with that part of the brain is expected to mature. The mounting evidence that young children may be more rather than less vulnerable than older people in certain critical areas of functioning is

sobering and should motivate rehabilitation professionals to redouble their efforts for this group.

Long-Term Outcome

Because children are a work in progress and because their long-term development is a product of a large number of interacting factors, predictions of long-term outcome are most often hazardous. Ben's experience, described by Ylvisaker and Feeney in Chapter 13, vividly illustrates the unpredictability of outcome. The location and severity of his injury led many to predict that his long-term cognitive and behavioral outcome would be severely compromised. In fact, his behavior fluctuated between severely challenging (including physical aggression and self-injury) and admirably compliant over the years after his injury, depending largely on the behavior-management system as well as cognitive and social supports available to him at any given time. Furthermore, at 10 years postinjury, he is successfully employed, an outcome many would have considered impossible during the first year or two after his injury. In Chapter 11, Ylvisaker and colleagues describe a young man whose cognitive and academic performance dramatically fluctuated over the school years after brain injury, depending on the cognitive supports and teaching practices available to him at the time.

These and other individual histories, together with the growing body of evidence that family, school, and social supports have a powerful impact on long-term outcome, should inspire rehabilitation and education professionals, and at the same time foster a sense of profound obligation to positively influence outcome. Outcome is not the inevitable unfolding of biological consequences of the injury. It is rather an ongoing journey, powerfully influenced by intelligent decisions made by many people along the way. Professionals who serve children and families in the early weeks and months after the injury should interpret these realities as conferring on them the responsibility of ensuring that the long road before the child is paved as effectively as possible. This includes ensuring that the people who make the greatest difference in the long run, including family, school personnel, and friends, are fully oriented, trained, and supported so that they can play their role as effective supports for the child. This theme is elaborated in Chapter 20.

Assessment Themes

Several chapters in this book present technical issues in assessment from varied professional perspectives. While acknowledging the importance of technically sophisticated assessments, professionals should also work collaboratively with everyday people (including family members, paraprofessional staff, and others) and with the child or adolescent in completing these assessments. The goal of functional assessment is to determine what needs to be done and what can be done to help the child succeed. That is, the focus of assessment is not merely the underlying, neurologic impairment, but the functional disability associated with that impairment, the real-world handicap created by that disability, and all of the strengths that the child and significant others bring to the task of overcoming the disability and social handicap. This assessment is best accomplished in collaboration with everyday people, in the context of everyday activities, and using the procedures of contextualized hypothesis testing. Assessment understood in these practical terms helps to overcome the serious challenges to the validity of office-bound assessments. These challenges are described in Chapter 10.

Collaboration with Everyday People

In Chapters 10 and 20, Ylvisaker, Gioia, and Feeney describe some of the benefits associated with organizing assessment as a collaborative process that includes the contributions of everyday people. In most cases, collaborating with real-world people not only enriches the assessment, it also confers collegiality and a shared sense (among professionals and everyday people) of ownership of intervention programs that have an important payoff in consistency and intensity of intervention. Furthermore, actively engaging family members and others in practical assessment tasks may be one of the most efficient ways of educating them about brain injury and management of the child.

Collaboration with the Child

In Chapter 12, Ylvisaker and colleagues describe procedures for self-assessment and discuss collaboration with the child or adolescent in assessment as a critical component of ongoing intervention in the area of executive functions. That is, if professionals jealously guard their monopoly on such activities as evaluating the child's abilities, setting goals for the child, monitoring progress, and making revisions in the intervention when necessary, they are depriving the child of exactly those experiences needed to facilitate growth in the area of executive functions and self-determination.

Intervention Themes

The nature and intensity of rehabilitation services, as well as the settings in which they are delivered, may differ dramatically among children with TBI, depending on a host of factors. It is difficult to think of any approach to intervention that is not useful for some children with TBI, at some stage of recovery, and with some profile of needs. However, the experience of clinicians since the 1970s underscores the importance of the following general intervention themes—themes that have been lived by the young people and parents whose first-person accounts opened this chapter.

Prevention of Injuries

The only truly effective intervention for TBI is prevention of the injury. This important truism is dictated by the fundamental reality that rehabilitation interventions for people with chronic brain injury are rarely curative. Good rehabilitation holds the promise of reducing impairment—and associated disability and handicap—and of helping people achieve their goals as effectively as possible despite ongoing disability. However, there is no cure.

People concerned with brain injury in children are, therefore, motivated to be as active as possible in prevention efforts. Legislation and social practices related to highway safety (e.g., increasing use of airbags in automobiles) along with increasing use of bicycle helmets have prevented a large number of brain injuries in children in recent years. Unfortunately, these epidemiologic gains have been counterbalanced by a growing number of injuries associated with assault and abuse. Injury prevention remains a top priority for rehabilitation professionals.

Prevention of Academic Failure

Before the implementation of TBI as an official educational disability, many children returned to school with a profile of academic abilities that did not seem to qualify them for special services or supports. In many cases, the result of early inattention to genuine educational needs was academic failure that increased over time, inevitably mixed with growing social and emotional challenges associated with that failure. After many months or years of failure, a child's downward developmental trajectory is difficult to reverse. On the other hand, appropriate educational supports implemented proactively hold the promise of preventing long-term failure and easing the long-term burden on schools, child, and family alike. Educational services and supports commonly used with children with TBI are discussed in Chapters 17 and 18.

Prevention of Social Failure

After a life-altering injury, it is difficult for children and adolescents to maintain a sense of competence and create satisfying social lives for themselves. Old friends often go their separate ways. Potential new friends may not fit the injured child's sense of social acceptability. Previously satisfying social activities may be ruled out by the new disability. Isolation and crushing loneliness are often a consequence. In Chapter 15, Sherwin and O'Shanick address the myriad issues associated with social success and satisfaction, and how professionals may help children and adolescents with TBI achieve satisfying social lives.

Prevention of Behavioral Failure

Prevention of growing behavior problems over the years after TBI depends in large part on preventing academic and social failure. In addition, people who serve children with behavior problems associated with brain injury should be familiar with a neuropsychological profile that mandates a focus on antecedent or proactive behavior management as opposed to the more typical contingency or consequence management. Positive, antecedent-focused approaches to behavior are discussed in Chapter 13, along with their neuropsychological and empirical rationale. Serious brain injury may also result in *primary*, neurologically based behavior problems that are best managed pharmacologically. In Chapter 5, O'Shanick discusses some of the special considerations in psychopharmacology for children with acquired brain injury.

Functional and Contextualized Intervention

Accumulated evidence from decades of intervention research with other disability groups combines with more recent studies of intervention for people with TBI to underscore the importance of a functional and richly contextualized approach to rehabilitation. Gains in performance achieved under laboratory or purely clinical training conditions rarely transfer without great effort to everyday activities in everyday contexts. Providing rehabilitation in the context of functional activities is an important step in the direction of addressing the classic problem of transfer of training. This theme is emphasized by Russell and colleagues and by Chester and colleagues in their discussions of physical rehabilitation in Chapters 6 and 8, respectively. The same themes are emphasized by Ylvisaker and colleagues in all chapters that address cognitive and communication intervention.

Ironically, the hard economic realities imposed by managed care may have the positive effect of forcing professionals to seek functional, everyday activities as the context for ongoing rehabilitation. For example, when appropriately trained and supervised, physical education teachers or health club personnel may provide ongoing physical therapy in a context that is natural and motivating for young people and may therefore support more efficient transfer of new skills to everyday life than does ongoing therapy in a medical setting. Similarly, attention to voice and speech improvement in the context of the school chorus or drama class may have analogous benefits, while consuming fewer health care dollars. Cognitive and executive system intervention may be more effectively pursued in a classroom, with appropriately trained and supported school staff, than in isolated therapies where the constant threat of failure of transfer looms large. Practical guidance in contextualizing intervention is offered by most of the chapters in this book.

Integrative Intervention

Many of the common themes in pediatric brain injury rehabilitation require tireless collaborative efforts. The most serious problems faced by children and adolescents with TBI are typically the domain of several rehabilitation or educational professionals. Rather than serving as the occasion for territorial skirmishes or exhausting efforts at careful role delineation and separation, recognition of this fact should lead professionals to embrace collaboration and integration of services. Furthermore, because family members and paraprofessionals are often the people whose skill and competence make the largest difference for the child with chronic disability, they must be viewed as critical members of the team of collaborators. This theme echoes through the parents' statements earlier in this chapter. Most of the chapters in this book are collaboratively written by people from diverse professional backgrounds, whose experience in the trenches has been enriched by intense cross-disciplinary collaboration.

Engagement of Everyday People in Pediatric Rehabilitation

Collaboration between rehabilitation professionals and everyday people in the child's life, mentioned above, deserves its own heading. After TBI, children are ideally surrounded by competent, optimistic, creative, and flexible people who know how to turn every activity and interaction with the child into one with rehabilitative value. A quick survey of the lives of children with disability in medical or home and school settings reveals that the majority of their time is spent with people who either have no training in rehabilitation or, as aides or paraprofessionals, have very little training. This fact should motivate rehabilitation professionals to focus much of their time and energy on helping these everyday people to become the best caregivers and teachers they can be for children with TBI. It should also encourage systems of care and third-party payers to increase their recognition of the critical importance of training and support for everyday people. This theme is further explored in Chapter 20.

Long-Term Focus in Rehabilitation

Earlier, I emphasized the difficulty of predicting long-term outcome and needs in children with TBI. Many do surprisingly well and achieve a level of success one would not dare predict early after the injury. Others experience developmental struggles over time that are more intense than suggested by the severity of the injury. Others, like Ben described in Chapter 13, have a developmental course best described as a roller coaster ride.

This central theme in pediatric TBI mandates an ongoing safety net for these children and adolescents. The safety net includes trained adults sensitive to the developmental problems that are possible consequences of the injury and sufficiently flexible to adjust services and supports over time, as the child experiences greater or lesser need. Just as errors can be made on the side of insufficient supports, they can also be made on the side of a system of supports that is too intense and leads to learned helplessness in the child and a failure to facilitate the level of development that is possible.

A long-term focus also mandates early attention to dimensions of development that may not seem, on the surface, relevant early in life. For example, in their chapter on rehabilitation for preschoolers, Ylvisaker and colleagues emphasize the importance of focusing on early development of executive functions, often thought to be late developmental acquisitions. The reality is that children with no identified disability have many years of developmentally normal "rehearsal" of executive functions before they are expected to be mature, self-regulated and self-determined young adults. Children with disability are often denied these rehearsal experiences, which can only jeopardize their development in this critical area of human function. Similarly, in Chapter 19, Fraser emphasizes the importance of an early focus on prevocational activities to prevent the all-too-common phenomenon of students with disability entering the world of work without the critical work habits and attitudes that dictate success in most jobs.

Funding Environment and Resources for Rehabilitation

In Chapter 6, Russell and colleagues describe draconian reductions in the average length of stay in their pediatric TBI rehabilitation program. Their experience is not unique. Managed care and other forces have resulted in serious reductions in resources available for brain-injury rehabilitation. At the same time, funding for regular and special education has been cut or threatened in many parts of the United States.

Several of the authors in this book acknowledge this changing environment for rehabilitation and call for an intensified focus on empowering nonspecialists, including community professionals, school staff, family members, aides, and other support people. Highly trained rehabilitation professionals are increasingly called on to distribute their expertise so that the child who has limited interaction with specialists may nevertheless benefit from that expertise over the long run. In Chapter 20, Ylvisaker and Feeney describe a rationale for collaborating with everyday people in the child's life and offer procedures for creating this collaboration and empowering everyday people so that they are in a position to play their role effectively over the years following the injury.

Creating a Satisfying Life: Personal Meaning

When all is said and done—when the last page is written and read—we return to individual human beings working to create meaningful, satisfying lives for themselves.

Therefore, this introduction to TBI in children and adolescents ends with John's rules. John knows this world—the world of young people struggling to create meaning in their lives after brain injury—as well as anybody. He has experienced it all—all levels and types of medical care, rehabilitation, and special education, the best and the worst—over the course of the 15 years since his injury at age 14. Those who would be of assistance to John and people like John are well advised to think deeply about his rules and the orientation to rehabilitation—and to life with other human beings—that these rules embody.

10 Rules for People Who Work with Children and Adults with TBI

1. *Treat people with respect.* I repeat that: Treat people with respect. Do not embarrass someone in front of others.
2. *Give people as much responsibility as they can handle.* We are not helpless.
3. *Be patient.* Give people time to express themselves. Do not butt in with your own ideas and words. Do not rush them.
4. *Listen to people and what they really are saying.* Do not do anything until you know exactly what people mean to say.
5. *Help people to laugh,* especially when they really are angry about something, such as being unable to drive.
6. *Have animals around.* Programs that serve people with brain injury should have cats and dogs for us to take care of. Gardening is good, too.
7. *Let people handle their own money.* I repeat: Let people handle their own money.
8. *Let people have their own space to be alone and to cool off.* That's important in a rehabilitation environment, living with so many strangers and with so much to be angry about. And always knock on the door first.
9. *Celebrate success.* Have a little party. It's important to have a little celebration of success every now and then.
10. *Help people to find meaningful things to do with their lives.* I'm a clown, a real clown, and this gives me all sorts of fun times in different places. I also deliver mail and ice cream three times a week at a nursing home. This is real work; real work is an important part of a real life. I want a real life.

Chapter 2

Neuropsychological Sequelae After Pediatric Traumatic Brain Injury: Advances Since 1985

Linda Ewing-Cobbs, Harvey S. Levin, and Jack M. Fletcher

Traumatic brain injury (TBI) is the leading cause of death in people younger than 45 years. In children, TBI contributes significantly to the spectrum of disability that occurs in relationship to brain injury. Epidemiologic studies have reported that approximately 10 per 100,000 children die as a result of TBI, the overall prevalence being 180–220 per 100,000 children (Annegers, 1983; Kraus, 1995). These figures demonstrate that TBI is a major public health problem.

Outcomes after TBI range from death to persistent vegetative states to significant physical and cognitive disabilities. Outcomes are clearly are related to severity of the injury. Children in whom significant injury is identified by Glasgow Coma Scale scores (Teasdale and Jennett, 1974) of less than 8, failure to follow commands within 24 hours, or posttraumatic amnesia of 7 days or more are at significant risk for persistent disability. At times, the disabilities are subtle, reflecting problems with motor coordination, attention, memory, or problem-solving skills, and arc apparent only on formal neuropsychological examinations. Problems of this sort lead to difficulties with adaptation in the family and other social environments as well as with learning and adaptation at school.

This chapter reviews neurobehavioral outcomes after TBI in children. A range of outcomes are covered. Specific attention is devoted to newer areas of outcome research, including infants and preschoolers, discourse, and executive functions. Data are reported in terms of results of group studies; therefore, a group mean reflects the *average* performance of members of different severity groups. Considerable variation is present within any group.

Intelligence Outcomes

Infants and Preschool-Aged Children

Studies of intellectual function after TBI have uniformly reported significantly lower scores in children who sustain severe brain injuries than in those with mild and moderate injuries. However, the relationship between age at injury and intellectual outcome after pediatric TBI has been evaluated infrequently. In an early study of recovery from TBI in children aged 2–18 years at injury, Brink and coworkers (1970) identified a direct relationship between coma duration and IQ scores after brain injury in 52 children rendered comatose for at least 1 week—longer coma duration was associated with lower IQ scores.

Brink and colleagues (1970) identified greater intellectual impairment in children who were younger than 8 years at the time of injury than in older children. Similar findings were reported by Lange-Cosack and coworkers (1979), who investigated long-term intellectual impairment 4 –14 years after severe closed head injury. These investigators found that the consequences of acquired brain injury were more severe in infants and young children than in school-aged children and adolescents. However, physically abused children were included in the samples followed by Brink and colleagues (1970) and Lange-Cosack and associates (1979). Inflicted injuries secondary to physical abuse commonly subject the brain to significant rotational acceleration-deceleration forces, which likely contributed to the poorer outcome in the younger children (Ewing-Cobbs et al., 1995).

Ewing-Cobbs and coworkers (1989) examined developmental quotients (IQ scores) prospectively in 21 children, ranging in age from 4 months to 5 years, who

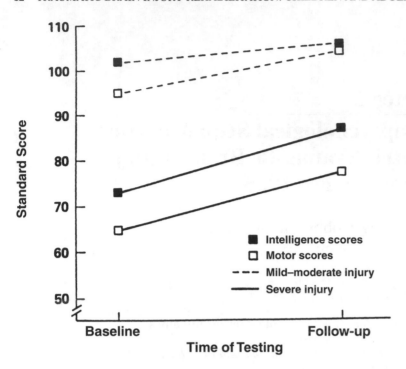

Figure 2-1. Change in intelligence and motor scores of infants and preschoolers who sustained mild to moderate and severe closed head injury, from baseline until follow-up at 8 months after the injury. Motor performance remained significantly below intellectual performance by the follow-up assessment. (Reprinted with permission from L Ewing-Cobbs, ME Miner, JM Fletcher, HS Levin [1989]. Intellectual, motor, and language sequelae following closed head injury in infants and preschoolers. J Pediatr Psychol 14;540.)

sustained noninflicted TBI. Because standard scores were adjusted for age, the scores for infants and preschoolers were combined. Children with severe TBI scored below those with mild and moderate injuries on both baseline and follow-up evaluations. At 8 months after injury, the children with severe TBI scored an average of 21 points below those with mild and moderate injuries. In children with severe injuries, the average score at baseline was 75.3, and the score at follow-up was 86.7. As indicated in Figure 2-1, the line depicting change in scores over time was steeper in the severely injured children than in those with mild to moderate injuries, indicating greater initial deficit and a greater increase in scores over time after severe TBI. Within the age range of this sample, age at injury was not significantly related to baseline or follow-up IQ scores.

The studies just reviewed largely excluded TBI due to penetrating injuries. In a study evaluating neuropsychological outcome 3 years after cerebral gunshot wounds, Ewing-Cobbs and coworkers (1994) identified greater intellectual deficit in children younger than 5 years at the time of the gunshot wound in comparison to older children and adolescents. Three-fourths of the younger children had IQ scores in the mentally deficient range at follow-up; in contrast, IQ scores of children aged 7–14 years all recovered to the average to low-average ranges. Therefore, these findings, in conjunction with those of Brink and coworkers (1970) and Lange-Cosack and coworkers (1979), suggest greater vulnerability of younger children to intellectual deficit after both closed and penetrating brain injuries.

School-Aged Children and Adolescents

Levin and Eisenberg (1979) evaluated intellectual function at least 6 months after closed head injury using the age-appropriate Wechsler scale in 30 children and adolescents aged 6–18 years. Intelligence test scores of less than 70, which indicated intellectual deficiency, were present in only a subgroup of the most severely injured patients. Children with mild to moderate closed head injuries did not exhibit deficient IQ scores 6 months or more after injury. Median Verbal and Performance IQ scores in the average range were obtained in all severity groups.

To evaluate intellectual recovery further after TBI, Levin and coworkers (1982a) examined IQ scores in school-aged children and adolescents matched for severity of TBI. At 1 year after the injury, these investigators reported a greater proportion of severely injured children than adolescents with residual intellectual deficit defined by an IQ score of less than 80. The Full Scale IQ score of one-third of the severely injured children was lower than 80; in contrast, IQ scores from all the severely injured adolescents recovered to at least the low average range. Consistent with findings by Brink and colleagues (1970), the greater proportion of children than adolescents with residual intellectual impairment was postulated to reflect more significant effects of diffuse cerebral insult on the developing brain relative to the mature brain.

Other studies of intellectual recovery after TBI in school-aged children and adolescents have identified particular vulnerability of the Performance IQ score as compared to the Verbal IQ score. In a prospective study, Chadwick and coworkers (1981a) identified reductions of Wechsler Verbal (mean, 96.1) and Performance (mean, 76.8) IQ scores at baseline assessment in severely injured children in comparison to orthopedic controls. Despite improvement to the average range 1 year after the injury, the mean Performance IQ score (mean, 102.3) was significantly lower than the Verbal IQ score (mean, 107.4) and remained lower through a 2-year follow-up.

Similarly, Winogron and coworkers (1984) retrospectively assessed intellectual outcome in children ranging in age from 2.5 to 17.3 years at the time of TBI who were assessed approximately 1 year after injury. Mean IQ scores were in the average range after mild and moderate TBI and in the low average range after severe TBI. The Verbal and Full Scale IQ scores were similar in children with mild, moderate, and severe TBI. However, the Performance IQ scores varied according to the severity of injury, being lower in the severe group than in the mild or moderate group and lower in the moderate group than in the mild group.

The prospective longitudinal follow-up studies of Jaffe and coworkers (1992) evaluated a cohort of TBI children aged 6–15 years who were consecutively admitted to two regional hospitals. To control for premorbid and demographic factors, each of the 98 TBI cases was individually matched with a control for age, gender, school grade, behavior, and academic performance. Initial evaluations were completed within 3 weeks after full orientation was achieved. Wechsler Full Scale, Verbal, and Performance IQ scores declined significantly with mild, moderate, and severe TBI. In comparison with scores from controls, Full Scale IQ scores of children with mild, moderate, and severe TBI were lower by 3, 14, and 21 points, respectively. Performance IQ scores were lower than Verbal IQ scores after moderate to severe injuries. At 1 year after injury, Jaffe and coworkers (1993) identified significant correlations between injury severity and IQ scores. Relative to matched case controls, Full Scale IQ scores of patients with mild, moderate, and severe TBI were lower by 2, 9, and 13 points, respectively. Mean scores for all severity groups were in the average range.

Anderson and Moore (1995) compared the recovery of Verbal and Performance IQ scores in children with moderate to severe TBI who were injured between the ages of 4 and 6 (early-injury group) with the recovery of children injured at ages 7–14 (late-injury group). Analysis of variance did not reveal differences in Verbal or Full Scale IQ scores at either 4 months or 2 years after the injury in the early- and late-injury groups. Moreover, no significant change in these scores was noted over the follow-up period. Although it did not differ according to age at injury, the Performance IQ score did increase more in the late-injury group than in the early-injury group by the 2-year follow-up. When the Full Scale IQ scores were grouped into below-average or deficient, average, and above-average categories, the distribution of scores was similar in the early- and late-injury groups at the initial assessment. However, more children in the late-injury group improved over time. Of the early-injury group, 60% had Full Scale IQ scores lower than 90 (less than the twenty-fifth percentile), as compared to 15% of the late-injury group. Anderson and Moore (1995) suggested that the IQ scores showed relative stability over a 2-year period; moderate to severe TBI sustained in early childhood was associated with a smaller increase in IQ scores, particularly the Performance IQ score, over time than was TBI sustained in later childhood.

In 96 children aged 6–16 years who had sustained TBI with loss of consciousness and who were evaluated within 12 months after the injury, Donders (1993) evaluated subtest patterns on the revised Wechsler Intelligence Scale for Children (WISC-R). The mean Verbal IQ score was 92.8, and the mean Performance IQ score was 91.1. Using cluster analytic methods, Donders (1993) identified four distinct profiles of subtest scores: Cluster 1 had relatively better scores on Verbal than on Performance subtests. However, the average difference between Verbal and Performance IQ scores was less than 8 points. Clusters 2 and 3 differed in terms of the global level of performance. Cluster 2 had a globally depressed level of functioning, with borderline to deficient mean performance on all subtests. Cluster 2 contained a significantly higher proportion of children with a preinjury special education background and the longest coma duration. Cluster 3 was associated with reduced efficiency on several Verbal subtests in addition to a poor score on the coding subtest. Cluster 4, which was the largest group and included 36% of the patients, had subtest scores uniformly within normal limits. Given these findings, Donders (1993) inferred that it is important to avoid over-reliance on the use of IQ test scores when assessing the range of sequelae after TBI.

All studies of intellectual recovery in school-aged children and adolescents have used the Wechsler scales. The frequent finding of lower Performance IQ than Verbal IQ scores after severe TBI may, in part, be an artifact of the subtest format of the Verbal and Performance scales. The Verbal scale generally assesses previously learned information such as vocabulary, fund of knowledge, mental arithmetic computation, and social reasoning. Owing to the highly structured tasks and relatively limited response requirements of the Verbal scale, children with significant acquired language impairments might score within normal limits. In contrast, the Performance scale consists of five timed subtests that require the child to problem solve using novel materials; additional points are given for rapid response times. Consequently, when lower Performance than Verbal IQ scores are obtained, additional assessment is necessary to identify whether lower scores are related to task demands for visuospatial analysis, problem solving, attention, motor skills, or response speed. Due to these factors, IQ scores should be used cautiously and should be integrated with multidisciplinary assessments and classroom observation when used to make decisions about child placement and services after TBI.

Language and Communication Outcomes

Despite infrequent aphasia and relatively subtle language disturbances after TBI, difficulties using language in a broader communicative context characterize the language behaviors of many children after TBI. Clinical descriptions of language production in children with TBI emphasize tangential, disorganized speech (Ylvisaker, 1993).

Structural Language

Early studies of language competence after TBI in children used standardized instruments such as aphasia batteries to identify patterns of strength and weakness. Linguistic deficits have been reported most frequently on indices of expressive language functions involving naming, word retrieval, and oral fluency. Children and adolescents evaluated within 4–6 months after severe TBI had lower scores on measures of object-naming latency and verbal fluency than did children with mild or moderate TBI (Chadwick et al., 1981b), dysnomia for objects presented visually or tactually to the left hand (Levin and Eisenberg, 1979), description of object function, confrontation naming of objects, verbal fluency, writing to dictation, and copying sentences (Ewing-Cobbs et al., 1987). Infants and preschoolers sustaining severe TBI showed significant reductions in both receptive and expressive language scores at baseline and 8 months after injury in comparison to children who sustained mild to moderate TBI. In addition, expressive language scores were lower than receptive language scores and indicated significantly more expressive deficits in children aged 4–30 months at injury in comparison with children aged 31–64 months at injury (Ewing-Cobbs et al., 1989).

The latter finding might reflect either actual differences in receptive and expressive language or differences in the specific tasks used. The expressive tasks used in this age range might require more organization and initiation of response than the receptive tasks. If receptive tasks required comprehension of rapidly presented speech or comprehension of extended discourse, a different pattern of findings might emerge. Similar to discrepancies in IQ scores, the relative vulnerability of expressive versus receptive language functions may be related more to the test content than to the actual language function being tested.

Studies examining linguistic outcomes at least 1 year after TBI revealed persistent deficits on measures of verbal fluency (Winogron et al., 1984) and object-naming latency (Chadwick et al., 1981b) in children and adolescents with severe TBI in comparison to patients with

mild injuries. In addition, a reduction in global language quotients derived from tests of general language development was noted (Jordan et al., 1988). Even though lower scores were obtained on traditional tests of language development, Jordan and Murdoch (1990) did not report a reduction on scores from either a standardized aphasia battery or a measure of dysarthria at a follow-up evaluation.

Discourse

Campbell and Dollaghan (1990) compared samples of spontaneous conversation, from sessions spanning a 13-month period, among a group of school-aged children and adolescents who sustained TBI and a group of age-matched controls. The initial assessment 2–16 weeks after injury indicated significant differences on measures of expressive language, including total number of words, total number of different words, the mean length of utterance in morphemes, and percentage of complex utterances. At the final follow-up, however, the TBI group produced fewer utterances than controls but did not differ from the controls on the other outcome measures, indicating substantial improvement in the TBI patients. Campbell and Dollaghan (1990) noted significant variations in the individual patterns of deficit and recovery in their patients.

Studies of discourse after severe pediatric TBI have revealed reductions in the quantity of speech, the amount of information conveyed, and alterations in the overall structure of narratives. Young children may be particularly vulnerable to perturbations in the development of communicative language. More recent investigations of language and communication skills have emphasized the evaluation of discourse, which refers to the use of communicative language in context (Dennis and Lovett, 1990). Discourse involves the effective production and understanding of text and reflects the integration of lexical, grammatical, cognitive, and pragmatic linguistic elements.

Chapman and coworkers (1992) evaluated discourse using a story-retelling task at least 1 year after mild to moderate or severe TBI in children aged 9–18 at assessment. In comparison to controls matched for age as well as children with mild to moderate injuries, children with severe TBI produced fewer words and sentences. However, measures of the length and syntactic complexity of sentences did not differ across the three groups. The children with severe TBI produced less information than did controls. Analysis of story grammar indicated that the severe TBI group lost significant core information, failed to signal a new episode with setting information, and did not produce essential action information as compared to the other groups. Despite these differences on measures of information and story grammar, the groups did not differ on measures of language production, including fluency or hesitational phenomena.

Because they require many other cognitive abilities such as planning, sequencing, word retrieval, working memory, and goal regulation, discourse tasks may provide sensitive measures of real-world information-processing abilities. For example, Dennis and Barnes (1990) identified significant discourse deficits an average of 3 years after TBI in children and adolescents. Although the patients demonstrated average performance on measures of verbal intelligence and language abilities, they displayed difficulty in interpreting ambiguous sentences and metaphors, drawing inferences, and developing sentences from words.

Ewing-Cobbs and coworkers (in press) conducted a study investigating narrative discourse after closed and penetrating brain injury in children aged 1–8 years at the time of injury. These workers evaluated narrative story retelling an average of 3 years after TBI in nine children with language deficits identified within the first month of recovery from injury and in eight children with TBI who lacked evidence of early language impairment. In comparison to siblings, the children with TBI who exhibited early language impairment had lower Verbal and Full Scale IQ scores. On the story-retelling task, they produced fewer words, utterances, different words, and demonstrative and personal pronouns conjoining meaning across sentences than did the sibling comparison group. Importantly, the children with TBI who exhibited acute language impairment recalled less than half of the key information needed to maintain the story theme and made more errors in sequencing story components than did the other groups.

However, the language-impaired TBI group did not differ from either the TBI or sibling comparison groups on measures of Performance IQ, rate and fluency of speech production, or naming errors. Their difficulty in retelling stories was characterized by recall of only one-third of the essential story components, failure to introduce characters, and difficulty manipulating pronouns to indicate the role changes of characters. The language-impaired TBI group incompletely described specific actions and intentions of different characters. The degree of disruption in story retelling was striking, as the task entailed retelling a well-known fairy tale, which placed fewer demands on organizational strategies and memory for novel information.

Brain injury acquired during infancy, preschool years, or early elementary years appears to be associated with persistent deficits on measures of discourse. Chapman and coworkers (in press) reported that severe TBI sustained between the ages of 1 and 7 years was associated with impairment in discourse assessed at ages 6–8. Story retelling by subjects with severe brain injury, as compared to controls, was characterized by reduction in (1) the amount of information retained, (2) the completeness of retelling different elements of the story, and (3) the production of the meaning or central theme of the story. These difficulties were present in follow-up intervals from 1 to 5 years after the injury. Children aged 1–4 years at injury demonstrated a trend to produce fewer T-units (sentences) and less information than did children aged 5–7 at the time of injury. The narratives produced by injured and control children were similar in terms of the use of cohesive markers conjoining meaning across text (e.g., referential pronouns, temporal connectives).

Visuomotor and Visuospatial Outcomes

Visuomotor and visuospatial functions frequently have been described as areas of particular difficulty after TBI. Motor slowing has been reported by several investigators. In their 1-year retrospective follow-up study of children with mild, moderate, and severe brain injury, Winogron and associates (1984) identified motor slowing in both hands and decreased manual dexterity only in the dominant hand in severely injured patients. Similarly, Chadwick and colleagues (1981b) reported deficits on a manual dexterity task requiring manipulation of pegs; these deficits persisted for more than 2 years after severe brain injury. The basis for persistent motor slowing and reduced dexterity are unclear. The impact of nonspecific motor slowing versus consequences of more specific lateralized lesions remains to be investigated.

Winogron and coworkers (1984) reported deficits on the Tactual Performance Test time-to-completion variable, which suggested inefficiency and slowing on a complex visuospatial task. Chadwick and colleagues (1981b) reported persistent difficulties in severely injured patients 1 year after injury on the Matching Familiar Figures Test, which is a motor-free test of visual perception.

To determine whether children with severe brain injury had a global deficit on tasks with visuospatial components, Bawden and coworkers (1985) categorized tests from the Halstead-Reitan Neuropsychological Test Battery into those requiring high speed, moderate speed, and low to no speed. Children with severe TBI were significantly slower than patients with either mild or moderate TBI on a variety of tests of motor speed as well as on a test requiring motor speed and visuospatial processing. When tests were grouped on the basis of the requirements for motor speed (Figure 2-2), children with severe TBI scored significantly lower on the summary measure for high-speed tasks than on the summary measure for low-speed motor tests. Bawden and colleagues (1985) interpreted these findings as indicating that the severely injured patients did not sustain a generalized deficit in motor or visuospatial areas. Group differences related to the severity of brain injury were not identified on other measures of motor strength, motor control, or visuospatial abilities. The summary measure for high-speed motor

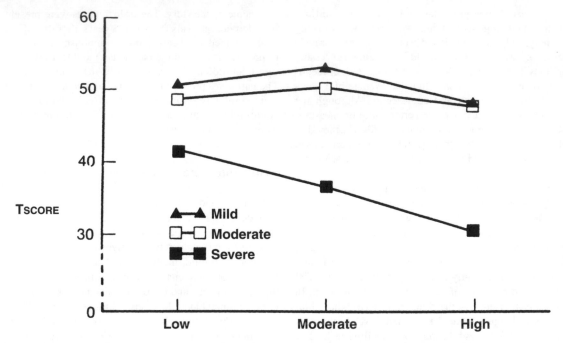

Figure 2-2. Children with severe brain injury performed significantly below patients with mild and moderate injuries on a summary score reflecting performance on tasks with high requirements for rapid motor performance. (Reprinted with permission from HM Bawden, RM Knights, HW Winogron [1985]. Speeded performance following head injury. J Clin Exp Neuropsychol 7;49.)

tests included scores from finger- and foot-tapping tests, pegboard tests, and the coding subtest from the WISC-R.

Jaffe and colleagues (1992) reported significant case-control discrepancies on a variety of measures of finger-tapping speed and on parent ratings of fine and gross motor functioning obtained at baseline assessment. Severe TBI was associated with a decline in all assessed areas of motor functioning with the exception of hand strength. One year after the injury, however, no significant relationships were obtained between injury severity and speed of finger tapping, name writing, or the Wechsler coding subtest reflecting psychomotor speed. Severity of injury continued to be associated with parental report of fine and gross motor dysfunction and speed of psychomotor problem solving (Jaffe et al., 1993).

Using analysis of individual growth curves, Thompson and coworkers (1994) evaluated longitudinal change in motor, visuospatial, and somatosensory skills in 49 children and adolescents aged 6–15 who sustained TBI of varying severity. Slower rates of change (recovery) were found for younger than for older children on measures of drawing, a timed pegboard task, and a timed tactile recognition task. Differences attributable to age were not identified on tests assessing motor-free visual perceptual functions. Overall, the severely injured young children showed slower recovery rates than did less severely injured young children (Figure 2-3). In contrast, recovery

curves were similar in the older patients, regardless of injury severity. Thompson and colleagues (1994) inferred that the slower growth of visuospatial and motor tasks in younger children supported the hypothesis of increased vulnerability of rapidly emerging skills to disruption by brain injury.

Attention

Despite the importance of attentional functions for successful completion of both cognitive and socially based tasks, few studies have examined attentional abilities after TBI. The few available findings regarding the type and persistence of attentional disturbance have been inconclusive. Chadwick and coworkers (1981b) reported attentional impairment in children in whom posttraumatic amnesia persisted for at least 2 weeks on measures of focused and sustained attention, including the Stroop test and a continuous performance test, at the baseline assessment. However, at the 4-month follow-up assessment, these children who had been severely injured scored lower than orthopedic controls only on the continuous performance task. Assessment of attention at 1 and 2 years after injury indicated comparable performance by children with severe injury and by controls on both measures.

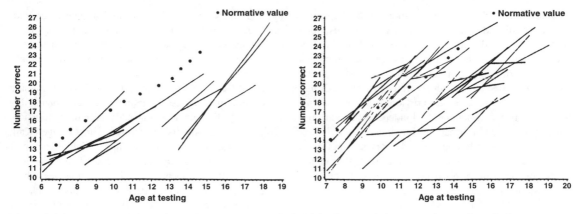

Figure 2-3. Estimated individual linear change curves are depicted for the test of visuomotor integration relative to age-normative values as a function of both age and Glasgow Coma Scale (GCS) scores. The right panel indicates that the improvement in most children with mild and moderate injuries paralleled normative expectations as indicated on the figure. The left panel shows the linear change curves of children with severe injuries having GCS scores of less than 9; the rate of change of younger children with severe injuries lagged behind their less severely injured age-matched mates. (Reprinted with permission from NM Thompson, DF Francis, KK Steubing, et al. [1994]. Motor, visual-spatial, and somatosensory skills after closed head injury in children and adolescents: a study of change. Neuropsychology 8;339.)

Kaufmann and coworkers (1993), using a computer-assisted adaptive-rate continuous performance test, evaluated 36 patients aged 7–16 years at the time of injury. This continuous performance test required the subjects to press a key at the onset of a target and not to respond to distracters presented on the computer screen. The rate of target presentation was increased after a series of correct responses was made within a given time limit. After either errors or responses with a long latency, the computer slowed the rate of presentation. Therefore, the mean interstimulus interval for each of the four trial blocks provided an index of attentional efficiency. Six months after TBI, patients with severe injuries scored lower than those with mild or moderate injuries. Young, severely injured children had the greatest impairment on the continuous performance test. Kaufmann and coworkers (1993) did not identify a relationship between injury severity and performance on the Wechsler digit-span subtest. The digit-span test has generally been insensitive to the residual effects of closed head injury in adults (Levin et al., 1982a).

Memory

The duration of confusion and amnesia immediately after TBI often is regarded as an indicator of the severity of TBI (Russell, 1932). This period of posttraumatic amnesia is the time during which a patient is unable to store and recall ongoing events in memory. We developed the Children's Orientation and Amnesia Test to evaluate orientation and memory objectively in children and adolescents, aged 3–15, after TBI (Ewing-Cobbs et al., 1990). The Children's Orientation and Amnesia Test consists of 16 items designed to assess three areas: (1) general orientation to person and place (recall of biographical information), (2) orientation to time, and (3) indices of immediate, short-term, and remote memory. Normative data are available for school and hospital controls (Baryza and Haley, 1994; Ewing-Cobbs et al., 1990).

To assess the predictive validity of this test, we examined the relationship between the length of time that scores on this test were below expected levels after TBI and the subjects' performance on memory tests 6 and 12 months after injury. In children and adolescents with posttraumatic amnesia that persisted for at least 3 weeks, both verbal and nonverbal memory scores were significantly more impaired at 6 and 12 months after injury than in patients whose orientation, confusion, and gross amnesia resolved more rapidly. Children's Orientation and Amnesia Test scores obtained at serial time points during the early stages of recovery provide an objective means of monitoring cognitive changes during the early stages of recovery and of timing the initiation of complex cognitive rehabilitation efforts (Ewing-Cobbs et al., 1990).

Levin and Eisenberg (1979), on the basis of an analysis of composite scores in the areas of memory, language, motor and somatosensory functioning, and visuospatial ability, identified memory as the most frequently disrupted neuropsychological domain. To further characterize the types of memory difficulties seen after TBI, Levin and coworkers (1988) evaluated verbal and visual memory functions using the Verbal Selective Reminding (Buschke, 1974) and Continuous Recognition Memory

(Hannay et al., 1979) tests in 58 children and adolescents who were injured at ages 6–15 and who had sustained either mild to moderate or severe TBI. The Verbal Selective Reminding test is a list-learning test that requires a child to learn and retain new verbal information. The child is reminded on subsequent trials only of words that he or she did not recall on the previous trial, thus permitting assessment of when the child independently and consistently retrieved information from memory.

The Continuous Recognition Memory test requires a child to discriminate target pictures from distracters. Scores obtained from this measure are *hits*, or the number of times that a previously viewed picture was correctly identified, and *false alarms*, the number of times a picture was identified incorrectly as having been previously presented.

Scores from Verbal Selective Reminding and Continuous Recognition Memory tests were transformed into standard scores on the basis of normative data for age, to enable comparison of scores across ages. Irrespective of the age of the child at injury, visual recognition memory scores were impaired in patients who were severely injured as compared to those with mild to moderate injuries. The mean consistent long-term retrieval score from the Selective Reminding test, which reflects the retrieval of newly learned information from memory, was lower in patients with severe TBI than in patients with mild to moderate injuries. Although the consistent long-term retrieval scores obtained from the adolescents were below those obtained from the children at the baseline evaluation, at the 1-year follow-up there were no significant differences between the performance of children and adolescents.

In an attempt to identify selective changes in aspects of learning and memory, several investigators have administered the California Verbal Learning Test (Delis et al., 1986) to children and adolescents with TBI of varying severity. On this list-learning task, patients with severe injury showed a slower rate of learning and acquired less information over the trials than did either controls or patients with mild TBI when assessed at baseline (Jaffe et al., 1992), 9 months after the injury (Yeates et al., 1995), and 1–2 years after injury (Levin et al., 1994b). Severity group differences on measures of word recognition were identified by Yeates and colleagues (1995) but were not isolated by Jaffe and coworkers (1992). One-year longitudinal follow-up by Jaffe and colleagues (1993) revealed persistent group differences only on measures of free and cued recall. Interestingly, learning characteristics such as clustering words semantically to enhance recall and the consistency of recall over trials did not vary with injury severity (Yeates et al., 1995).

Age-at-injury interactions were not obtained by either Yeates's group (1995) or Levin's group (1994a); the influence of injury severity on performance was similar for children and adolescents. The lack of interaction between age and injury severity differs from that in previous studies (e.g., Levin et al., 1988), yet the basis for the difference remains unclear. Variation in tests administered and characteristics of the samples studied may differentially affect test results.

The differences in outcomes for the list-learning and recognition memory tests might reflect developmental factors. Recognition memory is an early-developing function, typically being established before 5 years of age (Kail, 1979). Therefore, acquired brain injury might disrupt performance to a similar degree in young children and adolescents. In contrast, semantic organization strategies, which increase recall of a word list, develop throughout childhood into adolescence. The poorer performance of adolescents than children on the Selective Reminding task after severe TBI suggests that the effects of brain injury acquired during early childhood initially might be less disruptive than the effects of a similar injury during adolescence on tasks with a prolonged developmental trajectory indicating continued acquisition over a number of years. However, it is possible that as younger children mature, they will "grow into" neuropsychological deficits. Additional research is needed to determine whether there are long-term differences in the eventual level of development of complex functions. In other words, is the impact of a particular type of TBI on a given cognitive function the same in a child injured at age 2, 8, or 13 when that child is evaluated at age 15? An important area for further investigation involves the identification of possible delayed deficits that would likely be manifested as a failure to develop new abilities at age-appropriate rates. These types of developmental effects are clearly documented in primates after focal damage to prefrontal regions but have not yet been identified after pediatric TBI (Goldman, 1974).

Executive Functions in Children

Executive functions are defined broadly by constructs including inhibition, planning, working memory, resource allocation, and the development and implementation of strategies for problem solving (Pennington et al., 1996). The prefrontal lobes and interconnected regions currently are conceptualized as the primary anatomic substrate for executive function (Stuss and Benson, 1986). Pennington and coworkers (1996) noted that the term *executive function* is general and provisional and often used to describe the function of the prefrontal cortex.

The frontal lobes are vulnerable to focal damage after closed head injury (Mendelsohn et al., 1992). Magnetic resonance imaging findings in children sustaining severe closed head injuries disclosed focal lesions restricted to or primarily involving the frontal lobes in 40% of the sample (Levin et al., 1993). Gray matter lesions were seen most frequently in orbitofrontal and dorsolateral areas; frontal white matter lesions were also commonly visualized (Levin et al., 1993). Given the frequent injury to frontal regions after TBI, the investigation of executive function deficits is critically important to our understanding of posttraumatic cognitive and behavioral changes.

Experimental studies in nonhuman primates (Goldman, 1974), case studies of adults who sustained frontal lobe injury during childhood (Price et al., 1990), and studies concerning the neurobehavioral sequelae of traumatic frontal lobe lesions in children secondary to TBI (Levin et al., 1993, 1994a, b) have reported a wide range of impairments characterized by investigators as executive function deficits. This diversity in cognitive and behavioral sequelae may be related to heterogeneity in the neuroanatomic distribution of lesions across subregions of the prefrontal area. Variation in the age at injury and, by inference, the functional commitment of specific subregions of the prefrontal area also contributes to the wide variety of sequelae that have been reported after brain injury in the pediatric population.

The range of skills attributed to executive functions is broad, leading to problems with characterization of the domain of executive functions. Although there is no consensus on the definition of executive functions in children, important dimensions could include (1) self-regulation, (2) planning, (3) flexibility in problem solving, (4) temporal organization of behavior, (5) resource allocation, and (6) inhibition. We discuss research pertaining to the first three dimensions to illustrate the application of these constructs to the study of pediatric TBI.

Metacognition, which refers to the knowledge of one's own cognitive abilities, is an exemplar of the category of self-regulation. Metacognition includes self-assessment of memory performance and the understanding of how task variables affect the efficiency of memory. By monitoring the semantic features common to several words on a list, children can enhance their recall by clustering items from the same category (e.g., recalling all the fruits, then the vegetables). Use of the semantic clustering strategy implies verbal regulation and monitoring prior to recall.

Levin and coworkers (1991) studied use of semantic clustering in 52 normal children and adolescents by administering the children's version of the California Verbal Learning Test (Delis et al., 1986), which consisted of 15 words representing three categories of items (e.g., fruits). Levin and colleagues (1991) found an interaction of age with gender: The increased semantic clustering after age 7–8 years was exhibited primarily by girls rather than boys. Intrusion of extralist words also was lower in girls (mean, 1.7%) than in boys (mean, 5.1%). In comparison with 7–8 year olds, 13–15 year olds exhibited a higher level of semantic clustering, reflected by their recall of a string of items belonging to the same category before they proceeded to the next category.

Metacognition has also been studied by using the 20-Questions Task of Denny and Denny (1973). This task assesses the capacity to ask higher-level questions that reflect processing of the semantic properties common to a subgroup of animate and inanimate objects, which are presented to the child in a pictorial display. By verbalizing a feature such as a "living thing," older children can ask primarily constraint-seeking questions that eliminate several alternatives (e.g., a fish, dog, tree). In contrast, young children tend to ask hypothesis-type questions (e.g., "Is it the dog?"), which pertain only to a single item, thus failing to reflect verbal mediation of features common to two or more of the items. In a cross-sectional study (Levin et al., 1991), the percentage of constraint-type questions asked by normal children increased more than threefold from age 7–8 years to age 13–15 years. Analysis of developmental changes disclosed a corresponding decline in the percentage of hypothesis-type questions in these age ranges. Pseudoconstraint questions (e.g., "Is it the one that barks?"), which also eliminated only a single alternative, declined with age in normal children.

Another example of an executive function is *planning*, which refers to the capacity for setting goals and the ability to maintain an action sequence in working memory (i.e., maintaining a representation of the goal in working memory). The capacity for planning can involve breaking down a complex problem into subsidiary goals, monitoring the attainment of each subsidiary goal, and maintaining the overall solution in working memory. The Tower of London, a test developed by Shallice (1982) to investigate planning, involves rearranging beads on three vertical rods to match a model. The complexity of the problems composing this task is determined by the minimum number of moves necessary for a solution. The percentage of problems solved by normal children on the first trial increases with age. While administering the Tower of London, the examiner reminds the child of the rules, such as picking up only one bead at a time. Levin and associates (1994b) found that children who had sustained a severe brain injury tended to break the rules despite reminders by the examiner. This tendency to break the rules was particularly notable in the children with TBI who were 6–10 years old at the time of testing. The initial planning time, which is the time from presentation of the problem until the child initiates the first move, may be construed as reflecting impulsivity. However, Levin and coworkers (1994b) found that the initial planning time declines with age and is prolonged in children who have sustained a severe brain injury.

Flexibility in problem-solving skills and the ability to profit from environmental feedback are also examples of executive functions. The Wisconsin Card Sorting Test (Heaton, 1981) is a classic measure of flexibility in problem solving that involves shifting response strategy by sorting cards according to changes in the salient dimension (i.e., color, shape, number). Changes in the salient dimension are discovered by the child through attending to the examiner's feedback. Divergent reasoning, which

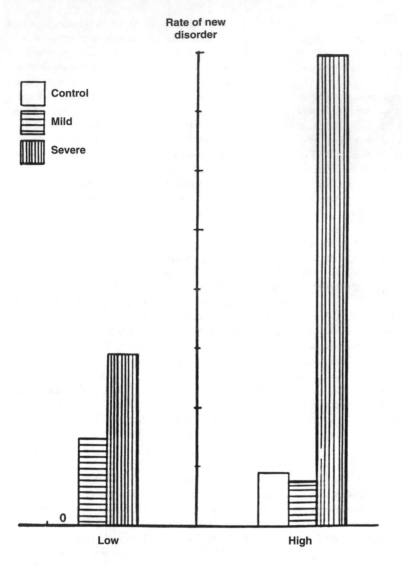

Figure 2-4. High rates of psychosocial adversity were associated with the development of significantly more new psychiatric disorders after traumatic brain injury only in children with severe closed head injury. (Reprinted with permission from M Rutter, O Chadwick, D Shaffer [1983]. Developmental Neuropsychiatry. New York: Guilford Press, 101.)

is exemplified by producing exemplars of a category, also involves flexibility in reasoning. Levin and coworkers (1993, 1996) found that children with severe TBI performed less well on these tasks as compared to children with mild to moderate TBI.

Behavioral and Family Functioning

Early studies of behavioral disturbance after closed head injury noted that children who sustained mild injuries had a higher incidence of preinjury behavioral disturbances than did children with moderate to severe brain injuries (Brown et al., 1981). However, after severe brain injury, children and adolescents developed new psychi-

atric disorders at a rate two to three times higher than in the mildly injured children. Brown and colleagues (1981) also noted that the likelihood of developing new behavioral problems was increased significantly in children residing in homes experiencing significant psychosocial adversity. The relationship between new psychiatric disorders and psychosocial adversity is depicted in Figure 2-4. The type of psychiatric or behavioral disturbance observed after injury commonly reflected an exacerbation of preinjury behavioral tendencies. With the exception of social disinhibition, behavioral changes associated with severe TBI were not characterized by specific features (Brown et al., 1981).

Behavioral sequelae during the first year after injury were examined by Fletcher and coworkers (1990) in children and adolescents with mild, moderate, or severe TBI categorized on the basis of the lowest Glasgow Coma Scale score and initial computed tomographic scan findings. The Vineland Adaptive Behavior Scales (Sparrow et al., 1984) and the Child Behavior Checklist (Achenbach, 1991), which used the parents as informants, were completed as soon after the injury as possible and again at 6 and 12 months after the injury. The baseline assessment was completed to indicate the child's level of functioning before the injury. Children with any known neuropsychiatric disorder, developmental delay, or special academic placement in school were excluded from the study. The preinjury adaptive behavior composite score from the Vineland test and the preinjury Child Behavior Checklist internalizing and externalizing scores did not differ significantly across the groups with differing injury severity. Patients with severe TBI developed adaptive behavioral disturbances during the first 6 months after injury, and these persisted over the 12-month follow-up interval on the Vineland scales. In contrast, the internalizing and externalizing scores from the Child Behavior Checklist did not show significant change from the preinjury to postinjury period in any injury severity group. The investigators (Fletcher et al., 1990) suggested that the rating-scale format of the Child Behavior Checklist and the item content were less sensitive in identifying posttraumatic behavioral changes than was the interview format and content of the Vineland scale.

Fletcher and coworkers (1996) replicated these findings using the revised Personality Inventory for Children and the Vineland. As with the Child Behavior Checklist, the behavioral adjustment scales of the revised Personality Inventory for Children did not separate TBI severity groups. However, scales related to cognitive functions as well as the Vineland scales indicated more concerns on the part of parents of children with severe TBI.

Perrott and coworkers (1991) evaluated cognitive, behavioral, academic, and family functioning in 18 children with TBI an average of 40 months after these children sustained TBI. In comparison to sibling controls, children with TBI demonstrated little residual cognitive impairment. However, significant behavioral and functional problems persisted through the follow-up period. Parents reported more behavioral problems and lower academic performance in the TBI children. Moreover, the children with TBI experienced more difficulties adapting to the demands of daily living and placed greater stress on the parent-child relationship in comparison to their siblings. In addition to placing greater demands on their parents, children with TBI tended to be more active and distractible than their siblings. Because no preinjury measures were obtained for this sample, Perrott and coworkers (1991) hypothesized that either functional problems displayed by the children with TBI predated their injuries or dysfunctional behavior became evident after the period of cognitive recovery.

In a longitudinal, prospective evaluation of family functioning during the first year after TBI, Rivara and coworkers (1992) evaluated 94 children, aged 6–15, and their families using interview ratings and psychometric measures of family and child functioning. The TBI severity groups were comparable on all measures before the injury. Most families had adequate to good levels of functioning and coping resources before the injury, as indicated by questionnaire scores that fell within population norms. On the basis of interviewer ratings, however, more than half of the families were determined to have high levels of stress and to be at risk for family relationship problems.

The best predictor of behavioral outcomes at 1 year after injury, irrespective of injury severity, was the preinjury level of family and child functioning. Similar to Fletcher and colleagues (1990), Rivara and coworkers (1994) found that changes in behavioral functioning over time were not detected by standardized measures and behavioral ratings but were apparent using an interview format. The global level of family functioning did not change significantly in families of children who sustained mild to moderate injuries; however, families of children with severe injuries were more likely to experience deterioration. The authors emphasized that most families adjusted well during the first postinjury year. Families of severely injured children were likely to experience higher levels of stress and stressed family relationships than were families with mild to moderately injured children.

Rivara and coworkers (1994) noted that academic and cognitive performance were predicted by preinjury family functioning as well as the severity of injury. In contrast, behavioral outcomes were associated more closely with preinjury family functioning than with the severity of injury. Overall, injury severity was a better predictor of academic and cognitive outcomes than of behavioral outcomes. Alternatively, preinjury measures of family function were a better predictor of behavioral problems. This sample may not be characteristic of TBI samples, as the socioeconomic status of the patient population was comparatively high. Moreover, attrition is greater in lower socioeconomic families and families with psychosocial problems.

Taylor and colleagues (1995) also reported strong relationships between child and family functioning before TBI and the quality of the child's outcome 6 months after TBI. In addition, more adverse child outcomes 6 months after TBI were associated with greater parental psychological distress, greater impact of the injury on the family, and more negative family interactions.

Additional research needs to be conducted to identify any systematic associations between behavioral outcomes and age at injury. In the studies by Fletcher and coworkers (1990, 1996), no differences attributable to age were apparent in severely injured patients younger than 7 years in comparison with patients aged 7–15 years on measures of either internalizing or external-izing behavior disorders or on measures of adaptive behavior. In contrast, Michaud and coworkers (1993) examined the history of occurrences of TBI in children receiving special education services for behavior disorders and in controls receiving regular education. Children with a history of TBI sustained during the preschool years were at significantly increased risk for development of behavioral disorders that were severe enough to necessitate special education assistance.

Developmental Issues

Age and Neurobehavioral Outcome

Within the pediatric age range, studies of neurobehavioral outcome after TBI in children and adolescents have frequently noted higher rates of death and disability in infants and preschoolers than in school-aged children and adolescents. Within the infant and preschool age group, it is unknown to what extent the less favorable outcomes are related to a higher incidence of inflicted injuries secondary to physical child abuse, which might be associated with more severe initial brain injury (Ewing-Cobbs et al., 1995).

Michaud and coworkers (1992) assessed survival and severity of disability in 75 children, aged birth to 16 years, with severe brain injury who were consecutively admitted to a level-one trauma center. Using the Glasgow Outcome Scale (Jennett and Bond, 1975), children who were 2 years of age or younger had a 50% mortality rate; only 17% recovered well. Children aged 3–14 had a 35% mortality rate, and 27% evidenced a good recovery. Michaud and associates (1992) noted that mortality and severity of disability tended to increase with decreasing age, whereas functional recovery increased with increasing age. Similarly, Levin and coworkers (1992) reported very severe injuries sustained by children aged birth through 4 years were associated with a 62% mortality rate, and 20% had either a good recovery or moderate disability 1 year after the injury.

In general, studies evaluating neurobehavioral outcome in younger and older children have identified more adverse neurobehavioral outcomes in infants and preschoolers who sustained severe TBI (Jennett et al., 1979; Levin et al., 1992; Luerssen et al., 1988; Michaud et al., 1992; Raimondi and Hirschauer, 1984). Although some investigators have reported similar outcomes in different age groups within the pediatric population (Braakman et al., 1980; Bruce et al., 1979), most studies examining specific age ranges have identified high death rates and less favorable neurobehavioral outcomes in infants and preschoolers. The high frequency of inflicted injuries secondary to physical child abuse might account for the increased rates of death

and disability in younger children as compared to school-aged children and adolescents.

Age and Cognitive Outcome

The relationship between age at the time of TBI and subsequent cognitive outcome is controversial. Although some investigators have noted that age at injury was not predictive of long-term outcome in severely injured patients (Costeff et al., 1990), less favorable outcomes were reported in other studies that used rating scales to assess the quality of cognitive, academic, and adaptive behavior outcome in children aged birth to 6 years in comparison to those aged 7–14 (Filley et al., 1987) and in children aged birth through 5 years than in children aged 6–18 (Kriel et al., 1989). In psychometric studies, age at injury was not identified as being related either to the severity of cognitive sequelae or to the rate of cognitive recovery (Chadwick et al., 1981a, b; Klonoff et al., 1977).

Our own studies have identified more severe expressive language deficits in children younger than 31 months than in those aged 32–64 months at injury (Ewing-Cobbs et al., 1989). Written language, attentional disturbance, visuomotor integration, fine-motor speed, and speed of tactile recognition were more impaired in school-aged children than in adolescents with comparable injury severity (Ewing-Cobbs et al., 1987; Kaufmann et al., 1993; Thompson et al., 1994). Adolescents initially performed less well than children on verbal memory tasks (Levin et al., 1988). It is important to note that the few intellectual outcome studies that have included infants or preschoolers have identified more severe long-term intellectual deficits in younger children (Brink et al., 1970; Ewing-Cobbs et al., 1994; Kriel et al., 1989; Lange-Cosack et al., 1979). However, all three studies of patients with closed head injury included physically abused children, which might account for the less favorable outcome.

It is possible that different skills are more vulnerable to impairment at different points during development. Some of our studies of language and memory after TBI of differing severity were consistent with the hypothesis that skills in a rapid stage of development at the time of brain injury were more adversely affected than more automated and overlearned skills (Ewing-Cobbs et al., 1987, 1989; Levin et al., 1988). Because rates of skill acquisition vary with development, different skills may be more affected by acquired brain injury depending on the child's level of development at the time of injury (Ewing-Cobbs et al., 1994). Acquired brain injury sustained during early childhood might be associated with more widespread cognitive impairment, as many skills develop rapidly during these years. In the area of behavioral functioning, whereas some studies have not identified any relationships of outcome in children aged birth to 7 years as compared to those aged 8–15 years at injury (Fletcher et al., 1990), Michaud and colleagues (1993) reported that children with a history of TBI during the preschool years were at significantly increased risk, later in their school years, for the development of behavioral disorders that were sufficiently severe to require special education intervention.

Executive functions might also show relationships between age at injury and age at assessment. Because executive functions represent complex cognitive constructs subsuming functions such as self-regulation, planning, and flexibility in problem solving, it is possible that relationships between age at injury and performance on executive function tasks will also follow a developmental progression. Developmental delays after a frontal lobe lesion is sustained during childhood have been most prominently reported in case studies rather than in larger-scale studies of children injured at varying ages (e.g., Price et al., 1990). Developmental consequences of early brain injury might include the failure of more complex cognitive abilities to develop at age-appropriate rates, which may be manifested as a failure to develop specific skills at expected ages. However, no longitudinal group studies of executive functions have been completed to support or contradict the occurrence of delayed deficits after pediatric TBI.

Clearly, more longitudinal neuropsychological, psychosocial, and educational studies that evaluate outcome are needed to address the important possibility of delayed deficits. In particular, social and behavioral domains may be more likely than cognitive domains to be characterized by delayed acquisition of normal functions over several years. It will be important to discriminate between a lowering or reduction in specific areas that is stable over time versus a delay in a specific area that becomes more pronounced over time. Given the lack of data regarding delayed deficits, it is essential that the developmental progress of each pediatric TBI patient be monitored closely in all areas so that rapid intervention and prevention of secondary deficits can be accomplished.

Assessment Issues

Because many decisions regarding school reentry, school placement, and need for educational and rehabilitation services are based on speech and language, psychoeducational, and neuropsychological assessment, knowledge of the strengths and weaknesses of traditional approaches to assessing children with TBI is very important. Most individuals working with children with TBI have received instruction in assessment of children with developmental disabilities, most notably specific developmental learning disabilities. The hallmark approach for diagnosing the presence of specific developmental learning disabilities is to identify a discrepancy between a child's intellectual

functioning and his or her performance on measures of academic achievement.

Application of a similar paradigm to assessment of children with TBI is inappropriate for a variety of reasons. First, most developmental disabilities are associated with a relatively constant level of functioning over time in different areas. In contrast, individuals with TBI often undergo very significant improvements in cognitive and behavioral functioning, particularly in the first 6–12 months after return to consciousness. Sampling behaviors at any given time might be misleading and may only highlight the child's functioning within a narrow time range, because significant improvement might occur rapidly. Therefore, assessments need to take into account the chronicity of the injury.

Second, the pattern of test scores obtained in assessing developmental disabilities is a relatively good predictor of actual classroom performance. In contrast, many tests of complex cognitive functions do not assess or highlight the types of information-processing deficits noted after TBI; children with significant functional deficiencies may score within the average range on a variety of standardized, normed tests. Therefore, tests that specifically assess areas that are more likely to be affected by TBI are essential. For example, IQ scores are likely to be reduced owing to the demands for information processing and speed of response after TBI, whereas more overlearned skills such as word decoding, spelling single words, and performing mathematic calculations are significantly less likely to be immediately affected by brain injury (Ewing-Cobbs et al., 1985). It is very common for a child with severe TBI to score within normal limits on traditional psychoeducational assessment despite significant deficiencies apparent in that child's management of the daily cognitive and social activities within the classroom. Because the Individuals with Disabilities in Education Act asserts that children must be evaluated in areas of potential deficiency, it is essential to include in assessment batteries evaluation of attention, memory, rapid motor performance, complex language, problem solving, and cognitive flexibility.

Moreover, children may function reasonably well in a structured one-on-one situation but might have significant difficulty within a classroom environment. Most commercially available standardized tests of academic functioning, language skills, and memory assess discrete cognitive functions. A child with TBI may or may not have difficulties on structured measures of specific cognitive abilities. However, it is much more likely that deficits will be apparent in situations requiring generalization of previously learned information, retention of information over units of time ranging from days to weeks, and focusing and monitoring attention. Although assessment of specific cognitive abilities is very important, classroom observation of more contextually valid behaviors is essential to highlight the type, nature, severity, and impact of information-processing deficits on daily functioning. After multidisciplinary assessment and direct classroom observation are complete, appropriate curriculum modifications and instructional methods can be implemented.

Assessment of the rate of development over time is essential to identify alterations in the acquisition of skills resulting in developmental lags or delayed deficits after severe TBI. As noted by Fletcher and coworkers (1987), a developmental analysis of behavior involves assessment of the rate, sequence, onset, and degree of development of a particular ability. Concepts of developmental delay, lag, and deficit are crucial to identifying the characteristics of skill development. Concepts of delay and lag imply that the skill develops later than expected but will eventually catch up and normalize over time. In contrast, the concept of deficit indicates a persistent impairment. Developmental analyses that include evaluation of the rate of change and eventual level of development of a specific skill are particularly valuable.

Assessment of the impact of moderator variables on cognitive and behavioral outcome should be emphasized. Age at injury, family environment, and socioeconomic background are examples of moderator variables. Given the persistence of behavioral difficulties and changes in family functioning after TBI (Perrott et al., 1991; Rivara et al., 1992, 1994; Taylor et al., 1995), assessment of psychological functioning, adaptive behavior, and family functioning—as well as interactions of these variables with cognitive and sociodemographic variables—is essential.

Conclusions

In this chapter, a range of outcomes after pediatric TBI is reviewed. Relative to our previous chapter on this topic in the last edition of this book (Ewing-Cobbs et al., 1985), it is clear that studies of outcomes have begun to shift from an emphasis on structured psychometric assessments to areas that involve language usage, problem-solving skills, planning and organization, and self-regulation. Although these outcome domains can be assessed using psychometric tests, assessment emphasizing language samples, structured interviews, and observational measures might be more sensitive to these areas of functioning. Such assessments are critically important because of the more direct associations of these outcome domains with the child's everyday adaptation to home and school. A child's ability to deal with people, exercise good judgment, manage his or her behavior and learning, and retain information in school are critical areas of functioning that often are impaired after moderate to severe TBI.

The shift toward evaluation of executive functions clearly reflects an attempt to grapple with these complex assessment issues. Such assessments have direct and ecologically valid implications for rehabilitation and for educational practices in the school. It is hoped that intervention efforts—particularly in schools—will also begin to move away from an important but narrow preoccupation with educational outcomes toward a broader perspective on programming for the child with TBI. It is critically important at this juncture to begin to develop rehabilitation and educational plans that address cognitive, psychological, and adaptive behavioral aspects of the development of the child with TBI.

Acknowledgments

Preparation of this manuscript was supported in part by National Institute of Neurological Disorders and Stroke grant 29462, Accidental and Nonaccidental Pediatric Brain Injury, to Dr. Ewing-Cobbs; grant 21889, Outcome of Pediatric Head Injury, to Dr. Harvey Levin; and by National Institute of Child Health and Human Development grant 27597, Neuropsychological Sequelae of Pediatric Head Injury, to Dr. Jack Fletcher. We acknowledge the assistance provided by the University Clinical Research Center at Hermann Hospital and the support of National Institutes of Health grant M01-RR-02558. The assistance of Nancy Crouch in manuscript preparation is gratefully acknowledged.

References

Achenbach TM (1991). Manual for the Child Behavior Checklist and Profile. Burlington, VT: University of Vermont.

Anderson V, Moore C (1995). Age at injury as a predictor of outcome following pediatric head injury: a longitudinal perspective. Child Neuropsychol 1;187.

Annegers JF (1983). The Epidemiology of Head Injury in Children. In K Shapiro (ed), Pediatric Head Trauma. Mount Kisco, NY: Futura, 1.

Baryza MJ, Haley SM (1994). Use of the Children's Orientation and Amnesia Test at hospital discharge for children with neurological and non-neurological traumatic injuries. Brain Inj 8;167.

Bawden HN, Knights RM, Winogron HW (1985). Speeded performance following head injury in children. J Clin Exp Neuropsychol 7;39.

Braakman R, Gelpke GJ, Habbema JDF, et al. (1980). Systematic selection of prognostic features in patients with severe head injury. Neurosurgery 6;362.

Brink JD, Garrett AL, Hale WR, et al. (1970). Recovery of motor and intellectual function in children sustaining severe head injuries. Dev Med Child Neurol 12;565.

Brown G, Chadwick O, Shaffer D, et al. (1981). A prospective study of children with head injuries: III. Psychiatric sequelae. Psychol Med 11;63.

Bruce DA, Raphaely RC, Goldberg AI, et al. (1979). Pathophysiology, treatment and outcome following severe head injury in children. Childs Brain 5;174.

Buschke H (1974). Components of verbal learning in children: analysis by selective reminding. J Exp Child Psychol 18;488.

Campbell TF, Dollaghan CA (1990). Expressive language recovery in severely brain-injured children and adolescents. J Speech Hear Disord 55;567.

Chadwick O, Rutter M, Brown G, et al. (1981a). A prospective study of children with head injuries: II. Cognitive sequelae. Psychol Med 11;49.

Chadwick O, Rutter M, Shaffer D, Shrout PE (1981b). A prospective study of children with head injuries: IV. Specific cognitive deficits. J Clin Neuropsychol 3;101.

Chapman SB, Culhane KA, Levin HS, et al. (1992). Narrative discourse after closed head injury in children and adolescents. Brain Lang 43;42.

Chapman SB, Levin HS, Wenek A, et al. (in press). Discourse after closed head injury in young children: relationship of age to outcome. Brain Lang.

Costeff H, Groswasser Z, Goldstein R (1990). Long-term follow-up review of 31 children with severe closed head trauma. J Neurosurg 73;684.

Delis DC, Kramer JH, Kaplan E, Ober BA (1986). The California Verbal Learning Test (research ed). New York: Psychological Corporation.

Dennis M, Barnes MA (1990). Knowing the meaning, getting the point, bridging the gap, and carrying the message: aspects of discourse following closed head injury in childhood and adolescence. Brain Lang 39;428.

Dennis M, Lovett MW (1990). Discourse Ability in Children After Brain Damage. In Y Joanette, HH Brownell (eds), Discourse Ability and Brain Damage: Theoretical and Empirical Perspectives. New York: Springer-Verlag, 199.

Denny DR, Denny NW (1973). The use of classification for problem solving: a comparison of middle and old age. Dev Psychol 9;275.

Donders J (1993). WISC-R subtest patterns in children with traumatic brain injury. Clin Neuropsychol 7;430.

Ewing-Cobbs L, Brookshire BL, Scott MA, Fletcher JM (in press). Children's narratives following traumatic brain injury: cohesion and linguistic structure. Brain Lang.

Ewing-Cobbs L, Duhaime AC, Fletcher JM (1995). Inflicted and noninflicted traumatic brain injury in infants and preschoolers. J Head Trauma Rehabil 10;13.

Ewing-Cobbs L, Fletcher JM, Levin HS (1985). Neuropsychological Sequelae Following Pediatric Head Injury. In M Ylvisaker (ed), Head Injury Rehabilitation: Children and Adolescents. San Diego: College Hill, 71.

Ewing-Cobbs L, Levin HS, Eisenberg HM, Fletcher JM (1987). Language functions following closed head injury in children and adolescents. J Clin Exp Neuropsychol 9;575.

Ewing-Cobbs L, Levin HS, Fletcher JM, et al. (1990). The Children's Orientation and Amnesia Test: relationship to severity of acute head injury and to recovery of memory. Neurosurgery 27;683.

Ewing-Cobbs L, Miner ME, Fletcher JM, Levin HS (1989). Intellectual, motor, and language sequelae following closed head injury in infants and preschoolers. J Pediatr Psychol 14;531.

Ewing-Cobbs L, Thompson NM, Miner ME, Fletcher JM (1994). Gunshot wounds to the brain in children and adolescents: age and neurobehavioral development. Neurosurgery 35;225.

Filley CM, Cranberg LD, Alexander MP, Hart EJ (1987). Neurobehavioral outcome after closed head injury in childhood and adolescence. Arch Neurol 44;194.

Fletcher JM, Ewing-Cobbs L, Miner ME, et al. (1990). Behavioral changes after closed head injury in children. J Consult Clin Psychol 58;93.

Fletcher JM, Levin HS, Lachar D, et al. (1996). Behavioral outcome after pediatric closed head injury: relationships with age, severity, and lesion size. J Child Neurol 11;283.

Fletcher JM, Miner ME, Ewing-Cobbs L (1987). Age and Recovery from Head Injury in Children: Developmental Issues. In HS Levin, HM Eisenberg, J Grafman (eds), Neurobehavioral Recovery from Head Injury. New York: Oxford University Press, 279.

Goldman PS (1974). An Alternative to Developmental Plasticity: Heterology of CNS Structures in Infants and Adults. In DG Stein, JR Rosen, N Butters (eds), Plasticity and Recovery of Function in the Central Nervous System. New York: Academic, 149.

Hannay HJ, Levin HS, Grossman RG (1979). Impaired recognition memory after head injury. Cortex 15;269.

Heaton RK (1981). Wisconsin Card Sorting Test (WCST). Odessa, FL: Psychological Assessment Resources.

Jaffe KM, Fay GC, Polissar NL, et al. (1992). Severity of pediatric traumatic brain injury and early neurobehavioral outcome: a cohort study. Arch Phys Med Rehabil 73;540.

Jaffe KM, Fay GC, Polissar NL, et al. (1993). Severity of pediatric traumatic brain injury and neurobehavioral recovery at one year—a cohort study. Arch Phys Med Rehabil 74;587.

Jennett B, Bond M (1975). Assessment of outcome after severe brain damage: a practical scale. Lancet 1;480.

Jennett B, Teasdale G, Braakman R, et al. (1979). Prognosis of patients with severe head injury. Neurosurgery 4;283.

Jordan FM, Ozanne AO, Murdoch BE (1988). Long-term speech and language disorders subsequent to closed head injury in children. Brain Inj 2;175.

Jordan SM, Murdoch BE (1990). Linguistic status following closed head injury in children: a follow-up study. Brain Inj 4;147.

Kail R (1979). The Development of Memory in Children. San Francisco: Freeman.

Kaufmann PM, Fletcher JM, Levin HS, et al. (1993). Attentional disturbance after pediatric closed head injury. J Child Neurol 8;348.

Klonoff H, Low MD, Clark C (1977). Head injuries in children: a prospective five year follow-up. J Neurol Neurosurg Psychiatry 40;1211.

Kraus JF (1995). Epidemiological Features of Brain Injury in Children: Occurrence, Children at Risk, Causes and Manner of Injury, Severity, and Outcomes. In SH Broman, ME Michel (eds), Traumatic Head Injury in Children. New York: Oxford University Press.

Kriel RL, Krach LE, Panser LA (1989). Closed head injury:

comparison of children younger and older than six years of age. Pediatr Neurol 5;296.

Lange-Cosack H, Wider B, Schlesner HJ, et al. (1979). Prognosis of brain injuries in young children (one until five years of age). Neuropadiatrie 10;105.

Levin HS, Aldrich EF, Saydjari C, et al. (1992). Severe head injury in children: experience of the Traumatic Coma Data Bank. Neurosurgery 31;435.

Levin HS, Benton AL, Grossman RG (1982a). Neurobehavioral Consequences of Closed Head Injury. New York: Oxford University Press.

Levin HS, Culhane KA, Fletcher JM, et al. (1994a). Dissociation between delayed alternation and memory after pediatric head injury: relationship to MRI findings. J Child Neurol 9;81.

Levin HS, Culhane KA, Hartmann J, et al. (1991). Developmental changes in performance on tests of purported frontal lobe functioning. Dev Neuropsychol 7;377.

Levin HS, Culhane KA, Mendelsohn D, et al. (1993). Cognition in relation to magnetic resonance imaging in head-injured children and adolescents. Arch Neurol 50;897.

Levin HS, Eisenberg HM (1979). Neuropsychological impairment after closed head injury in children and adolescents. J Pediatr Psychol 4;389.

Levin HS, Fletcher JM, Kusnerik L, et al. (1996). Semantic memory following pediatric head injury: relationship to age, severity of injury, and MRI. Cortex 32;461.

Levin HS, High WM, Ewing-Cobbs L, et al. (1988). Memory functioning during the first year after closed head injury in children and adolescents. Neurosurgery 22;1043.

Levin HS, Mendelsohn D, Lilly MA, et al. (1994b). Tower of London performance in relation to magnetic resonance imaging following closed head injury in children. Neuropsychology 8;171.

Luerssen TG, Klauber NR, Marshall LF (1988). Outcome from head injury related to patient's age: a longitudinal prospective study of adult and pediatric head injury. J Neurosurg 68;409.

Mendelsohn D, Levin HS, Bruce D, et al. (1992). Late MRI after head injury in children: relationship to clinical features and outcome. Childs Nerv Syst 8;445.

Michaud LJ, Rivara FP, Grady MS, Reay DT (1992). Predictors of survival and severity of disability after severe brain injury in children. Neurosurgery 31;254.

Michaud LJ, Rivara FP, Jaffe KM, et al. (1993). Traumatic brain injury as a risk factor for behavioral disorders in children. Arch Phys Med Rehabil 74;368.

Pennington BF, Bennetto L, McAleer O, Roberts RJ (1996). Executive Functions and Working Memory. In GR Lyon,

NA Krasnegor (eds), Attention, Memory, and Executive Function. Baltimore: Paul H. Brookes, 327.

Perrott SB, Taylor HG, Montes JL (1991). Neuropsychological sequelae, familial stress, and environmental adaptation following pediatric head injury. Dev Neuropsychol 7;69.

Price BH, Daffner KR, Stowe RM, Mesulam MM (1990). The compartmental learning disabilities of early frontal lobe damage. Brain 113;1383.

Raimondi AJ, Hirschauer J (1984). Head injury in the infant and toddler: coma scoring and outcome scale. Childs Brain 11;12.

Rivara JB, Fay GC, Jaffe KM, et al. (1992). Predictors of family functioning one year following traumatic brain injury in children. Arch Phys Med Rehabil 73;899.

Rivara JB, Jaffe KM, Polissar NL, et al. (1994). Family functioning and children's academic performance and behavior problems in the year following traumatic brain injury. Arch Phys Med Rehabil 75;369.

Russell WR (1932). Cerebral involvement in head injury. Brain 55;549.

Shallice T (1982). Specific impairments of planning. Philos Trans R Soc London B Biol Sci 298;199.

Sparrow SS, Balla D, Cicchetti D (1984). The Vineland Adaptive Behavior Scales. Circle Pines, MN: American Guidance Services.

Stuss DT, Benson DF (1986). The Frontal Lobes. New York: Raven.

Taylor HG, Drotar D, Wade S, et al. (1995). Recovery from Traumatic Brain Injury in Children: The Importance of the Family. In SH Roman, ME Michel (eds), Traumatic Head Injury in Children. New York: Oxford University Press.

Teasdale G, Jennett B (1974). Assessment of coma and impaired consciousness: a practical scale. Lancet 2;81.

Thompson NM, Francis DF, Steubing KK, et al. (1994). Motor, visual-spatial, and somatosensory skills after closed head injury in children and adolescents: a study of change. Neuropsychology 8;333.

Winogron HW, Knights RM, Bawden HN (1984). Neuropsychological deficits following head injury in children. J Clin Neuropsychol 6;269.

Yeates KO, Blumenstein E, Patterson CM, Delis DC (1995). Verbal learning and memory following pediatric closed-head injury. J Int Neuropsychol Soc 1;78.

Ylvisaker M (1993). Communication outcome in children and adolescents with traumatic brain injury. Neuropsychol Rehabil 3;367.

Chapter 3
Rehabilitative Medical Management

Anna J.L. Chorazy, Patricia K. Crumrine,
Jeanne M. Hanchett, Phyllis-Ann Mandella,
Mary Louise Russell, and Cynthia L. Smith

Severe brain injury is one of the medical occurrences that catapults a healthy child into a state of chronic impairment. The damage done to the brain at the moment of injury cannot be cured. Consequently, disabilities resulting from severe brain injury are of great significance to the patient, to the family, and to others involved in the patient's care (Orsillo et al., 1991; Rivara et al., 1993). The cost of care following brain injury is substantial, depending on the severity and nature of the injury (Jaffe et al., 1993). In this chapter, we discuss rehabilitative medical problems of acquired brain injury in children, basing our observations on 35 years' experience of the staff at The Rehabilitation Institute (TRI), a freestanding regional rehabilitation facility located in Pittsburgh for children and adults (Chamovitz et al., 1985).

The goal of rehabilitative medical management is to provide the services necessary for patients to recover maximally and to compensate adequately for lost or impaired function while they continue to develop physically, cognitively, and socially to their fullest potential. Vital to meeting this goal is the prevention of complications that will interfere with rehabilitative treatment and lead to further disability and future disease. Ideally, rehabilitation should begin in the intensive care unit and continue in the acute-care setting until the child is transferred to a formal rehabilitation program (see Chapter 6).

The optimal time for transfer to a rehabilitation program is the point at which children begin to show some awareness of their environment and some ability to respond to it. This is called *rehabilitation readiness*. Occasionally at TRI, we admit children who are minimally responsive to the environment, particularly if they were injured within the last 3 months. Intensive therapy is provided for a 30-day trial period, and the patient is discharged at the end of that time if there is no improvement.

Changes in the delivery of health care, especially managed care, encourage earlier discharge from inpatient programming to home and outpatient programming,

which places added stress on the family. The scarcity or lack of expert pediatric therapists in some communities further adds to the burden. School systems primarily consider the educational aspects of disability and may not be familiar with or capable of meeting the medical or therapeutic needs of the child with brain injury. Educational professionals need to expand their awareness of the medical and therapeutic needs of children with brain injury and how these needs affect the educational outcome; this may require increased willingness of school systems to accommodate these children and training for educational professionals (Savage and Wolcott, 1988; Savage et al., 1995).

The capabilities of the rehabilitation facility are as important as the patient's readiness (Goldberg and Sachs, 1992; Osberg et al., 1990). Units that are an integral part of an acute-care hospital can effectively manage patients whose conditions are less stable medically. Many freestanding rehabilitation hospitals require that patients be medically stable, which includes the absence of infection and the ability to breathe independently. Hence, TRI does not accept children who are febrile or respirator dependent. We make exceptions to this rule when the acute-care hospital performs an extensive diagnostic investigation and finds that the fever is central in origin. Patients with tracheostomy, gastrostomy, or nasogastric tubes are admitted, and attempts are made to remove these tubes as soon as it is medically safe to do so. We also admit patients with orthopedic devices, such as stabilizing halos, body jackets, and braces.

The physician who cares for children in a rehabilitation setting must be familiar with all aspects of child development as well as with the pathologic sequelae related to brain injury and their effects on a dynamically changing nervous system. A comprehensive evaluation of children with traumatic brain injury (TBI) includes a detailed history, parts of which (e.g., a personal "Lifeline" [Polinko et al., 1985]) are obtained by other team mem-

Table 3-1. Customary Initial Orders for Patients with TBI on Admission to Rehabilitation

---

1. Diet
2. Vital signs
3. Tuberculin skin test
4. Laboratory studies: complete blood cell count
   a. Chemical screen, anticonvulsant blood levels (if indicated)
   b. Urinalysis and urine culture with colony count
5. Medications
6. Institution of seizure control record
7. Physiatry consultation
8. Ophthalmology consultation
9. Neurology consultation
10. Psychiatry consultation, if indicated
11. Neuropsychology consultation
12. Dental consultation, if indicated
13. Nutrition consultation
14. Orthopedic consultation, if indicated
15. Physical therapy evaluation
16. Occupational therapy evaluation
17. Feeding evaluation
18. Speech-language evaluation and hearing evaluation
19. Cognitive rehabilitative therapy evaluation
20. Social service consultation
21. Recreation therapy, if indicated
22. Neurosurgical follow-up with referring surgeon, when possible

---

bers (see Chapter 16). The physical examination must be thorough, containing all the elements of a good evaluation but with special emphasis on the neurologic and neuromuscular systems. Children must be considered individually in terms of their pretraumatic status, genetic background, stage of development, severity and location of brain injury, associated multiple system injuries, and complications before admission to the rehabilitation program (Molnar and Perrin, 1992).

The rehabilitative medical care of children and adolescents properly belongs to the experienced primary-care physician, who shares responsibility and works closely with appropriate medical and surgical specialists and health-related professionals (Freeman, 1986; Jacobson et al., 1986; Tyler et al., 1989). Customary initial orders are outlined in Table 3-1. Computed tomographic (CT) scanning, magnetic resonance imaging (MRI), electroencephalograms (EEGs), and evoked potentials are not ordered routinely; typically, these have been performed during the acute-care period. In the acute phase, accurate long-term neurodevelopmental outcome is difficult to prognosticate by any neuroimaging techniques (Bachman, 1992; Helfaer and Wilson, 1993). Although Cope and coworkers (1988) advocate serial computerized evaluation, repeat diagnostic procedures (e.g., CT, MRI, and EEG) generally are not recommended (Jaffe

and Hays, 1986). These diagnostic procedures are undertaken only when indicated by such events as unduly slow progression, deterioration in neurologic status, significant change in seizure pattern, or evidence of increased intracranial pressure, or according to the protocol of the referring neurosurgeon.

Initial orders for all patients include consultation with appropriate medical subspecialists, including a pediatric physiatrist, neurologist, and ophthalmologist. We maintain frequent communication with the referring neurosurgeon whenever possible. On admission to TRI, all patients are evaluated by a nurse, dietitian, physical therapist, occupational therapist, speech-language pathologist, cognitive rehabilitation specialist, neuropsychologist, and social worker. When, on admission or during the course of treatment, medical findings indicate that additional evaluations are needed, consultation may be obtained from a pediatric orthopedist, otolaryngologist, gastroenterologist, general surgeon, pulmonologist, urologist, endocrinologist, or dentist.

Medical Issues During Rehabilitation

A variety of medical issues—some life-threatening, others minor—can confront children with brain injury during their rehabilitation. Each requires appropriate diagnosis and care. We list here the most commonly encountered problems.

Airway Problems

Aspiration is always a concern in children with TBI, who might not chew or swallow effectively and who often lack the judgment necessary to eat safely. Each patient who is not independently eating a regular diet at the time of admission to TRI receives a complete feeding and swallowing evaluation by a feeding therapist (see Chapter 7). Despite such precautions, the possibility of aspiration continues to be a concern (Splaingard et al., 1988). Our experience indicates that aspiration pneumonia is rare if the evaluation of feeding is thorough and feeding dysfunction is managed with appropriate caution (Logemann, 1989; Morton et al., 1993; Ylvisaker and Weinstein, 1989; Zerilli et al., 1990). Certain food consistencies are particularly dangerous and should be avoided. Patients with neurogenic swallowing disorders often have the greatest difficulty with thin liquids. Patients with oral motor dysfunction should not be given difficult-to-chew foods (e.g., tough meats, raw vegetables, fruits with tough skins). Patients with judgment disorders should be monitored and should not have free access to foods that could cause choking.

The most severe emergency is tracheostomy malfunction in a patient who is dependent on the tracheostomy tube to breathe. Mucous plugs, tracheal granulomas, and displaced tracheostomy tubes are the most common causes of sudden respiratory distress in these patients. These problems demand immediate intervention by the closest competent clinician, be it a physician or a skilled nurse. When a mucous plug is suspected, suctioning of the airway should be done. If that does not relieve the distress, removal of the tube, resuctioning, and tube replacement may be life-saving. Proper lubrication of the tube helps to avoid difficulty with reinsertion. It may be necessary to reinsert a smaller tube initially. Routine changing of tracheostomy tubes in tracheostomy tube–dependent patients can be dangerous. Appropriate measures should be taken to prepare for emergencies, such as inability to reinsert a tube, bleeding, or acute respiratory distress. Such measures include the availability of an emergency cart, oxygen, suctioning equipment, and extra tracheostomy tubes of various sizes, as well as the ability to transport the patient rapidly to an acute-care facility, if necessary.

It is safest to assume that patients who have a tracheostomy may have a tracheal granuloma. We often request a direct bronchoscopic examination by a pediatric otolaryngologist before permanent removal of the tube. Before this referral, we carefully assess the patient's ability to breathe without the tracheostomy by gradually reducing the size of the tube or covering it for short periods of time while closely observing the patient. In frightened children, this sometimes must be done by the physician who stands by the bedside and observes respiratory effort with the tracheostomy tube open and closed. If necessary, we occlude the tube playfully, using the examiner's finger or the child's own finger. Using such methods, the physician usually can make a reliable judgment as to whether the patient is dependent on this airway (Stool and Beele, 1973). Additional problems related to infections, such as tracheitis, tracheobronchitis, and pneumonia with or without aspiration, are usually treated with the appropriate antibiotics. Regular chest percussion, postural drainage, and suctioning help to clear secretions and benefit patients who have atelectasis or are at risk for aspiration. Respiratory adequacy is closely monitored clinically by observing respiratory effort, rate, and oxygen saturation by pulse oximetry. Children with tracheostomies are given viral influenza vaccine, and those at risk for recurrent aspiration are also given pneumococcal vaccine. Late complications, such as tracheal granuloma, scars, stenosis, and vocal cord paralysis, must also be considered (Citta-Pietrolungo et al., 1993; Crysdale et al., 1988). These lesions usually present as changes in vocal quality, stridor, or crouplike symptoms. Studies such as lateral neck radiographs, pulmonary function tests, and bronchoscopy aid in diagnosis of these problems.

Nutritional and Gastrointestinal Problems

Metabolic homeostasis is disrupted after severe brain injury. Hypermetabolism, hypercatabolism, hypergly-

cemia, increased counter-regulatory horn depressed immunocompetence, altered gastromc function, and the acute-phase response (e.g., increased levels of positive acute-phase proteins, decreased levels of negative acute-phase proteins, varied alterations in trace metal plasma concentrations, and fever) can be identified during the first 2 weeks after injury (Young et al., 1991). Electrolyte imbalance due to antidiuretic hormone secretion may be present early after brain injury and usually has subsided by the time the patient is transferred to the rehabilitation program.

When children enter rehabilitation soon after brain injury, malnutrition can be expected because children with acute brain injury have high caloric needs. Nasogastric and gastrostomy tube feedings with appropriate nutrients and fluid content are essential. Prolonged nasogastric tube feedings are not only uncomfortable but may cause irritation to the soft palate and pharynx and ulceration of the nasal and esophageal mucosa. Therefore, gastrostomy or gastrojejunostomy tube placement is favored, especially as this may be done with relative ease by the percutaneous approach (Towbin et al., 1988; Gauderer, 1991).

Anemia might occur if there has been significant blood loss or prolonged nutritional problems. Occasionally, anemia might be associated with gastrointestinal bleeding caused by stress ulcer or reflux esophagitis. Evaluation with barium esophagogram, esophagomometry, esophageal pH probe, gastroesophageal scintiscan, and fiberoptic endoscopic evaluation may be indicated. Prophylaxis with histamine H_2-receptor antagonist and antacids should be considered (Ylvisaker et al., 1990).

Comprehensive evaluation by a registered dietitian and other members of the rehabilitation team is imperative to returning the patient to metabolic homeostasis, proper fluid balance, and nutritional status for growth (see later in this chapter). Constipation necessitates the addition of fiber to the feeding; diarrhea must be treated appropriately and assessed with a stool culture to rule out infection. A stool should be obtained to test for *Clostridium difficile* toxin, especially for those children who have had prolonged treatment with antibiotics. Obesity may become a problem in late stages of recovery, particularly among those who are nonambulatory and therefore require fewer calories to maintain their weight.

Hypertension

Transitory hypertension can occur after localized or diffuse brain trauma (Zulch, 1969). During the acute period of management of brain trauma, hypertension is a frequent occurrence and is often attributable to high levels of circulating catecholamines or intracranial hypertension (Sandel et al., 1986). In most cases, this is transitory and has resolved before the patient is transferred for rehabilitative services. A small number of patients continue to manifest elevation in diastolic pressure after the period of increased intracranial pressure has subsided. If paroxysmal hypertension is accompanied by signs of autonomic dysfunction, occult spinal cord injury, adrenal hemorrhage, pheochromocytoma, or hypothalamic-pituitary dysfunction should be ruled out as an etiology (Sandel et al., 1986). Several patients with hypothalamic-midbrain dysregulation syndrome, characterized by hypertension, hyperthermia, hyperventilation, and decerebration, have been described (Pranzatelli et al., 1991). A response to propranolol was noted.

When a patient is on antihypertensive medication at the time of admission to the rehabilitation facility, the medication should be continued initially and then tapered slowly if blood pressures remain normal. Most patients are not receiving antihypertensive medications at the time of admission to our facility or are safely tapered off these medications soon after admission. Rarely, in some patients, hypertension due to structural lesions in the hypothalamus might continue for months or years after injury.

Urinary and Urologic Problems

It is common for patients with severe brain injury to have a urinary tract infection during the course of treatment. Many of these infections are caused by an indwelling catheter, which is necessary during the acute management of injuries. Such catheters should be removed as early as possible to avoid infection and to prevent urethral strictures, which are a significant long-term problem in some male patients who have had Foley catheters for extended periods. External urine-collecting devices (condom-catheters) can replace indwelling catheters in adolescent male patients. However, there are no satisfactory urine-collecting devices for young boys or female patients. Prolonged bed rest and incomplete emptying of the bladder, which might occur in the severely injured, slowly recovering patient, increase the risk of infection.

Because urinary tract infections may be unaccompanied by fever, we routinely order periodic urine cultures. A high fluid intake is maintained as an additional means of preventing infection and urinary stones. When fever occurs and physical examination does not reveal an obvious cause, a urine culture should be obtained. Antibiotics are chosen on the basis of antibiotic sensitivities of the organism. Frequent repeated urinary tract infections or voiding difficulties might indicate a need for in-depth urologic evaluation (Hald and Bradley, 1982).

Premorbid developmental status and history of bladder training or enuresis must be obtained as part of the assessment of bowel and bladder problems. The cortical loss of control of bladder and bowel function requires that patients be toileted regularly to regain these functions. A small percentage of the most severely involved patients never regain urinary or bowel continence. Many children have a prolonged period of enuresis but ultimately do achieve day and night continence.

Fever and Infection

Fever is a common occurrence in children and requires appropriate investigation in the child with TBI just as in a healthy child. The most common causes are viral infections of the upper respiratory tract and bacterial infections of lungs, urinary tract, ears, and skin (McCarthy, 1991). In the child with TBI, there are additional considerations. Open head injuries or pneumocephalus place a child at particular risk for central nervous system infection. Persistent rhinorrhea or otorrhea may indicate an undetected basilar skull fracture and spinal fluid leak. Because meningitis is a substantial risk, neurosurgical evaluation is indicated as soon as possible. Bone and soft-tissue infection should be suspected in patients who have orthopedic devices for complicated fractures. Patients who have required a splenectomy because of abdominal trauma are at an increased risk for unusual infection and should be monitored closely. Pneumococcal vaccine should be administered, accompanied by an explanation to the family regarding the risk of infections. Careful evaluation of the febrile patient, including physical examination, cultures, and assessment of change in central nervous system functioning, usually will indicate the cause of a fever. White blood cell count and x-rays may be helpful. Thrombophlebitis and pulmonary emboli pose a significant problem in adult patients but are seen rarely in children.

An unusual but important cause of fever in a child with TBI is hypothalamic injury. This fever of central origin is a diagnosis of exclusion, and a complete evaluation is required to rule out treatable causes. It usually occurs in patients who have had severe cerebral injury and tends to be recurrent. As the patient improves, the fever resolves.

Agitation and Irrational Behavior

As children with severe TBI move through the stages of recovery, agitation and irrational behavior may be a natural part of that progression. Three methods of management are used: (1) behavioral intervention, (2) medication, and (3) physical restraints. Informed staff members are usually able to handle episodes of agitation without pharmacologic or physical restraint by providing a secure environment, lowering the level of sensory stimulation, using a reassuring voice, rocking or patting, and redirecting. A family member's voice can be very calming. Patients who are ambulatory and agitated might be helped if they are allowed to walk, accompanied by a parent or a staff member, for extended periods.

Medication usually can be avoided but might be necessary when a patient is in danger of hurting himself or herself or others (Cardenas and McLean, 1992; Jaffe and Hays, 1986; Molnar and Perrin, 1992). It is important to remember that some tranquilizing agents can cause agitation and therefore will further complicate management (Mysiw and Sandel, 1997). Currently, we sometimes find small doses of lorazepam (Ativan) or chloral hydrate helpful. Caution should be exercised in using any psychoactive medication; the lowest effective dose given a few times is usually adequate to help a patient through this stage of recovery. Physical restraints are rarely indicated. An enclosed bed such as the Optima 300 bed (Val Products, Inc., Toledo, OH) is helpful for patients who have marked agitation. More information on dysfunctional behavior in head-injured children appears in Chapter 5.

Orthopedic Problems

Most children admitted to an inpatient rehabilitation facility after brain injury have been involved in motor vehicle accidents, either as passengers or pedestrians. Often they have sustained multiple injuries, including fractures. At the time of their rehabilitation admission, their fractures may not be fully healed and might require ongoing monitoring and care.

The long bones are fractured most frequently in pediatric victims of brain injury, the clavicle being the second most frequent site of fracture (Tepas et al., 1988). Neurologic dysfunction might complicate fracture healing: Flaccid paralysis from nerve injuries such as a brachial plexus injury may delay fracture healing. With spasticity, there is an increased risk of malunion from abnormal muscle forces (Hoffer and Brink, 1975).

Internal fixation is often used to manage long-bone fractures (Ziv and Rang, 1983). External fixator devices, such as the halo vest and Hoffman apparatus, are awkward and uncomfortable for the child. The pin sites of these devices require frequent cleaning and diligent monitoring for signs of infection. Fractures in limbs suffering flaccid paralysis require rigid internal fixation with a compression device, whereas fractures in spastic limbs require either rigid internal fixation or a well-applied cast (Guanche and Keanan, 1992).

Heterotopic ossification occurs less frequently in children than in adults (Hoffer et al., 1971). Most commonly, it occurs in children older than 10 years and it shows a propensity for long-term coma patients or patients with spasticity (Hurvitz et al., 1992; Nelson, 1992). Heterotopic ossification is suspected clinically when a patient's joint shows decreased range of motion, pain with range of motion, and swelling (Varghese, 1992). A bone scan will be positive 2–3 weeks before x-ray findings appear. Deceptively elevated alkaline phosphatase levels occur in growing children and in patients who have sustained fractures. The most commonly affected joints are, in decreasing order of frequency, hip, shoulder, elbow, and knee, with the highest incidence of ankylosis occurring in the elbow.

Treatment of heterotopic ossification includes passive range of the affected joint to the point of resistance. Etidronate disodium (Didronel) is used to treat only proved cases of heterotopic ossification in children, as rachitic bone changes have been reported in a pediatric patient who had been treated with etidronate disodium (Silverman et al., 1994). Surgical excision of calcification can be considered at approximately 2 years after the first appearance, because the calcifications are postulated to be mature at this time. Mital and coworkers (1987) reported successful surgical excision of immature calcification when postoperative salicylates at a dose of 60 mg/kg per day were used.

Skin Problems

In general, the incidence of decubitus is lower in children than in adults, possibly because of the relatively lower body weight of pediatric patients. Possible sources of decubitus in children who have sustained brain injuries include ill-fitting casts, splints, or braces. Based on transducer pressure studies, Solis and coworker (1988) postulated that in small children, whose head size is relatively large, the occiput is the most likely site for decubitus formation. In older children, the sacrum is the most common site. Prevention of decubitus includes frequently changing the child's position, monitoring equipment fit, and padding the surfaces on which the child is placed. Treatment of established decubitus includes positioning the child so that no weight is placed on the affected area and using a protective dressing such as Op-Site (Acme United Corporation, Bridgeport, CT) or DuoDerm (Convatec, Princeton, NJ).

Acne occurs frequently in adolescents. Steroids, used during the acute phase, or phenytoin (Dilantin) may aggravate this condition. Treatment of acne might include topical abrasives, drying agents, topical vitamin A, or antibiotics.

Headache and Pain

The incidence of posttraumatic headache is lower in children than in adults. Children who have sustained severe brain injuries experience posttraumatic headaches more frequently than do children with mild or moderate brain injuries. Mild analgesics, such as acetaminophen or ibuprofen, are helpful.

Other possible causes of pain include healing fractures, nerve injuries, muscle spasms, or previous surgical procedures. Usually mild analgesics are sufficient for treatment, although occasionally a combination of acetaminophen and codeine is needed. For short-term relief of severe muscle spasms, small doses of diazepam (Valium) are the most effective.

Cranial Nerve Impairment

Any of the cranial nerves may be damaged in severe brain injury, although those most commonly affected are the nerves involved in vision, hearing, balance, facial expression, and swallowing (Bruce, 1990). Olfactory and gustatory dysfunction frequently are underdiagnosed or misdiagnosed and should be suspected if there are changes in appetite or behavior (Zasler et al., 1992). Problems affecting olfaction should also be suspected when there is injury to the cribriform plate or when a cerebrospinal fluid leak occurs.

Vision Problems

Because most of our patients have one or more ophthalmologic problems, all patients undergo a comprehensive examination by an ophthalmologist. Vision problems can be caused directly by trauma to the brain, but it is not uncommon for visual impairment to result from associated eye injuries, which are usually detected and treated in acute care. Associated eye injuries might include eyelid lacerations, injury to the lacrimal collecting system, rupture of or injury to the globe, hyphema, corneal injuries, injury to the iris and ciliary muscles, injury to the lens, and neurosensory retinal damage and detachment (Catalano, 1993). The most common problems seen in rehabilitation are cranial nerve palsies, trauma to the optic nerve and chiasm, and visual field defects due to injury to the visual pathways or occipital cortex. Diplopia may be a symptom of fracture of the orbit. Retinal hemorrhages are seen often with injuries that result from child abuse (Duhaime et al., 1992).

Strabismus and ptosis usually resolve spontaneously in the first 6 months after injury; therefore, surgical correction should be postponed to allow spontaneous recovery. Judicious injection of botulinum toxin type A by an experienced ophthalmologist for cranial nerve palsy in selected patients may be of benefit to weaken the normal ipsilateral antagonist muscle during the time the nerve is healing (Biglan et al., 1989; Osako and Keltner, 1991).

The patient suffering low vision caused by injury may benefit from consultation with a low-vision specialist (Weiss and Soden, 1992). Visual evoked potential studies will aid in diagnosis.

Hearing Problems

Hearing problems sometimes occur in children with TBI (Jaffe et al., 1990). Therefore, hearing always is assessed. Brain stem auditory evoked potentials might be needed to make a diagnosis. Problems might be related to basilar skull fracture, temporal bone fracture, auditory nerve damage, or cochlear contusion and damage (Hall et al., 1993). Ossicular displacement or disruption is rare. Children are also prone to middle-ear infections and serous otitis media, which can result in conductive hearing problems, as can hemotympanum.

Uncommon Problems

A growing skull fracture is occasionally observed. This is a fracture that tears the dura at the fracture site, allowing the arachnoid and brain to protrude, thereby preventing healing of the fracture. A leptomeningeal cyst may result. Skull x-rays aid in the diagnosis. Cerebrospinal fluid fistula might be a late sequela if a defect in the pia-arachnoid has caused a cerebrospinal fluid leak (Mendizabal et al., 1992). Traumatic intracranial aneurysm is rare, and its diagnosis requires that the caregiver maintain a high index of suspicion in a child who fails to improve as expected or who manifests delayed neurologic deterioration (Ventureyra and Higgins, 1994).

Although children with severe brain injury can experience permanent impairment of hypothalamic-pituitary function, in our experience permanent impairment with resulting panhypopituitarism and traumatic diabetes insipidus is rare. Tanner staging is essential to monitor future sexual maturation or problems that might arise; rapid onset and progression of puberty is seen after severe brain injury.

Nutritional Assessment and Evaluation

The nutritional needs of the pediatric patient with brain injury have not been well researched (Phillips et al., 1987). Even less documentation exists concerning such patients' nutritional needs during the rehabilitation phase of recovery. Our approach to the nutritional management of the pediatric patient includes a comprehensive evaluation, development and implementation of a treatment plan, ongoing monitoring, and family education, including discharge and follow-up recommendations.

An outline of our assessment protocol at TRI is presented in Table 3-2. It includes a review of the metabolic responses to brain injury that have been identified in the adult patient (Young et al., 1991).

In the extremely malnourished child or adolescent, assessment of serum prealbumin and urinary urea nitrogen excretion might be indicated. Because it has a half-life of 2–3 days, serum prealbumin better indicates the current protein stores than does serum albumin. Serum prealbumin and urinary urea nitrogen tests are used to determine nitrogen balance and the need for additional protein in the diet.

Energy requirements are estimated using the Seashore formula (Seashore, 1984): Energy needs (calories per day) = [55 − (2 × age in years)] × weight (kg) × 1.5 (for maintenance, growth, and anabolism). If the child's weight is below the tenth percentile or above the ninety-fifth percentile on the growth charts of the National Center for Health Statistics, weight-age rather than chronologic age is used in the energy needs calculation. If sepsis is present, additional calories of 13% for each 1°C above normal (calculated energy needs × 0.67) are added.

Maintenance fluid requirements are estimated based on weight (Hazinski, 1984): Body weight of 0–10 kg requires 100 ml fluid/kg per day. (If renal and cardiac function is adequate, this may be increased to 150 ml/kg.) Body weight of 11–20 kg requires 1,000 ml fluid + 50 ml × (weight – 20 kg) per day. Body weight in excess of 20 kg requires 1,500 ml fluid + 25 ml (weight – 20 kg) per day.

Protein requirements during the rehabilitation recovery phase are estimated at the recommended daily allowance levels: for infants younger than 1 year, 2 g/kg body weight per day; for children, 1.0–1.5 g/kg per day of ideal body weight. Decubitus, infection, and steroid administration indicate an increase in protein needs to 1.5–2.0 g/kg per day.

One hundred percent of the recommended daily allowance for vitamins and minerals is required for children with brain injury. Additional supplementation might be needed due to the interaction of medications, wound healing, or food allergies.

Nutritional Treatment Plan

The development of a nutritional treatment plan is an interdisciplinary team task, involving the physician, registered dietitian, feeding therapist, nurse, and family. The dietitian determines calorie, protein, fluid, vitamin, and mineral requirements. The feeding therapist determines appropriate food and fluid consistencies, positioning requirements, and feeding techniques (see Chapter 7). The nursing staff monitors the patient's response to the feeding program, recording intake and output, feeding time, fatigue level, and tolerance of food consistencies (see Chapter 4). Family involvement in the nutritional care plan has several benefits:

- Families are extremely interested in feeding activities.
- Families can personalize a portion of the child's treatment, such as suggesting favorite foods, meals, and snacks.
- Family cooperation is imperative for safety reasons. Choking or aspiration resulting from improper food consistencies, positioning during food consumption, or feeding technique can occur when families are uninvolved in the child's current feeding program.
- Weight-control programs are ineffective without family support.

The physician coordinates and supervises the team's activities, using as a foundation the entire clinical picture of the patient.

Nutritional Treatment Plan Implementation and Monitoring

During rehabilitation, the interdisciplinary team meets frequently to assess and revise the treatment plan as the patient's status changes. Ongoing monitoring tools for determining nutritional status include weekly weights, creatinine height index (when desired intake level is achieved), monthly serum albumin levels, hematocrit and

Table 3-2. Nutritional Assessment

I.   History
     A. Age
     B. Gender
     C. Usual weight before injury
     D. Present activity level
     E. Feeding in acute-care hospital
        1. Type of feeding (texture)
        2. Method of delivery (oral, tube, or both)
        3. Amount consumed in 24 hours
     F. Food allergies and strong dislikes
     G. Presence or absence of decubitus, fever
II. Present medications
III. Anthropometric measurements
     A. Present height
     B. Present weight
IV. Laboratory data
     A. Hematocrit
     B. Hemoglobin
     C. Serum albumin
     D. Blood urea nitrogen

hemoglobin levels, and analyzed food intake records (Letson et al., 1981).

Nutritional requirements change during the rehabilitation process. Adjustments in calorie and protein levels may be necessary once an anabolic state is achieved. Maintaining nonambulatory patients at slightly less than their ideal body weight is beneficial in preventing impaired blood circulation, which may lead to pressure sores (Hargrave, 1979).

Tube feedings require additional monitoring plans. In our experience, the following considerations are important for tolerance and overall rehabilitation programming:

- Most patients do not have altered gastric emptying 2 weeks after injury. Enteral feedings maintain gastrointestinal tract integrity, which may be beneficial for immunocompetency and for reducing the metabolic response to stress (Ott et al., 1991). Therefore, enteral feedings are used most commonly in our facility.
- Intermittent drip and bolus feedings at night decrease the amount of time for daytime feedings, allowing additional time for therapies. Intermittent drip and bolus feedings may be dispensed via pump or gravity feed. They run 30 minutes to 1 hour and are followed by a 30-minute period of bed rest. This feeding method decreases the amount of vomiting and diarrhea and prepares the stomach for the introduction of meal-size volumes.
- Intermittent drip and bolus feedings while the patient is in an upright position may reduce gastroesophageal reflux and resultant aspiration (Podell, 1989).

Table 3-3. Incidence of Early and Late Seizures in Children After TBI

Study	Number of Early Seizures (%)		Number of Late Seizures (%)	
Hendrick and Harris, 1968	4,000	(6.5)		(1.3)
Stowsand and Bues, 1970		(7.0)	—	
Black et al., 1975	1,000	(15.0)	—	
Jamison and Kaye, 1974		(5.0)	—	
Jennett, 1975		(5.0)		(5.0)
Mises et al., 1970		(1.4)		(6.8)
Kollevold, 1976		(5.6)		(19.0)
Foulon and Noel, 1977	11		—	
Annegers et al., 1980	1,132	(2.6)	18	(1.6)
Hahn et al., 1988	937	(9.8)	2	(0.21)

- If the gastrointestinal tract has received no insult or if the insult is well healed, nonelemental formulations are useful in improving gastrointestinal tract function.
- Antidiarrheal medications may eliminate the need to change feeding formulations or the strength of formulation in the presence of loose stools.
- If diarrhea persists, tube feedings formulated from a combination of strained foods (i.e., Complete or tube feedings made from pureed baby foods, finely pureed table foods, milk, etc.) decrease the occurrence in some patients.
- When the patient can tolerate a transition from tube to oral feedings, the rehabilitation team works closely to maintain nutritional status. The dietitian provides information on total fluid and caloric needs for a 24-hour period and analyzes oral intakes to determine reductions in tube feedings. The responsibilities of the feeding therapist and nursing staff are described in Chapters 7 and 4, respectively.

Some patients experience hyperphagia. Our experience indicates that this phase is usually transient. Recording the time, amount, and types of food eaten in a logbook can serve as a cueing device for the patient; making low-calorie snacks (e.g., carrots, celery sticks, sugar-free drinks, and gelatin) easily accessible for staff to serve between meals reduces agitation and perseveration. Family members need detailed information concerning the hyperphagia treatment plan so that they can become active participants in this process. Family members also require nutritional counseling regarding appropriate food textures and specific food and drug interactions.

Discharge From and Follow-Up After Nutritional Treatment

Nutritional status is a component of discharge planning and follow-up. Families are counseled near discharge concerning hyperphagia, obesity prevention, possible food and drug interactions, and adequate intake for maintenance and growth. Guidelines may be given for meal and snack patterns and energy-expending activities. Families are encouraged to have their pediatrician monitor the patient for appropriate height and weight changes.

Posttraumatic Epilepsy

Epidemiologic Features

Seizures after brain injuries in young children are common. Pertinent issues include the timing of the seizure relative to the injury, the appropriate treatment approach, and the duration of treatment. Few studies have addressed these issues in children. The largest study (Annegers et al., 1980) was retrospective and included 1,132 children younger than 15 years. In this population, 2.6% had an early seizure and 1.5% developed late seizures. Hahn and coworkers (1988) followed up 937 children after brain injuries and found a high incidence of early seizures in children but a lower number of late seizures than that usually found in adults.

Time of onset of seizures in relation to the injury may have prognostic significance for later or recurrent seizures. Impact seizures are a form of early seizures, occurring at the time of injury. Early seizures present within the first week after the injury, and late seizures occur after the first week. Posttraumatic epilepsy is defined as two or more seizures after the first week of injury.

Early Seizures

Studies of seizures after TBI in children are summarized in Table 3-3. Early seizures have been reported to occur in 1.4–15.0% of children. Younger children have generally experienced a higher incidence of early seizures. However, Hahn and colleagues (1988) reviewed the course of 937 children with acute brain injury who were admitted to a large children's hospital and found that a younger age did not make a difference.

Most early seizures develop within the first 24 hours after injury. Pathophysiologic changes believed to contribute to seizures in this period include irritation from blood, systemic and central metabolic changes, and cellular disruption from the injury. These changes are not the same as those that contribute to late epilepsy. The more severe the injury and the lower the Glasgow Coma Scale (GCS) score, the greater is the chance that early seizures will occur.

Other factors associated with both early and late seizures include depressed skull fractures, dural penetration, posttraumatic amnesia, prolonged loss of consciousness, intracerebral hemorrhage, and epidural and subdural hematomas. Hahn and colleagues (1988) found that a GCS score of 8 or less correlated well with development of early posttraumatic seizures in adults. Lewis and coworkers (1993), in a retrospective study of 194 patients, noted that a GCS score of 3–8, an abnormal CT scan, and a loss of consciousness were associated with posttraumatic seizures. However, if these three factors were considered simultaneously, only the low GCS score was predictive for posttraumatic seizures: Of those patients with a low GCS score, 38.7% developed posttraumatic seizures, as compared to 3.8% with a GCS score of 8 or higher.

Seizures are classified according to the International Classification of Epilepsies (Commission on Classification and Terminology of the International League Against Epilepsy, 1981). Early seizures are usually partial, with features that might be clonic, tonic, dystonic, hemi-clonic, or tonic-clonic. The seizures usually involve facial and head areas. Hauser (1983) reported partial features in 40% of cases of early seizures. Partial seizures imply onset in a localized area of brain; however, the seizure focus might spread to other areas and become secondarily generalized. Impact seizures are usually single events, but seizures occurring after the injury often cluster. Status epilepticus, defined as a seizure lasting longer than 30 minutes, occurs in 1–5% of patients and is more common in children than in adults (Jennett, 1975). Status epilepticus tends to consist of partial seizures. Absence, myoclonic, atonic, and primary generalized tonic-clonic seizures are uncommonly seen after trauma.

Late Seizures and Epilepsy

Seizures that develop after the first posttrauma week are called *late seizures*. Late seizure types do not differ from early seizure types and are simple partial or complex partial with and without secondary generalization. If the patient experiences two or more seizures, the patient is said to have posttraumatic epilepsy.

Timing of the late period has varied. Hauser (1983) noted that seizures can still occur within the first few weeks after trauma because of acute changes related to the trauma, such as reaccumulation of the hematoma, development of infection, or systemic metabolic changes.

Whether these seizures should be considered early or late is debatable. Most authors define a late seizure as that developing after the first posttraumatic week. Those factors that appear to increase the risk for late seizures include the presence of an intracranial hematoma, depressed skull fracture, prolonged posttraumatic amnesia and, questionably, early seizures.

In children, the figures for posttraumatic epilepsy range from 0.21% to 19.0% (Annegers et al., 1980; Hahn et al., 1988; Kollevold, 1976) (see Table 3-3). Whereas early seizures are more common in children than in adults, late seizures and posttraumatic epilepsy are less common than in adults. Most seizures develop within the first year after the trauma. In adults, there appears to be a correlation between early seizures and posttraumatic epilepsy, but the data are less clear in children. Jennett (1975) and Hendrick and Harris (1968) noted an increased risk of later epilepsy after early seizures, although the incidence was one-half that found for adults. Annegers and colleagues (1980) found no correlation between early and late seizures.

The etiology of late seizures is different from that of early seizures. Willmore (1992) noted the impact of oxygen free radicals on cellular membrane and organelle functions in the development of seizures. These free radicals are the result of oxidation of hemosiderin and subsequent reaction with polyunsaturated fatty acids to form various free radical groups that damage cell membranes and organelles. Experimental studies have shown that these effects can be prevented with prior administration of alpha-tocopherol and selenium (Willmore, 1992). Other damaging mechanisms might include the production of excitatory amino acids such as glutamate, which is produced in mild to severe injuries involving frontothalamic and reticulothalamic pathways (Salazar, 1993).

The importance of a positive family history for epilepsy is uncertain (Hauser, 1983; Willmore, 1992). However, Willmore (1992) suggested that decreased levels of haptoglobin, which have been found in patients with familial epilepsy, might be significant as these are the glycoproteins that form stable complexes with free hemoglobin (Panter et al., 1985).

Weiss and coworkers (1983) developed a formula for predicting posttraumatic epilepsy for a population of Vietnam veterans. Predictions were based on the initial injury as categorized by (1) scalp, skull, or single-lobe injury without loss of consciousness; (2) features of scalp, skull, or single-lobe injury with impairment of consciousness; (3) multiple-lobe injury or wound crossing the midline without impairment of consciousness; and (4) features of multiple-lobe injury or wound crossing the midline with loss of consciousness. Those patients in category 4 developed earlier onset of seizures than those in category 1. The patients who did develop posttraumatic epilepsy did so within the first 12 months after the brain injury.

Seizures developing 4 or more years after the injury are more likely to persist (Jennett, 1975). Remission for 2 years does not guarantee that seizures will not recur (Caveness, 1963). Furthermore, the EEG does not appear to be predictive for determining those who will develop posttraumatic epilepsy (Jennett, 1975; Jennett and Teasdale, 1981; Thomaides et al., 1992). For example, Jennett (1975) found that 20% of patients with normal EEGs early after the injury still developed late epilepsy.

Treatment of Posttraumatic Seizures

Treatment issues differ for those children with acute seizures and those with late epilepsy. Patients with acute brain injuries with and without seizures are generally treated with anticonvulsants to prevent early seizures and the accompanying systemic complications such as aspiration pneumonia, further intracranial damage, and instability of vital signs (including blood pressure and respirations). Phenytoin has been the most commonly used drug. Well-controlled, double-blind studies of adults using phenytoin and placebo have demonstrated the efficacy of phenytoin in preventing the development of seizures within the first week after brain injury (Temkin et al., 1990). Temkin and colleagues (1990) showed that 3.6% of patients older than 16 years who were treated with phenytoin and 14.2% of those treated with placebo developed seizures. Phenytoin levels were maintained at 10–20 µg/ml throughout the first week. Others have found no differences between phenytoin and placebo at similar blood levels (Young et al., 1983a, b, c).

Lewis and colleagues (1993) reviewed the effect of prophylactic phenytoin in a retrospective study of 194 patients. In their high-risk group (GCS score, 3–8), 53% of those who received no anticonvulsants developed posttraumatic seizures, whereas only 15% of those who received anticonvulsants developed such seizures. These investigators concluded that the data obtained from the Temkin study could be applied to a pediatric population.

Current recommendations are that phenytoin loading be completed intravenously at a dose of 20 mg/kg and at a rate of 25 mg per minute. Intramuscular administration is not recommended because of poor drug absorption from muscle tissues and the potential for muscle necrosis secondary to high tissue pH. Measurements of phenytoin-free levels, as well as total serum levels, may be important in preventing the development of drug toxicity. Griebel and coworkers (1994) reported changes in protein binding of phenytoin in children after acute injuries, with progressive increases in the free fraction of phenytoin from day 1 to day 5. These workers did not note any signs of clinical toxicity, even with free levels of phenytoin of 8.5 mg/liter.

Despite its efficacy in the prevention of acute seizures, phenytoin does not affect the development of later seizures. Temkin and colleagues (1990) demonstrated that 21.5% of the phenytoin-treated group and 15.7% of the placebo-treated group developed seizures. By 2 years after brain injury, the figures were 27.5% and 21.1% for the phenytoin and placebo groups, respectively. Young and coworkers (1983b) also found that the prophylactic use of phenytoin did not prevent the development of late posttraumatic seizures.

Current recommendations are that antiepileptic drugs be used only during the acute phase of the injury and be discontinued as soon as possible if late seizures have not developed. These recommendations contradict recommendations from earlier studies that suggested that antiepileptic medication be continued for at least 1 year after the brain injury is sustained (Jennett and Teasdale, 1981).

Phenytoin has been the most frequently used drug for maintenance. Other commonly used antiepileptic drugs, such as phenobarbital and primidone, have effects on cognition and behavior (Trimble and Thompson, 1983). No studies compare the neurobehavioral side effects of phenytoin, carbamazepine, and valproic acid in a pediatric population with TBI. In her comprehensive review, Massagli (1991) did not draw any conclusion as to which drug is best for maintenance but suggested that cognition and behavior should be closely monitored during antiepileptic drug therapy and that, if clinical changes do occur, the physician should consider alternative drugs.

Wroblewski and coworkers (1989) replaced sedative drugs such as phenobarbital, primidone, and phenytoin with carbamazepine. Although their patients were switched to carbamazepine monotherapy, they were not evaluated for cognition and behavior before and after the change in medication.

Smith and coworkers (1994) demonstrated that both phenytoin and carbamazepine have negative effects on cognition in patients with brain injury. These authors noted that the effects were small and most evident in tasks requiring speed and motor skills.

Once they develop, late seizures usually persist. However, many patients do establish good control with the appropriately selected antiepileptic drug and with careful monitoring of the total and free serum levels of the drug. For maintenance, sedating drugs such as phenobarbital, primidone, and phenytoin should be avoided when possible. Although some sedation might occur with carbamazepine, studies indicate that these effects are less pronounced than with the other drugs mentioned. As most posttraumatic seizures are partial or complex partial, carbamazepine is an effective drug.

Alternatives include valproate, gabapentin, or lamotrigine. The latter two antiepileptic drugs were recently approved by the U.S. Food and Drug Administration for partial seizures. Gabapentin is an adjunctive drug that can be added to a primary antiepileptic such as carbamazepine without significant drug interaction. Side effects are minimal. Lamotrigine can be used as monotherapy for partial seizures. Side effects include drug rash, drowsiness, nausea, dizziness, and headache. Serious rash is more frequent in children who are taking sodium valproate when the dose of lamotrigine is rapidly escalated.

Once therapy is initiated, it should be maintained for a period of 2 years. If a patient remains seizure-free on medication for 2 years, the patient can be evaluated for drug discontinuation. Patients with a history of a penetrating injury, persistence of abnormality on head imaging, family history of epilepsy, and presence of epileptiform discharges on the EEG may be at greater risk for recurrence after withdrawal of medication.

In summary, children are more likely to have impact and early seizures but less likely to have posttraumatic epilepsy than are adults. Those factors that increase the risk of posttraumatic epilepsy include initial intracranial hematoma, depressed skull fracture, prolonged posttraumatic amnesia and, possibly, early seizures. It appears that the risk might be greater if several of these factors are involved. Treatment should be initiated for those children who have had a seizure or have any one of the cited risk factors. Phenytoin should be administered at a loading dose of 20 mg/kg intravenously and maintained at 5 mg/kg per day for the first week after trauma. If late seizures have not developed, the drug should be discontinued when the patient is believed to be clinically stable and ready to enter a rehabilitation program. Posttraumatic epilepsy, if it develops, is likely to be persistent and necessitates chronic antiepileptic therapy.

References

Annegers JF, Grabow JD, Groover RV, et al. (1980). Seizures after head trauma: a population study. Neurology 30;683.

Bachman DL (1992). The diagnosis and management of common neurologic sequelae of closed head injury. J Head Trauma Rehabil 7(2);50.

Biglan AW, Burnstine RA, Rogers GL, Saunders RA (1989). Management with strabismus with botulinum A toxin. Ophthalmology 96;935.

Black P, Shepard RH, Walker AE (1975). Outcome of head trauma: age and post-traumatic seizures. Ciba Found Symp 34;215.

Bruce DA (1990). Head injuries in the pediatric population. Curr Probl Pediatr 20(2);61.

Cardenas DD, McLean A Jr (1992). Psychopharmacologic management of traumatic brain injury. Phys Med Rehabil Clin North Am 3;273.

Catalano RA (1993). Eye injuries and prevention. Pediatr Clin North Am 40;827.

Caveness WF (1963). Onset and cessation of fits following craniocerebral trauma. J Neurosurg 20;570.

Chamovitz I, Chorazy AJL, Hanchett JM, Mandella P (1985). Rehabilitation Medical Management. In M Ylvisaker (ed), Head Injury Rehabilitation: Children and Adolescents. San Diego: College Hill Press, 119.

Citta-Pietrolungo TJ, Alexander MA, Cook SP, Padman R (1993). Complications of tracheostomy and decannulation in pediatric and young patients with traumatic brain injury. Arch Phys Med Rehabil 74;905.

Commission on Classification and Terminology of the International League Against Epilepsy (1981). Proposal for revised clinical and electrographic classification for epileptic seizures. Epilepsia 22;489.

Cope ND, Date ES, Mar EY (1988). Serial computerized tomographic evaluations in traumatic head injury. Arch Phys Med Rehabil 69;483.

Crysdale WS, Feldman RI, Naito K (1988). Tracheostomies: a 10-year experience in 319 children. Ann Otol Rhinol Laryngol 97;439.

Duhaime AC, Alario AJ, Lewander WJ, et al. (1992). Head injury in very young children: mechanisms, injury-types, and ophthalmologic findings in 100 hospitalized patients younger than 2 years of age. Pediatrics 90;179.

Foulon M, Noel P (1977). Epilepsie post-traumatic precoce dans l'efance: significance et prognostic à court terme. Neurol Belg 77;276.

Freeman JM (1986). Acute medical care of severe head injury is not enough. Pediatrics 77;251.

Gauderer MLW (1991). Percutaneous endoscopic gastrostomy: a 10-year experience with 220 children. J Pediatr Surg 26;288.

Goldberg AL, Sachs PR (1992). A guide to evaluating residential post-acute programs for children and adolescents with brain injury. J Cogn Rehabil 10;2.

Griebel ML, Kearns GL, Fiser DH, et al. (1994). Phenytoin protein binding in pediatric patients with acute traumatic injury. Crit Care Med 18;385.

Guanche C, Keanan MA (1992). Principles of orthopedic rehabilitation. Phys Med Rehabil Clin North Am 3;417.

Hahn YS, Fuchs AM, Flannery AM, et al. (1988). Factors influencing post-traumatic seizures in children. Neurosurgery 22;864.

Hald T, Bradley WE (1982). The Urinary Bladder: Neurology and Dynamics. Baltimore: Williams & Wilkins.

Hall JW III, Bratt GW, Schwaber MK, Baer JE (1993). Dynamic sensorineural hearing loss: implication for audiologists: case reports. J Am Acad Audiol 4;339.

Hargrave M (1979). Nutritional Care of the Physically Disabled. Minneapolis: Sister Kenny Institute.

Hauser WA (1983). Post-Traumatic Epilepsy in Children. In K Shapiro (ed), Pediatric Head Injury. Mount Kisco, NY: Futura, 271.

Hazinski MF (1984). Nursing Care of the Critically Ill Child. St. Louis: Mosby.

Helfaer MA, Wilson MD (1993). Head injury in children. Curr Opin Pediatr 5;303.

Hendrick EB, Harris L (1968). Post-Traumatic epilepsy in children. J Trauma 8;547.

Hoffer MM, Brink J (1975). Orthopedic management of acquired cerebral spasticity of childhood. Clin Orthop 110;244.

Hoffer MM, Garrett A, Brink J, et al. (1971). Orthopedic management of brain-injured children. J Bone Joint Surg Am 53;567.

Hurvitz AE, Mandac BR, Davidoff G, et al. (1992). Risk factors for heterotopic ossification in children and adolescents with severe traumatic brain injury. Arch Phys Med Rehabil 73;459.

Jacobson MS, Rubenstein EM, Bohannon WE, et al. (1986). Follow-up of adolescent trauma victims: a new model of care. Pediatrics 77;236.

Jaffe KM, Brink JD, Hays RM, Chorazy AJL (1990). Specific Problems Associated with Pediatric Head Injury. In M Rosenthal, E Griffith, M Bond, JD Miller (eds), Rehabilitation of the Adult and Child with Traumatic Brain Injury (2nd ed). Philadelphia: Davis, 539.

Jaffe KM, Hays RM (1986). Pediatric head injury: rehabilitative medical management. J Head Trauma Rehabil 4;30.

Jaffe KM, Massagli TL, Martin KM, et al.(1993). Pediatric traumatic brain injury: acute and rehabilitation costs. Arch Phys Med Rehabil 74;681.

Jamison DL, Kaye HH (1974). Accidental head injury in childhood. Arch Dis Child 49;376.

Jennett B (1975). Epilepsy and acute traumatic intracranial haematoma. J Neurol Neurosurg Psychiatry 38;378.

Jennett B, Teasdale G (1981). Management of Head Injuries. Philadelphia: Davis.

Kollevold T (1976). Immediate and early cerebral seizures after head injuries (part I). J Oslo City Hosp 26;99.

Letson AP, Ma KM, Stollar CA, Hain WF (1981). A Guide to Nutritional Care. Chicago: Mead-Johnson.

Lewis RN, Lee L, Imkelis SH, Gilmore D (1993). Clinical predictors of post-traumatic seizures in children with head trauma. Ann Emerg Med 22(7);132.

Logemann JA (1989). Evaluation and treatment planning for head injured patient with oral intake disorders. J Head Trauma Rehabil 4;24.

Massagli TL (1991). Neurobehavioral effects of phenytoin, carbamazepine, and valproic acid: implications for use in traumatic brain injury. Arch Phys Med Rehabil 72;219.

McCarthy PL (1991). Fever in Infants and Children. In PA Mackowiak (ed), Fever: Basic Mechanisms and Management. New York: Raven, 219.

Mendizabal GR, Moreno BC, Flores CC (1992). Cerebral spinal fluid fistulas: frequency in head trauma. Rev Laryngol Otol Rhinol 113;423.

Mises J, Lerique-Kochlin A, Rimoot P (1970). Post-traumatic epilepsy in children. Epilepsia 11;37.

Mital MA, Garber JE, Stinson JT (1987). Ectopic bone formation in children and adolescents with head injuries: its management. J Pediatr Orthop 7(1);83.

Molnar GE, Perrin JCS (1992). Head Injury. In GE Molnar (ed), Pediatric Rehabilitation. Baltimore: Williams & Wilkins.

Morton RE, Bonas R, Fourie B, Minford J (1993). Video fluoroscopy in the assessment of feeding disorders of children with neurological problems. Dev Med Child Neurol 35;388.

Mysiw WJ, Sandel ME (1997). The agitated brain injured patient. Part 2: pathophysiology and treatment. Arch Med Rehabil 78;217.

Nelson VS (1992). Pediatric head injury. Phys Med Rehabil Clin North Am 3;461.

Orsillo SM, McCaffrey RJ, Fisher J (1991). The impact of head injury on the family. J Head Inj 2(4);19.

Osako M, Keltner JL (1991). Botulinum A toxin (Oculinum) in ophthalmology. Surv Ophthalmol 36(1);26.

Osberg JS, DiScala C, Gans BM (1990). Utilization of inpatient rehabilitation services among traumatically injured children discharged from pediatric trauma centers. Am J Phys Med Rehabil 69(2);67.

Ott L, Young B, Phillips R, et al. (1991). Altered gastric emptying in the head injured patient; relationship to feeding intolerance. J Neurosurg 74;738.

Panter SS, Sadrzadeh SM, Hallaway PE, et al. (1985). Hypohaptoglobinemia associated with familial epilepsy. J Exp Med 161;748.

Phillips R, Ott L, Young B, Walsh J (1987). Nutritional support and measured energy expenditure of the child and adolescent with head injury. J Neurosurg 67;846.

Podell SK (1989). Intermittent tube feedings and gastroesophageal reflux control in head injured patients. J Am Diet Assoc 89(1);102.

Polinko PR, Barin JJ, Leger D, Bachman KM (1985). Working with the Family. In M Ylvisaker (ed), Head Injury Rehabilitation, Children and Adolescents. San Diego: College Hill Press, 103.

Pranzatelli MR, Pavlakis SG, Gould RJ, DeVivo DC (1991). Hypothalamic-midbrain dysregulation syndrome: hypertension, hyperthermia, hyperventilation, and decerebration. J Child Neurol 6;115.

Rivara JB, Jaffe KM, Fay GC, et al. (1993). Family functioning and injury severity as predictors of child functioning one year following traumatic brain injury. Arch Phys Med Rehabil 74;1047.

Salazar A (1993). Pathology of traumatic brain injury [abstract]. Epilepsia 34;1.

Sandel ME, Abrams PL, Horn LJ (1986). Hypertension after brain injury: case report. Arch Phys Med Rehabil 67;469.

Savage RC, Lash M, Bennett K, Navalta C (1995). Special education for students with brain injury. TBI Challenge 3;2.

Savage RC, Wolcott GF (eds) (1988). An Educator's Manual: What Educators Need to Know About Students with Traumatic Brain Injury. Washington, DC: National Head Injury Foundation.

Seashore JH (1984). Nutritional support of children in the intensive care unit. Yale J Biol Med 57;111.

Silverman SL, Hurvitz EA, Nelson VS, Chiodo MD (1994). Rachitic syndrome after disodium etidronate therapy in an adolescent. Arch Phys Med Rehabil 75;118.

Smith KR, Goulding PM, Wilderman D, et al. (1994). Neurobehavioral effects of phenytoin and carbamazepine in patients recovering from brain trauma: a comparative study. Arch Neurol 51;653.

Solis I, Kroskoup T, Trainer N, Maurburger MS (1988). Supine interface pressure in children. Arch Phys Med Rehabil 69;524.

Splaingard ML, Hutchins B, Sulton LD, Chaudhuri G (1988). Aspiration in rehabilitation patients: videofluoroscopy vs. bedside clinical assessment. Arch Phys Med Rehabil 69;637.

Stool SE, Beele JK (1973). Tracheostomy in infants and children: current problems. Pediatrics 3(5);1.

Stowsand D, Bues E (1970). Fruhanfalle und ihre ver laufe nach hirntramen im kindesalter. Z Neurol 198;202.

Temkin NR, Dikmen SS, Wilensky AJ, et al. (1990). A randomized, double-blind study of phenytoin for the prevention of post-traumatic seizures. N Engl J Med 323;497.

Tepas JJ, Ramenosky ML, Mollitt DL, et al. (1988). The pediatric trauma score as a predictor of injury severity: an objective assessment. J Trauma 28;425.

Thomaides TN, Kerezoudi EP, Chaudhuri KR, Cheropoulos C (1992). Study of EEGs following 24-hour sleep deprivation in patients with post-traumatic epilepsy. Eur Neurol 32;79.

Towbin RD, Bell WS Jr, Bissett GS III (1988). Percutaneous gastrostomy and percutaneous gastrojejunestomy in children: antegrade approach. Radiology 168;473.

Trimble MR, Thompson PJ (1983). Anti-convulsant drugs, cognitive function, and behavior. Epilepsia 24(Suppl 1);55.

Tyler JS, Mira MP, Hollowell JG (1989). Head injury training for pediatric residents. Am J Dis Child 143;930.

Varghese G (1992). Heterotopic ossification. Phys Med Rehabil Clin North Am 3;407.

Ventureyra ECG, Higgins MJ (1994). Traumatic intracranial aneurysms in childhood and adolescents. Childs Nerv Syst 10;361.

Weiss B, Soden R (1992). Head trauma and low vision: clinical modifications for diagnosis and prescription. J Am Optom Assoc 63;559.

Weiss GH, Feeney DM, Caveness WF (1983). Prognostic factors for the occurrence of post-traumatic epilepsy. Arch Neurol 40;7.

Willmore LJ (1992). Post-traumatic epilepsy. Neurol Clin 10;869.

Wroblewski BA, Glenn MB, Whyte J, Singer WD (1989). Carbamazepine replacement of phenytoin, phenobarbital and primidone in a rehabilitation setting: effects on seizure control. Brain Inj 3(2);149.

Ylvisaker M, Chorazy AJL, Cohen SD, et al. (1990). Rehabilitative Assessment Following Head Injury in Children. In M Rosenthal, E Griffith, M Bond, JD Miller (eds), Rehabilitation of the Adult and Child with Traumatic Brain Injury (2nd ed). Philadelphia: Davis, 558.

Ylvisaker M, Weinstein M (1989). Recovery of oral feeding after pediatric head injury. J Head Trauma Rehabil 4;51.

Young B, Ott L, Phillips R, McClain C (1991). Metabolic management of the patient with head injury. Neurosurg Clin North Am 2;301.

Young B, Rapp RP, Norton JA, et al. (1983a). Failure of prophylactically administered phenytoin to prevent early post-traumatic seizures. J Neurosurg 58;231.

Young B, Rapp RP, Norton JA, et al. (1983b). Failure of prophylactically administered phenytoin to prevent late post-traumatic seizures. J Neurosurg 58;236.

Young B, Rapp RP, Norton JA, et al. (1983c). Failure of prophylactically administered phenytoin to prevent post-traumatic seizures in children. Childs Brain 10(3);185.

Zasler ND, McNeny R, Heywood PG (1992). Rehabilitative management of olfactory and gustatory dysfunction following brain injury. J Head Trauma Rehabil 7(1);66.

Zerilli KS, Stefans VA, DiPietro MA (1990). Protocol for use of videofluoroscopy in pediatric swallowing dysfunction. Am J Occup Ther 44;441.

Ziv I, Rang M (1983). Treatment of femoral fraction in the child with head injury. J Bone Joint Surg 65;276.

Zulch K (1969). Medical Causation. In EA Walker, WF Caveness, M Critchely (eds), The Late Effects of Head Injury. Springfield, IL: Thomas, 453.

Chapter 4

The Recovery Continuum: A Nursing Perspective

June Marshall

The pediatric trauma continuum presents nurses with a challenging diversity of professional roles and practice settings. Although some groups of children and adolescents with traumatic brain injury (TBI) might fare better than their adult counterparts due to enhanced physiologic and developmental resilience, two groups that have not fared as well are children with frontal lobe injuries and infants. Despite historically optimistic perceptions regarding outcomes, these children, adolescents, and their families face a long, obstacle-strewn road to recovery. Overcoming the obstacles faced by these individuals and their families demands the brightest and best that nursing has to offer. Therapeutic nursing strategies in today's changing health care environment must be flexible, cost-effective, developmentally and culturally sensitive, and family centered.

Nursing Roles and Responsibilities in the Trauma Continuum

To meet their biopsychosocial needs, children and adolescents with TBI demand a broad range of nursing expertise. Professional nursing services and roles along the pediatric trauma continuum run the gamut from prevention education to acute-care and rehabilitative management and culminate in school and community-based settings. Few areas of pediatric subspecialty practice require such a vast array of nursing knowledge and skills as does the care of children and adolescents with TBI.

TBI Prevention Education

TBI prevention programs range from organized efforts (such as those sponsored by hospitals, local chapters of the Brain Injury Association, and SAFE KIDS) to anticipatory safety education carried out during the course of routine primary care visits. The National SAFE KIDS Campaign, via local grassroots coalitions, provides injury-prevention education and awareness programs focusing on bicycle, helmet, vehicle, pedestrian, and playground safety. SAFE KIDS also focuses efforts on media outreach and national, state, and local legislation regarding many aspects of childhood safety and injury prevention. Additional information on the services and resources of the National SAFE KIDS Campaign can be obtained by writing to their headquarters at 1301 Pennsylvania Avenue NW, Suite 100, Washington, DC, 20004-1707 or calling 202-662-0600.

Health care and community screening can identify risk factors associated with TBI in pediatric populations and create a sound basis for the development and implementation of appropriate preventive education. These risk factors include poor parenting techniques, family stress, substance abuse, firearm possession, evidence of home or community violence, lack of knowledge regarding safety devices (e.g., bicycle helmets, child safety restraints), and presence of any other risk-taking behaviors. Nurses play an important role in the assessment and identification of risk factors and in family education aimed at injury prevention. Prevention education must target specific risk factors identified through the assessment process and must also provide developmentally sensitive anticipatory guidance for high-risk populations. Leisure and vehicle safety, healthy parenting skills, alternatives to violent behavior, and issues regarding substance abuse are key elements of brain injury–prevention education programs.

Acute-Care Management

Acute-care nursing management of children and adolescents with TBI focuses primarily on prevention of secondary injury. Acute care of pediatric populations with severe injuries involves lifesaving measures initiated during the course of ground or air transport or in emergency departments. Survival and physiologic stabilization, including establishment and maintenance of airway, breathing, and circulation, are the foundations of this initial phase of nursing management. Depending on the severity of injury, the child or adolescent is then transferred to either a critical care or an inpatient hospital unit, where the goal continues to be prevention of secondary physiologic injury. In addition to the promotion of biopsychosocial recovery, nursing responsibilities during the acute-care phase include child advocacy, family support, and education. As the child or adolescent progresses through the acute-care phase, the nursing staff assists the family in making the transition to rehabilitative services.

Acute-care nursing management for children with mild to moderate brain injuries involves initial assessment and observation in a variety of health care settings and might also involve referral to community-based programs for rehabilitative services. The child or adolescent discharged from an emergency or ambulatory care setting without a hospital stay might experience significant short-term sequelae related to the brain injury. In these settings, the nursing staff shoulders an immense responsibility to educate parents, notify schools, and identify resource networks that can assist in managing these brain injury sequelae. Nurses in the acute-care setting also play an important role in identifying neglect or abuse and referring children to protective services when circumstances surrounding the injury are suspicious in nature.

Rehabilitation

The role of nurses in pediatric brain injury rehabilitation is the most diverse, with regard to responsibilities and practice settings, of any nursing roles described thus far. Nursing practice directly involved in pediatric brain injury rehabilitation might include working in an inpatient rehabilitation unit, in homes through a home care agency, in a long-term care facility, or in an infant intervention program. Other roles that involve specific aspects of rehabilitation nursing practice include case managers, school nurses, nurses in ambulatory health care settings, nurses in residential treatment facilities, or consultants to attorneys regarding life care planning.

Nurses are key members of collaborative interdisciplinary teams during the rehabilitation phase of recovery from pediatric TBI (Brillhart and Sills, 1994). The nurse directly manages identified nursing needs and supervises rehabilitation aides or assistants in providing delegated nursing tasks. The rehabilitation nurse might also serve as case manager for select patient populations. Primary nursing responsibilities involved in rehabilitation include promotion of recovery, advocacy, education, support, and empowerment for children, adolescents, and their families. In any therapeutic milieu, the rehabilitation nurse participates in the development, implementation, evaluation, and revision of the multidisciplinary treatment plan. The rehabilitation nurse serves as advocate, educator, consultant, and coach, not only for individuals with brain injuries and their families but also for a variety of personnel from community-based agencies and educational programs.

Theoretical Framework for Nursing in Pediatric TBI Cases

Pediatric nurses must draw on a vast array of biopsychosocial knowledge and skills when planning and providing care for children and families. The brain injury continuum, however, requires the sophisticated synthesis and integration of nursing theory and practice in a unique manner. This unique aspect of nursing practice draws on theories grounded in family systems and in individual and family development. Although family systems and developmental theories are relevant for many aspects of pediatric nursing, these theories often are stretched or redefined with regard to the alteration in functional domains (e.g., physiologic, cognitive, social, emotional) experienced by populations that sustain brain injuries.

Several theorists have created frameworks that are particularly relevant to nursing care of children and adolescents with TBI. Hymovich (1979) described one developmental framework that can be used for family assessment and identification of needs related to chronic conditions. Her framework focuses on domain-specific needs of both individual and family and on developmental tasks of the family in light of family strengths. Hymovich defined individual and family needs in terms of physiologic, cognitive, social, and emotional domains. Her model uses a family systems approach to enable individual family members to reach full potential and ultimately to function effectively within the community. The model recognizes the need for adaptations in family organization and management necessitated by the injured individual's chronic condition and defines a hierarchy of developmental issues that influence individual and family outcomes. In essence, if the family cannot meet its basic physical needs, the stresses of supporting the family's cognitive, emotional, and social development seem insurmountable. Building on the family's developmental strengths while ensuring that basic needs are met can facilitate the accomplishment of higher-level skills such as adaptation to injury and successful community reintegration.

Family-centered care principles create the cornerstone of healthy pediatric nursing practice and must be acknowledged and combined with other theoretical tenets when care is being provided for children, adolescents, and their families. These principles, published by the Association for the Care of Children's Health (Shelton et al., 1987), include the following essential components:

- The family is the constant in the child's life, whereas service-related systems and personnel change.

- Parent-professional collaboration must be facilitated at all levels of care.
- Unbiased and complete information regarding the child's care should be shared with the child's parents in a supportive manner on an ongoing basis.
- Appropriate policies and programs that provide emotional and financial support should be implemented to meet the needs of families.
- Family strengths and individuality should be recognized, and diverse methods of coping should be respected.
- Developmental needs of infants, children, adolescents, and their families should be understood and incorporated into health care.
- Parent-to-parent support is encouraged.
- Health care delivery systems should be designed to be accessible, flexible, and responsive to family needs.

Imogene King's (1981) open systems model and theory of goal attainment seem especially pertinent to rehabilitation nursing in pediatric populations with TBI. Her model uses an open systems framework that defines the individual as a personal system composed of concepts related to perception, the self, body image, growth and developmental factors, time, and space. This personal system then interacts individually with interpersonal systems and groups of interpersonal systems to form a social system. These interacting systems are combined with concepts related to health and the environment and, finally, to nursing. In King's model, the client and nurse interact with a focus on mutually establishing goals aimed at achieving optimal health, which leads to successful functioning in family and community roles. The nurse, patient, and family collaborate as team members to identify strategies for successful goal attainment.

Dorothea Orem (1985) defines prerequisites for self-care as those basic physiologic and psychological needs of all human beings. Her intervention model for nursing focuses on the level of support required from nurses to assist individuals or family members in meeting those basic needs. The levels vary from complete dependence on nurses in performing self-care tasks to an intermediate level in which the nurse assists in self-care and finally to a system whereby the nurse educates and facilitates independence in self-care. The major limitation in this model is that the ability to direct care independently in the face of severe disability, while being totally dependent on others to perform these aspects of care, is not recognized by Orem as a level of independence. The strength of Orem's model, however, is in the conceptualization of the nurse as a coach in empowering the child, adolescent, and family toward independence in self-care skills that preserve life and promote health and well-being. Both parents and novice professionals often require education regarding developmentally appropriate self-care goals for children and adolescents who are physically, cognitively, and socially impaired by neurologic insult.

The Acute-Care Phase

The acute-care phase of survival and recovery from TBI in childhood and adolescence necessitates skillful implementation of the nursing process. Astute nursing judgment, problem solving, and intervention strategies may prevent or minimize secondary injury, influence patient survival, and improve patient outcomes. The nurse's role during this crucial phase of recovery involves tremendous communication and collaboration with multiple medical specialists and other members of the multidisciplinary team. The nurse functions interdependently to identify problems, implement therapeutic interventions, evaluate response to treatment, and revise the plan of care accordingly. Johnson and Roberts (1996) suggest strategies that encourage hope for families during the acute recovery phase. The strategies include providing information, controlling decision making, enhancing the environment, promoting proximity of nurse and family to patient, fostering interpersonal relationships, and providing emotional support.

Important Aspects of the Assessment

Pediatric brain injury is a developmental phenomenon with regard to mechanism and nature of injury. Approximately 25% of brain injuries in children younger than 2 years result from physical abuse (Duhaime et al., 1992; Michaud et al., 1993a). Other common causes of TBI are motor vehicle collisions, falls, leisure- or sports-related injuries, and violent crimes. Factors associated with increased risk of TBI include male gender, nonwhite race, low socioeconomic status, family instability, peak periods for outdoor recreation, and living in congested areas (Johnston and Gerring, 1992; Kraus et al., 1990; Rivara, 1994).

Primary brain injuries can occur as the result of a direct blow to the head or from forces associated with acceleration-deceleration phenomena. Secondary injuries from loss of blood flow and oxygen to the brain might be caused by a number of factors ranging from hypoxia to hemorrhage (Ghajar and Hariri, 1992; Johnston and Gerring, 1992; Kaufman and Dacey, 1994; Michaud et al., 1993b; Noah et al., 1992). Nurses must have an understanding of mechanisms and types of injury and the pathophysiology of secondary injury, because nurses play a vital role in the initial assessment process. Often the assessment can identify factors that more clearly delineate the injury as traumatic or anoxic or hypoxic (or a combination of these). Duhaime and colleagues (1992) described a biomechanical profile that highlights the following salient aspects of initial assessment of the child in pediatric brain injury:

- Narrative description of the incident
- Time of incident
- Witnesses to the incident
- Child's position and location before and after the incident
- Instrument or object involved if head was struck directly
- If motor vehicle collision, speed of all vehicles involved, point of impact, and any other relevant information (e.g., use of restraints)
- Pressure or compression of chest or abdominal cavities
- Time (estimate) between incident and first observation
- Immediate response after the incident—subject's responsiveness, eyes open or closed, sounds (e.g., speech or crying), seizure activity, color
- Manipulation after the incident, such as resuscitation or shaking

Additional assessment of the child is completed after initial resuscitation in an emergency or critical care setting using the Glasgow Coma Scale (GCS) (Teasdale and Jennett, 1974) or the Modified GCS (James and Trauner, 1985). These scales quantify ocular, verbal, and motor responses and assist the practitioner in establishing and monitoring severity of injury during the acute phase. Patients with GCS scores of 8 or less are generally said to have severe injuries; those having scores of 9–12 fall into the moderate category, and scores in the 13–15 range are classified as mild (Langfitt and Gennarelli, 1982). Michaud and colleagues (1992) found that respiratory status in the emergency department and the motor component of GCS scores 72 hours after injury were most predictive of quality of survival. Ongoing assessment cannot be emphasized strongly enough in light of possible secondary injury, such as hemorrhage, cerebral edema, hypertension, or hypoperfusion, which may result in neurologic deterioration. Initial and ongoing family assessments provide insight into events surrounding the child's injury, coping styles, family functioning, and future concerns.

Intervention Strategies

Nursing interventions during the acute phase of brain injury recovery focus on resuscitation, stabilization, and prevention of secondary injury. The ABCs of care for any critical injury or illness in childhood—airway, breathing, and circulation—must be supported to sustain life and preserve brain function after brain injury. In addition, nursing strategies during the acute phase focus on management of increased intracranial pressure (ICP); hemodynamic homeostasis; appropriate fluid, electrolyte, and nutritional support; and administration and monitoring of pharmacologic agents. Acute nursing management promotes psychophysiologic comfort and initial recovery while facilitating family support and education.

Successful management of increased ICP is a critical element in recovery from the acute-care phase. ICP monitoring can be accomplished by a variety of techniques and devices. Some authors (e.g., Ghajar and Hariri, 1992) maintain that ventricular monitoring is the optimal method because of fluid coupling transduction and the ability to reduce ICP via cerebrospinal fluid drainage. Other methods used to reduce increased ICP include positioning the head in midline and 30-degree head elevation (in patients without spinal cord injury), sedation, controlled hyperventilation, dehydration (including use of osmotic agents), steroid administration, hypothermia, sensory deprivation, and barbiturate coma (Ghajar and Hariri, 1992; Noah et al., 1992). Studies evaluating the early use of hyperventilation have concluded that it must be used selectively and monitored carefully because of adverse side effects, including ischemia, increased ICP, and cerebral hypoxia (Crosby and Parsons, 1992; Stringer et al., 1993). Successful management of increased ICP may prevent cerebral herniation, preserve cerebral perfusion, and minimize secondary brain insult.

Respiratory management is another important aspect of care in patients with brain injury. Cerebral oxygenation is essential for preservation of brain tissue and function. Intubation and mechanical ventilation may be required. The respiratory care usually administered to critically ill patients, however, may be significantly decreased in patients with increased ICP because of the ill effects produced by activities such as endotracheal suctioning and chest physiotherapy. Any reduction in aggressive respiratory care may place the patient at risk for atelectasis or pneumonia. To prevent increased ICP, patients can be premedicated with lidocaine or thiopental sodium before suctioning.

Adequate cerebral perfusion without hyperemia or cerebral edema are the goals of hemodynamic monitoring and fluid and electrolyte therapy. Much controversy surrounds fluid restriction or dehydration as a means of preventing or treating cerebral edema (Noah et al., 1992; Prough, 1990; Shackford, 1990). Kaufman and Dacey (1994) argue that dehydration can lead to hypoperfusion and should be avoided. Two complications associated with fluid and electrolyte imbalances can occur, and both may be evidence of deteriorating outcome. The first, diabetes insipidus, might initially be managed by carefully maintaining fluid balance; if this therapy fails, however, pharmacologic intervention with vasopressin is indicated (Noah et al., 1992). The second, the syndrome of inappropriate excretion of antidiuretic hormone, can best be treated with fluid restriction. Common hematologic complications include anemia and disseminated intravascular coagulation (Noah et al., 1992).

Gastrointestinal system complications and nutritional support require careful attention in children and adolescents with brain injury. The most common gastrointestinal complication is stress ulcer. Pharmacologic prophylaxis is aimed at altering gastric pH but might not prevent gastric ulceration (Noah et al., 1992). Two other gastrointestinal sequelae include pancreatitis and gastroesophageal reflux (McLean et al., 1995). Nutritional support in pediatric brain injury is based on developmental requirements as well as on baseline and estimated nutrient needs. Brain injury creates significant stress and thereby increases metabolic demand, though the actual increase in metabolic need has been argued by several investigators (Chioléro et al., 1989; Creasey et al., 1989; Kaufman and Dacey, 1994; Moore et al., 1989; Phillips et al., 1987). Appropriate nutritional support should begin immediately after the patient's general condition and fluid and electrolyte status have stabilized. Nutrition may be provided either enterally or parenterally, depending on whether the patient's gastrointestinal tract is usable. Glucose intolerance is frequently associated with parenteral alimentation administration and might limit adequate provision of nonprotein calories, thereby necessitating insulin therapy (Noah et al., 1992).

In addition to the many physiologic aspects of nursing management, the acute phase involves the implementation of many therapeutic nursing strategies aimed at promoting cognitive, emotional, and social recovery. Brain injury is a stressful and disorienting phenomenon. Pediatric patients awaken from coma, often surrounded by strangers, in overstimulating, unfamiliar environments. Family members can enhance orientation, familiarity, and early recovery by their presence and involvement in the child's care. The family can provide helpful cues to the nursing staff regarding the individual's interests, developmental strengths and weaknesses, and baseline behavior patterns. The nurse can provide, on the basis of an understanding of the pathophysiologic insult and patient's status, family education regarding the stages of brain injury recovery. Ongoing assessment of both patient and family can assist the nurse in individualizing education and anticipatory guidance. Factors the nurse should consider when developing the education plan include family and patient needs, cultural issues, learning styles, family values, and readiness to learn. Activities such as making audiotapes or videotapes and bringing pictures or favorite objects from home might be suggested to distraught parents during early phases of recovery, when sensory input is limited. As the child or adolescent improves, the family can be more involved in social interaction and certain aspects of care such as bathing, range-of-motion, or sensory stimulation activities. Depending on the child's oral motor abilities, the family might also be involved in oral feeding activities.

During the course of the patient's recovery from the acute insult, the nurse might also assume a primary role of referral to other interdisciplinary team members on the basis of specific patient and family needs. Among these team members are physical, occupational, or speech therapists; a child life specialist; a psychologist; a social worker; a nutritionist; a teacher; a respiratory therapist; a chaplain; and a case manager or discharge planner. Family members may require much education and anticipatory guidance as they make plans for the transition to the rehabilitation phase of the child's recovery. The nurse's primary roles as the acute phase ends are often those of facilitator, liaison, and advocate.

The Rehabilitation Phase

The transition to rehabilitation is fraught with mixed emotions for many families. Although thankful for their child's survival, parents must now face the future with a child who is very different from the person they knew and who might have many special needs. Improvement from this point forward can range from minute gains to nearly complete recovery. The vast array of emotions experienced along this recovery continuum can include frustration, anger, guilt, denial, sadness, joy, relief, grief, and hope. These emotions are rarely static, and each family has its own means of coping with the prospects of permanent disability or impairment in a child. Developmental expectations can change significantly as a result of limitations imposed by the neurologic insult. Despite attempts to predict outcomes on the basis of factors associated with severity of injury (e.g., low initial GCS scores, prolonged coma, severe extracranial injury, prolonged increased ICP, hypoxic or ischemic injury, diffuse axonal injury, and mass lesions), children have been known to defy statistics and achieve remarkable recoveries. By the same token, deficits related to higher cognitive functions of abstract thought, reasoning, and judgment may not be readily apparent until adolescence or young adulthood, many years after the initial injury. In children and adolescents in whom impairments are not obvious, parents and professionals might deny the need for special services in the community. Therefore, the nursing staff must skillfully adapt its strategies to the ever-changing rehabilitative needs of the child or adolescent.

Nursing management during the rehabilitation phase must be individualized according to the child's or adolescent's specific physiologic, developmental, cognitive, social, and emotional needs. The nurse and physician team may focus heavily at times on physiologic needs, whereas there is much interdisciplinary collaboration regarding therapeutic management in all other domains. Supporting the family through the stages of coma recovery while educating and empowering the parents as caregivers becomes the central theme of family-centered care during the rehabilitation phase. Major problem areas for nurses during this phase of recovery are described in the following sections. Common nursing diagnoses related to TBI are outlined in Table 4-1.

Table 4-1. Common Nursing Diagnoses Related to Pediatric TBI

Potential for secondary injury related to agitation, confusion, combative behavior, or posttraumatic seizure disorder

Nutritional alterations—specifically, inappropriate nutrient intake (greater than or less than requirements, depending on success of early management on the basis of metabolic demand; undernutrition as a result of inadequate oral intake secondary to dysphagia; overnutrition as a result of hyperphagia secondary to poor impulse control, growth hormone stimulation, or pituitary insult)

Potential for aspiration related to absent protective reflexes (e.g., gag and cough reflexes), poor oral motor function, or gastroesophageal reflux

Fluid volume deficit related to inadequate oral intake or inability to meet estimated fluid demands secondary to increased insensible losses

Impaired skin integrity related to undernutrition, immobility, or shearing forces associated with agitation

Hypothermia or hyperthermia related to alterations in central neurologic control of temperature or infection

Incontinence of bowel or bladder (or both) secondary to upper motor neuron insult, concurrent spinal cord injury, or altered cognitive function

Caregiver strain related to stress, inadequate support systems, and increased demands on caregiver

Impaired physical mobility related to upper motor neuron insult, peripheral nerve injury, concurrent spinal cord injury, or movement disorder

Self-care deficit related to altered physical mobility, agitation, altered cognition, developmental delay, or lack of appropriate assistive devices

Ineffective airway clearance secondary to cranial neuropathy

Sleep pattern disturbance secondary to pain, agitation, unfamiliar or overstimulating environment, or interruptions for provision of nursing care

Chronic pain secondary to headache, heterotopic ossification, contractures, or spasticity

Sensory and perceptual alteration related to coma recovery, cranial neuropathy, or specific insult to visual, olfactory, auditory, tactile, or taste structure and function

Knowledge deficit related specifically to brain injury, to related aspects of care after brain injury, and to expectations for the future

Impaired social interaction related to aphasia, apraxia, impulsivity, poor insight, social isolation, or self-care deficits

Self-esteem disturbance related to altered self-perception and body image owing to injury-imposed disability or impairment

Impaired verbal communication related to aphasia or apraxia resulting from brain insult

Altered family processes related to changing roles and expectations resulting from the child's or adolescent's injury

Sexual dysfunction related to disinhibition, impulsivity, lack of insight, neurologic insult, or pharmacotherapeutic side effects

Source: AE McCourt (ed) (1993). The Specialty Practice of Rehabilitation Nursing: A Core Curriculum (3rd ed). Skokie, IL: Rehabilitation Nursing Foundation.

Nutrition

The nutrient needs of many children who sustain severe TBI and enter rehabilitation are inadequately met due to unpredictably high metabolic demands or to gastrointestinal or other multisystem complications. In contrast, some children, on entering rehabilitation settings, may receive greater nutritional supplementation than their current levels of activity demand. Because growth hormone stimulation often occurs as a result of injury, many children with TBI undergo tremendous growth spurts during coma recovery.

Provision of appropriate nutrients must be based on individualized assessment and knowledge of the patient's developmental requirements in light of both current needs and expected neurologic outcome. The goal of nutritional therapy during the rehabilitation phase is provision of nutrients in the most physiologically and economically acceptable method. Family realities and resources must be considered when the specifics of nutritional support in the home are decided. Long-term nasogastric tubes can be a source of both agitation and infection. If long-term enteral supplementation is anticipated, a percutaneous or surgical gastrostomy feeding tube may be indicated. In the child with poor oral motor function in whom nutrient needs are unlikely to be met by oral feeding, enteral nutrient supplementation can often alleviate parent-child struggles surrounding feeding issues. Home care plans for feeding must be made with the primary caregiver in mind. If the nursing staff spends 45 minutes to 1 hour feeding a child a mere fraction of the total nutrient needs for that meal, it is highly unlikely that a primary caregiver will succeed in meeting the child's nutrient needs by oral feedings on a daily basis at home.

Respiration

On entry into rehabilitation facilities, children with severe injury may have compromised respiratory function. Children who required mechanical ventilation for prolonged periods during the acute-care phase often require tracheostomies. Respiratory dysfunction in these populations most often involves the upper airway unless the child has aspirated, developed atelectasis, or acquired an infection that has affected the lower respiratory system. Assessment of protective cough and gag reflexes and the presence of a patent airway without residual tracheal stenosis are key factors in deciding whether to remove the tracheostomy before the patient's discharge from rehabilitation. Citta-Pietrolungo and colleagues (1993) recommend the following criteria for successful decannulation: (1) maintenance of adequate oxygenation and ventilation, (2) provision of intact mechanisms for managing secretions, (3) treatment of infections or other systemic abnormalities that increase the work of breathing, (4) maintenance of adequate nutritional status, and (5) airway protection and aspiration prevention. If the patient must be discharged to home with a tracheostomy in place, the primary caregiver and day-care or school personnel must be instructed in cardiopulmonary resuscitation and all aspects of tracheostomy care. The involved skills are suctioning, ventilating (bagging), providing site care, changing tracheostomy ties and tubes, administering humidified air (or oxygen), performing chest physiotherapy and postural drainage (if indicated), administering aerosolized medications (if indicated), performing emergency procedures related to respiratory distress, cleaning equipment and supplies, and preventing aspiration.

In children without tracheostomy tubes who may be at risk for aspiration, atelectasis, or pulmonary infection, protection of the airway through positioning, careful feeding techniques, pulmonary toilet, or suctioning may be indicated.

Bowel and Bladder Function

Bowel and bladder management during the acute-care phase is aimed at developmentally appropriate acquisition or reacquisition of continence and the prevention of urinary retention or constipation. Toileting programs may be initiated as soon as is cognitively appropriate. The use of timed voiding routines, verbal and physical cues, and accessible toileting devices may improve the child's chances at continence. Recognizing that injury, immobility, diet, and pharmacologic side effects can all affect urine and stool voiding and retention is the first step in creating a successful toileting program. Establishing normal bowel routines related to meal times can be difficult during the course of a busy treatment schedule. Stool softeners, toilet sitting after meals, and suppository programs are sometimes necessary to re-establish normalcy.

Skin Integrity

Assessment of skin integrity is a key component of all rehabilitative nursing practice. Specific risk factors for skin problems present in some individuals with brain i include poor nutritional status, diaphoresis, immobility, contractures, spasticity, urinary and fecal incontinence, combative or agitated behavior, upper- and lower-extremity orthoses, or inhibitory casts and surgically created or traumatic wounds. Acne vulgaris might be problematic after TBI and necessitates treatment with topical agents (McLean et al., 1995). Careful monitoring and early attention to erythematous skin can often prevent and certainly minimize breakdown. Use of positioning techniques or specialized pressure relief devices may be indicated.

Pharmacotherapeutics

An important interdependent nursing responsibility is the administration and monitoring of responses to pharmacologic agents in patients with TBI. Anticonvulsants may be given in patients with posttraumatic seizures and may also be used prophylactically (although their efficacy in this setting is controversial) (Aicardi, 1990; Temkin et al., 1990). Pharmacologic intervention may also be used to stimulate neurotransmitter production, manage depressive symptomatology, improve sleep and rest cycles, and treat behavior or attention disorders (Joseph and Wroblewski, 1995; Richelson, 1990). Careful assessment, monitoring, and documentation of agent-specific therapeutic effects and adverse reactions are essential elements of any successful treatment program.

Some neuropharmacologic agents are costly and have potentially harmful side effects. The risks and benefits should therefore be weighed carefully before their long-term use is recommended. Nursing input regarding patient response is important in evaluating efficacy of pharmacologic agents, as nurses observe the patients over larger windows of time than do other team members.

Sleep, Rest, and Comfort

Children and adolescents who enter rehabilitation facilities have generally come from frightening, overstimulating, and disorienting environments. Activities required to sustain life and promote recovery in intensive care and acute-care inpatient settings are often incompatible with normal patterns of sleep and rest. Creative scheduling of therapy sessions in a rehabilitation facility necessitates consideration of the developmental and physiologic needs of children and adolescents while satisfying payer requirements for daily hours of therapy. Normalizing naptime and bedtime rituals and scheduling appropriate time allotments for naps and sleep facilitate more effective therapy sessions while promoting recovery.

Communication

Communication is a basic human need often altered by brain injury. Nurses in pediatric rehabilitation settings are required to have not only an understanding of the developmental acquisition of communication skills but also a working knowledge of pathologic insult to communication functions caused by brain injury. Various augmentative or alternative communication systems or devices can be used in assisting patients to communicate their needs (Ried et al., 1995). Nonverbal, altered verbal, and assisted communication are often the norm during the rehabilitation phase. Assistance from parents regarding a child's language skills and terms for wants and needs, as well as meanings of nonverbal cues, can guide nursing staff to effective understanding of patient communication. Constant technological advances in augmentative and alternative communication systems necessitate strong collaborative relationships between speech and language pathologists, nurses, and patients' families to facilitate successful communication with the child or adolescent. Short, simple instructions or requests coupled with careful attention to patient response are the basic building blocks of therapeutic communication for nurses caring for children with TBI.

Activities of Daily Living and Self-Help Skills

The occupational therapist and nurse work closely together to identify patient deficits and set goals for the patient's accomplishment of self-care activities while trying to foster appropriate levels of independence. This aspect of care is among the most challenging tasks faced by rehabilitation team members and requires tremendous team collaboration to achieve success.

The nursing staff often bears an enormous responsibility for continuing multidisciplinary treatment plans during evening and weekend hours. Institutions that have the foresight to implement flexible scheduling of physical, occupational, and speech therapy staff experience the value of interdisciplinary collaboration and therapeutic intervention virtually continually. In many environments, however, nursing personnel are responsible for assisting clients with self-help goals, monitoring progress, and providing feedback to the team of therapists.

Discharge planning around self-help skills must take the real world into account. Parents' schedules, financial resources, community and family support, family values, and expectations for the child's outcome all influence the family's willingness and ability to promote independence in the child's self-care activities in the home environment.

Mobility

Nurses and physical therapists work closely together to facilitate the patient's independent mobility. Interventions aimed at preserving musculoskeletal function while preventing or treating complications (e.g., contractures, skin breakdown, and heterotopic ossification) foster the patient's return to independent mobility. Safe transfer techniques, application of lower-extremity orthoses, and use of assistive devices require team effort in getting patients to and from therapy sessions and about the unit.

Cognitive and Psychosocial Functioning

Cognitive impairment is one of the problematic deficits associated with TBI (Hall et al., 1990; Johnston and Gerring, 1992; Michaud et al., 1993a; Rivara et al., 1994). In individuals with severe injury, these deficits are readily apparent, whereas cognitive impairment can appear subtle in the face of mild injury. Short-term memory, judgment, reasoning, and higher-level executive functions are the cognitive functions most often affected in less severe injuries. Severe injury often produces devastating permanent cognitive disabilities. In addition to these cognitive changes, individuals with TBI often experience social and emotional changes such as impulsivity, disinhibition, lack of insight, altered attention span, irritability, poor anger control, aggression, anxiety, low frustration tolerance, and sleep disorders (Carney and Schoenbrodt, 1994; Hall et al., 1990; Johnston and Gerring, 1992; Michaud et al., 1993a, b).

The goals for nursing management of these cognitive, social, and emotional changes center around injury prevention, safety education, improvement in orientation and memory function, behavior management, social skills training, developmental stimulation, and emotional support. Providing a structured, consistent, and therapeutic milieu is crucial to a patient's cognitive, social, and emotional recovery. Incorporating play techniques, social interaction, child and adolescent interests, leisure skills, cultural values, and group techniques into treatment strategies is often more effective than are individual therapy sessions, which can be interpreted by the patient as boring and repetitious work.

Community Reintegration

The ultimate goal of every team member is successful community reintegration of the child or adolescent and the patient's family. The nurse actively participates in this process from the first day of the individual's rehabilitation stay. Family education is initiated very early in the child's stay to empower family members to meet the child's biopsychosocial home care needs. (See Table 4-2 for discharge criteria.) As inpatient hospital stays become increasingly limited, the team must often depend on community-based resources to implement portions of the patient-family education and treatment plan. Interdisciplinary collaboration and assessment are crucial to both the identification of family needs and the development of relevant educational strategies. Therapeutic leave and community outings offer opportunities

Table 4-2. Discharge Criteria in Pediatric Brain Injury Biopsychosocial Care

1. The family is able to demonstrate successfully all aspects of care related to the child's needs, including
   Nutrition: nutritional supplementation, oral feeding, or a combination
   Respiration: tracheostomy care, protection of airway, prevention of aspiration
   Activities of daily living: bathing, hygiene, grooming, dressing, and use of assistive devices
   Communication: use of verbal and nonverbal cues and alternative or augmentative communication systems
   Mobility: range of motion, positioning techniques, application of orthoses, and use of assistive devices
   Cognitive functions: appropriate sensorimotor stimulation and memory techniques
   Physiologic status: medication administration and wound care
   Bowel and bladder functions: continence program, such as scheduled voiding and bowel routine
   Skin integrity: strategies for prevention of skin breakdown, skin assessment techniques, and treatment measures for actual breakdown
   Safety: knowledge of safety measures in home and community environment, aimed at injury prevention
   Social-emotional functions: behavior management and social skills strategies, coping measures, and realistic family system expectations
2. Community referrals are established, including
   Educational services
   Vocational and independent living programs (if age-appropriate)
   Financial services
   Legal services
   Multidisciplinary therapy services
   Medical care
   Day care or respite services (or both)
   Leisure programs
   Family support networks
   Client advocacy resources
   Home health care
3. Therapeutic leave goals are met.
4. Case management plan is established: Case manager is assigned and follow-up plans are made.

for individual and family practice of newly acquired skills in a supportive environment.

Referral to community resources and educational programs is a precursor to successful community re-entry. The establishment of positive working relationships among hospitals, rehabilitation settings, and school systems is crucial to the success of any child's or adolescent's return to school. Protocols such as that outlined by Ylvisaker and colleagues (1995b) offer useful strategies that create a safety net for students after TBI. Important elements are positive family education, notification of the school nurse or other designated school representative regarding the student's injury and special needs, and implementation of flexible programming so that the student's needs are met as they evolve or resolve. Educational interventions are most successful in the context of usual academic settings and routines (Ylvisaker et al., 1995a).

The nurse, in collaboration with other team members, has a responsibility to inform families of and to advocate for patients' rights under the law with regard to public programs, including educational, financial, and vocational resources. Managed care continues to govern referrals to health care providers, but the nurse plays an important role in helping families gain access to appropriate com-

munity-based services that best meet their children's needs. Finally, the nurse has a responsibility to facilitate skill mastery, to monitor patient and family outcomes, and to revise plans of care across the recovery continuum.

Relevant Nursing Research and Future Trends

Several topics in the nursing literature have sparked investigation. The first centers around prevention of secondary injury and management of increased ICP during the acute-care phase. Although most of the research has been carried out in adults with brain injury, investigators have studied various aspects of endotracheal suctioning with regard to the impact of those activities on ICP. The aspects of endotracheal suctioning that have been studied include manual hyperventilation, negative pressure, catheter size and depth, duration, number of passes, and head position. On the basis of research findings in adult studies (Kerr et al., 1993), the following guidelines regarding endotracheal suctioning have emerged:

- Midline head positioning
- Preoxygenation

- Cautious hyperventilation
- Suction duration of approximately 10 seconds
- Suction passes, approximately two per procedure
- Negative pressure not to exceed 120 mm Hg
- Catheter diameter approximately one-half the internal diameter of endotracheal tube

Other investigators have focused on patient and family outcomes. Hall and coworkers (1992) reported reduced lengths of stay in an acute-care setting after the implementation of a multidisciplinary team approach to acute brain injury management. Carson (1993) examined parental experience in caring for children who survived brain injury. The investigator identified three phases in the recovery process, labeled *centering on, fostering independence,* and *seeking stability*. During the first phase, attention is focused primarily on the injured child. The second phase focuses on promotion of the child's independent functioning. In the final phase, family system homeostasis is the primary goal, promoting the injured individual's optimal abilities while minimizing family stress.

Baker (1990) studied families of children who had sustained TBI. Using the Family Adaptation to Medical Stressors instrument (Koch, 1985), Baker found statistically significant correlations ($p < 0.05$) between the variables compared in the following sets:

- Depression and family rules that permit emotional expression
- Trust and parental perceptions of available assistance
- Illness anxiety and number of people available for assistance (outside the nuclear family)
- Trust and patient's age
- Depression and increased expression of negative emotions
- Depression and family role flexibility

Baker (1990), who did not note significant differences between the findings in mild and severe brain injury, followed administration of the Family Adaptation to Medical Stressors instrument with interviews in a small subset of subjects. The families interviewed reported family changes that especially involved developmental changes in siblings. Parents of children with mild injury voiced concerns and frustration at the lack of knowledge on the part of professionals in understanding brain injury treatment. Parents in Baker's study also expressed concern regarding their child's future and their need to ensure developmental independence.

Strohmyer and her colleagues (1993) studied young adults who had sustained TBI. She reported good outcomes with regard to functional independence but cited problems in psychosocial adaptation. The small sample studied makes it difficult to generalize findings to other populations or to identify specific factors responsible for poor psychosocial adaptation after brain injury. This study does, however, support a common finding in pediatric populations after brain injury—namely, that functional independence far exceeds psychosocial adaptation.

Another area of interest in the nursing literature again focuses on outcome data. DiDonato and Schaffer (1994) published findings related to a multitude of patient outcomes. These authors contacted 82 adult clients after discharge from a rehabilitation facility. Patient outcomes reported included living arrangements, use of support services, use of substances (alcohol and drugs), vocational status, recreational and leisure activities, and life satisfaction. On the basis of their findings, the facility with which these researchers were affiliated implemented corrective action plans that included family and payer education, substance abuse programming, and several improvements in discharge-planning strategies. Their discussion regarding determination of facility-based cost savings has tremendous implications for the future in light of the current economic environment in health care. Factors such as program flexibility, availability of after-care continuity, client gains over time, other patient outcome data, and the matching of facility resources with specific needs may, in the future, influence rehabilitation facility selection and reimbursement on the part of payers.

As clinical pathways and other models of care are implemented, accompanied by limited resources and reduced lengths of stay, case managers and payers will rely increasingly on outcome data when making treatment and funding decisions (Lang, 1995). The proactive implementation of such outcome studies may prove crucial to the long-term survival of rehabilitation programs. In addition, many studies that have been carried out in adult populations should be adapted appropriately and replicated in pediatric populations and vice versa. Future trends in pediatric nursing research related to populations who have survived TBI must continue to address the prevention of secondary injury and to define intervention strategies that improve long-term outcomes for children, adolescents, and their families. Investigators must focus on designing studies that measure whether rehabilitation produces outcomes that are worth the cost of providing care (Hall and Cope, 1995). In the face of changing health care environments, continued development, implementation, and evaluation of objective outcome measures in pediatric populations are essential to the credibility of future nursing research efforts.

Acknowledgments

I extend my thanks to the many children and adolescents and their families who have survived TBI and enlightened me in my practice; to Dr. Janice Cockrell, for immense education and guidance in the field of pediatric rehabilitation; to Dr. Kathy Sawin, who remains my mentor in pediatric rehabilitation nursing; to Debbie Calligaro, MS,

RN, Kim Davies, BS, RN, and Regina Muir, MS, RN, for reviewing the nursing content of the chapter; and, finally, to Sara Luoma and Kimberly White for their tremendous secretarial support.

References

Aicardi J (1990). Epilepsy in brain injured children. Dev Med Child Neurol 32;191.

Baker JE (1990). Family adaptation when one member has a head injury. J Neurosci Nurs 22;232.

Brillhart B, Sills F (1994). Analysis of the roles and responsibilities of rehabilitation nursing staff. Rehabil Nurs 19;145.

Carney J, Schoenbrodt L (1994). Educational implications of traumatic brain injury. Pediatr Ann 23;47.

Carson P (1993). Investing in the come back: parent's experience following traumatic brain injury. J Neurosci Nurs 25;165.

Chioléro R, Schutz Y, Lemarchand T, et al. (1989). Hormonal and metabolic changes accompanying severe head injury or noncranial injury. JPEN J Parenter Enteral Nutr 13(1);5.

Citta-Pietrolungo TJ, Alexander MA, Cook SP, Padman R (1993). Complications of tracheostomy and decannulation in pediatric and young patients with traumatic brain injury. Arch Phys Med Rehabil 74;905.

Creasey L, Johnson A, Decker M (1989). Caloric requirements in the traumatically brain-injured pediatric population. Top Clin Nutr 4(4);56.

Crosby LJ, Parsons LC (1992). Cerebrovascular response of closed head-injured patients to a standardized endotracheal tube suctioning and manual hyperventilation procedure. J Neurosci Nurs 24;40.

DiDonato BA, Schaffer VL (1994). The importance of outcome data in brain injury rehabilitation. Rehabil Nurs 19;219.

Duhaime AC, Alario A, Lewander WJ, et al. (1992). Head injury in very young children: mechanisms, injury types and ophthalmologic findings in 100 hospitalized patients younger than 2 years of age. Pediatrics 90(2);79.

Ghajar J, Hariri RJ (1992). Management of pediatric head injury. Pediatr Clin North Am 39;1093.

Hall DM, Johnson SL, Middleton J (1990). Rehabilitation of head injured children. Arch Dis Child 65;553.

Hall KM, Cope DN (1995). The benefit of rehabilitation in traumatic brain injury: a literature review. J Head Trauma Rehabil 10(1);1.

Hall M, Brandys C, Yetman L (1992). Multidisciplinary approaches to management of acute head injury. J Neurosci Nurs 24;199.

Hymovich DP (1979). Assessment of the Chronically Ill Child and Family. In DP Hymovich, MU Bernard (eds), Family Health Care. New York: McGraw-Hill, 280.

James HE, Trauner DA (1985). The Glasgow Coma Scale. In HE James, HG Aras, RM Perkin (eds), Brain Insults in Infants and Children. Orlando, FL: Grune & Stratton, 181.

Johnson LH, Roberts SL (1996). Hope facilitating strategies for the family of the head injury patient. J Neurosci Nurs 28;259.

Johnston MV, Gerring JP (1992). Head trauma and its sequelae. Pediatr Ann 21;362.

Joseph AB, Wroblewski B (1995). Depression, antidepressants, and traumatic brain injury. J Head Trauma Rehabil 10(2);90.

Kaufman BA, Dacey RG (1994). Acute care management of closed head injury in childhood. Pediatr Ann 23;18.

Kerr ME, Rudy EB, Brucia J, Stone KS (1993). Head injured adults: recommendations for endotracheal suctioning. J Neurosci Nurs 25;86.

King I (1981). A Theory for Nursing: Systems, Concepts, Process. New York: Wiley.

Koch AA (1985). "If only it could be me." The families of pediatric cancer patients. Fam Relat 34;63.

Kraus JF, Rock A, Hemyari P (1990). Brain injuries among infants, children, adolescents and young adults. Am J Dis Child 144;684.

Lang GE (1995). Quality benchmarks for brain injury rehabilitation services. Rehabil Nurs 20;310.

Langfitt TW, Gennarelli TA (1982). Can the outcome from head injury be improved? J Neurosurg 56;19.

McLean DE, Kaitz ES, Keenan CJ, et al. (1995). Medical and surgical complications of pediatric brain injury. J Head Trauma Rehabil 10(5);1.

Michaud LJ, Duhaime AC, Batshaw ML (1993a). Traumatic brain injury in children. Pediatr Clin North Am 40;553.

Michaud LJ, Rivara FP, Grady MS, Reay DT (1992). Predictors of survival and severity of disability after severe brain injury in children. Neurosurgery 31;254.

Michaud LJ, Rivara FP, Jaffe KM, et al. (1993b). Traumatic brain injury as a risk factor for behavioral disorders in children. Arch Phys Med Rehabil 74;368.

Moore R, Najarian MP, Konvolinka CW (1989). Measured energy expenditure in severe head trauma. J Trauma 29;1633.

Noah ZL, Hahn YS, Rubenstein JS, Aronyk K (1992). Management of the child with severe brain injury. Crit Care Clin 8(1);59.

Orem D (1985). Nursing: Concepts of Practice (3rd ed). New York: McGraw-Hill.

Phillips R, Ott L, Young B, Walsh J (1987). Nutritional support and measured energy expenditure of the child and adolescent with head injury. J Neurosurg 67;846.

Prough DS (1990). Fluid resuscitation in head-injured patients: unsolved issues. J Intensive Care Med 5;53.

Richelson E (1990). Antidepressants and brain neurochemistry. Mayo Clin Proc 65;1227.

Ried S, Strong G, Wright L, et al. (1995). Computers, assistive devices, and augmentative communication aids: technology for social inclusion. J Head Trauma Rehabil 10(5);80.

Rivara FP (1994). Epidemiology and prevention of pediatric traumatic brain injury. Pediatr Ann 23(1);12.

Rivara JMB, Jaffe KM, Polissar NL, et al. (1994). Family functioning and children's academic performance and behavior problems in the year following traumatic brain injury. Arch Phys Med Rehabil 75;369.

Shackford SR (1990). Fluid resuscitation in head injury. J Intensive Care Med 5;59.

Shelton TL, Jeppson ES, Johnson BH (1987). Family-Centered Care for Children with Special Health Care Needs. Washington, DC: Association for the Care of Children's Health.

Stringer WA, Hasso AN, Thompson JR, et al. (1993). Hyperventilation-induced cerebral ischemia in patients with acute brain lesions: demonstration by xenon-enhanced CT. Am Soc Neuroradiol 14;475.

Strohmyer LL, Noroian EL, Patterson LM, Carlin BP (1993). Adaptation six months after multiple trauma: a pilot study. J Neurosci Nurs 25;30.

Teasdale GM, Jennett B (1974). Assessment of coma and impaired consciousness: a practical scale. Lancet 2;81.

Temkin NR, Dikmen SS, Wilensky AJ, et al. (1990). A randomized double-blind study of phenytoin for the prevention of post-traumatic seizures. N Engl J Med 323;497.

Ylvisaker M, Feeney T, Maher-Maxwell N, Meserve N (1995a). School re-entry following severe traumatic brain injury: guidelines for educational planning. J Head Trauma Rehabil 10(6);25.

Ylvisaker M, Feeney T, Mullins K (1995b). School re-entry following mild traumatic brain injury: a proposed hospital-to-school protocol. J Head Trauma Rehabil 10(6);42.

Chapter 5
Pharmacologic Intervention

Gregory J. O'Shanick

Although the role of pharmacologic intervention in the neurorehabilitation of adults with traumatic brain injury (TBI) now is well accepted (Gualtieri, 1988; Stein et al., 1994; Sutton et al., 1987), past efforts of neurorehabilitation of brain injuries in children and adolescents have not involved pharmacologic intervention to a significant extent (Parmelee and O'Shanick, 1987). Recent advances in psychopharmacology of childhood and adolescent psychiatric disorders have increased clinicians' comfort level regarding the use of medications in concert with psychotherapeutic interventions (Hyman, 1988). Similarly, the strategy of combining appropriate pharmacologic management and neurorehabilitation therapy provided by the occupational therapist, speech-language pathologist, physical therapist, and others holds the potential to optimize recovery (Hayes and Dixon, 1994).

This chapter addresses current trends in the use of pharmacologic agents in the TBI population. It is intended to introduce the reader to the types of agents, their clinical uses, and their risks and benefits. References for pediatric neurobehavioral studies are cited where they exist. In most cases, the use of these agents is an extrapolation either from the non-TBI pediatric and adolescent psychiatric literature or from the adult neurobehavioral literature.

Readers not familiar with pediatric or adolescent dosages are advised to consult either the *Physicians' Desk Reference* (1997) or the *Harriet Lane Handbook* (Barone, 1996) for further information. In many situations, the neurobehavioral syndromes outlined in this chapter are not listed among the indicated uses for these medications in the *Physicians' Desk Reference*. Although using medication for a nonapproved indication is acceptable medical practice, the prudent professional will obtain informed consent from the parent or legal guardian after full disclosure of a drug's known risks and benefits.

Some agents also may not be approved for use in children or adolescents (as of the publication of this chapter). Again, the reader is encouraged to consult the foregoing references in that regard. The reader having any doubt or misgivings about the prescribing of these agents should obtain referral to or consultation from a pediatric psychopharmacologist.

Treatment Issues

TBI in children and adolescents is not a random event. Studies suggest that environmental chaos, familial disruption, and psychiatric diagnosis may predispose toward brain injury in children (Ewing-Cobbs et al., 1995). Population studies have also found that the major vector for injury in adolescent years is "typical" active, risk-taking adolescent activity rather than a predilection toward substance abuse or acting out, as had been thought previously.

In the adolescent age group, injury characteristics are related to mode of injury: Injuries in those younger than 4 years are primarily the result of physical assault (e.g., child abuse), whereas falls and motor vehicle accidents assume a greater proportion of the etiology with advancing age (McLean et al., 1995). The literature on injury severity has been skewed toward more severe injuries that require inpatient treatment. Studies indicate that the more common injury in this age group (as with adults) is so-called mild brain injury evaluated in the office by primary-care physicians (pediatricians and family practitioners). In school-based samples, this under-reporting phenomenon may account for the misdiagnosis of psychiatric conditions other than brain injury.

Comprehensive evaluation involves the assessment of physical, psychological, social, and developmental characteristics of the child who has sustained a brain injury. From this broad-based foundation, the clinician can define the most appropriate medication intervention. Medical evaluation should provide the answers to critical questions regarding site(s) of injury in the brain, severity of any deficits, preexisting medical conditions, current developmental stage (and the expected neurobiological correlates), and the familial and genetic risk factors for the child.

Site of Injury

Assessment of injury site is commonly performed in severely injured children (McLean, 1995). In such situations, neuroanatomic studies (computed tomography and magnetic resonance imaging) and electrophysiologic studies (electroencephalography, evoked responses) are used routinely for both treatment and prognostic purposes. When milder injuries are encountered, observational data may be the only assessment obtained. Duration of unconsciousness, memory discontinuity episodes, or changes in behavior (e.g., agitation) can provide some insight into the injury severity. When combined with external injury location (e.g., abrasions on chin, forehead) and characteristics of the accident (e.g., height of fall, speed of impact, use of protective equipment), an indirect measure of force and direction can be surmised. This impact information can then be extrapolated to define the site of injury.

The utility of neuroanatomic imaging procedures in milder forms of brain injury is controversial. Functional neuroimaging procedures (e.g., single photon emission computed tomography, positron emission tomography scanning) may define areas of perfusion deficit or lowered metabolic activity not revealed by anatomic means (Worley et al., 1995). The findings can then be used to employ pharmacologic interventions rationally.

Combining functional assessment information (obtained from physical, occupational, and speech and language therapists and neuropsychologists) with functional neuroimaging provides a basis for multidimensional localization of the injury areas. Preinjury and postinjury developmental assessment sets the contextual stage for the problems that are defined. Family history and genetic predisposition must be evaluated to understand the child's expected medical future and the likely course of recovery. Site of injury can be correlated with information about the neurotransmitter most prominent in the region and enable rational medication intervention.

Agents Available

Anticonvulsants

Anticonvulsants (e.g., carbamazepine, valproic acid, phenytoin, phenobarbital, gabapentin, lamotrigine) act to prevent abnormal neuronal firing patterns. Such activity can occur as a result of direct injury to the cell or to chem-

ical changes around the cell. These seizures can be either focal or generalized events. Focal seizures may involve sensory, motor, or behavioral regions of the brain (Post and Uhde, 1983). One way in which anticonvulsants (e.g., benzodiazepines, barbiturates, valproic acid) may prevent seizures is by increasing the activity of the inhibitory neurotransmitter gamma-aminobutyric acid (GABA). These anticonvulsants (e.g., carbamazepine) may also decrease the firing rates by preventing the snowball effect of seizure production called *kindling*. Valproic acid, carbamazepine, and lamotrigine can be used not only to prevent seizures but to decrease irritability, improve frustration tolerance, decrease headache, and stabilize mood swings. Balance problems may also respond to valproic acid.

Once these agents are prescribed, follow-up blood testing is required to ensure that the concentration of the medication in the blood is in the therapeutic range, the level required to inhibit seizures in 95% of patients. These tests may also involve assessment of liver function and blood counts (complete blood cell count) to monitor potential toxicity of these agents. Side effects commonly encountered with these agents include fatigue (barbiturates, benzodiazepines), dizziness (phenytoin, carbamazepine), and gastrointestinal irritation (valproic acid).

Antidepressants

Antidepressants were first developed in the 1940s, and many refinements have occurred subsequently. Types of antidepressants include monoamine oxidase inhibitors (MAOIs), tricyclic antidepressants (TCAs), heterocyclics, and specific serotonin-reuptake inhibitors (SSRIs). Novel antidepressants having combination effects (e.g., amoxapine, venlafaxine) have also been developed (Richelson, 1996).

MAOIs (e.g., phenelzine, tranylcypromine) act by slowing the breakdown of neurotransmitters at the synapse. The agents currently available require strict dietary control to prevent toxic reactions that will elevate blood pressure to lethal levels. MAOIs tend to increase energy and may cause insomnia even at low dosages. Prescription of these agents must be supervised closely to prevent accidental drug-drug interactions (e.g., avoiding meperidine, decongestants, diet pills).

TCAs (e.g., amitriptyline, imipramine, desipramine, nortriptyline, protriptyline, clomipramine) are closely related to antihistamines and possess similar characteristics (Mysiw and Jackson, 1987). They act by decreasing the resorption of neurotransmitter into the releasing neuron. No dietary restrictions are necessary with TCAs. They act to increase two neurotransmitters, serotonin and norepinephrine. Onset of action is generally 2–4 weeks after treatment is started, due to the need to achieve certain blood concentrations and then for the agent to cross into the neuron. Periodic assessment of blood level is useful to ensure an effective concentration. Side effects with TCAs are due largely to their antihistaminic and anticholinergic properties. They tend to be more sedating and induce initial sleep improvement. They also tend to cause dry mouth, delayed urination, constipation, and light-headedness due to orthostatic hypotension. The anticholinergic side effects can assist in alleviating some types of posttraumatic dizziness. Some cardiac changes can be seen, including increased heart rate and (rarely) skipped beats. TCAs can also lower the seizure threshold after TBI. These medications can be used for explosive episodes, emotional incontinence, headache relief, chronic pain management, and insomnia in addition to typical depressive symptoms.

SSRIs (e.g., fluoxetine, fluvoxamine, sertraline, paroxetine, nefazodone) are the newest agents in the antidepressant class. They prevent the resorption of serotonin into the releasing neuron and increase its availability to the next neuron downstream. These powerful medications have a more rapid onset of action. They usually have no cardiac side effects. Principal side effects include nausea, dizziness, fatigue, and (occasionally) tremor. The SSRIs can also cause sexual dysfunction. Interaction with anticonvulsants can influence seizure threshold.

Novel antidepressants combine serotonin-reuptake inhibition with norepinephrine-reuptake inhibition (e.g., venlafaxine) or dopamine blockade (e.g., amoxapine). Side effects are similar to other similar agents. However, amoxapine can cause involuntary movements, as can neuroleptics.

Antianxiety Agents

Antianxiety agents (e.g., lorazepam, diazepam, alprazolam) exert their effect by increasing GABA (Hyman, 1988). This activity then slows the firing rates of all neurons in the region. Historically, agents that increase GABA have been used (in the form of alcoholic beverages) to reduce stress in society for thousands of years. Currently used agents are primarily benzodiazepines, although barbiturates are still prescribed. The effect of these agents is to reduce the individual's awareness of environmental stress and to disrupt memory of the events. Another class of agents (typified by buspirone) acts to decrease the impact of environmental events through interference with serotonin activity in the hippocampal (memory-processing) regions of the brain. Buspirone is also used to decrease aggressive impulses.

Side effects of GABA-potentiating agents include sedation, short-term memory disruption, and muscle relaxation. In addition, some users develop drug tolerance. These agents act to raise the seizure threshold and have some use as secondary anticonvulsants. They cannot be withdrawn without medical supervision, to prevent severe withdrawal delirium, including potentially lethal seizures. The use of ethanol with these agents greatly increases their sedating properties and can result in slowing or cessation of breathing. Short-term use is appropriate if closely supervised by the physician.

Neuroleptics

Neuroleptics (e.g., chlorpromazine, haloperidol, thioridazine, thiothixene) act by blocking the transmission of dopamine-stimulated nerve impulses (Black et al., 1985). Generally, they are used infrequently for agitation and aggressive behavior, as studies have shown that they may slow the recovery rate after brain injury. They may be required in severe cases of delusional thinking or hallucinations. Other similar medications are used to decrease nausea and vomiting and to enhance the effect of narcotic analgesics.

Side effects include abnormal involuntary movements, low blood pressure, lowered seizure threshold, and decreased memory. Permanent movement disorders can be seen. Newer agents, such as clozapine, are less likely to cause movement problems, although lowered production of blood cells might be observed (Jibson and Tandon, 1996).

Antiparkinsonian Agents

Antiparkinsonian agents (e.g., levodopa, amantadine, bromocriptine, pergolide, benztropine) act to increase dopamine activity or decrease cholinergic activity at the synapse (Cedarbaum, 1987). This capacity may be beneficial in certain types of amotivational syndromes and initiation deficits. These agents are used to increase endurance (both cognitive and physical) and to improve swallowing for certain patients. They can also improve initiation and mood.

Side effects include agitation, nausea, blood pressure changes, and headache. High dosages also may induce hallucinations or paranoid delusions (Birkmayer, 1978).

Psychostimulants

Psychostimulants (e.g., methylphenidate, dextroamphetamine, pemoline) are used to decrease daytime drowsiness, increase attention and concentration, and increase mood temporarily (Wilens et al., 1995). They act by increasing the release of already-produced norepinephrine and dopamine from storage areas of the neuron (Coper and Herrmann, 1988). Their onset of action is within hours, and their duration usually is less than 24 hours (with the exception of pemoline). Long-term use must be monitored closely by a physician, because of the abuse potential of psychostimulants and their potential influence on the seizure threshold. Paranoid thoughts and insomnia can also be triggered by the unmonitored use of these agents.

Anticholinergic Agents

Anticholinergic agents (e.g., meclizine, scopolamine) can be used to increase tolerance for certain types of dizziness, to increase endurance, and to relieve initial insomnia. Their ability to lower seizure threshold and cause dry mouth, constipation, and confusion at high doses mandates medical monitoring of these agents.

Antihypertensives

Antihypertensives are used for headache management, aggressive behavior, and impulsivity. Beta-blockers (e.g., propranolol, atenolol) were the first of this class to be used successfully (Grendyke and Kanter, 1986).

Their side effects include lowered heart rate and blood pressure. They cannot be used for patients at risk for hypoglycemia, as they mask the physical complaints.

Certain agents (e.g., propranolol) may also increase depressive symptoms. Alpha-blocking agents (e.g., clonidine) are used to decrease impulsivity and blood pressure (McIntyre and Gasquoine, 1990). Calcium channel blockers (e.g., verapamil) have been used to treat migraine headaches after TBI. Their primary side effects include lightheadedness and constipation (Childs, 1986).

Narcotic Antagonists

Narcotic antagonists (e.g., naltrexone) are a class of medications that block the brain's naturally produced opiates (endorphins) from attaching at receptor sites in the brain. These agents can be used to decrease self-injurious behavior, bulimic symptoms, and suicidal tendencies (Buzan et al., 1995). Their side effects include potential liver irritation, confusion, and headache.

General Concepts in Pharmacologic Treatment

Medications prescribed after a brain injury improve the brain's natural ability to produce and use neurotransmitters. The medications act as a cast for the neuron to allow more normal activity during recovery. When the neuron fails to recover its function, medications are used as splints to allow the most normal neuron function possible (O'Shanick, 1987).

Medication selection is based on four concepts:

1. Target symptom. What is the problem to be addressed by drug intervention? Problems could include headache, insomnia, dizziness, depression, and impulsivity. On the basis of a specific definition of the problem, medication effect can be weighed against the likelihood of spontaneous improvement. Also, the underlying neurochemical problem can be addressed if the region of the involved area is known or if the problem has a known neurochemical deficiency.

2. Route of administration. How is this medication best administered: orally, by injection, by inhalation, or by some other route? The speed of absorption is determined largely by the route of administration. Problems associated with toxic levels can be accelerated, too.

3. Onset of action. How much time does the medication require to work? This factor depends on the speed at which the medication crosses from the blood stream into the neuron and, then, the speed with which it alters the neurotransmitter activity.

4. Side effect profile. What are the medication's side effects? All medications have side effects, and the risk-benefit ratio must be considered. This evaluation includes determining whether the side effects are permanent (e.g., tardive dyskinesia) or temporary (e.g., dry mouth).

Clinical Syndromes and Medication Strategies

Sleep Disorders

Evolution of changed sleep patterns after TBI is well documented. Classifying these changes into disorders of sleep initiation, sleep maintenance, and sleep quality is useful in treatment planning. Evaluation consists of a child's detailed sleep history obtained from both patient and parent and, occasionally, nocturnal studies (either oximetry or polysomnography). A positive family history can also increase the clinical suspicion of these problems.

Disorders of sleep initiation may occur secondary to pain or impulse control deficits. Sleep onset delays due to ruminative worrying are seen (Conn and Sanders-Bush, 1987; Grahame-Smith, 1988). Primary treatment is focused on sleep hygiene (e.g., limiting beverages, avoiding caffeine and high sugar loads, effecting cooler ambient temperatures, providing white noise) (Girardi et al., 1995). When such treatment is insufficient, the use of a sedating antihistamine (e.g., diphenhydramine) or trazodone can augment initial sleep.

Sleep maintenance disorders can arise from multiple etiologies, including autonomic excitability as seen in posttraumatic stress disorder, periodic leg movements and nocturnal myoclonus, depressive sleep disorder, obstructive sleep apnea, and hypothalamic dysfunction with associated nocturia or enuresis. Sleep-precipitated seizures are a rare but possible cause. Treatment of these sleep disorders is predicated on the underlying neurophysiology. For autonomic excitability, the use of desipramine or nortriptyline may assist in reducing the heightened autonomic tone that disturbs sleep architecture. Periodic leg movements and nocturnal myoclonus may respond to a combination of dopamine-agonist therapy (e.g., carbidopa-levodopa) and a benzodiazepine (e.g., clonazepam). Treatment of depressive sleep disorder consists of primary antidepressant therapy to alleviate the full constellation of neurovegetative symptoms. Sleep apnea syndromes require mechanical nocturnal ventilation assistance but are uncommon in this population. Hypothalamic dysfunction, specifically diabetes insipidus, may be modified through the use of intranasal desmopressin acetate (DDAVP). Seizures and generalized sleep architecture disruption after TBI may respond to the sedating effects of gabapentin.

Attention and Concentration Deficits

Alterations in focused attention may adversely influence all other traumatic deficits (Mack, 1986). Careful identification of vigilance and simultaneous processing difficulties allows intervention with pharmacologic agents that increase catecholamine activity in the central nervous system. The use of such stimulants as methylphenidate, dextroamphetamine, and pemoline is well described in the literature (Glenn, 1987). Shorter-acting agents such as methamphetamine may also improve attention and concentration. Trials of dopamine agonists such as amantadine may also be beneficial if the reaction to declining stimulant blood levels creates increased irritability. Concurrent use of a serotoninergic agonist (e.g., fluoxetine) may attenuate irritability while potentiating attention improvement (Sommi et al., 1987).

Apathy and Amotivation

Disturbances of initiation are among the most devastating encountered after TBI. Deficits of motor initiation are well recognized as reflecting a deficiency of dopamine in the basal ganglia. Behavioral deficits of initiation may also share this deficiency and consequently improve with dopamine-agonist therapy (Koller and Herbster, 1988). Amantadine, carbidopa-levodopa, and bromocriptine are the agents most commonly prescribed in this setting (Chandler et al., 1988; Eames, 1989). Some effect from more traditional stimulant therapy may be obtained. In severe TBI with extensive subcortical damage, initiation deficits may be improved with the use of anticholinergic agents to reduce the relative excess of cholinergic activity-inhibition.

Low Frustration Tolerance and Impulsivity

Defining age-appropriate frustration tolerance in children and adolescents after TBI is a major challenge. Behavioral regression to a style characteristic of an earlier developmental stage may respond to behavioral or environmental manipulation. When this fails, pharmacologic structuring with agents that potentiate serotonin and reduce catecholamine activity is beneficial. Many of these agents can also be effective in more overtly aggressive or violent behaviors. However, early detection of and intervention in impulsivity may prevent the emergence of more fulminant explosive episodes. Frustration tolerance can be improved by the use of lithium, buspirone, and SSRIs to increase serotonin (Glenn and Joseph, 1987; Levine, 1988; Stanislav et al., 1994) either alone or in combination with catecholamine-inhibiting agents such as propranolol and clonidine (Jenkins and Maruta, 1987). When intraparenchymal hemorrhaging has occurred with the potential deposition of hemosiderin, anticonvulsant therapy with carbamazepine or valproic acid may reduce impulsivity and irritability (Bouvy et al., 1988).

Aggression and Violence

Aggressive and violent behaviors result from multiple factors including biological, psychological, and social antecedents. Predatory and territorial aggression syndromes have been described and attributed to serotonin deficiencies or catecholamine excesses. Although pharmacologic treatment in this setting parallels that of low frustration tolerance, acute episodes may require the use of sedating neuroleptics (e.g., perphenazine and droperidol) to obtain rapid behavioral control (Rao et al., 1985). In general, chronic use of neuroleptics is discouraged except when this behavior reflects an underlying psychotic disorder. Sexual aggressiveness in either gender may respond to high-dose progesterone therapy or SSRI administration.

Appetite Disturbance

Hypothalamic injury can result in bulimic symptoms that may be persistent or intermittent. Organic bulimia has been described as responding to opiate-antagonist therapy (naltrexone) (Childs, 1987). Oral stimulation syndromes such as those seen in bitemporal anterior injury (e.g., Klüver-Bucy syndrome) have been reported to respond to carbamazepine (Stewart, 1985).

Loss of appetite may be associated with a primary disorder of smell and taste sensory dysfunction. Swallowing difficulties (silent aspiration) may produce a behavioral paradigm in which food and liquids are avoided as a learned response to this frightening situation. Primary treatment of these deficits is indicated. Severely injured patients may use feeding situations to demonstrate their control, albeit fragile, over themselves and their destiny. Behavioral techniques to facilitate appropriate autonomy are the primary intervention.

Self-Injurious Behavior

Self-inflicted injury must be evaluated in the context in which it occurs. Self-stimulation in a perseverating patient may result in repetitive injuries that are not intended to be self-injurious. Conversely, purposeful self-mutilation and overt suicidal tendencies require rapid intervention to extinguish these behaviors. Use of narcotic antagonists in more primitive forms of self-mutilation is well described and efficacious (Buzan et al., 1995). Use of narcotic antagonists in ruminative suicidal thoughts may be beneficial either alone or in tandem with SSRIs (e.g., fluvoxamine) more typically prescribed for obsessive-compulsive syndromes (Richelson, 1996).

Misperception Syndromes

Disturbances of perception and information processing (e.g., paranoia, hallucinosis) may appear overtly as more traditional psychotic syndromes. Hallucinosis that occurs after TBI must be evaluated thoroughly to eliminate the possibility that an underlying seizure disorder exists. Even in the face of a negative evaluation, the use of anticonvulsants (e.g., phenytoin, carbamazepine, valproic acid, gabapentin, lamotrigine) is often beneficial in alleviating these symptoms (McAllister, 1985). Atypical antipsychotics (e.g., clozapine, risperidone) may provide a greater therapeutic response than do traditional neuroleptics (Duffy and Kant, 1996; Elovic, 1996).

Organic paranoia may result from sensory deprivation syndromes or injuries to the associational cortex of the brain that prevent precise and accurate appraisal of environmental situations. Prosodic dysfunction may exacerbate this phenomenon. The combined use of clonazepam and impulse-controlling agents may alleviate this syndrome.

Conclusion

Treatment of neurobehavioral disturbance after TBI may benefit from a combination of traditional therapies and pharmacologic manipulation. These agents may be necessary either for brief periods or chronically as an adaptive aid in maximizing functional independence in the community. Evaluation of need must be balanced against risks of ongoing side effects. Parental knowledge of these risks and benefits is mandatory to minimize anxiety, which could compromise compliance.

References

Barone A (ed) (1996). The Harriet Lane Handbook: A Manual for Pediatric House Officers (14th ed). St. Louis: Mosby.

Birkmayer W (1978). Toxic delirium after L-dopa medication. J Neural Transm 14(suppl);163.

Black JL, Richelson E, Richardson JW (1985). Antipsychotic agents: a clinical update. Mayo Clin Proc 60;777.

Bouvy PF, van de Wetering BJM, Meerwaldt JD, Bruijn JB (1988). A case of organic brain syndrome following head injury successfully treated with carbamazepine. Acta Psychiatr Scand 77;361.

Buzan RD, Thomas M, Dubovsky SL, Treadway J (1995). The use of opiate antagonists for recurrent self-injurious behavior. J Neuropsychiatr Clin Neurosci 7;437.

Cedarbaum JM (1987). Clinical pharmacokinetics of antiparkinsonian drugs. Clin Pharmacokinet 13;141.

Chandler MC, Barnhill JL, Gualtieri CT (1988). Amantadine for the agitated head-injury patient. Brain Inj 2(4);309.

Childs A (1986). Calcium channel blockers in psychiatry. P.E.N. Online, January 10–12.

Childs A (1987). Naltrexone in organic bulimia: a preliminary report. Brain Inj 1(1);49.

Conn PJ, Sanders-Bush E (1987). Central serotonin receptors: effector systems, physiologic roles and regulation. Psychopharmacology 92;267.

Coper H, Herrmann WM (1988). Psychostimulants, analeptics, nootropics: an attempt to differentiate and assess drugs designed for the treatment of impaired brain functions. Pharmacopsychiatrica 1;211.

Duffy JD, Kant R (1996). Clinical utility of clozapine in 16 patients with neurological disease. J Neuropsychiatr Clin Neurosci 8;92.

Eames P (1989). The use of Sinemet and bromocriptine. Brain Inj 3(3);319.

Elovic E (1996). Atypical antipsychotics: risperidone and clozapine. J Head Trauma Rehabil 11(3);89.

Ewing-Cobbs L, Duhaime A-C, Fletcher JM (1995). Inflicted and noninflicted traumatic brain injury in infants and preschoolers. J Head Trauma Rehabil 10(5);13.

Girardi NL, Shaywitz SE, Shaywitz BA, et al. (1995). Blunted catecholamine responses after glucose ingestion in children with attention deficit disorder. Pediatr Res 38;539.

Glenn MB (1986). CNS stimulants: applications for traumatic brain injury. J Head Trauma Rehabil 2(4);74.

Glenn MB, Joseph AB (1987). The use of lithium for behavioral and affective disorders after traumatic brain injury. J Head Trauma Rehabil 2(4);68.

Grahame-Smith DG (1988). Serotonin (5-hydroxytryptamine, 5-HT). Q J Med 254;459.

Grendyke RM, Kanter DR (1986). Therapeutic effects of pindolol on behavioral disturbances associated with organic brain disease: a double-blind study. J Clin Psychiatr 47;423.

Gualtieri CT (1988). Review: pharmacotherapy and the neurobehavioral sequelae of traumatic brain injury. Brain Inj 2(2);1.

Hayes RL, Dixon CE (1994). Neurochemical changes in mild head injury. Semin Neurol 14(1);25.

Hyman SE (1988). Recent developments in neurobiology: part II. Neurotransmitter receptors and psychopharmacology. Psychosomatics 29;254.

Jenkins SC, Maruta T (1987). Therapeutic use of propranolol for intermittent explosive disorder. Mayo Clin Proc 62;204.

Jibson MD, Tandon R (1996). A summary of research findings on the new antipsychotic drugs. Psychiatr Forum 16;i.

Koller WC, Herbster G (1988). D1 and D2 dopamine receptor mechanisms in dopaminergic behaviors. Clin Neuropharmacol 11;221.

Levine AM (1988). Case report: buspirone and agitation in head injury. Brain Inj 2(2);165.

Mack JL (1986). Clinical assessment of disorders of attention and memory. J Head Trauma Rehabil 3;22.

McAllister TW (1985). Carbamazepine in mixed frontal lobe and psychiatric disorders. J Clin Psychiatr 46;393.

McIntyre FL, Gasquoine P (1990). Case study: effect of clonidine on post-traumatic memory deficits. Brain Inj 4(2);209.

McLean DE, Kaitz ES, Keenan CJ, et al. (1995). Medical and surgical complications of pediatric brain injury. J Head Trauma Rehabil 10(5);1.

Mysiw WJ, Jackson RD (1987). Tricyclic antidepressant therapy after traumatic brain injury. J Head Trauma Rehabil 2(4);34.

O'Shanick G (1987). Clinical aspects of psychopharmacologic treatment in head-injured patients. J Head Trauma Rehabil 2(4);59.

Parmelee DX, O'Shanick GJ (1987). Neuropsychiatric interventions with head injured children and adolescents. Brain Inj 1(1);41.

Physicians' Desk Reference (51st ed). (1997) Montvale, NJ: Medical Economics.

Post RM, Uhde TW (1983). Treatment of mood disorders with antiepileptic medications: clinical and theoretical implications. Epilepsia 24(suppl 2);97.

Rao NB, Jellinek HM, Woolston DC (1985). Agitation in closed head injury: haloperidol effects on rehabilitation outcome. Arch Phys Med Rehabil 66(1);30.

Richelson E (1996). Synaptic effects of antidepressants. J Clin Psychopharmacol 16(suppl 2);l.

Sommi RW, Crismon ML, Bowden CL (1987). Fluoxetine: a serotonin-specific, second generation antidepressant. Pharmacotherapy 7;1.

Stanislav SW, Fabre T, Crismon ML, Childs A (1994). Buspirone's efficacy in organic-induced aggression. J Clin Psychopharmacol 14;126.

Stein DG, Glasier MM, Hoffman SW (1994). Pharmacologic treatments for brain-injury repair: progress and prognosis. Neuropsychol Rehabil 4;337.

Stewart JT (1985). Carbamazepine treatment of a patient with Klüver-Bucy syndrome. J Clin Psychiatr 46;496.

Sutton RL, Weaver MS, Feeney DM (1987). Drug-induced modifications of behavioral recovery following cortical trauma. J Head Trauma Rehabil 2(4);50.

Wilens TE, Biederman J, Spencer TJ, Prince J (1995). Pharmacotherapy of adult attention deficit/hyperactivity disorder: a review. J Clin Psychopharmacol 15;270.

Worley G, Hoffman JM, Paine SS, et al. (1995). 18-Fluorodeoxyglucose positron emission tomography in children and adolescents with traumatic brain injury. Dev Med Child Neurol 37;213.

Chapter 6
Intervention for Motor Disorders

Mary Louise Russell, Susan I. Krouse, Amy Karas Lane, Daniel Leger, and Carol Ann Robson

In this chapter, we discuss evaluation and treatment for children and adolescents with motor disorders after traumatic brain injury (TBI). Acquired central nervous system dysfunction may impede motor skills necessary for functional task performance or may render caregiving more laborious. Efforts to improve the motor functioning of children with TBI involve collaboration of a variety of professionals, family members, and school personnel.

A presentation of detailed therapeutic intervention programs is beyond the scope of this chapter. However, we hope that medical professionals who care for children with TBI and resultant motor dysfunction will find useful guidelines for their own practice and information they can share with pediatric patients and their caregivers. In this chapter, we outline interventions for the acute-care hospital, the inpatient rehabilitation facility, and outpatient treatment. Suggestions for transition of therapy services, from the inpatient to the outpatient setting, are also provided.

General Considerations

Enduring Principles

Neurodevelopmental Maturation

One enduring principle governing the assessment and treatment of motor disorders of all children, including those with TBI, is that children are in a process of neurodevelopmental maturation. Children's age-expected motor milestones should be determined accurately to establish proper therapeutic goals. Therapeutic approaches are modified according to the level of cognitive maturation. Most young children are far more motivated to cooperate with play activities than to repeat a seemingly endless series of exercises. The two major goals of therapeutic interventions for

the child with TBI are (1) to maximize age-appropriate independent function and (2) to minimize the degree of assistance required from caregivers.

Various Domains Affected

TBI may affect a child's functioning negatively in a number of domains, and dysfunction in one domain can adversely affect functioning in another. For example, visual-perceptual problems may render safe, independent mobility difficult. Cognitive dysfunctions, such as shortened attention span or memory deficit, in children with TBI may limit the effectiveness of therapies. For example, a child with poor sequencing skills may have difficulties with dressing himself or herself. A child with a poor attention span may not hear all the directions given by a therapist. Later, we suggest and discuss some strategies to use during therapy sessions for those children with cognitive dysfunction. Cognitive rehabilitation is discussed in Chapters 9–12.

Family and School Personnel Education

Most children with TBI are discharged to the care of family members and return to an education setting, albeit a modified one. Such children may demonstrate new impairments that require more involved levels of care than that needed previously. Consequently, their caregivers—usually family members—will need to learn new skills. These skills are often beyond normally expected parenting abilities, and make caregiver training a goal of rehabilitation. Once the child is discharged from an inpatient hospital, school personnel become involved in the goals of maximizing age-appropriate independence and minimizing the level of care required. In addition to that provided by school-based therapists, assistance with the child's ongoing rehabilitation may be provided by teachers, physical education instructors, aides, school nurses, art instructors, music instructors, and bus drivers. Before

Table 6-1. Physical Outcome for Children with TBI

Study Authors	Number of Subjects	Age Range	Patients Selected	Postinjury Time	Outcome
Boyer and Edwards (1991)	220	6 mos– 21 yrs	Admitted to an inpatient reha- bilitation hospital	1–3 yrs	Function at 1 yr after injury: 21% mobility dependent; 64% communication disorders; 79% perceptuocognitive defects Recovery status (Glasgow Coma Scale at 1 yr; n = 178): 48% good recovery; 19% moderate disability; 16% severe disability; 16% vegetative; 1% deceased
DiScarla et al. (1992)	598	>7 yrs (average age, 13)	Subjects of National Pediatric Trauma Registry, phase 2; with impairment in one or more func- tional domains present at discharge from acute care	Variable; children assessed at discharge from acute care	Average portion of complete independence (an extrapolated % score based on FIM raw score): Group A (n = 463) with recovery expected in <7 months, mean = 87%; Group B (n = 66) with recovery expected in 7–24 months, mean = 63%; Group C (n = 69) with recovery expected in >2 years, mean = 46%.

the child's discharge from inpatient hospitalization, recommendations for outpatient therapies—whether school based or at an outside facility—should be made, with consideration for the child's educational, social, and emotional needs. Currently, inpatient rehabilitation hospitalizations are of increasingly shorter duration. Consequently, family members and school personnel now perform functions formerly handled by inpatient nurses and therapists, leading to an increasing need for inpatient nurses and therapists to train and educate home and school caregivers for children with TBI.

Current Issues

Outcome

Knowledge of recent physical outcome studies for children with TBI is useful in counseling families and planning therapeutic interventions. Of course, making specific detailed predictions for any child based on studies of large groups of children is difficult. However, outcome studies do provide general information regarding patterns of functional recovery. Table 6-1 summarizes data from two physical outcome studies for children with TBI.

In general, the outlook for recovery of motor function in children with TBI is more favorable than that for recovery of cognitive and behavioral function. At 1 year after TBI, 21% of the 220 children assessed by Boyer and Edwards (1991) were dependent for mobility. In comparison, 64% had communication disorders and 79% had per-

ceptuocognitive defects (see Table 6-1). In a study of 344 children with TBI, Brink and colleagues (1980) found that 73% of the subjects regained independence and self-care. In studies completed in 1992 and 1993, Jaffe and coworkers assessed 94 children with TBI, initially at 3 weeks after achievement of full orientation and again at 1 year after the initial testing. Overall, they found that the greatest degree of measurable improvement occurred in tests of motor performance.

Injury severity does appear to be inversely related to ability to function independently; that is, children assessed as having the most severe injuries are the least likely to perform age-appropriate self-care tasks. In a study by DiScarla and associates (1992), 598 children with TBI were evaluated at discharge from acute care hospitalization. A clinician assessed each child in terms of time expected for recovery after discharge from acute care: The group judged to have the mildest injuries (n = 463) received, on average, a percentage FIM score of 87%. Children placed in the middle severity group (n = 66) received, on average, a percentage FIM score of 63%. Children placed in the highest severity of injury group (n = 69) received, on average, a percentage FIM score of 46% (see Table 6-1).

It should be noted that although children with TBI may recover basic motor and independence functions, potentially handicapping qualitative deviations in their performance may remain. This point is documented in a study by Chaplin and colleagues (1993) comparing the gross- and fine-motor performances of 14 children with TBI with that of 14 noninjured children. Analysis of the subtests showed that when speed was a component of either fine- or gross-motor tasks, significant differences were found. Speed of eye-hand coordination appeared to be particularly sensitive to the effects of TBI. Such findings have been corroborated by neuropsychological studies (Knights et al., 1991). Deficiencies in eye-hand coordination speed may impair the ability of a child with TBI to keep up with note taking and timed tests in school. Such difficulties with higher-level motor function may cause children with TBI to fall increasingly behind their peers in schoolwork and recreational activities.

Reduced Inpatient Stays

One current trend is toward decreasing inpatient rehabilitation stays for children with TBI. Data from Table 6-2 indicate that at one rehabilitation facility in 1993, the average length of an inpatient stay for a child with TBI was approximately one-fourth the average length of stay in 1983. Such shorter inpatient rehabilitation hospitalizations necessitate timely yet accurate assessment of the child's deficits and prognosis for recovery as well as the family's ability to cope with needs for ongoing care, therapies, and supervision. In the face of shorter inpatient stays, the inpatient therapist functions as an educator for family members, school personnel, and outpatient therapists and provides direct interventions for the child. Communication and collaboration among the inpatient therapist, the family, and those who will be providing interventions after discharge are essential.

Outcome Assessment

Third-party payers often request documentation of the efficacy of the therapeutic services being reimbursed. Reports with quantitative data are easier to interpret than are those with qualitative descriptions. Standardized adaptive behavior tests for children have been developed, including the Wee FIM and the Pediatric Evaluation of Disability Index (Lord et al., 1991). In addition to being used for documentation to obtain insurance reimbursement, these adaptive behavior tests may be used for research data collection.

Acute-Care Intervention

Often, the first evaluation and intervention for motor dysfunction of children with TBI occur in the acute-care hospital. In this setting, rehabilitation personnel must be aware of the child's medical condition and neurologic status. Interventions may include complication prevention, positioning, and cognitive and communication remediation. Therapeutic efforts in the acute-care hospital prepare the child for the next step of recovery and are helpful in

Table 6-2. Comparative Census of Children* with TBI at an Inpatient Rehabilitation Hospital

	1983	1993
No. of patients	24	35
Total patient days	2,412	1,184
Average length of stay in days	121	34

*Patients aged 18 years or younger.
Source: Unpublished data from medical record review, The Rehabilitation Institute of Pittsburgh.

determining the requirements for services once the child is medically stable and ready for discharge.

Evaluation

Medical Condition

Any questions about a child's limitations that may affect therapies should be addressed to the responsible physicians and nurses. Immobilization of extremities or particular joints may be necessary because of intravenous lines or fractures. Fractures or other injuries may limit weight-bearing activities. Occasionally, therapies may excessively agitate a child with elevated intracranial pressure (ICP). In such cases, it may be necessary to postpone therapies until the ICP has stabilized. Reports have demonstrated that placing a patient in a position that inhibits posturing may decrease elevated ICP (Cowley et al., 1994). Medical complications such as infections and recent procedures requiring sedation may hinder the child's ability to respond to therapies.

Neurologic Status

Neurologic assessment for children with TBI includes evaluation of tone, spontaneous movement, oral-motor functioning, and cognitive status. The presence of decreased or increased tone and the influence of positioning on tone should be noted. A child with decorticate posturing, for example, may demonstrate less spasticity in a side-lying than in a supine position. Spontaneous movements should be noted, with attention paid to less active movement of one limb relative to the contralateral extremity. Evaluation of oral-motor function includes assessment of tongue movement and the patient's apparent ability to manage oral secretions. Cognitive status evaluation includes assessment of the child's level of alertness, ability to follow commands, and tolerance for stimulation. Evaluation of these various domains will assist therapists in providing both appropriate interventions and useful information to families, nurses, and physicians.

Treatment

Complication Prevention

In the acute-care hospital, decubiti and contractures are significant complications to be prevented. Attempts to avoid decubiti include frequently changing the child's position, monitoring the fit of splints, and padding the surfaces on which the child is positioned. Because of their relatively large head size, younger children appear to be at greatest risk for developing pressure breakdowns at the occiput. The sacrum appears to be the site of greatest risk for older children (Solis et al., 1988). Contracture formation should be prevented by passive range of motion (ROM) and the use of resting splints.

Positioning

As stated previously, frequent position changes may prevent decubitus development. Positioning in side-lying or prone positions may inhibit primitive posturing patterns. When possible, placing the child in a sitting position and assisting in maintaining that position as necessary will promote greater environmental awareness, assist in clearing secretions, prevent pulmonary atelectasis, and assist oral-motor functioning. Splinting will assist in proper positioning. For the child with ankle plantar flexor spasticity, for example, splints holding the ankles at 0 degrees of dorsiflexion will promote proper plantigrade foot alignment for sitting and transfers. It may be helpful for physical and occupational therapists to collaborate with nurses on a positioning schedule for the child with TBI.

Cognitive and Communication Functions

The noisy, busy environment of the acute-care hospital, particularly of the intensive care unit, may hinder the already compromised cognitive functioning of the child with TBI. Visiting family members and all personnel working with the child can orient the child to the surroundings, time, and so forth. The child may have a regularly occurring, relatively alert time; ideally, therapeutic interventions would be attempted at this time.

In the acute-care hospital, speech-language pathologists often work with physical and occupational therapists in treating a child with TBI. Often, the child is aroused by the activity involved in physical and occupational therapy and will be maximally responsive to communication intervention at that time. One of a speech-language pathologist's first tasks is to establish a consistent means of expression for the child. Response systems may be eye blinks, finger or foot movements, or hand squeezes. With improved cognitive function, the child may be able to use head shakes, a picture board, writing, or mouthing of words. Enabling the child to communicate basic needs, such as pain, hunger, thirst, cold, or hot, is the focus of early communication intervention.

If the speech-language pathologist can establish a reliable means of response for the child, therapy can focus on language and cognitive dysfunction. The child with TBI may show the greatest response to familiar people and places. Family members can speak to the child during the speech and language therapy sessions, or taped recordings of their voices can be incorporated. Pictures of siblings, friends, pets, and significant locales, such as home and school, may assist with orientation tasks (Cowley et al., 1994).

Inpatient Rehabilitation Criteria

Deciding whether a child requires inpatient rehabilitation hospitalization after discharge from acute care or whether outpatient monitoring or therapies will be adequate is crucial. Possible criteria to use in determining whether a child with TBI requires an inpatient rehabilitation admission include injury severity, medical condition, cognitive functioning, and need for caregiver training.

Injury Severity

Severity of TBI is often assessed using the Glasgow Coma Scale (GCS) or the Abbreviated Injury Scale for head injuries (AIS-head). A GCS of 3–8 is defined as severe, and an AIS-head score of 5 is defined as critical. Most often, children who have sustained serious or critical TBI are admitted to inpatient rehabilitation facilities (Massagli and Jaffe, 1994). Such children are also most likely to demonstrate a significant number or degree of functional impairments. In a 1991 study of 4,870 cases of children with TBI, DiScarla and coworkers found that 42% of patients with four or more functional impairments were discharged to inpatient rehabilitation or to extended care. Only 2.9% of patients with one to three impairments were discharged to such facilities.

Medical Condition

Often, medical stability is noted as a criterion for admission to an inpatient rehabilitation facility. A child with TBI could be determined to be medically stable once continuous monitoring of neurologic, pulmonary, and cardiac status is no longer necessary. Many rehabilitation centers regard as desirable the ability to tolerate 3 hours of therapy per day. Medical problems such as fractures or poor cardiopulmonary endurance may necessitate treatment modifications once the child is admitted to an inpatient rehabilitation facility.

Cognitive Functioning

To benefit maximally from inpatient rehabilitation, children with TBI should be awake for several hours per day and capable of following commands (Massagli and Jaffe, 1994). Children with less cognitive functioning may be given a short trial of rehabilitation in anticipation of their becoming more alert. Discharge from an acute-care to an extended-care facility has been mentioned as an option for the nonresponsive child. It has been our experience that finding appropriate subacute units or long-term care settings for children with severe TBI is very difficult.

Need for Caregiver Training

Even without minimally desired cognitive functioning, children with TBI may be considered for inpatient rehabilitation admission for caregiver training. In the absence of suitable extended-care facilities, such children are discharged to the home to be cared for by family members. Their medical needs may be so complex that concentrated caregiver training in a rehabilitation facility is necessary. Family members can be instructed in tasks, such as positioning and passive ROM, that will prevent the complications of decubiti and contractures. A program of ongoing environmental stimulation can be established. Careful postdischarge follow-up by a physiatrist is essential for such children. With improvements in cognitive function, such children may require readmission to an inpatient rehabilitation facility to maximize their recovery.

Specific Types of Motor Dysfunction and Their Treatment

Rigidity

Rigidity, a consistent resistance to passive ROM, may be the initial motor finding for children with severe TBI on admission to inpatient rehabilitation (Jaffe et al., 1985). Despite the demonstrated, great resistance to passive stretch, affected children seem to have less propensity to develop soft-tissue contractures than do children with spasticity. As children with rigidity are influenced by disinhibited tonic neck and labyrinthine reflexes, they may benefit from positions that decrease primitive reflex influence, such as sitting with the neck flexed or lying with flexed knees and hips (Table 6-3). For most, rigidity gradually resolves, except in children who remain in persistent vegetative state. As time passes, such children tend to demonstrate decreasing resistance to passive stretch, but purposeful motor function may not yet be developed (Molnar and Perrin, 1992).

Spasticity

Clinical Findings

Spasticity, defined as velocity-dependent resistance to passive stretch, most often occurs in a pattern of hemi-

plegia. Occasionally, a pattern of double hemiplegia occurs, with one side more affected than the other and with the arm more involved than the ipsilateral leg. Hemiplegia may be associated with a pattern of sensory neglect for the affected side and a visual-field cut (see Table 6-3). Dysarthria may accompany spasticity (Molnar and Perrin, 1992).

Treatment

Passive Range of Motion and Positioning.   The simplest therapeutic intervention for spasticity is passive ROM. The therapist may need to alter the child's position so that the influence of primitive reflexes does not contribute to increased spasticity. Children in emerging stages of cognitive recovery may become agitated further with stretching, and a means of distracting them may be necessary. A sustained stretch to the legs may be provided through the use of a tilt table or stander. Flexion contractures of the wrist may be prevented by using resting-hand splints. Plantar flexion contractures of the ankles are prevented through the use of resting-foot splints, most often set at neutral. Table 6-4 provides guidelines for using casts and splints, and Table 6-5 describes positioning techniques.

Activities to Gain Strength and Control.   As the child attains the ability to move spastic extremities voluntarily, therapists and staff can proceed with activities designed to encourage gains in strength and control. Motor recovery for hemiplegic patients usually proceeds from proximal to distal; therefore, efforts should be directed first toward proximal strengthening and control. For patients with a hemiplegic arm, a preliminary voluntary motor function goal is the attainment of volitional shoulder, scapular, and trunk control (Tomas et al., 1993). Therapists may encourage hemiplegic children to use both arms through two-handed play activities, such as riding a tricycle or bicycle or catching a large ball. Even as they regain proximal motor strength, spastic hemiplegic patients may demonstrate weakness, easy fatigability, and lack of dexterity of the affected limbs (i.e., the negative symptoms of spasticity). Loss of motor control is secondary to lack of sequential recruitment and discrete differences in transmission rate of motor neurons and to changes in firing of a muscle relative to its agonists and antagonists. Thus, even with gains in motor strength, patients may still be disabled by deficits in motor control (Katz, 1992). Such deficits may explain why children with seemingly minor weakness of an arm will switch hand dominance (Molnar and Perrin, 1992).

Serial and Inhibitory Casts.   Serial casting is indicated for children who are losing passive ROM despite optimal therapeutic and nursing interventions. Serial casting may also be used to increase joint ROM to a critical level for positioning and the performance of functional activities.

Table 6-3. Motor Sequelae and Functional Implications

Probable Dysfunction	Site of Damage	Functional Implications
Rigidity	Extrapyramidal lesions, rigidity in antigravity muscles; causes decerebrate posturing; rigidity in extensor muscles causes decorticate posturing	Prevents active movements and good positioning
Spasticity (hypertonicity)	Extrapyramidal tract, cerebral cortex, internal capsule, brain stem, or spinal cord; upper motor neuron syndrome, with release of cortical inhibition	Limits full range; can lead to contractures; interferes with purposeful movements; clonus interferes with weight bearing over extremities; often the major problem in brain injury
Hypotonicity	Cerebellum or muscle; impaired muscle proprioception or motor innervation	Prevents initiation of balanced muscle contraction for stability
Ataxia		
Limb	Cerebellum	Limits equilibrium control to regain balance during movement, limits graded control of trunk extremities
Truncal	Labyrinth, cranial nerve VIII, vestibular pathways	Possibly accompanied by vertigo and nystagmus
Tremors		
Resting	Basal ganglia	Hinders smooth, graded control of movements; may limit patient's gross-motor ability or only limit accuracy in fine-motor tasks
Cerebellar	Cerebellum for intentional activity	
Apraxia	Precentral gyrus or supramarginal gyrus of dominant cerebral hemisphere	May affect gross-, fine-, or oral-motor tasks; limits spontaneous movements
Dysarthria	Central or peripheral nervous system	May affect phonation, respiration, articulation, resonance, prosody, feeding, and swallowing; most severely dysarthric patients nonverbal; mildly dysarthric speech possibly intelligible although disordered

Table 6-4. Guidelines for Using Casts and Splints

Type of Cast or Splint	Purpose	Area	Materials	Wearing Schedule
Serial cast	Increase joint range of motion (ROM) to desired range and continuously decrease the negative influences of spasticity	Finger, thumb, hand, wrist, forearm, elbow, knees, ankles, and feet	Plaster, fiberglass, or a combination of both	Worn continuously in a series for 1–2 wks, with passive ROM to those joints between the cast changes
Inhibitory cast	Provide inhibitory input to specific areas to gain active control and increase ROM; to position joint at the most functional angle	Finger, thumb, hand, wrist, forearm, elbow, knees, ankles, and feet	Plaster, fiberglass, or a combination of both	Worn continuously 1–5 days, depending on patient's tolerance

Type of Cast or Splint	Purpose	Area	Materials	Wearing Schedule
Bivalved positioning cast	Maintain ROM in a functional position	Finger, thumb, hand, wrist, forearm, elbow, knees, ankles, and feet	Plaster and fiberglass	Upper extremities: typically worn 2 hrs on and off, gradually decreasing wearing time as functional control improves. Lower extremities: worn 2 hrs on and off, gradually increasing to 6–8 hrs/day, possibly decreasing wearing time as functional control improves
Resting-hand splints	Maintain proper wrist and hand position, prevent joint contractures, maintain ROM	Finger, hand, wrist, and forearm	Low- or high-temperature plastic	Typically worn 2 hrs on and off
Positioning splints	Maintain the extremity in a functional resting position, prevent joint contractures	Finger, thumb, hand, wrist, forearm, elbow, knees, ankles, and feet	Low- or high-temperature plastic, plaster, fiberglass, or dense foam	Worn as tolerated

Table 6-5. Positioning for Common Motor Dysfunction

Dysfunction	Position	Intervention
Flexor spasticity resulting in flexor pattern in arms, legs, and neck	Prone	Place child in prone position, turn head to desired side, attempt to extend legs fully (can place sandbags over hips and buttocks), attempt to abduct arms away from trunk (can place pillows under head and chest)
	Side-lying	Place child on desired side, position legs into extension (can use sandbags to block hips), align head and neck into neutral position (can place pillows in front of trunk and between arms)
Extensor pattern influence causing total extension of head, neck, trunk, arms, and legs	Side-lying	Place child on desired side, position in maximum possible trunk and leg flexion (can use sandbags or pillows to maintain position), position arms in shoulder and elbow flexion (using pillows for stabilization), align head and neck in neutral position
	Sitting	Position pelvis in a symmetric, neutral anteroposterior tilt; attempt to achieve 90-degree flexion at hips, knees, and ankles; use solid seat and back inserts in wheelchair; can use wedged seat to increase hip flexion (seat should provide support under the femur, with knee no higher than hip); position feet flat on the footrests (straps can be used to ensure foot position); position trunk in midline against solid back insert (can use lateral supports as needed); attempt to position arms at sides, in slight shoulder and elbow flexion, with palms resting on a full lap tray (blocks or padding can be added to tray as needed for positioning); maintain head in midline with slight chin tuck if possible; use supporting headrest
Shoulder retraction	Side-lying	Place child on desired side; move the more affected shoulder gently forward; support the position with pillows or sandbags behind the back and between the arms (if both shoulders are affected, the shoulder on the underside is placed forward)
	Supine	Guide the humerus and scapula forward so that the shoulder is flexed and gently abducted, support the arms and hand on a pillow with the elbow slightly flexed ahead of the shoulder and with the hand open

Table 6-5. *Continued*

Dysfunction	Position	Intervention
	Sitting	Position trunk in midline against solid back insert, attempt to position arms at the sides in slight shoulder and elbow flexion, place the elbows slightly anterior to the shoulders, support the arms with the palms resting on a full lap tray
Ankle plantar flexor(s) spastic	Sitting	Position feet flat on the footrests (straps can be used to ensure foot position; may use angle-adjustable footrests to facilitate foot position)
	Standing	Stand child on tilt table or in supine stander with three straps (across lower chest, across hips, and proximal to the knees), ensure that the feet are flat, directly under the hips

For example, serial casting is commonly used to increase ankle dorsiflexion to neutral. The ability to dorsiflex the ankle passively to neutral optimizes sitting position and facilitates transfers and standing. Inhibitory casts provide inhibitory input to specific areas, allowing children with spasticity to gain active control and increase ROM. Serial and inhibitory casts are described further in Table 6-4. During a course of casting, attention must be paid to skin integrity and neurovascular status. Casting may be accompanied by peripheral nerve blocks or motor point blocks (Lehmkuhl et al., 1990).

Neurolytic Blocks.   Neurolytic blocks, either of peripheral nerves or motor points, are indicated for short-term reduction of spasticity in a joint. For the child with extreme spasticity in one or a few critical joints, neurolytic blocks may prevent disabling contracture formation. If such a child is determined to be losing passive ROM, neurolytic blocks should be considered, perhaps with serial casting or systemic antispasticity drugs.

Neurolytic blocks may be used to improve passive positioning or active function. Commonly, spasticity of the following muscles adversely affects positioning, hygiene, and function: hip adductors, hamstrings, ankle plantar flexors, elbow flexors, wrist flexors, and finger flexors. A peripheral nerve trunk block usually results in a greater decrease in spasticity of a given muscle than does a motor point block. Many muscles have multiple motor end plates, and it can be difficult to block all the motor points to eliminate spasticity completely. Injecting a peripheral nerve entails some risk of dysesthesia secondary to possible involvement of the sensory fibers. The obturator nerve, which supplies the hip adductor muscles, is one peripheral nerve that carries few sensory fibers. Motor point blocks may be used when total elimination of spasticity in a muscle is undesirable, most often for the child demonstrating some active, voluntary control of the extremities (Ball, 1995). At our facility, motor point

blocks of the biceps, flexor digitorum sublimis, and gastrocnemius muscles have been performed.

Portable constant-current stimulators are now available, facilitating the performance of peripheral nerve and motor point blocks. To assess the effects of a proposed block, a short-acting block with a local anesthetic (e.g., lidocaine or bupivacaine) can be performed. Historically, an aqueous solution of phenol at a concentration of 3–6% has been used for relatively long-term blocks. Phenol motor point blocks have a duration of 3–6 months. Peripheral nerve blocks with phenol last longer, 6–12 months (Gans et al., 1990).

Botulinum toxin A, which is produced by the bacterium *Clostridium botulinum*, has gained interest as a neurolytic agent for localized spasticity control. It acts by inhibiting the release of acetylcholine at the neuromuscular junction. In 1994, Cosgrove and associates reported on its use in children with cerebral palsy, and application may be considered for children with TBI and spasticity. Investigators report that for the majority of subjects, botulinum toxin A requires 2–3 days after injection to manifest its desired effects, which then last 2–3 months. Botulinum toxin A can be injected into the muscle belly at random. One factor potentially limiting its widespread use is its high cost (Ball, 1995).

Systemic Medications.   Systemic medications for spasticity reduction are indicated for those children with diffusely increased muscle tone. For example, if positioning in a wheelchair proves to be impossible for patients with marked extensor posturing of the trunk and lower extremities, such patients would be candidates for systemic antispasticity drugs. Other indications for pharmacologic spasticity treatment are listed in Table 6-6.

For children, the most commonly used antispasticity drugs are dantrolene, diazepam, and baclofen. The sites of action, doses, and complications of these drugs are listed in Table 6-7. Many experts regard dantrolene as the drug of choice for treatment of spasticity of central nervous system origin (Katz and Campagnolo, 1994; Molnar and Perrin, 1992). Dantrolene and baclofen combined may demonstrate a synergistic effect (Molnar and Perrin, 1992). The use of diazepam is often limited by its accompanying sedating effect.

Long-Term Spasticity Reduction. For long-term reduction of spasticity in children who have sustained TBI, selective posterior rhizotomies or continuous intrathecal baclofen infusions may be considered. When the child's motor recovery appears to have maximized (usually at approximately 18 months after the initial injury), orthopedic surgery may be considered to ameliorate muscle contractures occurring secondary to spasticity. One of the most commonly performed procedures is percutaneous tendo-Achilles lengthening. The percutaneous method is used to avoid overlengthening of the tendon, which would result in a crouch gait from excessive passive ankle dorsiflexion (Pinzur, 1993).

Hypotonicity

Hypotonicity, or low resting muscle tone, most often occurs in the trunk. Children with hypotonic trunks have increased difficulty with active trunk control. Initially, they may require adaptive seating, with bilateral lateral trunk supports and anterior chest bibs or harnesses, to use their arms voluntarily. As they become able to participate actively in their therapies, their therapists may attempt to facilitate trunk extension (Table 6-8).

Ataxia

Ataxia with or without spasticity is the most frequently occurring motor dysfunction in children with TBI. It may become noticeable only as a child begins to move spontaneously or as spasticity resolves (Molnar and Perrin, 1992). Some children demonstrate spasticity in a hemiplegic pattern and ataxia of the contralateral limbs. Ambulators with ataxia show a wide-based gait, mid- to high-guard position

Table 6-6. Indications for Pharmacologic Spasticity Treatment

1. Interference with the patient's active movement
2. Contracture formation or progression in a posturing limb
3. Interference with appropriate positioning or hygiene
4. Self-inflicted trauma during muscle spasms
5. Excessive pain on range of motion or during muscle spasms
6. Excessive therapy time devoted to contracture prevention rather than to functional activities

Source: L Stine, DY Shin (1993). Management of hypertonicity using chemical denervation following traumatic brain injury. Phys Med Rehabil 7;527.

of the arms, and truncal sway (see Table 6-3). Children who frequently fall may require helmets for head protection. Therapists may use limb weights or provide proprioceptive input to the joints. A reverse-style walker (e.g., Kaye Posture Control Walker [Kaye Products, Inc., Hillsborough, NC]) is often the most suitable for ataxic children. Having to pull the walker behind the body encourages erect trunk posture and slows ambulation speed. Also, weights may be placed on the walker. Some ataxic children do relatively well with adapted tricycles.

Ataxia may be a manifestation of vestibular dysfunction. A surgically correctable cause of vestibular dysfunction is endolymphatic fistula (Molnar and Perrin, 1992). Physical therapy may ameliorate manifestations of uncorrectable causes of vestibular dysfunction. Specific treatment strategies are determined by the specific etiology of the dysfunction, which may be unilateral vestibular hypofunction, positional vertigo, or bilateral vestibular loss. Exercises may be used to encourage adaptation of the vestibular system or to improve the substitution of alternative approaches to promote gaze and postural stability. The incidence of vestibular dysfunction is greatest in patients who have sustained temporal bone fractures (Herdman, 1990).

Table 6-7. Drugs Used in Treatment of Spasticity

Name	Site of Action	Dose	Complications
Dantrolene (Dantrium)	Periphery, extrafusal muscle fibers	25 mg bid (maximum, 100 mg qid depending on size)	Drug hepatitis (rare), most common in women >25 yrs; weakness
Diazepam (Valium)	Spinal cord and supraspinal limbic system	1 mg bid (maximum, 5 mg qid depending on size)	Drowsiness; weakness; potentiates other drugs; paradoxical reactions
Baclofen (Lioresal)	Spinal cord and supraspinal	5 mg bid or tid (maximum, 20 mg qid)	Lethargy, hallucinations (rare); gradual increase or decrease of dose mandatory

Source: MB Jaffe, JP Mastrilli, CB Molitor, AS Valko (1985). Intervention for Motor Disorders. In M Ylvisaker (ed), Head Injury Rehabilitation: Children and Adolescents. San Diego: College Hill Press, 167. Copyright 1997, Butterworth–Heinemann.

Table 6-8. Functional Mobility Checklist

Functional	Limitations	Interventions
Bed mobility	Physical (e.g., fracture with weight-bearing precautions)	Provide compensatory strategies or equipment; use trapeze for adolescent; use elbows or uninvolved extremities to scoot, pull on bed rails; plan ahead (e.g., get onto bed with head toward pillow)
	Cognitive (e.g., decreased overall movements due to lethargy)	Use multisensory input (e.g., verbally describe patient's movements while initiating and providing weight bearing through the joints)
Supine (from-to) sit	Physical (e.g., decreased trunk control)	Target trunk control during components of supine to sit and sit to supine; have child explore various methods of rolling (e.g., pull on bed rail, initiate roll with hips or arms); side-lying on elbow (check to see whether patient can maintain this position while attempting to move other parts of the body); coordinate arm and leg movement as patient generates momentum to change position; sitting (facilitate trunk extension, emphasize moving from and returning to midline)
	Cognitive (e.g., decreased language processing for verbal direction)	Bypass cognitive limitations (model target movements with reduced verbalizations, physically guide patient through movements)
Sit (from-to) stand	Physical (e.g., decreased ankle range of motion secondary to increased plantar flexion tone; the resultant difficulty in active dorsiflexion limits the patient's ability to shift weight forward)	Use serial casting, standing program (tilt table, supine stander, prone stander, freedom stander), education program for passive range of motion as frequently as possible (by patient, family, and staff); work on reaching forward to floor in sitting; reinforce movements in all transfers
	Cognitive (e.g., increased impulsivity resulting in unsafe behaviors)	Reinforce safe behaviors (ask child to recite appropriate sequence for transfers prior to starting movements; prepare for or remind child of sit-to-stand sequence before task initiation; during actual task, slow the child down and use verbal cues)
Toilet transfer	Physical (e.g., predominant extensor pattern interfering with transfers)	Cue by verbal or physical means to maintain flexion during transfer (e.g., "Lean forward"; "Stay forward while you lift your hips off the chair and onto the toilet")
	Cognitive (e.g., decreased memory for sequence of movements)	Reinforce correct sequence (post correct transfer sequence in a highly visible location in the bathroom; reinforce correct sequence with the patient via overlearning; train family and staff in the correct sequence)
Ambulation	Physical (e.g., ataxic movement interfering with voluntary control)	Provide correct physical cues (apply weights to appropriate body parts: may need to experiment with placement; provide proprioceptive input through joints)
	Cognitive (e.g., left-side neglect-inattention resulting in decreased safety)	Offer multisensory input and cueing to increase patient's awareness and attention to the left side (e.g., visual, "Look and find your mom. She is on your left"; verbal, "Look to the left"; tactile, permit the patient to make contact with environmental obstacles on the left; stand on the walking patient's left—neglected—side)
Wheelchair mobility	Physical (e.g., decrease in coordination of extremities affecting patient's ability to propel wheelchair)	Train in necessary movement patterns (provide hand-over-hand or foot-over-foot assistance; emphasize the movement of one set of extremities at a time, such as arms, then legs; model the correct arm and leg movements; give verbal feedback during wheelchair propulsion)
	Cognitive (e.g., decreased problem-solving skills impairing mobility, as a result of which the patient may get stuck in a corner)	Provide decreasingly less obvious clues during wheelchair mobility training (e.g., wheelchair course with lateral boundary "markers," beginning with maximum structure, using portable wall dividers as lateral boundary markers,

Functional	Limitations	Interventions
		changing the lateral boundary markers to cones, changing the lateral boundary markers to masking tape, and removing all lateral boundary markers and verbally cueing the patient to propel wheelchair along a given course); proceed to more challenging and less structured mobility situations gradually, as patient's cognitive level permits (e.g., have patient propel the wheelchair in the cafeteria)
Stairs	Physical (e.g., decreased balance interfering with stair negotiation)	Explore means of improving balance and providing compensatory strategies (play appropriate games that improve unilateral stance and such weight-shifting skills as soccer, kickball, balance beam activities, hopscotch; teach patient and family such safety precautions and compensatory strategies as holding onto the railing, ensuring that an adult is with the patient on stairs)
	Cognitive (e.g., figure-ground deficit affecting the patient's ability to see the edge of the step)	Highlight stairwell surroundings by adding contrast (e.g., colored tape) to the edge of the step, adding tactile cue (e.g., rubber lip) to the edge of the step or to the handrail above each step, coloring alternating steps, ensuring that stairways are well-lit, reminding patient to search for step edge with foot before stepping and to use handrail for safety, and ensuring that an adult is with the patient on stairs
Floor (to-from) stand	Physical (e.g., hemiplegia and weakness on the less involved side)	Compensate for weakness by positioning the patient near a stable support surface (e.g., furniture), assisting the patient to tall kneeling, placing both of the patient's hands on the support surface, assisting the patient to shift weight onto the hemiplegic side while bringing the less involved leg forward into half kneeling, instructing the patient to lean forward and stand up
	Cognitive (e.g., poor organization and sequencing of steps involved)	Reinforce step sequence by identifying the correct sequencing, using age-appropriate visual cues (e.g., brightly colored numbers, hand and foot prints), reinforcing correct sequence with patient via overlearning, and training family and staff in the correct sequence

Tremor

Tremor is often seen with ataxia and frequently occurs with attempts to initiate movements, particularly those requiring a high degree of fine-motor coordination (see Table 6-3). In one study of 131 children with TBI and tremor, the tremor was found to have subsided spontaneously in half the cases (Johnson and Hall, 1992). Limited success has been found using drug treatment for children with tremor after TBI. For children aged 7–12 years, propranolol (Inderal), 20 mg three times daily, has been effective in some cases (Ellison, 1978).

Apraxia

Apraxia, or motor-planning problems, may affect children's voluntary movements. Despite seemingly adequate strength, apraxic children cannot perform a given motor task. Functionally, they appear worse than the results of

manual muscle testing would seem to indicate. They may be able to perform a given movement automatically but not on command (see Table 6-3). Therapeutic strategies for such children include multiple repetitions of a task, so that it becomes automatic to them, and breaking a task down into its component parts.

Motor Speech Dysfunctions

Speech dysfunctions that may occur in children with TBI are outlined in Table 6-9. Details are supplied in the following sections.

Dysarthria

Dysarthria is a term for a group of motor speech disorders. Its most frequent symptoms in pediatric patients with TBI are articulatory imprecision, phonatory weakness, and a slow rate of speech. Persistent dysarthria is more common in adolescents than in younger children.

Table 6-9. Motor Speech Dysfunction

Dysfunction	Probable Site of Damage	Functional Deficit	Corresponding Therapeutic Invention for Functional Deficit
Dysarthria: lack of control of volitional and automatic oral motor actions; chewing, tongue, and jaw movements possibly affected	Central nervous system, possible damage to motor cortex area controlling oral movement; cranial nerves V, VII, IX, X, or XII possibly damaged	Impaired speech production secondary to tone abnormalities	Provide gross- and fine-motor treatments designed to normalize tone. Note any vocalizations that occur spontaneously during yawning, sighing, and other physical activities. Reinforce and shape any vocalizations that may be used for communication purposes. Use electromyography for biofeedback to relax shoulder and facial muscles, if patient is able to cooperate. Provide alternatives for verbal communication purposes.
		Soft and breathy voice	Teach patients to control timing of breathing. Encourage patient to vocalize during physical activities. Instruct patient in use of voice amplifier for noisy situations, such as the classroom.
		Inaccurate articulation	Instruct patient in formation of proper mouth movements using a mirror. Provide opportunities for systematic skill practice and drill, if patient is able to cooperate.
		Monotonous voice pitch	Provide the patient with opportunities to increase voice inflection, using singing, dramatic readings, poetry.
		Slow rate of speech	Instruct the patient to minimize the number of words required for successful message transmission. Train the patient to eliminate inspiratory pauses within utterance.
Apraxia: impaired ability to motor-plan articulatory positions and to sequence movements (respiratory, laryngeal, and oral) for volitional speech	Precentral gyrus or supramarginal gyrus of dominant hemisphere	Diminished or absent vocalizations, usually for severely affected patients	Facilitate patient's phonation by oral movements (e.g., chewing, grunting, humming, or imitating animals or inanimate objects), gesturing, stimulation of larynx with a vibrator, application of rapid pressure beneath the ribs, automatic activities (e.g., counting, singing, or rhyming), cues via cloze technique (e.g., piece of ___). Provide substitutes for vocal output (e.g., switches or call signals; such signals for yes-no as eyeblink, pointing to yes-no sign, and shaking or nodding the head; gesturing; pantomiming; signing; drawing; writing; communication board; and other augmentative communication systems).

Dysfunction	Probable Site of Damage	Functional Deficit	Corresponding Therapeutic Invention for Functional Deficit
		Diminished intelligibility usually found in moderately affected patients; multisyllabic words often most difficult for affected patients	Train patient to reduce rate of speech (e.g., emphasis on visual modality, pacing board). Train patients to pause between words to allow time for motor planning and measured articulatory executions (e.g., contrastive stress drills, melodic intonation therapy, motor kinesthetic training).
Hypernasality: disproportionate nasal emission of vocal sounds, resulting in abnormal speech resonance	Central nervous system: cranial nerves V, VII, IX, X, or XII; peripheral nerves	Incomplete (weak) or inappropriate and uncoordinated action of velopharyngeal mechanism, hypertonicity or hypotonicity in the muscles of the articulators, abnormal tongue positioning	Evaluate using videofluoroscopy, with possible interventions (e.g., palatal lift prosthesis, surgery, Teflon injection, pharyngeal flap placement). Consider these interventions on a highly individualized basis, but generally not until 1 yr after injury.

Sources: MM Hodge, SD Hall (1994). Effects of Syllable Characteristics and Training Rate in a Child with Dysarthria Secondary to Near Drowning. In JA Till, KM Yorkston, DR Beukelman (eds), Motor Speech Disorders: Advances in Assessment and Treatment. Baltimore: Paul H. Brookes, 229; and MB Jaffe, JP Mastrilli, CB Molitor, AS Valko (1995). Intervention for Motor Disorders. In M Ylvisaker (ed), Head Injury Rehabilitation: Children and Adolescents. San Diego: College Hill Press, 167.

The speech of severely affected patients may be unintelligible. Improvements in dysarthria may be noted as the patient's overall motor function ameliorates, particularly in such domains as sitting posture, head control, and breath support. Any spontaneously occurring vocalizations are reinforced. The speech-language pathologist attempts to provide the patient with a basic vocabulary of easily articulated words. Mirrors may be used to provide visual feedback of mouth movements.

The speech of mildly affected patients is understandable. A monotonous vocal pitch may be noted for these children. For those with sufficient attention span and ability to cooperate, systematic drill and practice can be used. Encouraging the affected child to shout during vigorous physical activity may increase the reduced vocal volume present in some mildly dysarthric patients (Jaffe et al., 1985).

Apraxia of Speech

Apraxia of speech is impaired ability to motor-plan articulatory positions and to sequence movements (respiratory, laryngeal, and oral) for volitional speech. Apraxia of speech is more common in younger children than in adolescents. Apraxic patients may mouth words initially, then whisper without phonation. They may produce sounds spontaneously during sighing, laughing, or yawning. Speech-language pathologists can draw a patient's attention to any spontaneous sounds produced, alternate in making sounds with the patient, and encour-

age sound repetition. Oral movements such as chewing, grunting, coughing, and humming may facilitate phonation. Progressive approximation of sounds and movements that the patient is capable of producing may be used to teach new ones. In the key-word technique, the speech-language pathologist uses a word that the child has mastered to assist in transferring the target sounds to other words (Jaffe et al., 1985).

Hypernasality

Hypernasality of speech is caused by nasal emission of vocal sounds, resulting in abnormal speech resonance. Causes include deficits in the action of the velopharyngeal mechanism, spasticity or low tone of the muscles of the articulators, and abnormal tongue positioning. Videofluoroscopy is needed for thorough evaluation of possible palatal insufficiency. In severe cases, a lifelong palatal prosthesis or surgery is considered: The soft palate is raised to the posterior pharyngeal wall by a palatal lift, producing a mechanical obstruction between the oral and nasal cavities. Sufficient cognitive recovery is needed before the child can participate in fitting and training with the prosthesis. For operative intervention, Teflon injection or pharyngeal flap surgery is a possibility. Patients with respiratory problems are not candidates for palatal surgery. Children with TBI are not usually considered for either a palatal prosthesis or surgical intervention until at least 1 year after trauma (Jaffe et al., 1985).

Functional Goals of Intervention

Awareness of the child's preinjury and current levels of developmental and cognitive function is necessary to set appropriate treatment goals and to use proper means for attaining those goals. Children may require interventions to regain previously attained milestones and to achieve new milestones not attained before the injury. Impairments in one domain may affect the attainment of milestones in another. For example, difficulties in the gross-motor skill of adequate trunk control may impede a child's ability to use the hands for fine-motor skills secondary to a lack of proximal stability.

Age-Related Functional Goals

Infants

The motor assessment of infants with TBI may be complicated by the presence of age-appropriate findings associated with a physiologically immature neuromuscular system. Even noninjured infants may have hyperactive deep-tendon reflexes. The influence of primitive reflexes may be persistent in infants 3–6 months old (Gans et al., 1990). These factors render tone abnormalities in infants difficult to determine. Even in children with congenital cerebral palsy, tone abnormalities such as spasticity may not be obvious until ages 1–2 years.

Infants with TBI lack previously acquired motor skills (Ylvisaker et al., 1990). Therapy to elicit age-appropriate motor functions includes play activities, such as having an infant reach for an attractive object. Small children first acquire floor mobility, such as creeping and crawling. As infancy is a period of relatively rapid growth, particular attention should be given to contracture prevention (Gans et al., 1990). Oral-motor functioning, such as feeding, should be assessed (see Chapter 7). The mean age for producing the first meaningful word is 1 year. Speech-language pathologists can facilitate prelanguage skills (e.g., babbling and turn taking) with infants functioning below a cognitive level of 1 year.

Preschool-Aged Children

Therapeutic interventions for preschoolers with TBI are based on play activities, as children of this age learn through playing and exploring their environment. Some children may require repeated demonstrations of the proper use of toys and equipment. For severely affected children without functional ambulation, alternative means of mobility may be necessary to permit them to explore the environment. For normally developing youngsters, the preschool period is the time for refinement of gross- and fine-motor skills. If possible, further refinement of motor skills already present should be attempted for preschoolers with TBI (Ylvisaker et al., 1990). Ambulation patterns can be improved to render gait more efficient and less energy consuming.

School-Aged Children

Most school-aged children with TBI return to an educational environment after discharge from an inpatient rehabilitation facility. Their ability to function in such an environment must be assessed and treated. An important skill for academic functioning is handwriting. As the child advances in grade level, a greater volume of handwriting at a greater speed is necessary. To avoid compromising their academic functioning, some children may require alternatives for handwriting, such as typewriters, tape recorders, computers, or oral testing. To cover distances efficiently within the school building, children who are marginal ambulators may require wheeled mobility devices (e.g., wheelchairs or scooters) (Ylvisaker et al., 1990). To enhance the child's self-esteem and acceptance among peers, involvement in sports and extracurricular activities should be encouraged. Horseback-riding programs for children with physical disabilities are becoming more widespread. Activities such as martial arts or swimming can be modified to accommodate a child's motor dysfunction.

Teenagers

Teenagers with TBI are often concerned with career choices and peer acceptance. For older teenagers with TBI, a referral to the bureau of vocational services during inpatient rehabilitation should be considered. The driving ability of such teenagers requires careful assessment. As teenagers are greatly concerned about their physical appearance and acceptance by peers, prescribed equipment and devices should be as cosmetic and unobtrusive as possible (Ylvisaker et al., 1990).

Task-Related Functional Goals

More than one specific means may be available to attain a given rehabilitation goal for a child with TBI. For example, the goal of independent mobility may be attained by unassisted ambulation, by ambulation with assistive devices such as a cane or a walker, or by use of a wheelchair or scooter. As previously stated, an overriding goal of rehabilitation is to maximize patient independence. Attaining this goal for children with TBI may be compromised by such cognitive deficits as impulsivity and lack of insight, which compromise safety. Naturally, some parents may be overprotective. Encouraging parents to allow their child the proper amount of independence is one function of the rehabilitation team (Gans et al., 1990). Specific functional domains for motor intervention for children with TBI include mobility, self-care, communication, age-appropriate play and sports, and vision. Goals within each of these domains are determined by chronologic age, level of cognitive functioning, and degree of motor dysfunction. Proper goal setting in an inpatient rehabilitation facility involves considering the level of support the child's caregivers will be able to provide after discharge. Input and feedback from the child and caregivers regarding goals and the means suggested to attain those goals are essential.

Mobility

To attain mobility—whether unassisted (e.g., crawling and walking) or assisted (e.g., using walkers or manual or electric wheelchairs)—children must be able to voluntarily control movement of some part(s) of their bodies. In general, the greater the number of skeletal muscle groups they can control voluntarily, the greater the degree of unassisted mobility they will attain. Therapists can train children to control voluntarily specific muscle groups, with the eventual goal of unassisted ambulation (e.g., by progressing them through the developmental sequence for ambulation: first crawling, then kneeling, then standing). Advanced activities to develop more refined neuromuscular control may include hopping, jumping, running, and navigating an obstacle course. Biofeedback can be used to train selected children in selective motor control (Cardenas and Clawson, 1990). Some children with either permanent or temporary TBI attain mobility by ambulating with assistive devices. To ambulate with (or without) assistive devices, children must be able to maintain static equilibrium in a seated position (i.e., they must be able to sit without hand support). The need for assistive devices and the type of device required can be determined by the presence or absence of equilibrium reactions. Children who can sit without hand support but who lack any equilibrium reactions will require a walker for ambulation. Those who have lateral equilibrium reactions but lack anterior (front) and posterior (back) equilibrium reactions will require crutches for ambulation. Those who possess lateral and anterior equilibrium reactions but lack posterior reactions are capable of walking without support (Rang et al., 1986).

As the motor capabilities of children with TBI may improve, their need for assistive-device support requires ongoing reassessment. Some children with severe motor dysfunction may require wheelchairs for mobility. Members of a subgroup of this group may function as household ambulators and require a wheelchair for long-distance mobility. Children's wheelchairs should feature cushioned supportive seats and backs. For children capable of independent transfers, wheelchairs should be constructed so as not to interfere with this activity. Children with poor sitting balance may require lateral trunk supports and anterior chest support, such as a bib vest or an H harness (Rang et al., 1986). A tilt-in-space wheelchair, which maintains a constant hip and knee flexion at 90 degrees, may be helpful for those who lack voluntary head control or who demonstrate mass lower-extremity extension (Gans et al., 1990). As a cognitively age-appropriate 3-year-old child can operate an electric wheelchair safely, such a mobility device should be considered for very severely physically involved children who desire independent mobility and possess ade-

quate safety knowledge, visual function, and judgment. Such children may require assessment for their most reliable site of control (Alexander, 1986). During an inpatient rehabilitation hospitalization, children with TBI can be evaluated for the most appropriate type of mobility device (mobile seating system). (See Chapter 8.) At our facility, recommendations for a mobility device to be purchased for a child are made near the end of the hospitalization, as improvements in motor function during the stay would change some of the mobility device's requirements.

Self-Care Skills

Expectations for appropriate self-care skills for children are age related: Much more is expected of a teenager than of a 3-year-old child. For a child in the initial stages of cognitive recovery, the beginning step in attaining the goal of independent self-bathing may be to have the child touch the face with a washcloth. Adaptive devices are provided as indicated, bearing in mind that children are quick to reject any device that they perceive to be unwieldy or that "slows them down." For dressing, clothing modifications such as Velcro and elastic openings and shoe laces may be helpful. For grooming and hygiene, some children with motor involvement require bath seats, bath chairs, and raised toilet seats. Obtaining measurements of doorway widths and bathroom dimensions and learning the number of steps to entrances and bedrooms in a child's home may be helpful for those for whom accessibility could be a difficulty. In dressing training for children with cognitive dysfunction, assistance may be rendered via posted checklists in the bedroom.

At our facility, inpatients with TBI attend instruction in a classroom, which provides the opportunity to evaluate independence in mobility and self-care in a school environment. Teenagers should be evaluated for safe operation of kitchen appliances and for performing household tasks. Community mobility should be assessed, as children with TBI may do relatively well in the comparatively quiet environment of a rehabilitation center but may decompensate on a crowded city street.

Communication

On admission to an inpatient rehabilitation facility, children with TBI may be incapable of verbal communication due to limited cognitive awareness, motor dysfunction, or the presence of tracheostomies or nasogastric feeding tubes. Attempts may be made to provide such patients with a call signal or a simple switch system to signal need. The ability to use yes and no responses consistently requires abstract reasoning and, initially, may be beyond the capabilities of a child with TBI. A more appropriate first communication goal may be to provide a means for the patient to express needs and emotions. A basic communication board could have pictures corresponding to needs, such as a glass for "I am thirsty." Simple drawings of facial expressions could allow the child to notify caregivers of physiologic pain or emotion. The appropriate number of pictures on an initial communication board is four to six. As cognitive recovery progresses, efforts can be made to establish gestures for yes and no responses. During the rehabilitation hospitalization, attempts are made to have patients ingest food orally (see Chapter 7). Children usually accomplish taking food orally before they accomplish speaking (Jaffe et al., 1985).

As children with TBI begin to attempt to speak, motor speech disorders may become noticeable. Apraxia may affect speech intelligibility. Moderately affected apraxic patients are usually more intelligible when they reduce their speech rate and pause between words, allowing time for careful articulation and motor planning. A pacing board may be useful. Some patients demonstrate a residual deficit of a breathy or weak voice. They are instructed in compensatory strategies such as phrasing, producing specific phonemes, intonation patterns, and motor planning (Jaffe et al., 1985).

Augmentative Communication

Severely dysarthric or apraxic patients may require augmentative communication devices (Jaffe et al., 1985). The speech-language pathologist and occupational therapist can work together to find the best method for device access. Possible means of accessing a system include direct selection, switch activation, and scanning. Direct selection is usually the most rapid means but also requires the greatest degree of motor control. The child's cognitive and perceptual capabilities must also be considered. The increase in cognitive and perceptual load needed for operation of an augmentative communication device may result in decreased performance (Levine et al., 1992). Patients with severe cognitive limitations are unable to use an augmentative communication device (Jaffe et al., 1985).

The Macaw (Prentke-Romich, Wooster, OH) and the Dynavox (Sentient Systems, Pittsburgh, PA) are appropriate augmentative communication devices for children with TBI in the early stages of recovery. The Macaw has an eight-picture display and programmable output. For example, a tape recording of a parent's voice can be made and used as the vocal output. The child may be more willing to use a device with a familiar human voice as output than one with a computer-generated voice. The access means for the Dynavox can be adjusted as the child's physical capabilities improve. Initially, one or more switches may be used for access; eventually, the child may progress to using a keyboard. Children with severe physical involvement may require advanced augmentative communication devices, such as those capable of using eye movement input to operate a scanning selection process and a computer monitor (Platts and Fraser, 1993).

Play

Children learn through playing. Efforts at improving the motor capabilities of children with TBI may involve care-fully structured and designed play activities. Children with motor dysfunction may require assistance to play more effectively and to avoid undue frustration in their playing attempts. Switch modifications can be fabricated for greater ease in operating battery-powered toys. Children with poor fine-motor control may find it easier to manipulate large-diameter crayons and pencils. Those with weak hand grips may be able to use magic markers. In terms of gross-motor activities, many children enjoy swimming, as the buoyancy provided by water may facilitate movement of weak extremities. Tricycles and bicycles can be modified to provide greater support to those with poor trunk control. Training wheels may furnish added stability for patients with poor balance. Those with difficulties in hand-eye coordination may be able to hit a ball mounted on a pole (as in T-ball) rather than a thrown ball. Horseback-riding programs and Challenger Little League teams are increasingly available for children with physical impairments. The availability of such programs in or near the child's hometown can be determined before discharge from an inpatient rehabilitation facility.

Vision

Visual function evaluation and treatment of children with TBI is both challenging and necessary. The challenge is in the difficulty of detecting vision problems, which may not be noticeable either to the patient or the casual observer. Because of a limited expressive vocabulary, children may find it difficult to describe their visual perceptions even if they recognize these perceptions as abnormal. Diagnosing and treating deficits in visual and perceptual function is so important because of the role these functions play in the independent and safe performance of activities of daily living. Delays in self-initiated movement, locomotion, and reaching in response to auditory cues have been documented in children with vision impairments (Murphy, 1991). Hyvärinen (1995) lists eight specific visual functions to be included in a comprehensive evaluation of children: (1) visual acuity, (2) contrast sensitivity, (3) visual field, (4) color vision, (5) adaptation, (6) visual sphere, (7) accommodation, and (8) oculomotor functions.

Visual acuity in adults is assessed by determining recognition acuity. Government regulations are based on acuity measured by line tests. These tests necessitate a developmental age equivalent of at least 18–30 months.

In children, visual acuity is determined most often by grating acuity tests. In such tests, the subject detects parallel lines of diminishing width. Data from these tests should be supplemented by clinical observations from therapy sessions (Hyvärinen, 1995).

Gianutsos and Matheson (1987) stated that in assessing visual acuity, both near-point acuity (from 16 in.) and far-point acuity (from 20 ft) should be measured. For children, the near point roughly corresponds to reading distance, and the far point corresponds to the distance from a school desk to the blackboard. Providing corrective lenses for children with diminished acuity may result in improvements in cognitive and motor tasks.

Contrast sensitivity is the skill of appreciating small differences in the luminance between adjacent surfaces. Most environmental objects have low to medium (as opposed to high) contrast. Visually impaired children have been found to show greatest attention to objects of high contrast (Hyvärinen, 1995).

The visual field is the area that can be seen when the child looks straight ahead. Modified confrontation techniques can be used to assess visual-field area in children. An important differential diagnosis is to be made between neglect of one-half of the body (inattention) and actual visual-field loss (Hyvärinen, 1995).

Compensatory training, such as teaching patients to turn the head toward the side of vision loss, has been advocated. In citing research on adults who have sustained TBIs, Warren (1993) noted that such training has not been found to diminish the size of visual-field loss. What has been determined is that such training does improve the efficiency, accuracy, and scope of visual search patterns performed by adult patients (Warren, 1993). For children with visual-field losses, Hyvärinen (1995) advocated the use of activities that combine locating a specific toy or object with manipulating it. Using this technique, vision is combined and reinforced with motor input.

Often, color vision is diminished in children with visual deficits. It can be measured by sorting tests. Recognition of color is an important component of object recognition. Children with cortical blindness may have difficulties in identifying objects via visual assessment of shape and form. For such children, color can be used as a compensatory coding system (Hyvärinen, 1995).

Visual sphere is the distance within which children are able to respond to an object of given contrast, size, color, and speed of movement. Children's responses may be influenced by their interest in the object presented. The visual sphere parameter determines ability to detect landmarks for orientation in both familiar and unfamiliar environments (Hyvärinen, 1995).

The eye keeps objects in focus by changing the refractive power of the lens through the process of accommodation. For accommodation deficits, reading glasses may be necessary. For children, such reading glasses must be strong, as focal distances are short. For obtaining the proper degree of accommodation via corrective lenses, close cooperation with an ophthalmologist or optometrist is necessary (Hyvärinen, 1995).

Oculomotor function evaluation often reveals difficulties with binocular vision resulting from a lack of proper synchronization and coordination of both eyes. Children with TBI may complain of double vision, often describing what they see as blurry. Other symptoms may include eye strain, diminished depth perception, or difficulties in

adjusting focus easily between far and near targets (Gianutsos and Matheson, 1987). Prism glasses have been advocated for treating adults with diplopia. Children may have difficulty using such glasses properly. At our facility, patching of one eye has been used to provide temporary relief for children with diplopia.

Collaborative Intervention

At our facility, one method for assisting the child with TBI to attain functional goals is team treatment, which requires that the child's therapists know each other. During team treatment, two or more therapists work together on a mutually agreed-on set of possible goals. Such sessions usually occur once or twice weekly. The specific therapeutic tasks and procedures undertaken are determined by the patient's abilities, level of fatigue, and motivation. Appendix 6-1 presents a case history and a sample team-treatment session.

During a team-treatment session, the therapists must determine how many activities the patient can comfortably perform at one time. For example, can the patient maintain sitting balance, use an arm to point to a communication board, and manage saliva? In the course of the session, the therapists can collect specific information to assist in goal setting for future sessions. They can observe firsthand the treatment approaches most effective for the patient.

Team-treatment sessions provide a unique opportunity for therapists to observe and treat the patient in a holistic manner. Goals pursued during these sessions are compatible with real life, in which patients will need to do two (or more) things at once. The total child is more likely to be kept in mind during individual treatment sessions as a result of information gleaned from team-treatment sessions. For example, physical therapists can become more aware of the importance of the cognitive and communication components in any activity, even one that is considered to involve primarily movement. During team-treatment sessions, the boundaries between various disciplines are blurred. The therapists work together to serve the total child best, while gaining increased respect for each other's area of expertise. Team-treatment sessions can be morale boosters for patient and family and for therapists themselves, providing a multisensory reminder to all concerned that no one is alone in seeking the patient's functional improvement.

Impact of Cognitive and Emotional Dysfunction

When children with TBI are admitted for inpatient rehabilitation, their progress in motor recovery may be hindered by their cognitive and emotional dysfunctions.

Table 6-10. Cognitive Interventions Commonly Used in Physical Rehabilitation

Area of Cognition	Possible Interfering Behavior	Possible Intervention
Attention-concentration	Becomes distracted, appears disinterested, interrupts frequently	Provide high degree of structure; reduce environmental distractions
	Becomes agitated with excessive external stimulation	Treat in a quiet area; reduce length of sessions; redirect frequently
	Is unable to complete tasks	Give instructions in short, simple sentences; provide visual cues (e.g., photo routines)
	Walks or looks away when addressed	Provide hand-over-hand guidance
Perception	Cannot identify common objects	Explore multimodality approach
	Does not know what to do with common objects	Talk through activity with child
	Cannot locate objects within view	Have the child explore environment and objects with hands
	Does not understand verbal messages	Have the child visually scan the environment for cues; identify and use child's optimum modality for processing information
Memory	Does not follow directions	Provide visual cues (e.g., photo cues or written cues) to guide the child through tasks
	Becomes disoriented	Use meaningful, familiar, functional objects, activities, and routines to achieve motor goals
	Forgets how and when to do daily tasks	Provide an easy-to-follow daily schedule (e.g., photos); label areas (e.g., drawers) to facilitate independent activities of daily living; avoid nagging
Cognitive organization	Actions and ideas are out of sequence	Provide visual cues and talk through the organization of tasks with the child
	Fails to group similar items, begins tasks without assembling needed materials	Help the child to group necessary items before beginning an activity
	Is unable to identify main ideas or purposes of activities	Have the child identify the purpose of activities before beginning and dictate a short summary of activities on completion
Judgment	Behaves in an unsafe manner (acts without recognizing possible consequences)	Redirect the child before beginning an activity; with a safety net in place, allow the child to experience the effects of unsafe behavior; have the child view personal unsafe behavior on videotape

Such dysfunctions may prevent children from attaining motor skills of which they are physiologically capable. Cognitive and emotional dysfunctions often require therapists to modify the treatment approach. Table 6-10 lists possible therapist interventions in the face of interfering cognitive deficits.

Therapists whose primary domain is maximizing motor recovery may pursue cognitive, behavioral, and academic goals. A physical therapist working on ambulation training may encourage a child with TBI to count the number of steps that have been taken. A speech-language pathologist or occupational therapist may work on sequencing task steps for instruction on self-feeding.

In dealing with children whose emotional dysfunction interferes with progress in therapy, input from a behavioral psychologist may be helpful.

When admitted for inpatient rehabilitation, many patients may be somnolent. For each child, a search for particularly motivating stimuli must be made. Usually, such stimuli are familiar persons and objects. Therapy sessions must be scheduled for patients' awake times and may have to be relatively short. As cognitive recovery progresses to the agitated state, a quiet environment for therapy sessions may be needed. While children are in the agitated state, energy-expending activities may be helpful.

When children have attained cognitive recovery sufficient to follow commands, they are able to participate actively in their therapeutic regimens (Michaud et al., 1993). During inpatient rehabilitation (and even after discharge), areas of ongoing cognitive difficulty may include attention and concentration, perception, memory, thought or task organization, and judgment (Nelson, 1992). Deficits in short-term memory are most common. Judgment deficits include lack of insight and impulsivity. Children with lack of insight will attempt to perform tasks for which they lack the physical capabilities. Children with impulsivity will attempt to perform a task immediately on command, without first taking necessary precautions. To ensure their patients' safety and maximize their recovery, therapists must be aware of the cognitive and emotional deficits of the children they are treating.

Transition to Outpatient Status

Establishing Appropriate Discharge Goals

Before discharge, children with TBI should be as prepared as possible for the surroundings they will be entering. A child's ability to navigate safely in school and community settings requires assessment. The family may require training to monitor unsafe behaviors. Before discharge, responsible caregivers may need to construct concrete supervision schedules. Therapists may need to assess a child's general level of endurance; for example, would this patient be able to ambulate throughout the school day, perhaps traveling relatively long distances within set limits of time? Caregiver input regarding any problems encountered during therapeutic weekend leaves may indicate how well a child is likely to function in the home environment.

Commonly, patients are discharged from an inpatient rehabilitation facility when they are considered no longer dependent on intensive therapy services. A determinant of time of discharge may be the availability of outpatient and school therapy services. Community outpatient and school therapists may have little or no training or experience in treating children with TBI. Consequently, before discharge, instructions from the inpatient therapists to these outpatient therapists are essential. The caregivers' ability to care for the child after discharge requires assessment. Some families possess greater physical, financial, and emotional resources than do others. Different families may have different discharge goals and requirements for the child with TBI. Ongoing family training sessions and regularly scheduled family conferences are an important part of an inpatient rehabilitation stay.

Establishing Therapy and Equipment Needs

Children's patterns of motor recovery and rates of progress will be useful in determining therapy needs after discharge. Provision for assisting them to achieve developmental milestones as they age may be necessary. Efforts to prevent avoidable complications, such as contracture formation in spastic patients, can be undertaken by caregivers with proper training.

Families

One discharge requirement is an environment that is ready for children on their return. Assessment of the home situation is thus vital. It may be accomplished by a therapist visit to the home or by the provision of the floor plan and measurements of the home to the therapists. To maximize independence and ease of care at home, bathroom modifications such as bath chairs, toilet rails, and tub grab bars may be necessary. Families should be introduced either personally or by phone to a wheelchair and equipment vendor in their area. They should be given a schedule for any necessary cast- or splint-wearing program and information as to where to obtain new casts or splints.

School

When a child with TBI returns to school, some creative approaches are necessary to meet outpatient therapeutic goals. The school may face limitations of time, physical environment, and personnel. The school day may not contain sufficient time in which to schedule therapies and to provide needed rest breaks and supplemental instruction. Also, because the typical school day provides significant peer socialization opportunities, time for interaction with others may be sacrificed if every minute of the school day for the child with TBI is scheduled for instruction or therapy. Modifications in the physical environment of the school, such as bathroom railings, may be necessary. The child in the process of motor recovery may require that all classes be on one floor or may need extra time to change classes. Therapists with experience in treating children with TBI may not be available locally.

In the face of such limitations, it may be necessary to identify and contact school personnel who would be available to assist in meeting outpatient therapeutic goals. School nurses, teachers, specialized instructors, and teachers' aides can help. A trained aide could assist or supervise transfers and ambulation. An exercise program could be given to the physical education instructor. During music period, the goal of improving vocal volume and breath support could be pursued. Ameliorating fine-motor dysfunction could be one goal for the child during art class, computer instruction, or writing and penmanship lessons.

Communicating with Community Care Providers

Before and after discharge, communication with the child's community care providers is essential. The primary-care physician should be given ongoing information about the rehabilitation course and progress as well as a copy of the discharge summary. This physician should receive documentation of the necessity for outpatient therapies and specialized equipment.

Also before discharge, a conference with caregivers, therapists, and school personnel with recommendations for therapies and proper classroom placement is beneficial. The inpatient therapists can visit the school, or school staff can come to the rehabilitation facility. In the rehabilitation facility, school staff can observe the child's treatment sessions and obtain any needed information and training from the therapists and nurses. Videotapes of treatment sessions are important supplements to visits or telephone conversations. The inpatient therapist can send a copy of the therapy discharge summary to the corresponding outpatient therapist.

Treatment of Outpatients

In planning outpatient treatment regimes for children with TBI, time limitations and financial reimbursement constraints must be considered. Patients may struggle with fatigue as they attempt to balance the demands of school and outpatient therapies. Also, many insurance carriers currently limit the number of outpatient therapy hours to be reimbursed. Outpatient therapy frequencies can be reduced through the use of home and school programs. Additionally, alternatives to traditional therapies can be sought. However, as some children with TBI will have long-term motor sequelae, ongoing outpatient monitoring and treatment in some form may be necessary.

Long-Term Motor Problems

As children with TBI age, they change physically (e.g., grow larger and heavier), as does their environment. Families of children with severe physical involvement may require more equipment to provide care in the face of increasing height and weight. The transfer-dependent patient who, as a young child, could be picked up and carried easily may require a Hoyer lift as a teenager with greater body mass. Those who were marginal ambulators with relatively low centers of gravity as young children may become wheelchair dependent as teenagers with greater body weights and higher centers of gravity (Gans et al., 1990). With growth, equipment will require adjustment and replacement. With age, children's environments also change. The marginal ambulator who could "get around" in a relatively small elementary school may require a wheelchair in a larger junior or senior high school. The intellectual demands of school increase with age. The child who as a preschooler could spend many hours per week in therapeutic regimens simply may not have the time to do so in later years, when advancing through school.

Spasticity may diminish for some children with TBI. In others, as they attain large physical size, their spastic-

ity may seem to worsen as their relatively larger muscles produce relatively greater resistance to passive stretch. The continuing need for antispasticity drugs, such as dantrolene, requires ongoing assessment. Soft-tissue contractures that develop may be ameliorated by surgical lengthening, transfers, or release of the affected muscles (Pinzur, 1993). Spastic adolescents should be monitored for the development of scoliosis (Gans et al., 1990).

Possible Alternatives to Traditional Therapeutic Regimens

Some children with TBI experience motor recovery sufficient to render them functional (e.g., to be able to ambulate without assistive devices). Of these, many will continue to experience difficulties with higher-level motor skills, such as balance and coordination. Such children may benefit from alternatives to traditional therapeutic regimens, including developmental dance classes, martial arts classes, and modified circuit courses in health clubs. Horseback riding and swimming can be modified to be enjoyed by children with severe motor involvement. Alternative activities, such as voice lessons or drama instruction, may benefit those with residual motor speech dysfunction.

Continued Patient, Family, and School Education

As children with TBI grow older, one goal is their increasing independence. In our society, independence is often affected by the speed with which one performs tasks; in other words, with increasing maturity comes an increasing emphasis on efficiency. For children who have TBI and residual motor deficits, the use of environmental modifications and equipment may result in greater efficiency. For example, a child with slow, laborious handwriting may have more efficient written output using a typewriter or computer. The use of such devices should not be seen as a failure but rather as provision for greater self-sufficiency. Providing guidance regarding age-appropriate functional goals for children with TBI and motor involvement is an ongoing task for physicians and therapists.

References

Alexander MA (1986). Orthotics, Adapted Seating and Assistive Devices. In GE Molnar (ed), Pediatric Rehabilitation. Baltimore: Williams & Wilkins, 158.

Ball KR (1995). The use of neurolytic blocks for the management of spasticity. Phys Med Rehabil Clin North Am 6;885.

Boyer MG, Edwards P (1991). Outcome one to three years after severe traumatic brain injury in children and adolescents. Injury 22;315.

Brink JD, Imbus C, Woo-Sam J (1980). Physical recovery after severe traumatic brain injury in children and adolescents. J Pediatr 97;721.

Cardenas DD, Clawson DR (1990). Management of lower extremity strength and function in traumatically brain-injured patients. J Head Trauma Rehabil 5(4);43.

Chaplin D, Deitz J, Jaffe KM (1993). Motor performance after traumatic brain injury. Arch Phys Med Rehabil 74;161.

Cosgrove AP, Corry IS, Graham HK (1994). Botulinum toxin A prevents the development of contractures in the hereditary spastic mouse. Dev Med Child Neurol 36;386.

Cowley RS, Swanson B, Chapman P, et al. (1994). The role of rehabilitation in the intensive care unit. J Head Trauma Rehabil 9(1);32.

DiScarla C, Grant CC, Brooke MM, Gans BM (1992). Functional outcome in children with traumatic brain injury: agreement between clinical judgment and the functional independence measure. Am J Phys Med Rehabil 71(3);145.

DiScarla C, Osberg JS, Gans BM, et al. (1991). Children with traumatic head injury: morbidity and post acute treatment. Arch Phys Med Rehabil 72;662.

Ellison P (1978). Propranolol for severe post–head injury action tremor. Neurology 28;197.

Gans BM, Mann NR, Ylvisaker M (1990). Rehabilitation Management Approaches. In M Rosenthal, ER Griffith, MR Bond, JD Miller (eds), Rehabilitation of the Adult and Child with Traumatic Brain Injury. Philadelphia: Davis, 592.

Gianutsos R, Matheson P (1987). The Rehabilitation of Visual Perceptual Disorders Attributable to Brain Injury. In MJ Meier, AL Benton, L Diller (eds), Neuropsychological Rehabilitation. New York: Guilford, 202.

Herdman SJ (1990). Treatment of vestibular disorders in traumatically brain-injured patients. J Head Trauma Rehabil 5(4);63.

Hodge MM, Hall SD (1994). Effects of Syllable Characteristics and Training Rate in a Child with Dysarthria Secondary to Near Drowning. In JA Till, KM Yorkston, DR Beukelman (eds), Motor Speech Disorders: Advances in Assessment and Treatment. Baltimore: Paul H. Brookes, 229.

Hyvärinen L (1995). Considerations in the evaluation and treatment of the child with low vision. Am J Occup Ther 149;891.

Jaffe KM, Fay GC, Polissar NL, et al. (1993). Severity of pediatric brain injury and neurobehavioral recovery at one year. Arch Phys Med Rehabil 74;587.

Jaffe KM, Fay GC, Polissar NL, et al. (1992). Severity of pediatric brain injury and early neurobehavioral outcome: a cohort study. Arch Phys Med Rehabil 73;540.

Jaffe MB, Mastrilli JP, Molitar CB, Valko AS (1985). Intervention for Motor Disorders. In M Ylvisaker (ed), Head Injury Rehabilitation: Children and Adolescents. San Diego: College Hill Press, 167.

Johnson SLJ, Hall DMB (1992). Post traumatic tremor in head injured children. Arch Dis Child 67;227.

Katz RT, Campagnolo DI (1994). Pharmacologic management of spasticity. Phys Med Rehabil 8;473.

Katz RT (1992). Mechanisms, measurement and management of spastic hypertonia after head injury. Phys Med Rehabil Clin North Am 3;319.

Knights RM, Ivan LP, Ventureyra ECG, et al. (1991). The effect of head injury in children on neuropsychological and behavioral functioning. Brain Inj 5;339.

Lehmkuhl LD, Thoi LL, Baize C, et al. (1990). Multimodality treatment of joint contractures in patients with severe brain injury: cost, effectiveness, and integration of therapies in the application of serial/inhibitive casts. J Head Trauma Rehabil 5(4);23.

Levine SP, Horstmann HM, Kirsch NL (1992). Performance considerations for people with cognitive impairment in assessing assistive technologies. J Head Trauma Rehabil 7(3);46.

Lord J, Taggart PJ, Molnar GE (1991). Assessment instruments for evaluation of motor skills in children. Phys Med Rehabil 5;389.

Massagli TL, Jaffe KM (1994). Pediatric traumatic brain injury: prognosis and rehabilitation. Pediatr Ann 23(1);29.

Michaud LJ, Duhaime AC, Batshaw ML (1993). Traumatic brain injury in children. Pediatr Clin North Am 40;553.

Molnar GE, Perrin JCS (1992). Head Injury. In GE Molnar (ed), Pediatric Rehabilitation. Baltimore: Williams & Wilkins, 254.

Murphy F (1991). Motor development and the young visually impaired child. Crit Rev Phys Med Rehabil 3(1);13.

Nelson VS. (1992). Pediatric head injury. Phys Med Rehabil Clin North Am 3;461.

Pinzur MS (1993). Lower extremity complications following traumatic brain injury. Phys Med Rehabil 7;637.

Platts RGS, Fraser MH (1993). Assistive technology in the rehabilitation of patients with high spinal cord lesions. Paraplegia 31;280.

Rang M, Silver R, de la Gorza J (1986). Cerebral Palsy. In E Wood, RB Winter (eds), Pediatric Orthopedics. Philadelphia: Lippincott, 345.

Solis I, Krouskop T, Trainer N, Marburger R (1988). Supine interface pressure in children. Arch Phys Med Rehabil 69;524.

Stone L, Shin DY (1993). Management of hypertonicity using chemical denervation following traumatic brain injury. Phys Med Rehabil 7;527.

Tomas ES, Undzis MF, Shores EA, Sidler MR (1993). Nonsurgical management of upper extremity deformities after traumatic brain injury: the Ranchos Los Amigos comprehensive treatment program. Phys Med 7;649.

Warren M (1993). A hierarchical model for evaluation and treatment of visual perceptual dysfunction in adult acquired brain injury (part 1). Am J Occup Rehabil 47(1);42.

Ylvisaker M, Chorazy AJL, Cohen SB, et al. (1990). Rehabilitation Assessment Following Head Injury in Children. In M Rosenthal, ER Griffith, MR Bond, JD Miller (eds), Rehabilitation of the Adult and Child with Traumatic Brain Injury. Philadelphia: Davis, 558.

Appendix 6-1
Case Study with Team Treatment

Case History

CB, born April 13, 1980, was 13½ years old when he underwent the described treatment session on September 13, 1993. He was a right-handed Amish boy who sustained a traumatic brain injury on July 2, 1993, when he fell from a carriage while attempting to hitch a horse, and struck his head on a rock. Initially, he did not lose consciousness but reported to his mother that his head hurt. He vomited, then could not be aroused. At the referring acute-care hospital, he was posturing, and admission computed tomographic scan showed an acute left epidural hematoma. He underwent a left temporal frontal craniotomy and evacuation of the epidural hematoma. Evacuation of a residual hematoma was performed on July 5, 1993. On July 22, he underwent placement of a tracheostomy and a percutaneous endoscopic gastrostomy.

CB was admitted to our facility on August 2, 1993. On admission, he had decerebrate posturing and was assessed as functioning cognitively at level II on the Ranchos Los Amigos Scale. He underwent bilateral serial casting to increase passive ankle dorsiflexion. Within the first month of admission, he increasingly followed simple commands using his left arm; he appeared to have a right hemiplegia. By the end of the first month, he had accurate yes-no responses. He was decannulated on September 10, 1993. By September 13, he could say "Hi" and "Bye," could sit for 1 minute without assistance, and held his right arm in extension.

Sample Team-Treatment Session for Patient

The session takes place in a small gym area that offers diminished visual distractions.

The patient's physical therapist, occupational therapist, and speech therapist are present. Parents, family members, nursing staff, and school personnel may observe and interact during the session. (This is an efficient and effective way to facilitate family and staff training.)

The patient is out of the wheelchair and seated on a mat, with the occupational therapist behind him for stabilization and facilitation. The physical therapist and speech therapist are in front of him. Only one person at a time speaks to CB.

Session goals are as follows:

1. Improve transfers
2. Improve trunk control, sitting balance, and head and neck control
3. Improve functional use of upper extremities
4. Increase functional eye-hand coordination
5. Improve breath control and support for speech
6. Investigate best immediate augmentative communication options (e.g., potential switch activation, use of spelling board)
7. Increase oral-motor control (e.g., lip closure, consistent control of saliva)
8. Improve orientation
9. Demonstrate memory within a 30-minute session

During the session, a number of activities are accomplished:

1. Therapists ask patient to identify them by extended gaze, pointing, or head nodding.
2. Patient assists in transfer by helping to remove lap tray, splint, Velcro attachments, and the like; holding arm(s) up; preparing for transfer (i.e., leaning forward, scooting, lifting legs, etc.); and transferring (i.e., performing sit-to-stand, pivoting, scooting back, etc.).
3. Patient prepares for a sitting activity by positioning feet appropriately, aligning head and trunk, placing

hands in weight-bearing position, and swallowing saliva.

4. Patient participates in sitting activities that may include visually tracking a person moving throughout the room, pointing to a communication board in response to verbal questions, and reaching for a pencil in a variety of planes to complete a simple writing task.

5. Patient assists in a transfer back into wheelchair.

6. Patient participates in a review and wrap-up of the session by identifying session activities and verifying log-book notes (previously written by a therapist).

Chapter 7

Therapy for Feeding and Swallowing Disorders After Traumatic Brain Injury

Jeri A. Logemann and Mark Ylvisaker

The limited data available on the incidence of swallowing problems in adults and children with traumatic brain injury (TBI) indicate that incidence varies by type of health care institution (Cherney and Halper, 1989; Ylvisaker and Weinstein, 1989; Yorkston et al., 1989). The greatest incidence occurs when patients are in the acute-care setting, and incidence diminishes from acute rehabilitation through outpatient rehabilitation. Although there are no reported data on the incidence of feeding and swallowing problems after severe TBI in children, it is safe to say that transient impairments at an early stage of recovery are pervasive and that significant residual problems that require long-term therapeutic management are not uncommon. Swallowing disorders are singled out for special treatment in this book because these disorders can have serious medical implications and must be managed accordingly.

There is currently no general agreement regarding use of the terms *feeding* and *swallowing*. Following Logemann's usage (1983), in this chapter the term *feeding* includes (1) placement of food in the mouth; (2) manipulation of food in the mouth (e.g., chewing, tasting, and bolus formation); and (3) posterior movement of the bolus by the tongue. The term *swallowing* generally encompasses, in addition to these three feeding processes, triggering of the pharyngeal swallow and movement of the bolus through the pharynx and esophagus into the stomach. Occasionally, the word *swallowing* is used in a narrower sense to refer to the aspects of deglutition that commence with the triggering of the pharyngeal swallow.

Although treatment techniques for oral motor feeding disorders are listed in Appendix 7-1, this chapter focuses primarily on diagnosis and treatment of disorders of swallowing that occur after the oral phase of deglutition. These disorders generally require instrumental assessment techniques and are more serious medically than are oral-motor feeding problems. Oral-motor dysfunction alone, regard-

less of the severity, need not interfere with oral intake of food, as special placement techniques (e.g., syringe) or diet change (liquid only) can bypass the oral phase of swallowing entirely. The pharyngeal phase of the swallow cannot be bypassed and is critical to safe and efficient oral intake.

The ultimate goal of treatment for dysphagic patients is complete recovery of normal eating patterns while the patient's health and nutritional status are being maintained. Unfortunately, some children with severe TBI cannot achieve this goal because of apparently permanent impairments of deglutition. For these latter patients, more restricted goals might be identified, such as (1) oral feeding using compensatory techniques, or some degree of primitive or abnormal oral patterns or a restricted range of food consistencies; (2) combined oral and nonoral feedings, with nonoral feedings used primarily to maintain hydration; and (3) minimal "recreational" oral feeding (for long-term, severely involved patients). The dysphagia (swallowing disorders) program for a child with TBI in the early stages of cognitive recovery is part of the sensory stimulation program, which is designed to increase the child's alertness and adaptive responses. Improvement in oral feeding also heightens a child's motivation and sense of normalcy while providing a naturally pleasurable experience.

The objectives of this chapter are to describe neurogenic swallowing disorders, emphasizing those that are particularly common after TBI; to introduce anatomic and physiologic concepts relevant to an explanation of these disorders and their treatment; to describe evaluation, including radiographic procedures, and the purposes and limitations of these procedures; to emphasize special considerations for cognitively impaired patients who have feeding or swallowing disorders; and to present treatment options. Therapists responsible for the assessment and treatment of swallowing disorders should consult Logemann (1983, 1993) and other references for a more thorough discussion of the issues addressed in this chapter.

Disorders of Swallowing After TBI

Disorders of feeding and swallowing can result from anterior cortical (motor strip) lesions or from damage to the brain stem. With very severe brain injury, there is a strong possibility of combined focal, multifocal, and diffuse cortical, subcortical, and brain stem damage, making localization of the lesion responsible for a feeding or swallowing problem difficult. However, lower brain stem—especially medullary—damage usually results in significant problems with triggering of the pharyngeal swallow and its motor control.

Specific swallowing disorders are described according to the four stages of swallowing: (1) oral preparatory, (2) oral, (3) pharyngeal, and (4) esophageal. These stages and the corresponding disorders are discussed in greater detail by Logemann (1993).

Oral Preparatory Phase

General Description

The oral preparatory phase of swallowing includes placement of food in the mouth and oral manipulation for bolus preparation as well as for the pleasure of eating. This phase involves coordinated movement of the jaw, lips, tongue, cheeks, and palate. Graded and refined jaw movements are required to open the mouth to allow food to enter and to reduce food to a consistency ready for bolus formation by the tongue. Lateral tongue movements move the food particles to and from the molars for chewing and mix it with saliva. Refined lip movements are needed to form a seal on the cup, straw, spoon, or fork and to keep food in the mouth during the oral preparatory and oral stages. Cheek (buccal) tension keeps food out of the lateral sulci (space between teeth and the cheeks) during chewing and assists in posterior propulsion of the food for swallowing. Active downward, forward pressure of the soft palate against the back of the tongue creates a posterior seal and prevents food from trickling into the pharynx prematurely while food is held in the mouth. Posterior elevation of the tongue against the soft palate helps to create the posterior seal. With active chewing, this seal is not maintained, and there is frequently premature spillage of food into the pharynx. This is a normal phenomenon.

When oral preparation is complete, a variety of refined tongue movements collect the food particles from any location in the oral cavity to form a cohesive bolus prior to the beginning of the oral stage of the swallow. The tongue creates a bolus of appropriate size in relation to the viscosity of the food. Maximum volume of the bolus is reduced as the viscosity increases. The duration of the oral preparatory stage varies with food consistency as well as with individual style. The processes are voluntary in neurologically normal individuals beyond infancy. Normal breathing continues during this phase, and the airway is open.

Disorders

In the oral preparatory phase, a number of disorders commonly occur that are the result of central nervous system dysfunction after TBI:

1. *Primitive or pathologic reflexes:* Developmentally primitive or pathologic reflexes, including the rooting reflex, tonic or clonic bite, and food ejection, are often present after TBI and interfere with normal oral preparatory patterns.

2. *Abnormal muscle tone:* Muscle hypotonicity or hypertonicity of the lips, cheeks, jaw, and tongue interferes with the normal function of these structures during the oral preparatory phase.

3. *Abnormal sensation:* Hypersensitivity to touch can elicit pathologic reflexes or tonal changes, such as lip pursing or retraction or total head hyperextension or deviation. In contrast, as a result of hyposensitivity, food particles may be lost in the mouth, fall out of the mouth, or prematurely fall into the pharynx. The direction in which the food falls depends on head position and the consistency and amount of food.

4. *Movement disorders:* A combination of abnormal reflex, sensation, and muscle tone creates characteristic movement disorders after TBI: difficulty opening the mouth to receive food, difficulty closing the lips around a cup or utensil, loss of food from the mouth or into the pharynx before the swallow, and a suckle-swallow pattern that excludes tongue lateralization and bolus formation and often requires several suckle movements before a swallow can be initiated.

Disorders of sensation, muscle tone, and movement patterns can easily cause food to enter the pharynx before the pharyngeal swallow is initiated, with the possibility of aspiration before the swallow, despite an otherwise adequate swallow mechanism.

Oral Phase

General Description

The oral phase of swallowing begins when the bolus is picked up by the tongue, and the tip and lateral margins of the tongue maintain a seal with the anterior and lateral alveolar ridge. The bolus rests on the anterior tongue, and the midline of the tongue progressively elevates to squeeze or strip the bolus along the palate (Blonsky et al., 1975; Kahrilas et al., 1993; Miller, 1982;

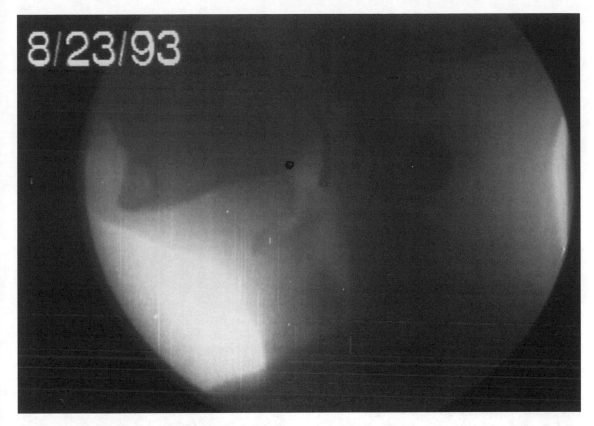

Figure 7-1. Lateral radiographic view of the head and neck, showing the location of the pharyngeal swallow trigger point. When the leading edge of the head of the bolus reaches the trigger point, the pharyngeal swallow should be initiated.

Shedd et al., 1961). The oral phase ends when the leading edge of the bolus passes the point at which the lower edge of the mandible crosses the tongue base (Figure 7-1) and the pharyngeal swallow is triggered. The oral phase is under voluntary neural control and normally takes approximately 1.0–1.5 seconds to complete (Blonsky et al., 1975; Mandelstam and Lieber, 1970).

Disorders

The tone, sensation, and movement disorders of the tongue already described can interfere dramatically with the oral phase of swallow. Suckle-swallow or munch patterns (Morris, 1982), which are not uncommon after TBI, result in bolus dispersion as well as inefficient and slow anterior to posterior movement of the midline of the tongue. Food can trickle over the back of the tongue before the swallow and either collect in the vallecular space or fall into the airway or pyriform sinuses, as shown in Figure 7-2. Premature spillage of material into the pharynx during active chewing is a normal phenomenon, except when liquid or pudding is being held before the swallow begins or during oral transit. Inadequate labial and buccal tension will also decrease the efficiency of this phase.

Pharyngeal Phase

General Description

The pharyngeal swallow is triggered as the leading edge of the bolus passes the base of the tongue. There is an age effect on pharyngeal triggering. In children and young adults (aged 20–30 years), the pharyngeal swallow is triggered when the bolus reaches the anterior faucial arch, whereas in older individuals (at least 60 years of age), the pharyngeal swallow is triggered as the leading edge of the bolus passes the tongue base.

The pharyngeal phase of the swallow starts when the hyoid and larynx begin to elevate and ends when the bolus passes through the cricopharyngeal sphincter (or pharyngoesophageal segment) and into the esophagus. Unless controlled voluntarily, the four physiologic processes that define the pharyngeal phase are triggered or programmed by the brain stem swallow center:

1. The nasopharynx is closed by active movements of the velum and pharyngeal walls to prevent food from entering the nose.

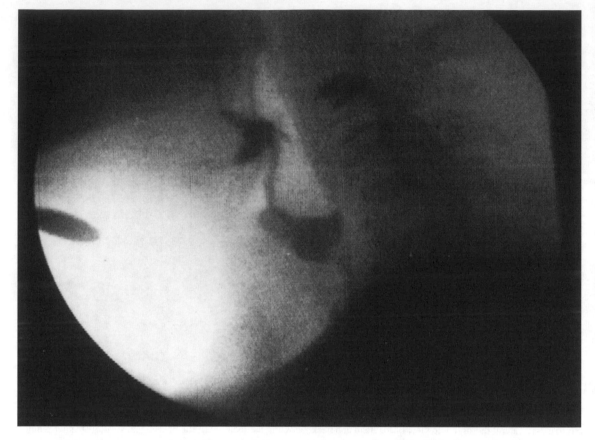

Figure 7-2. Lateral radiographic view of the oral cavity and pharynx, showing premature spillage of the bolus into the pharynx.

2. Food is propelled through the pharynx by oral tongue action followed by tongue base posterior movement and pharyngeal wall contraction (Kahrilas et al., 1992).
3. The airway is protected by the elevation of the larynx and by three valving actions: (a) closure of the true vocal folds, (b) tilting of the anterior arytenoid to contact the epiglottic base, and (c) contraction of the false vocal folds and downward folding of the epiglottis (Logemann et al., 1992).
4. The cricopharyngeal valve, normally closed to keep esophageal contents out of the pharynx, opens by anterior tugging of the hyoid and larynx and by bolus pressure, facilitated by relaxation of the cricopharyngeal muscle (Curtis et al., 1984; Jacob et al., 1989; Kahrilas et al., 1991).

During the pharyngeal phase, the bolus divides evenly as it passes around the epiglottis and through the two pyriform sinuses. In approximately 20% of normal swallowers, the bolus is directed down only one side of the pharynx. The coordination and duration of normal pharyngeal-stage events vary with the viscosity and volume of the food or liquid swallowed (Jacob et al., 1989; Kahrilas et al., 1991, 1992, 1993; Logemann et al., 1992).

The pharyngeal swallow is in part voluntary and in part automatic (Miller, 1982). The tongue propulsion in the oral phase represents the cortical or voluntary input to the triggering of the pharyngeal phase. The four above-mentioned neuromuscular functions characteristic of the pharyngeal phase occur under brain stem control, but most can be modified by voluntary control (Kahrilas et al., 1991; Martin et al., 1993). The pharyngeal phase of the swallow normally takes no more than 1 second, and respiration is temporarily halted for that portion of the pharyngeal stage when the airway is closed (Blonsky et al., 1975; Mandelstam and Lieber, 1970).

Disorders

If triggering of the pharyngeal swallow is delayed, the bolus may lodge in the valleculae or the pyriform sinuses or may enter the airway, which is open until the pharyngeal swallow is triggered. Most often, children with a pharyngeal delay have difficulty with liquids because liquids are more likely to splash into the airway during the delay than are other substances of thicker viscosities. Our experience and that of other clinicians suggests that, aside from oral disorders, the most common swallow disorder after TBI is a delayed or absent pharyngeal swallow (Lazarus, 1989; Lazarus and Logemann, 1987; Logemann, 1983). If the pharyngeal swallow is not delayed more than 3 or 4 seconds, and if very small quantities of food are given and the patient is well positioned (i.e., chin down), a delayed pharyngeal swallow simply means that food will collect in the vallecular space before the swallow. If larger quantities are given or if the patient's head is hyperextended, the food will enter the pharynx and is more likely to enter the airway, which, until the pharyngeal swallow is triggered, is less protected while the head is in the hyperextended position.

Inadequate velopharyngeal closure, if severe or if accompanied by uncoordinated pharyngeal contractions, will result in nasal regurgitation. However, failure of the airway protection mechanisms during the swallow is not, in our experience, a common swallowing disorder after TBI. Failure of airway protection can result in aspiration (i.e., entry of food or liquid into the airway) during the swallow. Children who can follow directions and are alert can facilitate airway protection by holding their breath immediately before and during the swallow and by coughing and spitting immediately after the swallow, and then swallowing again (a supraglottic swallow, described later).

Failure of the larynx to elevate can cause residue to remain on top of the larynx after the swallow and aspiration after the swallow, when the child opens the larynx to inhale. Unilateral or bilateral weak pharyngeal wall contraction results in an inefficient swallow, leaving residue in the pharynx and on one (unilateral) or both pharyngeal walls and possibly causing aspiration after the swallow. This problem is not uncommon after TBI.

Damaged cricopharyngeal opening usually results from reduced forward movement of the larynx and hyoid and limits the amount of bolus entering the esophagus, with the likelihood of significant aspiration after the swallow. Because the pharyngeal recesses are large enough to hold several cubic centimeters of food, this disorder is often misdiagnosed as fatigue. Affected children may not cough or sputter until after they have attempted to swallow four to five spoonfuls. Cricopharyngeal disorders are sometimes observed after head trauma, particularly if there is physical damage to the neck (Logemann, 1983), but they are not common. If food of the easiest-to-swallow consistency is served and combined oral and pharyngeal transit time of such food is greater than 10 seconds per swallow, supplementary tube feedings will probably be necessary to maintain nutrition, even if airway protection is not a problem (Logemann, 1983).

Esophageal Phase

The esophageal phase of swallow begins with the entrance of the bolus into the esophagus at the cricopharyngeal or upper esophageal sphincter and ends with passage of food through the gastroesophageal (lower esophageal) sphincter into the stomach. The esophageal phase is completely involuntary and normally takes 8–20 seconds (Mandelstam and Lieber, 1970). This phase is not discussed, as esophageal disorders are not assessed or treated by feeding-swallowing therapists, although such disorders occasionally masquerade as oropharyngeal swallowing disorders if they result in reflux (i.e., material from the stomach coming back up into the esophagus or pharynx) and potential aspiration.

Assessment of Swallowing

Assessment and treatment of swallowing disorders should be a team process. The attending physician—with a nutritionist and, if indicated, ear, nose, and throat; pulmonary; and gastroenterologic medical specialists—evaluates the child's medical history and current nutritional, physiologic, and general health status relevant to feeding decisions. The swallowing therapist (usually a speech-language pathologist, but occasionally an occupational or physical therapist or a nurse specifically trained in dysphagia management) should complete a bedside examination of oral structures and function and, indirectly, of laryngeal function and swallowing effectiveness (Linden et al., 1993). If pharyngeal-phase swallowing disorders or aspiration are suspected, a videofluorographic (VFG) swallowing study should be performed by a radiologist working with the swallowing therapist. The purposes of the VFG assessment are (1) to define the patient's swallowing physiology, thereby determining the reason for aspiration; (2) to introduce treatment strategies to assess the effectiveness of each; and (3) to design an effective treatment plan.

During the VFG study, treatment procedures, including postural changes, increasing sensory input, therapeutic strategies, and food consistency modifications, should be introduced to assess the immediate effects (Logemann, 1993). In some cases, the introduction and assessment of therapeutic procedures will enable the patient to begin at least limited oral intake immediately.

With all relevant information assembled, the dysphagia team makes a decision regarding the initial treatment regimen. The most common possibilities are as follows:

1. Nasogastric tube or gastrostomy feeding only, with a program of oral motor and swallowing therapy but no food provided orally.

2. Nasogastric or gastrostomy feeding for nutrition and hydration, and swallowing therapy that includes trial oral feedings of small quantities of food and close monitoring of response.
3. Combined oral and tube feeding, systematically decreasing the latter as oral intake increases with swallowing therapy.
4. Exclusively oral feeding, with a systematic normalization of methods of intake (e.g., from syringe to tongue blade to spoon to self-feeding) and of food consistencies.

If the fourth option is selected, pudding or applesauce may be easiest for patients with TBI; thick nectars and blenderized solid foods may also be appropriate. Dry or multi-textured solid foods are often difficult for dysphagic patients to swallow. Thin liquids may prove the most difficult to consume for patients with TBI because of bolus formation problems, a delayed pharyngeal swallow (if present), and the rapid movement of thin liquids through a slowly responding system. It is important to note, however, that the choice of food consistency for a particular patient will depend on knowledge of that patient's anatomic or physiologic swallowing disorder(s).

In making initial decisions regarding a treatment regimen, the team must remember that feeding and swallowing disorders can be treated as effectively, if not more effectively, with no food or very small quantities of food as with large quantities. There is no treatment advantage to a potentially dangerous and premature resumption of oral feedings. Nonetheless, the team should proceed aggressively with exercises directed at improving those neuromotor functions necessary for the patient's normal swallowing and with early trial oral feedings, as normalization of eating patterns might be foremost in the minds of patients and their families. This normalization may be related to behavior management and cognitive reorientation. Continuous family and patient counseling is critical throughout this initial decision-making process. Whenever possible, involvement of family in the treatment regimen is also critical.

Bedside Assessment

The swallowing therapist's bedside examination should include careful observation of the patient's overall postures, muscle tone, and reflex patterns, as well as the anatomy, reflexive and nonreflexive functioning, and sensation in the oral cavity (Logemann, 1983; Morris, 1978). Assessment of pharyngeal intactness and airway protection can be done only indirectly at the bedside, as inferences from gross observation of swallowing symptoms are known to be unreliable (Logemann, 1982; Linden and Siebens, 1983; Splaingard et al., 1988).

Oral and Laryngeal Reflexes

Three reflexes are triggered in the posterior oral cavity and larynx: palatal, gag, and protective cough. Each of these reflexes should be triggered, if possible, and the responses assessed for intactness of muscle contraction. A normal or functional swallow cannot be determined or predicted from any of these reflexes. However, muscle contractions involved in each response can be assessed. These reflexes are neurologically independent in that the presence or absence of one does not necessarily indicate the presence or absence of any of the others. Hence, it is unacceptable—although not uncommon—to draw strong conclusions regarding the status of the swallowing mechanism from the presence or absence of a gag reflex (Logemann, 1983; Leder, 1996; Aviv et al., 1996).

To stimulate the palatal reflex, the soft palate in the midline is touched just posterior to the hard palate juncture, preferably with something cold (e.g., a size 00 laryngeal mirror). The expected response is upward and backward movement of the velum, without pharyngeal wall movement. Several stimulations may be necessary to elicit this response.

To stimulate the gag reflex, the back or base of the tongue or posterior pharyngeal wall is touched. The expected response is strong contraction of the pharyngeal walls and soft palate and elevation of the larynx and pharynx with forward propulsion to clear the pharynx by bringing reflux, vomit, or other foreign material into the mouth.

Material in the airway should stimulate the protective cough reflex. The expected response to the presence of such material is cough (i.e., diaphragm contracts, larynx elevates, pharynx constricts). Note that the voluntary cough and the cough reflex are neurologically independent of one another. Many children who have suffered TBI have no reflexive cough in response to food entering the airway.

Swallowing Efficiency and Aspiration

Currently, all methods for bedside assessment of aspiration and the identification of the pharyngeal aspects of swallowing have a high error rate (approximately 40%). Four tests are described for use at the bedside. However, the clinician must be cautious in interpreting these tests for the pharyngeal phase of swallowing.

The swallowing therapist conducts the *four-finger test* at the patient's bedside. The production of secretions can be increased with oral stimulation (e.g., anything placed in the mouth, such as dampened gauze), and spontaneous swallowing can be observed. Alert children can also be instructed to swallow. When observing or assessing swallow, the therapist places an index finger lightly under the patient's chin anteriorly, a second finger on the hyoid bone, and third and fourth fingers above and below the thyroid cartilage. By such placement, the following information can be collected: (1) initiation of tongue movements, (2) number of tongue movements prior to a swallow, (3) initiation of hyoid and laryngeal movement with the pharyngeal swallow, and (4) timing and strength of laryngeal elevation. Such information provides a rough indication of the presence or absence of the pharyngeal swallow and oral transit time. It is *not* an indication of pharyngeal efficiency. A cough following the swallow indicates a cough reflex, but also is strongly suggestive of aspiration. Absence of a cough does not mean the patient is a safe swallower. Approximately half of all children with TBI who aspirate do not cough in response.

A second test of swallowing efficiency and aspiration is the blue-dye test (Manley, 1983). For patients with tracheostomy tubes, four drops of methylene blue dye can be placed on the tongue so that the colored saliva will not escape as drool. After several minutes, the patient should be suctioned. Alternatively, a larger amount of thin liquid can be dyed blue and given to the child to swallow, after which tracheal suction is undertaken.

The presence of a significant amount of dye in the suctioned material is positive evidence of aspiration but does not indicate the reason for the aspiration. Therefore, treatment cannot be planned from this test. In this case, a VFG study should be ordered. The absence of dye does not guarantee the absence of aspiration. The test should be repeated several times if the results are negative. If a tracheostomy tube is present, this test can be very useful during the initial stages of oral feeding, both for diagnostic purposes and for suctioning if the patient aspirates.

The phonation test is conducted by asking alert children to vocalize after a swallow. A wet, hoarse quality to the voice suggests aspiration (Linden and Siebens, 1983). If patients are unable to follow instructions, the therapist should listen for spontaneous breathing, vocalizing, and coughing. If breathing is noisy or if the voice or cough after trial oral feeding is hoarse or wet sounding, then aspiration should be suspected and a VFG study should be ordered for the patient.

Pneumonia, especially recurrent pneumonia, or suspicious lung sounds are further indication of possible aspiration of food or refluxed material. A positive pneumonia history in a child with TBI also warrants a VFG study. If reflux and aspiration of stomach contents are suspected, reflux assessments using scintigraphy should be completed.

Radiographic Assessment

Those children whose bedside examination or pathophysiologic and medical history indicate the possibility of aspiration or pharyngeal-phase dysfunction should undergo a VFG swallowing study known as the *modified barium swallow* or the *cookie swallow test*. The purpose of the study is to provide diagnostic information relevant to the following questions:

- Should oral feedings be reintroduced?
- How efficiently do the oral, pharyngeal, laryngeal, and upper esophageal structures function during swallowing, and what is the cause of the patient's aspiration or inefficient swallow?
- How adequate is the patient's airway protection under varying conditions?
- How is swallowing affected by changes in the patient's posture, increase of sensory input, introduction of swallowing maneuvers, modification of food consistency and amount, method of food presentation, physical prompts, and instructions?

A VFG swallowing study provides information that is otherwise unavailable but essential to effective dysphagia therapy. From a medical standpoint, the key goal is to determine the reason for and the amount of aspiration relative to the patient's posture, the food consistency provided, other therapeutic strategies, and the method of food intake. For swallowing therapists, it is equally important to identify the nature of any pharyngeal dysfunction in patients who may or may not aspirate and to document radiographically the effects of management strategies. Ideally, the swallowing therapist will have a good working relationship with the radiologist so that experimentation with the patient's positioning, food consistency, and method of food intake can occur during the radiographic study.

Because the questions to be answered by the VFG study of oral and pharyngeal aspects of swallowing differ dramatically from those at issue in standard barium swallow studies (i.e., esophageal anatomy and motility), the procedures also differ dramatically. Most important, the child should be seated in his or her normal eating position and very small quantities of food given initially. Positioning for neurologically impaired children often requires advance preparation, time, and ingenuity. Use of a tumble-form chair placed on a cart (Figure 7-3) may be the best way to position infants and young children during radiographic study. The child is given one-third to one-half teaspoon of barium liquid, followed by two swallows each of larger measured volumes of liquid as tolerated (3, 5, and 10 ml), plus cup drinking, and then two swallows of pudding or applesauce, followed by a small piece (one-fourth) of a barium pudding–coated cookie, if the child can chew.

The study begins with a lateral view to measure oral and pharyngeal transit times; to observe location of residual food in the oral cavity and pharynx, triggering and motor control of the pharyngeal swallow, and gen-

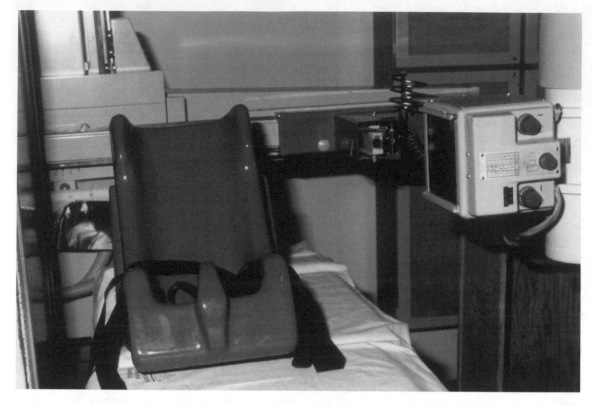

Figure 7-3. A tumble-form chair on a cart positioned in the videofluorographic equipment can be used to position infants and young children during the radiographic study of oropharyngeal swallow.

eral pharyngeal efficiency; and to determine amount of and reason for aspiration. One or two swallows are repeated in a posteroanterior view to detect possible unilateral pharyngeal disorders and to examine vocal fold functioning. To assess vocal fold movement, the patient's neck is hyperextended and the patient is asked to say, "Ah, ah, ah."

Radiographic swallowing studies are particularly important for cognitively impaired children suspected of having pharyngeal-stage swallowing disorders, as these children are rarely able to recognize or describe their swallowing problems (Arvedson and Brodsky, 1993). Children often benefit from having time to watch the x-ray study, see the room, and hear the sounds occurring during the study; given such an introduction, children are more likely to complete the test successfully. Taste experimentation prior to the study may be necessary to identify the taste that results in improved oral responsiveness and to avoid contamination of the results because of taste aversions. Logemann (1989, 1993) gives additional details on the procedures and purposes of this VFG swallowing study.

Treatment

Appendix 7-1 includes a large number of intervention procedures for feeding and swallowing disorders, organized according to the anatomic or physiologic dysfunction(s) they address. These procedures, which should be selected after a thorough team assessment and careful identification of the disorder, have been compiled from a variety of sources, including Morris (1978, 1982) and Logemann (1983, 1993). The treatment suggestions fall under five major categories:

1. *Neuromuscular treatment:* Neuromuscular treatment involves inhibitory and desensitizing stimulation for hypersensitivity, hypertonicity, and hyperreflexia and excitatory stimulation and strengthening exercises for hyposensitivity, hypotonicity, and hyporeflexia.

2. *Posture:* The best position of the total body and the head in relation to the body normalizes tone and reflexes, creates the most efficient movement of food, and maximizes patient safety (i.e., eliminates aspiration) (Logemann et al., 1994; Rasley et al., 1993; Shanahan et al., 1993).

Table 7-1. Guidelines for the Swallowing Therapist in Preparing for Treatment Sessions

Abnormal muscle tone	Consult occupational or physical therapist regarding procedures to normalize total body tone before proceeding with feeding or oral treatment.
Positioning	
Normal eating position	Seat patient upright: hips flexed 90 degrees, knees flexed 90 degrees, feet supported, shoulders relaxed, arms forward, head in midline and slightly flexed.
Dysphagic eating position	Severely involved children might need to be treated in a semiupright position in bed, head and knees propped with pillows. A chin-tuck position (head flexed forward) often is important for patients with traumatic brain injury, as it narrows the airway entrance, pushes the epiglottis backward, and widens the vallecular space, adding a dimension of safety for children with a delayed pharyngeal swallow. Tilting or turning the patient's head, or even side-lying, may be indicated for specific pharyngeal disorders (see Appendix 7-1).
Communication	Prepare all children with simple descriptions of what is to be done. Give specific instructions (e.g., "Lift your tongue now") only if the patterns cannot be re-established on an automatic basis. Similarly, feedback should remain general (e.g., "Nice job") rather than specific (e.g., "You swallowed too quickly that time"), unless a decision has been made to bring the process under voluntary control and the child can understand somewhat complex directions. Make the session pleasant and encouraging; discontinue temporarily in the face of agitation.

3. *Food:* The best consistency, taste, and temperature are used to control movement of the food, to effect efficiency of swallowing and airway protection, and to avoid taste aversions (Bisch et al., 1994; Logemann et al., 1995).

4. *Swallowing therapy techniques:* Alert children can learn compensatory food placement or compensatory swallowing therapy techniques to enhance food movement and airway protection.

5. *Medical and nutritional issues:* Issues to be considered include adequate nutrition and hydration, adequate airway protection and pulmonary function, prosthetic devices, and surgical intervention (Middaugh, 1989).

Treatment Sessions

It generally is preferable to have several short (10- to 15-minute) oral-stimulation swallowing therapy sessions per day rather than one or two extended sessions. We give written instructions to alert children who can read and exercise independently and ask them to exercise at least five times per day for 5–10 minutes each time. Exercises should be done in front of a mirror and followed by a functional task (e.g., facial expression, speech, eating).

With cognitively and motorically involved children, family members, nursing staff, and stimulation team members are sometimes included in the dysphagia program. However, because dysphagia treatment requires considerable skill and can be aversive and even frightening, treatment staff should be well trained and should establish a good relationship with each child. After intervention sessions, children must remain in an upright position and be observed for several minutes so that delayed responses can be monitored.

Family members often have strong feelings associated with oral feeding. Mothers of young children might feel an intense, but unspoken, need to feed the child as an act of nurturing. Consequently, careful and sympathetic counseling is necessary to gain parents' acceptance of what they may perceive to be a too-slow reintroduction of oral feeding (Hutchins, 1989). The therapist must explain the intervention process thoroughly at each stage of recovery. If a radiographic study has been completed, family members often benefit from seeing the videotape of the study and being told why the patient should not be fed by mouth.

Table 7-1 outlines principles of positioning and communication useful in preparing children for feeding or swallowing treatment sessions.

Treatment of Children with Severe Cognitive Deficits

Some decrease in cognitive functioning frequently accompanies disorders of feeding and swallowing after TBI (Yorkston et al., 1989). Cognitive impairment compounds the already difficult task of helping children to improve their feeding and swallowing patterns. Profound confusion and agitation, for example, may temporarily eliminate the possibility of swallowing intervention. Furthermore, intervention techniques that include verbal instructions may not be options for children in the early stages of cognitive recovery. Even relatively well-recovered patients may have difficulty acquiring compensatory swallowing techniques because of a depressed ability to learn new routines.

The following cognitive challenges are frequently encountered by the rehabilitating child with TBI:

- Impulsiveness and impaired judgment may require close monitoring; keeping food out of reach; cueing the child to chew, swallow completely, and eat slowly; and eliminating from the diet foods that could be dangerous if swallowed whole. Because feeding treatment can be unpleasant and even frightening for a child, the therapist must be skilled in preparing, reassuring, calming, and redirecting the child with TBI.
- Reduced initiation may require frequent cues to take food, chew, and swallow.
- Impaired monitoring may require examination of the child's oral cavity after every meal to ensure that the child has not stored potentially dangerous quantities of food in the lateral sulci.
- Weak attention and concentration, including agitation, may require that the child eat in nondistracting, low-stimulation environments and receive ongoing cues to focus on the task at hand. Treatment personnel should be familiar to the child and should schedule treatment sessions during times when the child is known to be most alert.
- Impaired new learning may require repeated instruction and ongoing cueing.

Patterns of Recovery of Oral Intake After TBI

The most common pattern of recovery of swallowing after TBI is slow, steady improvement over weeks or months until safe and efficient oral intake is achieved. Some children with severe TBI do not recover normal swallowing without chronic intervention such as thermal-tactile stimulation at every meal. This type of chronic maintenance therapy is usually designed by the swallowing therapist and is implemented by a caregiver. In a few severe cases, swallowing may not recover immediately and long-term nonoral feeding will be necessary. These children should be assessed at least yearly to determine whether later spontaneous recovery has occurred. Some children with TBI recover safe and efficient swallowing and oral intake years after their injury.

Behavioral Eating Disorders

Behavioral eating disorders, defined as developmentally inappropriate eating patterns attributable in part to motivational problems or skill deficits (versus physiologic dysfunction), are extremely common in children

(Babbitt et al., 1994a). It has been estimated that up to 25% of children experience behavioral eating difficulties at some point during infancy or childhood (Sisson and Van Hasselt, 1989). This estimate increases in the population of children with developmental disabilities (Palmer and Horn, 1978). In their sample, Budd and colleagues (1992) found that 26% of childhood feeding disorders were purely organic, 10% purely functional, and the remaining 64% a combination of organic and functional.

Although firm estimates of behavioral eating problems among children with acquired brain injury are not available, our experience suggests a frequency sufficiently high to merit careful professional attention. The typical natural history of behavior problems associated with eating in children with developmental disability suggests that children with severe TBI might be similarly vulnerable. What begins as an organically based difficulty with eating or swallowing might be maintained as a persistent food refusal or selectivity as a result of ill-conceived reinforcement contingencies (Budd et al., 1992). That is, caregivers who are understandably anxious about nutrition and nurturing may translate this anxiety into extreme attention to the child's eating-related behavior, reinforcement of the child's food refusals (e.g., by allowing the child to escape eating or to gain access to desired foods), or power battles that take place at mealtimes. It is easy to understand how parents of a child with TBI, actively grieving their child's recent injury and experiencing a strong desire to nurture the injured child, would be at risk for these negative eating-related dynamics. Training, counseling, and support for parents and other caregivers must, therefore, be directed in part at preventing the evolution of behavioral eating problems.

Behavioral Intervention Programs

Behaviorally oriented intervention programs for children with developmental disability or motivational eating problems unrelated to neurologic impairment have generally been designed according to principles of traditional applied behavior analysis (see reviews by Babbitt et al., 1994a, b). For example, positive eating behaviors (e.g., accepting and swallowing a bite of food) can be followed by reinforcement (e.g., praise, desirable food, toy), whereas negative behavior (e.g., refusal, crying) can be systematically ignored. Negative reinforcement paradigms are rarely used but have been reported in the case of two children with long-standing food expulsion or packing (Babbitt et al., 1992). In these cases, swallowing a bite of food was rewarded with escape from what had become an aversive feeding situation.

In the tradition of applied behavior analysis, antecedent manipulation has been restricted to immediate antecedents, including the taste and texture of the food (e.g., masking nonpreferred foods with the taste of preferred foods; alternating preferred and nonpreferred foods) and the nature of the presentation and instructions. Extinction of problem behaviors (e.g., food expulsion, crying) has been addressed by eliminating their reinforcer (e.g., parents are instructed to persevere in feeding in the face of resistance), by removing the child from a reinforcing situation contingent on the negative behavior (e.g., giving "time out"), and by punishing the negative behavior (e.g., following volitional vomiting with a noxious taste). Because extinction programs are potentially dangerous, they are recommended by behavioral psychologists only in extreme cases and with intensive behavioral supervision.

Modified Behavioral Intervention Programs

Our experience in pediatric TBI rehabilitation supports some modification of these intervention programs for motivational eating disorders. For example, because of the intensity of parental feelings associated with feeding a child with recent-onset brain injury, parental compliance with rigid behavioral programs is difficult to achieve. In addition, when children who had grown accustomed to considerable control in their lives emerge from coma with minimal control in all realms, such children learn that they can easily achieve control over adult behavior and reactions by manipulating their mealtime behavior. Therefore, behavioral programs that highlight the importance of accepting food can inadvertently sabotage resumption of normal eating by giving the child an irresistible control option (i.e., control adult behavior by refusing to eat).

An alternative that has been successful in many cases of prolonged food refusal or selectivity after childhood TBI features reduction in the amount of adult attention given to eating, combined with creative manipulation of background setting events. (Setting events and their manipulation in behavior management programs are discussed in Chapter 13). The following cases illustrate these principles. In each case, an organic basis for the feeding disorder—including pharyngeal swallowing disorder, gastroesophageal reflux and associated pain, oral hypersensitivity, seriously distorted sense of smell and taste, and absent feelings of hunger—had been ruled out. In other cases, intervention for these organic disorders may precede or accompany behavioral interventions.

Case Study: Jim

Jim was 14 years old when he was referred to a specialized inpatient brain-injury rehabilitation program six months after severe TBI. He had severe spastic quadriplegia, including moderate oral motor impairment, but normal pharyngeal swallowing physiology. He was physically capable of eating pureed and ground food and of drinking thickened liquids, but he consistently refused to eat or drink. His trial behavioral feeding program, which included presentation of presumably desirable foods, clear instructions to accept the food, and removal of attention after prolonged refusal, was completely unsuccessful. Examination of a videotape of a trial feeding session revealed that Jim smiled broadly when the therapist turned away contingent on Jim's refusal of the food offered. Because Jim apparently enjoyed the control he was able to exercise over others during dining times, the program was changed to focus on antecedents and setting events as opposed to consequences: (1) Only staff whom Jim liked were allowed to eat with him; (2) staff ate their meals with Jim, making dining primarily a social occasion; (3) conversations during dining times were pleasant and did not focus on eating; and (4) Jim was periodically invited to accept a bite of food, with no directives and no consequences for refusal. Under these circumstances, Jim began to eat in sufficient quantity to eliminate some of his gastrostomy-tube feedings. He was discharged with tube feedings for hydration and emergencies (e.g., illness) but typically taking three substantial meals orally per day.

Case Study: Jon

Jon was 4 years old when he incurred a severe closed head injury in an automobile crash. At 3 months after his injury, despite moderate gross motor impairment, he had normal swallowing physiology and oral motor function, including intelligible speech. However, he refused every feeding attempt, presumably because of power struggles that had evolved during early attempts to feed him in the acute-care hospital. Because of this history, feeding therapy highlighted removal of all adult attention to eating. Small amounts of food (e.g., crackers) and liquid (e.g., a washcloth soaked in fruit juice), along with toys, were left on Jon's lap tray during solitary play. Available playthings included toy eating utensils and some toys that were coated in honey or other sweet food. Over the course of several days, Jon progressed from playing with the utensils and food (e.g., crushing the cracker) to licking his fingers to placing the food or washcloth on his lips to swallowing small quantities of the food. After this self-paced desensitization, larger quantities of preferred foods were made available with an adult present (still with no direct attention to eating) and, finally, Jon accepted normal meals during social dining times.

Case Study: Bob

Bob was 13 years old and had been injured approximately 6 months earlier when he was admitted to a specialized pediatric rehabilitation program. He had moderate gross motor and mild oral motor impairment but normal swallowing physiology. When he began eating at approximately 3 months after his injury, his parents were his primary feeders and Bob succeeded in selectively refusing all foods with the exception of two or three favorites. Because of this extended history of succeeding in power battles with his parents, the feeding program in rehabilitation was designed to avoid all potential for such conflict. Rather, Bob was placed at a table with slightly older adolescents, all of whom ate. This group of "tough" male adolescents created rules for their table, one of which was "tough guys eat." Anybody who chose not to eat was told by the adult supervisor (who ate with the boys and played along with the tough-guy script) that this was an acceptable choice but that he would have to leave the table. The social and emotional appeal of being at the tough-guy table and being a member of a tough-guy group of adolescents was sufficient to reduce Bob's food selectivity to normal levels within a week.

Clearly, not all behavioral feeding disorders are treated as easily and quickly as those described in the preceding case studies. Furthermore, many disorders involve a tricky combination of organic and behavioral components. The important point we wish to make is that behavioral eating disturbances after childhood TBI can often be prevented by avoiding anxious confrontations and dangerous control battles centered around eating. Resumption of eating after severe TBI, with its complex physiologic and psychological components, holds the potential for generating such disturbances. Furthermore, traditional behavioral feeding programs may inadvertently heighten this potential by placing too much emphasis on the child's acceptance of food and by creating a negative eating context that involves rigid and unpleasant feeding procedures. Positive and indirect approaches to behavioral eating disorders, in contrast, are designed to reduce anxiety and rigidity around eating, eliminate power battles, and prevent the evolution of food aversions and manipulativeness, thereby reducing the threat of long-term motivational eating disturbances.

Integrating Social and Cognitive Rehabilitation with Dining Programs

Mealtimes are ideal occasions to target cognitive, communicative, and social goals in a contextually meaningful way. For example, requesting, commenting about, and rejecting food is a good context within which to practice speech or augmentative communication systems. Focusing on eating in the face of distractions can help the child gain control over attentional functions. Choosing foods and the order in which to eat them is a natural planning activity and can be emphasized as part of cognitive rehabilitation. Finally, as soon as possible, children should be grouped with peers during dining times: Targeting positive social interaction at mealtimes is more meaningful from social, cognitive, and behavioral perspectives than is similar teaching in an artificially devised social skills group. Dining programs in rehabilitation hospitals should, therefore, be collaborative, including physical, occupational, speech, and recreation therapists, psychologists, social workers, medical and nursing staff, and family members.

Parent Education and Support

Parents vary greatly in terms of their history with their children and with feeding, their ability to understand technical issues in pathophysiology and treatment, and their availability and willingness to work collaboratively with staff. However, most parents of children with TBI have a strong natural desire to see their children quickly resume normal eating and to participate in this process as a means of meeting their own needs to nurture their injured children. Furthermore, most parents are willing to work collaboratively with staff, assuming staff members respect the parents' unique knowledge and position and engage them in a respectful manner. Particularly in cases involving young children, staff must appreciate the extreme importance that parents attach to feeding and nurturing their children and the importance of the intimacy and bonding that are associated with feeding.

Creating a collaborative alliance between parents and staff begins with feeding assessment. In a rehabilitation hospital, parents should be asked not only about the child's preinjury history in relation to eating but also what they have learned about the child's current ability to eat. In addition, parents have important knowledge about the child's food preferences and about ways to handle and calm the child. Staff must receive parents' insights nonjudgmentally and engage them in subsequent assessment activities, including VFG studies if they are warranted. Even parents of children who are transferred from an acute-care setting to rehabilitation with a physician's order to avoid oral feeding may

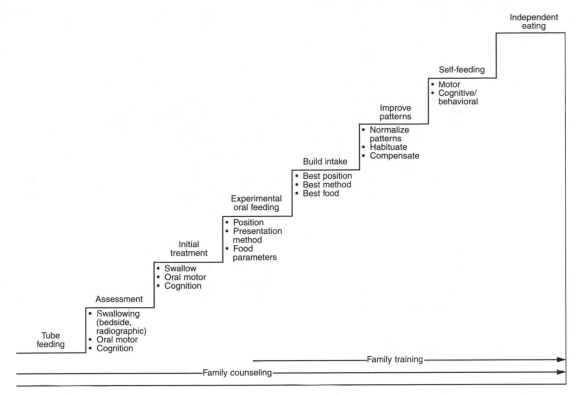

Figure 7-4. Stages of progression from tube feeding to oral feeding. (Modified with permission from The Rehabilitation Institute of Pittsburgh.)

have tried to feed the child. Parents who have observed x-ray procedures and to whom the results have been clearly explained tend to be more long-suffering allies in the therapeutic process than those who have simply been told to wait until a staff member instructs them that it is safe to feed the child.

Although recovery of oral feeding skills is not always predictable, there is a general progression through stages (Figure 7-4). Anxiety is reduced when parents know where their child is along a meaningful, logical continuum toward normal eating, even if no promises about outcome or no time estimates can be made. Furthermore, every effort should be made to enable parents to participate in prefeeding therapeutic activities, including oral stimulation for purposes of desensitization or normalization of oral motor patterns. Trained parents can significantly increase the intensity of the prefeeding program and simultaneously meet their own nurturing needs. If a child's swallowing problems persist for extended periods, there is value in identifying safe ways for parents to experiment with trial oral feeding, possibly with extreme safety precau-

tions in place. For example, parents might help their child chew on a washcloth soaked in nectar, with the child's head positioned in such a way that the liquid will fall safely forward out of the mouth. In this way, the child experiences some pleasure in tasting food, the parents feel they are doing whatever they can do to promote recovery, and the child practices chewing.

Summary

In this chapter, we have summarized the most common swallowing disorders experienced by children and adolescents after TBI, along with guidelines for assessment and intervention. Because of the seriousness of swallowing disorders, careful team decision making, possibly using radiographic assessment procedures, is critical. Intervention decisions are made after the problem has been precisely delineated. The importance of integrating cognitive, behavioral, social, and family intervention with treatment of physiologic swallowing disorders is highlighted.

References

Arvedson JC, Brodsky L (eds) (1993). Pediatric Swallowing and Feeding: Assessment and Management. San Diego: Singular Publishing Group.

Aviv JE, Martin JH, Sacco RL, et al. (1996). Supraglottic and pharyngeal sensory abnormalities in stroke patients with dysphagia. Ann Otol Rhinol Laryngol 105;92.

Babbitt RL, Hoch TA, Coe DA (1994a). Behavioral Feeding Disorders. In DN Tuchman, RS Walter (eds), Disorders of Feeding and Swallowing in Infants and Children. San Diego: Singular Publishing Group, 77.

Babbitt RL, Hoch TA, Coe DA, et al. (1994b). Behavioral assessment and treatment of pediatric feeding disorders. Dev Behav Pediatr 15;278.

Babbitt RL, Hoch TA, Krell D, Williams K (1992). Exit Criterion: Treating Motivational Absence of Swallowing. Poster presented at the Convention of the Association for Behavior Analysis, May, San Francisco.

Bisch EM, Logemann JA, Rademaker AW, et al. (1994). Pharyngeal effects of bolus volume, viscosity and temperature in dysphagic neurologically impaired patients and normal subjects. J Speech Hear Res 37;1041.

Blonsky E, Logemann J, Boshes B, Fisher H (1975). Comparison of speech and swallowing function in patients with tremor disorders and in normal geriatric patients: a cinefluorographic study. J Gerontol 30;299.

Budd KS, McGraw TE, Farbisz R, et al. (1992). Psychosocial concomitants of children's feeding disorders. J Pediatr Psychol 17;81.

Cherney LR, Halper AS (1989). Recovery of oral nutrition after head injury in adults. J Head Trauma Rehabil 4(4);42.

Curtis D, Cruess D, Berg T (1984). The cricopharyngeal muscle: a video recording review. Am J Radiol 142;497.

Davis J, Lazarus C, Logemann J, Hurst P (1987). Effect of a maxillary glossectomy prosthesis on articulation and swallowing. J Prosthet Dent 57;715.

Hutchins BF (1989). Establishing a dysphagia family intervention program for head-injured patients. J Head Trauma Rehabil 4(4);64.

Jacob P, Kahrilas P, Logemann J, et al. (1989). Upper esophageal sphincter opening and modulation during swallowing. Gastroenterology 97;1469.

Kahrilas PJ, Lin S, Logemann JA, et al. (1993). Deglutitive tongue action: volume accommodation and bolus propulsion. Gastroenterology 104;152.

Kahrilas PJ, Logemann JA, Krugler C, Flanagan E (1991). Volitional augmentation of upper esophageal sphincter opening during swallowing. Am J Physiol 260;G450.

Kahrilas PJ, Logemann JA, Lin S, Ergun GA (1992). Pharyngeal clearance during swallow: a combined manometric and videofluoroscopic study. Gastroenterology 103;128.

Lazarus C, Logemann JA (1987). Swallowing disorders in closed head trauma patients. Arch Phys Med Rehabil 68;79.

Lazarus CL (1989). Swallowing disorders after traumatic brain injury. J Head Trauma Rehabil 4(4);34.

Leder S (1996). Gag reflex and dysphagia. Head Neck 18;138.

Linden P, Kuhlemeier KV, Patterson C (1993). The probability of correctly predicting subglottic penetration from clinical observations. Dysphagia 8;170.

Linden P, Siebens A (1983). A dysphagia: predicting laryngeal penetration. Arch Phys Med Rehabil 64;281.

Logemann J (1983). Evaluation and Treatment of Swallowing Disorders. Austin, TX.

Logemann J (1993). A Manual for Videofluoroscopic Evaluation of Swallowing (2nd ed). Austin, TX: Pro-Ed.

Logemann J, Kahrilas P (1990). Relearning to swallow post CVA: application of maneuvers and indirect biofeedback: a case study. Neurology 40;1136.

Logemann J, Kahrilas P, Kobara M, Vakil N (1989). The benefit of head rotation on pharyngeal esophageal dysphagia. Arch Phys Med Rehabil 70;767.

Logemann J, Lazarus C, Jenkins P (1982). The Relationship Between Clinical Judgment and Radiographic Assessment of Aspiration. Paper presented at the annual meeting of the American Speech-Language-Hearing Association, November 20, Toronto.

Logemann JA (1989). Evaluation and treatment planning for the head-injured patient with oral intake disorders. J Head Trauma Rehabil 4(4);24.

Logemann JA, Kahrilas PJ, Cheng J, et al. (1992). Closure mechanisms of the laryngeal vestibule during swallow. Am J Physiol 262;G338.

Logemann JA, Pauloski BR, Colangelo L, et al. (1995). Effects of a sour bolus on oropharyngeal swallowing measures in patients with neurogenic dysphagia. J Speech Hearing Res 38;556.

Logemann JA, Rademaker AW, Pauloski BR, Kahrilas PJ (1994). Effects of postural change on aspiration in head and neck surgical patients. Otolaryngol Head Neck Surg 110;222.

Mandelstam P, Lieber A (1970). Cineradiographic evaluation of the esophagus in normal adults. Gastroenterology 58;32.

Manly CA (1983). Dysphagia Assessment. Workshop presented at the conference on Technology in the 80s: Impact on Speech and Language Services, October, New York.

Martin BJW, Logemann JA, Shaker R, Dodds WJ (1993). Normal laryngeal valuing patterns during three breath-hold maneuvers: a pilot investigation. Dysphagia 8;11.

Middaugh PA (1989). Early nutritional management post-head injury. J Head Trauma Rehabil 4(4);17.

Miller A (1982). Deglutition. Physiol Rev 62;129.

Morris S (1978). Oral-Motor Problems and Guidelines for Treatment. In JM Wilson (ed), Oral-Motor Function and Dysfunction in Children. Chapel Hill: University of North Carolina.

Morris S (1982). The Normal Acquisition of Oral Feeding Skills: Implications for Assessment and Treatment. New York: Therapeutic Media.

Palmer S, Horn S (1978). Feeding Problems in Children. In S Palmer, S Ekvall (eds), Pediatric Nutrition in Developmental Disorders. Springfield, IL: Thomas, 107.

Pouderoux P, Kahrilas PJ (1995). Deglutitive tongue force modulation by volition, volume, and viscosity in humans. Gastroenterology 108;1418.

Rasley A, Logemann JA, Kahrilas PJ, et al. (1993). Prevention of barium aspiration during videofluoroscopic swallowing studies: value of change in posture. AJR Am J Roentgenol 160;1005.

Shanahan TK, Logemann JA, Rademaker AW, et al. (1993). Chin down posture effects on aspiration in dysphagic patients. Arch Phys Med Rehabil 74;736.

Shedd D, Kirchner J, Scatliff J (1961). Oral and pharyngeal components of deglutition. Arch Surg 82;371.

Sisson LA, Van Hasselt VB (1989). Feeding Disorders. In JK Luiselli (ed), Behavioral Medicine and Developmental Disabilities. New York: Springer Verlag, 45.

Splaingard MK, Hutchins B, Sulton L, Chaudhuri G (1988). Aspiration in rehabilitation patients: videofluoroscopy vs. bedside clinical assessment. Arch Phys Med Rehabil 69;637.

Welch MW, Logemann JA, Rademaker AW, Kahrilas PJ (1993). Changes in pharyngeal dimensions effected by chin tuck. Arch Phys Med Rehabil 74;178.

Wheeler R, Logemann J, Rosen J (1980). A maxillary reshaping prosthesis: its effectiveness in improving the speech and swallowing of postsurgical oral cancer patients. J Prosthet Dent 43;491.

Ylvisaker M, Weinstein M (1989). Recovery of oral feeding after pediatric head injury. J Head Trauma Rehabil 4(4);51.

Yorkston KM, Honsinger MJ, Mitsuda PM, Hammen V (1989). The relationship between speech and swallowing disorders in head-injured patients. J Head Trauma Rehabil 4(4);1.

Appendix 7-1
Treatment Options

Key:
*Can be done regardless of the child's level of alertness, unless medically contraindicated. In some cases, the child must be sufficiently alert to be aware of food in the mouth.
†Requires the child to process simple instructions.
‡Requires the child to learn new procedures.

I. Oral or facial dysfunction
   A. Hypersensitivity to stimulation: Grimace, pathologic reflexes, hypertonicity of oral structures
      *1. Gradual desensitization: Apply firm pressure with a warm washcloth or gauze pad, gloved fingers, or other implement. Begin at some distance from the face. Gradually move closer to the mouth, always stopping short of eliciting pathologic responses.
      *2. Oral stimulation: Use a glycerin swab, gloved finger, or other implement (note infection control issues with finger stimulation). Use jaw control during stimulation, if needed.
         a. Techniques
            (1) Firmly rub gums (first upper, then lower) on one side and then the other. Start with one rub and increase to four per quadrant. Use pureed food on the swab or the finger if the child can swallow and if production of saliva is desired.
            (2) Firmly rub front to back on the palate first on one side, then the other, and then the midline. Stop short of a gag.
            (3) Firmly tap down on the tongue, front to back on the midline. Stop short of a gag.
            (4) Stimulate across the surface of the tongue for tongue flattening.
            (5) Stimulate lightly along the lateral edges of the tongue for lateralization.
            (6) Holding the tongue between gloved index and middle fingers, vibrate tongue side to side for range and tone reduction.
            (7) With gloved index finger inside and gloved middle finger outside the oral cavity, vibrate cheek muscles to reduce cheek tone.
         b. Precautions
            (1) Give the child time to swallow after each stimulation.
            (2) Always stop short of an abnormal response.
            (3) Do not overstimulate.
            (4) Gradually increase the amount of stimulation that the child can tolerate.
            (5) Be sensitive to the offensiveness of gloved fingers in the mouth. Use a swab or other implement if indicated.
            (6) Do not place gloved fingers or a fragile implement in the oral cavity of a child with a tonic bite reflex.
   B. Hyposensitivity or hypotonicity
      *1. Orofacial musculature: Several strengthening exercises are included for specific hypotonic structures. Most exercises for hypotonic muscles are facilitated by first stimulating the belly of the muscle being

exercised. Possible forms of stimulation are tapping firmly or flicking with gloved finger, quickly stretching the muscle, rapid brushing, or light application of ice. Sensory stimulation can be initiated before the child is cognitively capable of deliberately exercising the structures.

*2. Intraoral hyposensitivity: Experiment with food temperatures (especially cold) and tastes (especially sour or spicy). Place food on the more sensitive side of the oral cavity.

II. Lips
   A. Hypertonicity: Poor closure, loss of food, drooling
      *1. See hypertonicity suggestions in section I.A.
      *2. Apply firm pressure below the nose to lower tone. Do not pull down on a hypertonic upper lip.
      *3. Allow time for closure on the spoon or tongue blade or cup during feeding. Do not allow the patient to scrape food off the spoon using upper teeth.
      *4. Use a straw to encourage lip closure. This can initially be done using the straw as a pipette, with the therapist holding one end of the straw to control the amount of food or liquid taken.
   B. Hypotonicity: Weak closure, loss of food, drooling
      *1. See suggestions for hypotonicity stimulation in section I.B.
      †2. Place a button held by a string inside the child's lips in front of the teeth. Pull on the string and ask the child to hold the button by pursing his or her lips.
      †3. Have the child hold tongue blades between his or her lips and resist outward pull. As lip closure improves, decrease the number of blades to increase task difficulty.
      †4. Instruct the child to smile or pucker or raise or lower the upper or lower lip, all against finger resistance. Gradually increase resistance.
      †5. Instruct the child to suck on a straw (no food) with the end held closed to offer resistance. If the child can swallow, have the child practice sucking heavy liquids through a straw.
      †6. Have the child hold exaggerated facial expressions.
      †7. Instruct the child to alternate between an exaggerated smile (or "ee") and exaggerated pucker (or "oo"). Increase the length of time in each posture.
      †8. Gradually increase the amount of time the child is expected to maintain continuous, firm lip closure.
      †9. Have the child practice, with exaggerated articulation and in all word positions, words with bilabial consonants (m, b, p, w).
     *10. In feeding, wait for the child to bring the upper lip down on the tongue blade, spoon, or cup. Instruct the child to avoid scraping food off the spoon with the upper teeth. Do not simply pour liquid into the mouth. Use a tongue blade or shallow spoon before proceeding to a deep-bowl spoon.

III. Cheeks
   A. Hypertonicity: Grimace, pseudosmile, poor lip closure. See hypertonicity suggestions in section I.A.
   B. Hypotonicity: Loss of food in lateral sulci, weak facial expression
      *1. See suggestions for hypotonicity stimulation in section I.B.
      †2. Instruct the child to exaggerate facial expressions involving cheek muscles. Have the child hold the expressions for increasing periods or against finger resistance, or both.
      †3. Instruct the child to alternate rapidly between an exaggerated smile and an exaggerated pucker.
      †4. Instruct the child to puff out his or her cheeks by filling them with air. Gradually increase finger resistance against the puffed cheeks.
      *5. During feeding
          a. Apply external pressure on the affected cheek to keep food out of the sulcus.
          b. Place food on the unaffected side and tilt the patient's head slightly toward that side.

IV. Tongue
   A. Hypertonicity
      1. Tongue bunched; forward thrust to initiate the swallow
          *a. See suggestions for hypertonicity stimulation in section I.A.2.
          †b. Administer textured food and place it in a molar position when possible. Instruct the child in the use of jaw control unless the jaw control itself increases hypertonicity.
          †c. Mild to moderate tongue thrust: Instruct the child to position the tongue on the alveolar ridge and to initiate a swallow with upward or backward tongue movement, keeping the tongue tip in contact with the alveolar ridge.
      *2. Tongue retraction: Apply firm pressure on the belly of the tongue with a spoon or tongue blade; gradually bring the spoon or tongue blade farther forward on the tongue.

B. Reduced tongue lateralization
   *1. Stroke lightly along the lateral edges of the patient's tongue with a toothbrush, swab, or similar instrument.
   †2. Instruct the child to press the tongue laterally against a tongue blade.
   †3. Allow the child to practice chewing on a piece of gauze. First, place the dampened end of a gauze roll on the child's tongue at the midline. Then ask the child to move the end of the gauze to each side of the mouth, to chew on it, and to move it back to midline.
   *4. Begin feeding with pureed food; gradually add texture. Place small pieces of crunchy food on the molars to encourage lateralization; facilitate a chew.

C. Hypotonicity: Reduced tongue elevation
   †1. Instruct the child to elevate the front of the tongue as far as possible, hold for a second and release. Elevate the back of the tongue as far as possible, hold for a second and release.
   †2. Instruct the child to push the tongue up against a tongue blade.
   †3. Instruct the child to push up against a roll of gauze (juice-soaked gauze if the child can swallow). The therapist should hold the end of the gauze. The size of the gauze roll can be diminished as tongue elevation improves.
   †4. Have the child practice hard-contact consonant-vowel syllables beginning with /t/ and /k/.
   *5. During feeding, regularly check the child's palate for packed food.
   *6. If there is a residual tongue elevation impairment, consider consulting with a maxillofacial prosthodontist to discuss a prosthetic appliance that will lower the roof of the mouth (hard palate) to meet the tongue (Davis et al., 1987; Wheeler et al., 1980).

D. Reduced bolus formation and cupping of the tongue
   †1. Use a licorice whip, a long piece of gauze soaked in juice, or a Lifesaver on a string. Firmly hold one end of any of these items and place the other end in the child's mouth. Have the child move his or her end around in the oral cavity, retrieve it, and return to midtongue. Instruct the child to gradually increase range, accuracy, and speed of movement.
   †2. Give the child a small amount of pudding. Ask him or her to hold the bolus with the tongue, move the bolus around in the mouth, and then spit it out. Check for residue. When the child can manipulate the pudding bolus satisfactorily, gradually liquefy the material. Ask the child to hold each bolus with the tongue, move it around the mouth, bring it to the middle of the tongue, and hold it again. The child should then spit the material out, and the therapist should check the oral cavity for residue.

†E. Reduced anteroposterior tongue movement to start the swallow: Place a long piece of juice-soaked gauze front to back along the child's tongue. Have the child squeeze the juice out of the gauze by pressing the tongue against the gauze, in an anterior to posterior motion. The child should swallow at the end of the tongue movement.

F. General tongue dysfunction
   *1. If the tongue is mildly to moderately involved, tilt the child's head toward the stronger side to keep food from being lost on the weaker side.
   *2. If the tongue is severely involved but the pharyngeal swallow is adequate, use a syringe or straw to place the food directly in the back of the child's oral cavity.
   *3. Children with primitive suck-swallow or munch patterns should be able to eat pureed foods adequately (if the pharyngeal swallow is normal). However, a diet of nothing but pureed foods will not improve tongue patterns. Hence, textured and crunchy foods placed on the child's molars should be introduced as soon as possible, consistent with patient safety. Alternate placement on the sides of the mouth. If the child cannot safely manage textured or crunchy foods, gauze can be used for practice chewing and tongue lateralization, as described in section IV.C.3.
   *4. The drinking of thick liquids (thick nectar or fluids of milkshake consistency) may be easier for the child to manage. Also, such liquids usually are less likely to be aspirated and less likely to worsen the child's primitive oral patterns than are thin liquids. If excessive secretions are a problem, reduce the child's intake of milk and milk products.

V. Jaw
   A. Hypertonicity
      *1. Jaw thrust: Use the child's optimal positioning for his or her disorder and encourage jaw control during feeding and oral stimulation. Do not encourage jaw control if it increases the force of the thrust pattern. See suggestions for hypertonicity stimulation in section I.A.2.
      *2. Bite reflex (tonic)

a. See suggestions for hypertonicity stimulation in section I.A.2.

b. Press firmly on the belly of the child's masseters to release them. Massage in a rotary pattern. Do not try to pull the spoon out of the child's mouth during a tonic bite reflex, as this usually increases the reflex.

  B. Hypotonicity: Reduced range

    *1. See suggestions for hypotonicity stimulation in section I.B.

    †2. Have the child move his or her jaw in all directions (open lateralization to each side), hold for 1–2 seconds in each direction, and release. Add resistance.

  C. Weak vertical and rotary chewing movements

    *1. Place small pieces of fruit in a juice-soaked gauze sleeve and hold both open ends of the sleeve. Place the fruit between the child's molars and facilitate chewing movements.

    *2. Use a combination of pureed foods and easily crunched foods placed directly on the molars. Manually assist the child with chewing motions if necessary. When starting with pureed foods, gradually thicken them as the child progresses.

VI. Velum: Hyporeflexive, hypotonic

  *A. With a cold metal object (e.g., size 00 laryngeal mirror), lightly touch the child's soft palate on the midline, slightly posterior to the juncture of the hard and soft palates. Look for reflexive lifting.

  †B. Have the child repeat hard-attack "ah" sounds. This exercise can be preceded by thermal-tactile stimulation.

VII. Pharyngeal swallow delayed or absent (possible aspiration before the swallow)

  *A. With a cold, size 00 laryngeal mirror, rub the base of the anterior faucial arch vertically. Repeat 5–10 times while looking for some movement of the soft palate or larynx. Then immediately ask the child to swallow or (if safe) present a very small amount of ice water or ginger ale, held in a straw (used as a pipette), at the base of the anterior faucial arch. Place liquid in the same area that has been stimulated and ask the child to swallow. Repeat this procedure several times daily until the pharyngeal swallow is triggered and the delay decreases. Gradually increase the amount of liquid to be swallowed or switch to a liquid of thicker consistency presented at the faucial arches.

  *B. If the pharyngeal swallow continues to be mildly delayed when oral feeding is initiated, the child's head should be tilted forward to reduce the possibility that food will enter the airway before the swallow. If the delay is significant (more than several seconds), oral feeding should be avoided.

  †C. If the child is alert and the pharyngeal swallow is mildly delayed, the supraglottic swallow technique (see section VIII.B) should be used.

VIII. Larynx: Reduced airway entrance closure (possible aspiration during the swallow) or reduced glottic closure (possible aspiration during the swallow)

  †A. The optimum posture for the child may be chin tucked down or head rotated to the impaired side if there is unilateral laryngeal damage.

  †B. If airway entrance closure between the arytenoid cartilage and the base of the epiglottis is impaired, teach the child the super-supraglottic swallow (Logemann, 1993; Martin et al., 1993). Instructions are the same as for the supraglottic swallow (see section VIII.D) except that the child should bear down hard while holding his or her breath and swallowing.

  †C. Adduction exercises for vocal fold closure problems

    1. Instruct the child to hold his or her breath (requires glottic closure) while pushing down or pulling up on a chair.

    2. Instruct the child to hold his or her breath while pulling or pushing and producing a clear voice.

    3. Instruct the child to repeat short "ahs" with a hard glottal attack.

    4. Instruct the child to produce "ah" with a hard glottal attack and to prolong voicing for several seconds.

    5. Place hand on child's forehead and instruct the child to push his or her head against your hand while the child holds his or her breath or phonates.

  ‡D. If vocal fold closure is moderately to severely impaired, teach the child to use the supraglottic swallow (Martin et al., 1993). This process should be practiced without food and before food is introduced. Instruct the child to:

    1. Take a deep breath and hold it at the height of the inhalation.

    2. Keep holding breath while swallowing.

    3. Cough or clear throat immediately after swallowing (do not inhale before coughing).

    4. Spit or swallow again.

  ‡E. Train the child to cough or clear the throat and then to spit or to swallow whenever he or she notices a wet, hoarse quality to the voice. The child should phonate frequently during eating and after every swallow at the outset of therapy, to check for residue on the vocal folds.

IX. Pharynx
    A. Unilateral pharyngeal dysfunction: Residue or pooling on one side
        *1. Tilt the child's head toward the stronger side to encourage food to proceed along the more efficient channel. If the condition is severe, have the child eat in a side-lying position.
        *2. Turn the child's head toward the weaker side to close the pharynx and pyriform sinus on that side (Logemann et al., 1989).
        ‡3. Teach the child to clear the throat and to either spit or swallow again after every swallow.
        *4. Alternate solid and liquid swallows so that the liquid washes the solid food through the pharynx.
    B. Reduced pharyngeal contraction bilaterally
        *1. Alternate foods of semisolid and liquid consistencies.
        *2. Avoid serving solid and sticky foods.
        *3. Evaluate the child's swallow while the child assumes a supine position, to determine whether aspiration is eliminated.
        †4. Instruct the child to swallow several times with each presentation of food.
        ‡5. Teach the child to clear the throat and to either spit or swallow again if there is any suspicion of residue in the pharynx.
        *6. Re-evaluate the child's swallowing radiographically at 1- to 2-month intervals. Reduced peristalsis may recover within the first 6 months after the brain injury.
    C. Reduced tongue base movement
        *1. Tilt the child's chin down, which pushes the tongue base posteriorly (Welch et al., 1993).
        †2. Teach the child the effortful swallow (Logemann, 1993). Ask the patient to squeeze hard when he or she swallows (Pouderoux and Kahrilas, 1995).
        ‡3. Instruct the patient to practice the super-supraglottic swallow.
        †4. Ask the child to pull the tongue straight back in the mouth as far as possible, to hold this position for a second, and then to release. This is a range-of-motion exercise for the tongue base.
X. Cricopharyngeal dysfunction
    *A. Await spontaneous recovery. Cricopharyngeal dysfunction in children with brain injury will often recover spontaneously in 3–4 months. Children with this disorder should be re-evaluated radiographically every 1–2 months to assess recovery.
    ‡B. Voluntary control of cricopharyngeal sphincter: Teach the child the Mendelsohn maneuver (Kahrilas et al., 1991; Logemann and Kahrilas, 1990), which increases the extent and duration of laryngeal elevation and anterior movement and extends the width and duration of cricopharyngeal opening. Instruct the child to:
        1. Swallow and feel the Adam's apple lifting.
        2. Swallow again but, as the Adam's apple lifts, hold it up with your muscles (no digital pressure) for several seconds.
    ‡C. If the problem is mild, have the child consume only small amounts of food, using repeated swallows or the Mendelsohn maneuver.
    D. Cricopharyngeal myotomy (ear, nose, and throat procedure): This surgical procedure cuts the cricopharyngeal muscle along a vertical plane. Controversy exists as to its effectiveness. The procedure should not be done within 6 months of brain injury and should be done only if there is documented spasm in the cricopharyngeal muscle.

Chapter 8

Assistive Technologies for Children and Adolescents with Traumatic Brain Injury

Colleen Connolly Chester, Kim Henry, and Terri Tarquinio

For a young child or adolescent with traumatic brain injury (TBI), assistive technologies offer myriad possibilities for achieving greater independence and maximizing the use of residual skills and abilities. Throughout this chapter, the term *assistive technologies* is applied to a broad range of equipment and devices used for mobility, spoken and written communication, memory and cognition, environmental interaction, educational and vocational activities, and recreation and leisure. For the purposes of this discussion, *assistive technologies* will include also devices that may be characterized as rehabilitative or educational technologies because of their role as tools used to develop skills (Cook and Hussey, 1995).

One of the important aspects of applying assistive technologies to the needs of children with TBI is that a specific device may be used for both assistive and rehabilitative or educational purposes. Because it is desirable that an assistive device play multiple roles, additional considerations become part of the device selection process, as is clearly noted throughout this chapter.

The sections that follow highlight basic information about common types of assistive technologies. Also presented are relevant issues pertaining to the application of these technologies as options for a child with TBI.

The Past 30 Years

Although wheelchairs and other types of medical equipment have been available since the 1800s, it was not until the 1970s that equipment to enhance or augment a person's functional level became a standard component of TBI rehabilitation. These years were marked by active research and exploration in the field of rehabilitation for persons with TBI and in the fields of science and technology. When industrial and aerospace technologies were applied to the needs of people with disability, the fields of rehabilitation technology and assistive technology emerged. As the latter term implies, the fundamental goal was to use technology to *assist* a person in performing a task as efficiently as possible. Because all people have specific combinations of physical, sensory, and cognitive abilities, one of the primary challenges confronting the field of rehabilitation engineering is to offer technology that can be modified and customized easily to match each person's needs.

Selecting Assistive Technology

The capabilities of a particular piece of equipment are only one factor in a process leading to the successful integration, acceptance, and use of technology by children and adolescents with TBI. At the core of this process is a blend of interactions between a child and a device and the environment in which that child-device tandem functions (Reid et al., 1995; Scherer and McKee, 1989). Add to this selection process the influences of time and funding and it becomes apparent that the identification of appropriate assistive technology is a dynamic and sometimes complex task. Pointing out that selection of a specific device is not the end but a means to an end does not imply that the process must be difficult. However, the more knowledgeable, prepared, and open-minded each person involved in this process is, the greater the possibility for successful implementation of an assistive technology solution.

The process of selecting assistive technologies, along with strategies to support their application and integration into a child's everyday life, has been the focus of clinical practices and service delivery models that have grown with these technologies since the mid-1970s. Over the last 20 years, much has been written about the assistive technology evaluation process, including discussions about issues relevant to children and young adults with TBI (Bray et al., 1987; Scherer, 1993). Cook and Hussey (1995) present a comprehensive assistive technology service delivery model based on principles of human performance engineering.

To complement this body of information from research and clinical work, first-hand accounts are now available from adolescents and adults who have been using assistive technology for a number of years after incurring TBI as children. The experiences of these people offer unique perspective and insight into both the factors that influence successful integration of assistive device(s) and the effectiveness of the devices from a technological point of view. This chapter includes the stories of three young people who have used and continue to use assistive technology in their everyday lives. These clients shared their thoughts about the devices they have used in the past and use now, the benefits and shortcomings of having to rely on various technologies and, possibly most important, their feelings about needing to integrate assistive technology into their daily lives.

Before embarking on the journeys taken by young people during their childhood, it is worthwhile to review the various types of assistive technologies, particularly as they relate to the needs of children with TBI. Each section highlights (1) the characteristics and features of the technology itself, (2) assessment issues concerning the different types of technologies, and (3) rehabilitation and educational practices that create the framework supporting the integration of assistive technology into the lives of these children. Throughout this chapter, our goal is to elucidate the following themes:

- The integration of motor, sensory, cognitive, behavioral, social, and academic perspectives in team decisions about assistive technology options
- The need for active participation of the family and, when appropriate, the child or adolescent with TBI
- The child's acceptance and successful use of assistive technology
- The impact of assistive technology on a child's self-esteem, sense of empowerment, and motivation
- The application of assistive technology to address the temporary versus long-term needs of a child with TBI
- The need for flexible assistive technology options that can be modified or changed as a child's abilities change
- The importance of training and ongoing support for families and educators so that the child can best be served over time

Categories of Assistive Technologies: Assessment and Intervention Considerations

Seating and Mobility

In the choice of a seating system and wheelchair for a child with TBI, consideration must be given to the fact that, depending on the stage of recovery, physical, sensory, and cognitive changes are possible. Many children continue to make significant changes for months and even years after TBI. In addition, children with TBI experience growth spurts as part of their physical development. To respond effectively to the changing needs of a child with TBI, temporary seating systems and wheelchairs may be used initially. Equipment owned by a hospital, rehabilitation center, or distributor of durable medical equipment can be loaned or rented (Trefler et al., 1993). Because many wheelchair-funding sources provide conservative guidelines for the expected life span of a system, purchase of a permanent seating system and mobility base should not be a hurried process (Golinker and Mistrett, 1997). When specifications for a defined seating system and wheelchair are developed, components should have the potential to be adjusted to changes in a child's needs.

In addition to physical growth, many physical and tonal changes can occur in clients with TBI. For instance, a person may initially have a high degree of muscle stiffness, presenting with excessive extensor tone of the hips and spine. Therefore, the seating system must be durable and stable enough to withstand the amount of external force placed on it. A helpful technique for reducing this extensor tone is to wedge the seat surface so that the hip angle remains slightly closed (Jaffe et al., 1985). The client's physical status should be monitored regularly to assess whether adjustments should be made to the seating system.

For patients who have poor motor control and are unable to maintain an upright head or trunk position, a reclining or tilt-in-space wheelchair is often recommended (Gans et al., 1990). Providing proper head support is a common and sometimes difficult issue (Shaw and Monahan, 1989). In addressing the need for a tilt-in-space or reclining wheelchair, a patient's visual and vestibular senses must be considered. Reclining affects head position and may cause discomfort or compromise visual fields, resulting in a pulling forward of the head. Thus, the evaluating therapist, prior to making final recommendations, should always assess the patient carefully while he or she is using the recline or tilt-in-space feature. Over a period, the person's control may improve to the point at which these features no longer are needed.

Like other assistive technology, a wheelchair and seating system can be used to meet individuals' needs both therapeutically and functionally (Kanyer, 1992). For instance, therapeutically they can be provided with less lateral and anterior trunk support in their seating system so that they can work on increasing active trunk control. In some component seating systems, the lateral supports can be removed during a therapy session and then put back in place. However, care should be used to avoid interfering too much with function while trying to meet therapeutic goals. Too little support can compromise a patient's ability for upper-extremity functioning or can promote development of a spinal curvature. Each client should be evaluated carefully when these decisions are made.

Mobility is another important factor that can vary as a client changes. Provision of a means for independent mobility alters a person's entire world. Many people with TBI are highly motivated to become independently mobile but are unable to propel a manual wheelchair effectively, because they have poor upper-extremity strength or poor coordination that interferes with the ability to propel oneself with the lower extremities (or with a combination of upper and lower extremities) or because a manual wheelchair is not an efficient means for mobility. Therefore, a decision must be made about the feasibility of a power wheelchair.

Several factors come into play in considering power mobility for clients with TBI. First, patients' physical ability to access a power wheelchair controller is addressed, followed by an in-depth evaluation of the visual-perceptual abilities and cognitive skills needed to maneuver the wheelchair safely through their environment. Molnar and Perrin (1983) suggested that power mobility should be considered for children with TBI as young as age 3 who have the cognitive and visual-perceptual—but not the physical—skills to use other mobility devices.

A client may need extensive training and practice before a solid recommendation can be made for purchase of a power wheelchair. Power mobility training can also be used as a functional method to train a person's cognitive, visual-perceptual, and fine-motor skills in the middle phases of recovery. The patient can learn much about environmental awareness, visuospatial relationships, and safety and judgment issues while engaging in a functional and motivating activity such as driving a power wheelchair.

If a child will be using portable assistive devices (augmentative communication systems, environmental control units, etc.), a wheelchair frame attachment point for a mounting system must be determined. Depending on the positioning needs for the device(s), integrating other equipment so that it is readily available for use can influence the selection process significantly. Access and operation of multiple devices must also be considered. For some individuals, integrating access through a power wheelchair controller is an effective strategy (Caves, 1994; Guerette and Sumi, 1994).

Finally, the choice of a manual or power wheelchair must address accessibility issues. A patient's home, school, community, workshop, or workplace should be assessed to ensure that a wheelchair can be used and maneuvered within the environment. In addition, transportation of the wheelchair must be determined. Transport may be by car, van, public transportation, or school bus. For safety, adequate wheelchair tie-down systems must be considered.

Technology for Visual Impairments

In the consideration of any type of assistive technology, the patient's visual status is an important factor. People with TBI often have visual or perceptual problems, such as acuity impairments, visual-field deficits, a visual neglect, or the inability to discriminate visual information in a crowded display. A visual-field deficit may be suspected if abnormal posturing in a seating system is observed. For instance, individuals may present with forward trunk and head alignment and, possibly, rotation of the head in a sitting position. Initially, this posturing may be mistaken for a postural weakness when, in fact, it may be the only way that such individuals can see the information presented directly in front of them. It is important to compensate for this limitation so the user of the assistive device can position the head to see. Often, therapists are tempted to have children wear an anterior trunk support to maintain an upright position, but they must primarily be allowed to position the head so that they can see.

Another means for addressing visual-field deficits is to position any small visual materials in a location where they can be seen without compromising a child's postural alignment. Adaptive equipment that is commercially available to assist with positioning of items includes wedges, copy stands, and mounting devices.

A visual-field neglect should also be considered when recommending assistive technology. During the early stages of recovery from brain injury, it may be more important to provide visual or auditory cues to increase the patient's attention to the neglected side. However, in the later stages of recovery, function may be a higher priority. At this point, perhaps the school desk or workstation should be set up so that visual material is within the range at which the person visually attends. Figure 8-1 shows an example of a workstation layout that keeps visual stimuli in a midline position.

In the areas of reading, computer access, and augmentative communication, many options are available to assist the person with a visual acuity impairment. Enlarging materials on a monitor using software or using a closed-circuit television for reading and writing activities are two solutions. The ability to change the contrast of colors on a screen can also be helpful for a person with visual acuity problems. Auditory or spoken feedback can be used to supplement any visual information being presented. For example, screen-reading software combined with a speech synthesizer can provide access to standard computer application software. This solution is also good for patients who have difficulty with visual tracking or changing focus from a keyboard to the display or monitor. Instead of (or in addition to) looking at the screen, such people can listen to the auditory feedback to check their typing accuracy, thus increasing their efficiency. A less technical modification would be to provide tactile feedback to keyboards or displays.

Augmentative Communication

When and in what form to introduce communication technology are often complex questions. Many issues

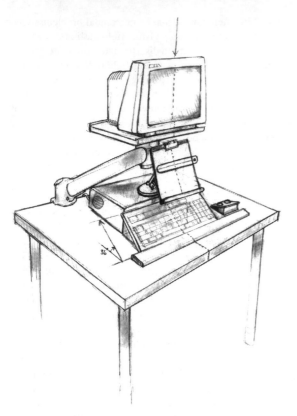

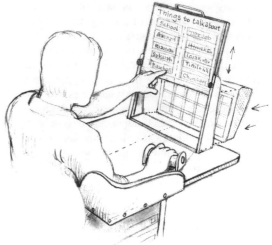

Figure 8-2. An augmentative communication system incorporating both a manual board and an electronic, digitized speech device set up for easy access. The manual board has conversation-topic choices, whereas the speech output device has more specific messages.

Figure 8-1. A computer workstation with components arranged so that visual information is presented in midline.

must be considered and skills evaluated before a decision in these matters can be made. DeRuyter and Kennedy (1991) provided a detailed discussion of specific assessment and service delivery issues relevant to nonspeaking persons with TBI. Each stage of recovery (i.e., early, middle, or late) is characterized by different communication needs (Blackstone, 1989). Timing is often critical. During the early stages of recovery, speech may be absent or unintelligible. It is crucial to introduce some form of communication to allow children to express their most basic needs, at the very least. Often, time may not allow formal determination of the optimal system. The goal is to give the patient some form of communication as soon as possible. However, the early stage of recovery may be marked by significant language, physical, and cognitive deficits. These deficits challenge clinicians in the selection and training of technology but, at the same time, technology may be therapeutically beneficial to the recovery of some of these impaired areas.

Technology may facilitate recovery of language and cognitive skills by providing visual and auditory feedback to the child with TBI. Language concepts can be reinforced by vocabulary programmed into a communication device that provides voice output and has an overlay with pictures or words. The consistency and repetition are valuable feedback that the child can control. Besides providing auditory and visual feedback, the system gives children an opportunity to communicate with people in their environment who can then provide feedback to the child through the uniqueness of their responses. The technology can offer excellent learning opportunities for the child by providing concrete visual information that is confirmed by the auditory feedback and the reaction of the communication partner. For example, the child selects a picture of a basketball, and the following message is spoken: "I'm a basketball fan. Is there a game on tonight?" The communication partner responds, "Oh, so am I. Let's check the TV listing. What team do you like?"

In deciding on the type of system to introduce at any stage of recovery, it is important to develop technology systems that meet the potential user's current cognitive, language, and physical abilities, while facilitating language and learning, word finding, and pragmatic development and challenging the user to improve these abilities. With the help of other team members, decisions should be made about how users will access the device. If children are physically able, it is preferable to introduce a direct-selection system in which they point to the picture, word, or letter that they desire. Direct selection is the most efficient way to make choices. Figure 8-2 shows an example of an augmentative communication system that blends a manual board and an electronic, digitized speech device set up for direct selection.

If physical deficits prevent direct selection, other methods of access may be options, depending on the child's current cognitive and sensory status. Physically, children may not be able to directly select the areas they wish, so a visual or auditory scanning system may be investigated. Scanning, however, can be a cognitive and sensory challenge under the best circumstances (Levine et al., 1992). For children with TBI and resultant impaired cognitive skills and (possibly) impaired visual or auditory senses, scanning may initially be an overwhelming or impossible task. As children begin to regain some function, however, the careful introduction of these access methods may lead to successful access to a functional communication system.

Recovery from TBI is a dynamic, ongoing process. The same description can be applied to communication and technology. For this reason, professionals should never be satisfied that a child's current system is the most appropriate form of technology. As children recover and regain function, their ability to access may change and, in turn, other types of technologies previously dismissed may provide options more suitable to the child's current physical and sensory abilities. The same capability applies to cognition and language. As these functions return or are relearned, the volume and diversity of the vocabulary that must be included will change. In some cases, the current technology may be adapted to meet the child's changing needs but, in other cases, the technology being used may not offer the sophistication that the child's cognitive skills now demand; thus, a new form of technology may have to be introduced. The job is rarely finished and the goals will change constantly, from (1) initially wanting to give children an opportunity to communicate basic needs in the most transparent manner to (2) using the technology to help them to reenter the classroom to (3) using technology that will enable them to communicate complex thoughts through written and vocal output (Ladtkow, 1993).

Computer Access and Applications

Personal computers have become commonplace and are an integral part of educational and academic settings, beginning with preschool and kindergarten. In addition, growing numbers of families have personal computers at home. Today's computers can be used as multimedia devices due to their advanced graphic, sound, and processing capabilities. Not only does this capacity greatly enhance the interactive qualities of a personal computer, it extends the application of this technology as an assistive device. Because of their range and flexibility, personal computers can serve as both assistive and therapeutic tools for a child with TBI.

For a child who has physical limitations resulting from TBI, access to a personal computer can be achieved through a range of alternative input devices. For example, software can permit single-finger input from a standard keyboard. Adapted keyboards that are either much smaller or much larger than standard types are available to facilitate

modified keyboarding skills. Trackballs, joysticks, or devices that respond to head movements can be substituted for a standard computer mouse. A child who can produce consistent vocalizations may be able to use a voice recognition system that responds to spoken commands.

Another method of computer access is based on the use of software that displays a keyboard on the computer screen. Selections can be made from this virtual keyboard by using a variety of input devices (e.g., a single switch). For example, a person can activate a switch and make selections by controlling the movement of a highlighting mechanism and stopping it on a specific keyboard location. This process is called *scanning*. When an efficient means of access has been developed and implemented, the application of computer technology can begin.

Just as a healthy child's educational experiences should not be delivered solely through computer-based learning, the cognitive rehabilitation program for a child with TBI should not center around or consist predominantly of exercises performed on a personal computer. As a therapeutic tool, however, a personal computer can be used to promote independent practice. Small-group activities that incorporate the use of a computer provide a setting in which children can practice social interactions through cooperative learning (Male, 1994). When computer-based cognitive retraining tasks are performed in a therapeutic environment that facilitates the bridging of skills to their application in everyday situations, computer technology can be a powerful tool for both the child and the therapist (Gianutsos, 1992; Ylvisaker et al., 1994). A computer can also be a valuable tool for a child who needs to work on fundamental cause-and-effect skills through higher-level cognitive tasks such as planning and organization. Retraining of visual-perceptual skills can also be enhanced through computer-based activities (e.g., tracking an object moving through a maze or choosing the object that differs from others in a set).

As children recover from TBI, they may need alternative methods for writing and completing schoolwork. By using a computer for word processing and other written tasks, children with upper-extremity motor involvement can participate in these activities with an appropriate level of independence. Cognitive processes involved in language development are stimulated and reinforced through many features available in word-processing, writing, and other language arts programs. The use of basic spell-checking, grammar-checking, and thesaurus options in most word-processing programs can be powerful language development tools. As adolescents reach the age at which vocational goals are established, computers can play a significant role in training activities and can serve as primary work tools. Educational software that simulates different environments and situations provides an opportunity for children and young adults to work on mathematic, critical-thinking, problem-solving, and other higher-level cognitive skills (Turnbull et al., 1995). For example, a program that requires a person to operate a store promotes development of counting skills (inventory), money skills (setting prices and making change), organizational skills (tracking multiple items), and decision-making skills (determining what supplies are needed and when to buy them).

Given the extent to which computers are integrated into our society, effective and meaningful access to this technology should be a goal for a child with TBI, if only to ensure that child's ongoing development of computer literacy skills. Dunn (1994) noted the impact of microcomputer technology on the development of life skills. In most instances, however, much more can be gained from the application of this technology. A computer can be one of the most powerful assistive and augmentative devices that children with TBI can use throughout their lives.

Cognitive Prostheses

The cognitive changes that often occur after TBI have been well observed and documented over the years. It has been shown that memory, new learning, organization, and problem-solving skills are often compromised. Loss or change in these areas can make reentry into the community a frustrating and anxiety-provoking experience. Inability to memorize or recall new information profoundly influences a child's capacity for functioning effectively in a traditional school environment. A decreased ability to organize one's thoughts can make it impossible to complete a routine task. These cognitive deficits may prevent a child from pursuing leisure activities or maintaining good peer relationships.

How could technology possibly make it easier to deal with such complex problems? Many methods can be used to address such issues. Most people use strategies to help them to remember assignments or appointments. For example, they write things down, use calendars, make lists, ask questions, or read books to help solve a problem. For the child who has TBI and is having difficulty processing written information, cue cards and other paper materials can be developed through the use of graphics (Doss and Reichle, 1991). The strategies listed above can also be implemented through common consumer-available technology. Children with TBI who may be unable to read the time on the clock might, if the time is spoken, be able to process and understand the information. Watches come equipped with alarms that remind people when they need to move to the next task. Electronic date books and address books come in pocket sizes and will beep as a reminder of appointments or display a phone number or address with the push of a button. Computers allow people to record notes, thoughts, and data in large volumes and with less effort. Through speech synthesizers, a computer can read back material in a way that can aid in the processing and organization

of information. All these strategies can be used by a child or adolescent with TBI and may make an important difference in everyday functioning. For some children, though, they may not be enough.

The application of computer-based systems with custom software modules is another approach that has demonstrated positive outcomes for people with TBI (Cole and Dehdashti, 1992; Cole et al., 1993; Kirsch et al., 1988; Levine and Kirsch, 1985; Napper and Narayan, 1994). The computer software is designed to present information and deliver prompts in a manner appropriate to the user's cognitive abilities. For example, these types of systems have been used to guide a person through a specific task, such as baking a cake. Before proceeding from one cue to the next, the computer presents instructions that require a response from the user to confirm that an action has been taken.

A topic of interest for many years has been the design and development of portable, electronic memory aids that are specifically intended to address the cognitive needs of people with TBI. Harris (1984) outlined features for a dedicated, electronic memory aid. He emphasized the need for a device with programmable, visual, and spoken cueing capabilities. Research efforts focused on the implementation of such memory aids have been presented (Friedman, 1993; Henry et al., 1989). As information technologies continue to be integrated into small packages, portable systems that can determine a person's location and provide needed information, such as directions to a given destination, will be available (Vanderheiden and Cress, 1992). This theme is elaborated in Chapter 11.

Environmental Control and Interaction

Many types of low- and high-technology appliances and other devices found in the home, school, and workplace are considered commonplace, everyday tools. People have grown so comfortable with some technologies that their functions are often taken for granted: stoves and microwaves for cooking; lamps and overhead fixtures to provide light; televisions, video cassette recorders, radios, and compact disc players to enable people to see and hear information. In general, people have come to accept and (in many ways) rely on these technologies in their lives. Most of these appliances require a specific (usually physical) manipulation of their controls for activation: How do children with TBI and associated physical and cognitive deficits access these everyday tools and interact with their environment?

In the spectrum of assistive technologies, devices termed *environmental control units* can provide a range of environmental control capabilities. Some environmental control units allow very basic on-off operation of electrical appliances. Others provide full control of the television, video cassette recorder, lamps, telephone, and almost any other electrical appliance. Most environmental control units are composed of a transmitter and receiver, which allow commands to be sent through wireless connections so that access is not restricted to specific locations in the immediate environment.

Besides augmenting and facilitating children's operation of many commonplace appliances found in their environment, environmental control technology can also be applied in a therapeutic manner. Some children possess a high degree of motivation to control things in the environment, and this drive can be used as the basis for switch-access training. If a child's present level of physical functioning requires accessing of assistive devices via a single switch, the development of these skills can be achieved through a basic environmental control unit that does nothing more than turn an appliance on or off. Building from one appliance to two, then to three or four presents an activity in which choices have to be made and causal associations are reinforced.

Other methods can be used to modify a child's environment to permit achievement of independent accessibility. Light switches can be changed so that they are activated by a gross touch. Automatic door openers and intercoms, along with other sensors and controllers, can be used to retrofit existing environments. Such structural modifications as building a ramp, widening doorways to provide clearance for a wheelchair, or changing the sink, tub, or shower and commode in a bathroom may also have to be considered as part of addressing a child's ability to move and interact with maximum safety and independence within a setting.

Recreation and Leisure

Often, it is easy to underestimate the importance of recreation and leisure-time activities in relation to other, apparently more critical aspects of a child's recovery from TBI. However, consideration should be given to identifying some activities that a child may have enjoyed prior to the brain injury and that can be enjoyed simply for pleasure and relaxation. In many instances, low-technology adaptations are needed for a child to be able to play with toys, read a book, listen to books on tape, or play board and card games. Books that can be read aloud with a scanner offer children the opportunity to independently perform an activity that might otherwise have been unfulfilling due to poor reading comprehension.

Children can participate in outdoor activities as well. Many types of adaptive recreational equipment are available for activities ranging from skiing to biking to swimming. As a child grows, involvement in sports or other recreational activities offers important experiences for socializing and maintaining good mental and physical health.

Experiences of Three People Using Assistive Technology

This section illustrates through personal thoughts and observations the impact of assistive technology in the lives of three young people who were injured as children. Each of their stories offers insight into the interplay between the person, the technology, and the environment.

Case Study: Bruce

Bruce is a 12-year-old middle-school student who has had the opportunity to use assistive technology after a TBI at age 8. However, because some of the technology was not integrated and monitored fully, it was not used to its full potential.

After acute-care hospitalization, Bruce was involved in a comprehensive rehabilitation program and continues to receive outpatient therapy services through his school. He now attends a regular education class with supportive services.

At the time of Bruce's initial rehabilitation, his brain injury left him with very limited control of his legs. Because of this impairment, he was not predicted to be a functional ambulator in the near future. Bruce also had a nonfunctional left arm and limited use of his right arm, compromising his ability to propel a manual wheelchair. To address mobility, Bruce and his rehabilitation team determined that he had the skills needed to use a power wheelchair.

In ordering Bruce's first power wheelchair, all aspects of his physical functioning, visual perception, and cognition-safety judgment were considered. The power wheelchair was to serve two purposes for Bruce: to facilitate independent mobility and to assist in improving the aforementioned areas of functioning. In addition, the environments in which Bruce was to use the power wheelchair were considered carefully for their accessibility and safety. Transport of the power wheelchair to and from school was also considered. The entire team was invested in providing Bruce with power mobility, and he showed motivation to use a motorized wheelchair. More importantly, Bruce's family was very involved in the selection process and was excited about the functional and therapeutic benefits of independent mobility.

Although mobility was clearly a priority for Bruce and his family, another area that had to be addressed was his ability to communicate, vocally and in writing. Because Bruce had some ability to vocalize and his family was able to understand his speech, an augmentative communication device was not a primary consideration. Familiar communication partners were able to understand him, but novel partners had difficulty. Bruce became reliant on his family to interpret his speech. When he returned to school, communication was problematic, due to the lack of an interpreter or any alternative communication system. Reentering school introduced another problem for Bruce. He had no means of writing effectively, because his fine-motor skills were affected by his injury. He was unable to use a pencil or a typewriter.

To solve Bruce's problems with speech and written output, he was given a portable laptop computer system fitted with a speech synthesizer. This device would serve as a means for typing messages and having them spoken; it would also serve as a writing device for completing homework assignments. Because Bruce had significant limitations with hand function, he found it difficult to reach all the keys on the keyboard; therefore, he was also given the software and equipment needed to enable him to use single-switch scanning to compose messages.

Approximately 1 year after Bruce received his computer, he and his mother were asked about his progress in being understood and completing his homework assignments. They both agreed that he used the computer initially but that it was just too slow for him. Bruce's fine-motor function also had improved, enabling him to access the keyboard. Using the single-switch scanning method slowed the typing process for Bruce, and he became frustrated. They said that interpreting for him was much quicker (as his teachers were getting better at understanding his speech), as was writing his homework assignments for him as he recited. When they were questioned further, they revealed that they received only a limited amount of initial training in the use of the system and that it was not always readily available for Bruce to use. A mounting system had been provided, so that the computer could be mounted on his wheelchair. However, it was not set up by someone knowledgeable in mounting systems. His mother stated that it was too cumbersome for her to figure out. For this reason, Bruce had abandoned the computer system.

Several important lessons can be derived from this case. With respect to the issue of easy access to his computer, valid reasons may have justified the delay in mounting the system. Possibly his wheelchair-driving skills had to develop, and his parents did not want the computer to be damaged. Once his driving skills improved, however, the mount could have been incorporated. If some follow-up intervention had occurred, he would have had access to his computer if it had been mounted properly to his wheelchair. Once that had been accomplished, he could have been trained in its basic operation and focused on a limited number of functions.

Second, too much was expected of Bruce's family in managing his technology. Because families have so much with which to contend when their loved ones return home from their initial rehabilitation, they can experience difficulty in retaining much of the information provided. Thorough training in how to use equipment may occur as part of the discharge process, but only a small percentage of it may be remembered and applied. Therefore, often it is beneficial to start out teaching and applying the basics and gradually to offer more information. A series of outpatient treatment sessions may be necessary.

It is also essential to complete an initial setup of the assistive devices that a patient will be using. For Bruce, this meant integrating the computer with the wheelchair and attaching all components so that the configuration was functional. Just getting through everyday tasks can be difficult; for a family, having to set up technology for accomplishing such tasks can be a substantial burden. It seems that many families are able to help their loved ones to apply technology much more effectively when there is little or no setup.

Over time, children with TBI can often perform tasks more effectively because either they improve in critical skill areas or they adapt to the situation. If Bruce's skills were monitored, he could have had the system grow with him, as the equipment is designed to be accessed via a variety of methods.

Overall, Bruce was given technology that was appropriate for him; however, his experience is an example of how monitoring, training, and follow-up is crucial in maintaining an optimal level of functioning through the use of technology. Table 8-1 summarizes several key points related to the provision and application of assistive technology illustrated by Bruce's experiences.

Case Study: Patrick

Patrick is a 16-year-old young man who will tell you that one of the things on his mind these days is the Scholastic Aptitude Test (SAT) he will be taking this school year. As Patrick is a junior in high school, the SAT is just one of the things on the academic schedule aside from his regular assignments. In addition, Patrick maintains a steady therapy and home-exercise program as he continues to meet both physical and cognitive challenges resulting from his TBI at age 9. Given that Patrick is a self-described "experimenter," it is not surprising to hear him, along with his mother, Pam, talk about a variety of assistive technologies that have played roles in his life.

Following his accident and treatment at an acute-care hospital, Patrick became an inpatient at a regional rehabilitation hospital. Technology was used early in his rehabilitation program. He and his

Table 8-1. Lessons in the Application of Assistive Technology (AT): Bruce's Experience

AT selection process

In the evaluation of a device for spoken or written communication, the capability of the device to support multiple selection methods may be very important. As a child's physical, sensory, and cognitive abilities change, the selection method may change. If so, evaluate the ease with which different input devices can be connected and selection methods set up.

Consider accessibility and safety issues in all the environments in which a child and family want a power wheelchair to be used. Discuss transporting needs during the evaluation process.

Training in the use of AT

Highlight sections of equipment manuals and, when necessary, provide written instruction sets ("cheat sheets"). If family members can find information quickly and easily, chances of using it will be greater.

Identify the most important device features and provide training around those first. Develop a plan for introducing new device features and applications.

Develop a realistic training plan. Build a consensus with all team members: the child using the technology, the parents and family members, educators, and clinicians.

Integration of AT into life situations

Introduce technology in stages if a child with TBI is going to use multiple forms of AT. The order in which specific technology is provided should be guided by the priorities of both child and family if no medical conditions are compromised.

Complete device mounting and placement before discharge. If not all the equipment is available before discharge, an appointment should be scheduled to coincide with its arrival.

Follow-up and monitoring of AT use

Maintain contact with the family after receipt of new technology. (Even brief phone calls provide a means of monitoring device integration.)

Assist the family in identifying supports beyond the clinical team: vendor and manufacturer support, literature, books, and the like.

---

mother are quick to recall how his speech-language, cognitive, and occupational therapeutic regimens included computer-based activities that supported and reinforced physical and cognitive skills that Patrick was relearning.

By age 10, Patrick was back to attending his community school, supplemented by outpatient therapeutic regimens. Even at that young age, Patrick was willing to integrate technology into his daily routine. He reported wearing a portable functional electrical stimulation device during school for perhaps a month so that certain muscle groups would be stimulated by an electrical impulse at specific times as he walked. Although Patrick did not use this device for very long, his (and his parents') willingness to try this device allowed a therapeutic technique to be explored. With that type of openness, Patrick and his family have approached the many assistive and therapeutic technologies that they have encountered. Patrick says, "Nothing [technology] was more trouble than it was worth."

Although Patrick takes notes by hand during class, he uses a personal computer to do homework and to work on programs that supplement his academic studies. For example, he has been studying for the SAT by using a program on his personal computer to work through sample mathematics and language questions. This allows Patrick to further develop his problem-solving skills through guided exploration of information and processes.

Although Patrick primarily uses only his right hand to type on the keyboard, he says that "work would be challenging" without the computer. His mother mentions how much easier it is to edit homework assignments (e.g., a research paper for a sophomore-year class) on the computer. Because of this, Patrick does not find the prospect of revising, making corrections, checking spelling, and other tasks that are part of completing an assignment so overwhelming.

It is not surprising that a 16 year old would use a computer to do his homework. However, for Patrick, several types of technologies have played a role in both his therapy and his daily living experiences. Patrick is still working hard to improve the function of his left arm and hand. For example, he now uses a biofeedback system during therapy sessions to work on further development of his left forearm and hand. He is learning to carry over the control of the muscle responses in his left forearm and hand through relaxation and visual cues that he practices. Patrick says he is "looking for a feeling."

Throughout these last 7 years, Patrick has approached the use of technology as a tool. All the technology he has used, regardless of the length of time, has been perceived as a true "assistive" device. Patrick sees himself as an experimenter and, with the support of his family, maintains an openness to technology that allows the dynamics between person and machine to play out. All the while, though, it is Patrick who is applying the technol-

Table 8-2. Lessons in the Application of Assistive Technology (AT): Patrick's Experience

---

AT selection process

Recognize when a child will use a combination of different technology and strategies for mobility, communication, and the like. Identify the settings in which the child will need to use technology and evaluate options appropriate to those environments.

Consider the capabilities of standard off-the-shelf software in developing computer-based solutions to address cognitive deficits or to supplement academic studies. Evaluate their effectiveness as tools along with specialized software packages.

Training in the use of AT

Family members' comfort level with technology has a significant impact on its use and effectiveness.

Introduction of computers or environmental control devices as therapeutic tools provides the opportunity for training of alternative access methods.

Integration of AT into life situations

The role of AT will change in the life of a child with TBI. As a child's skills and abilities are developed, the need for technology may fade or the application may change.

A child's self-esteem, independence, and control can be enhanced through the appropriate application of AT.

Follow-up and monitoring of AT use

When computer-based activities are integrated successfully into a therapy program, scores and other data generated by the software are more useful sources of information in relation to therapy goals.

Nothing can substitute for active family support and participation.

---

ogy to meet his objectives. When asked to think in general about the role played by technology in his life, Patrick's response was, "Technology has played about half the role. Most of it came from me." Patrick has integrated several types of technologies at different stages of his recovery, for varying amounts of time, and for different purposes. However, all were considered means to gaining greater independence and function. (See Table 8-2 for a summary of points raised by Patrick's approach to assistive technology.)

Case Study: Justin

Justin is 19 years old. In 1989, at the age of 14, he sustained a TBI as the result of a skateboarding accident. He was in a trauma unit at an acute-care hospital for 1 month and then spent 1 year at a rehabilitation facility. He has received physical, occupational, and speech-language therapy since his injury.

Justin's injury affected him in many ways. He is unable to walk, talk, or use either of his arms. Because of the severity of his injury, technology was introduced very early in his recovery, both as a therapeutic tool and as a means to augment or replace lost skills. When Justin began his rehabilitation, the first technology introduced was a laptop computer with specialized software designed to help him communicate both in writing and voice, through the use of voice-output technology. Justin said that he received training at the same time that his therapists were learning the equipment. Later, when he returned to school, he found that the staff there were more knowledgeable about the equipment and,

therefore, able to provide better training. He maintains that the training in both settings was very helpful for him, something he has proved by using his system efficiently whenever he chooses.

Power mobility was also introduced during the course of Justin's rehabilitation, but this element has been an uphill battle for Justin and his family. Although he is capable of operating a power wheelchair, the system originally obtained for him failed to meet his seating needs and never functioned properly. For these reasons, it has not been used. Justin believes that wheelchairs in general often are too big and "sometimes don't get you where you want to go."

Justin attends regular high school classes in his home town. A full-time educational assistant is assigned to be with him throughout the school day. Justin says his computer system has helped him tremendously in high school: "I can do homework faster." However, he also says that he does not like taking it to school functions. "It's bulky, and we are always worried about weather at football games." At home or with close friends, Justin chooses to use his nontechnological systems, such as a letter board, to communicate. This is because "my parents are very fast with my letter board and signals. Having the computer on [the wheelchair] does get in the way of tables and corners."

Justin is an active teenager who likes to do everything. He goes to the mall, church, movies, and school functions. He sings the praises of the technology he has used and how it has helped him to keep up with his schoolwork. He admits, however, that it is not how he chooses to communicate outside of school. When asked what he would change

Table 8-3. Lessons in the Application of Assistive Technology (AT): Justin's Experience

AT selection process

Evaluating a child with TBI for a seating system may occur in stages. Given the probability that a child's physical status will change through the early and middle stages of recovery, final seating and wheelchair base recommendations should not be rushed.

Backup and alternative systems should be identified along with the primary system whenever possible.

Training in the use of AT

Whenever possible, children should participate in staff and family training sessions regarding their AT devices. These experiences contribute to their sense of ownership and empowerment.

When technology is used in an educational setting, multiple staff members should receive some level of training. Sharing the equipment setup and maintenance responsibilities renders the process less overwhelming.

Integration of AT into life situations

Developing a transition plan that includes important operational and application information about each assistive device helps to minimize the amount of time required for a child to begin using existing technology in a new setting.

Durability and strength of an assistive device are as important as its operational features.

Follow-up and monitoring of AT use

As children with TBI mature, they may have increasingly strong preferences about where they will use certain assistive devices.

Decreased use of a device does not always imply abandonment of the technology. The decrease in use may be due to an improvement in physical, sensory, or cognitive skills or to other strategies proving to be more effective in particular settings.

about the technology he is using, he said that he wishes it were "more compact and less delicate." When technology fails (and even when it is working), Justin relies on his manual system for social communication and mobility.

Justin's experiences are a good example of all that can be positive—and, at the same time, limiting—about the use of assistive technology. Technology has been a crucial element in his successful return to school but, at times, use of technology would prohibit him from enjoying an activity fully. His own determination, in conjunction with the support of his family and teachers, has helped to make the use of technology successful. Technology is not responsible for Justin's accomplishments but, without it, his road back to health would have been longer and harder. Table 8-3 summarizes points about the use of assistive technology demonstrated through Justin's story.

Summary

In this chapter, the various types of assistive technology were discussed, as were selection and application issues particularly relevant to children with TBI. Through the experiences of three children who have been using assistive technology since their TBI, both the benefits and pitfalls of assistive technology use were brought to light. Those of us involved in the process of facilitating the integration of assistive technology into people's lives should acknowledge the significant contribution that such technology can make toward recovery from TBI. We should recognize also the strong interaction between a person and technology and environment and the balance that must be achieved for a successful outcome. Appendices 8-1 and 8-2 list resources for further exploration of assistive technology.

Acknowledgments

The authors thank Eric G. Canali for the illustrations included in this chapter.

References

Blackstone SW (1989). Clinical news. Augmentative Communication News 2(6);4.

Bray LJ, Carlson F, Humphrey R, et al. (1897). Physical Rehabilitation. In M Ylvisaker, E Gobble (eds), Community Re-Entry for Head Injured Adults. San Diego: College Hill, 25.

Caves KM (1994). Integrated Interface Systems. Presented at the First International Symposium on Controls for Access and Powered Mobility, September 16–18, Memphis, TN.

Cole E, Dehdashti P (1992). Prosthetic Software for Individuals with Mild Traumatic Brain Injury: A Case Study for Client and Therapist. Proceedings of the Rehabilitation and Assistive Technology Society of North America 1992 Annual Conference. Washington, DC: Rehabilitation and Assistive Technology Society of North America, 170.

Cole E, Dehdashti P, Petti L, Angert M (1993). Design Parameters and Outcomes for Cognitive Prosthetic Software with Brain Injury Patients. Proceedings of the Rehabilitation and Assistive Technology Society of North America 1993 Annual Conference. Washington, DC: Rehabilitation and Assistive Technology Society of North America, 426.

Cook AM, Hussey SM (1995). Assistive Technologies: Principles and Practice. St. Louis: Mosby–Year Book.

DeRuyter F, Kennedy MRT (1991). Augmentative Communication Following Traumatic Brain Injury. In DR Beukelman, KM Yorkston (eds), Communication Disorders Following Traumatic Brain Injury: Management of Cognitive, Language, and Motor Impairments. Austin, TX: PRO-ED, 317.

Doss LS, Reichle J (1991). Using Graphic Organization Aids to Promote Independent Functioning. In J Reichle, J York, J Sigafoos (eds), Implementing Augmentative and Alternative Communication: Strategies for Learners with Severe Disabilities. Baltimore: Paul H. Brookes, 275.

Dunn K (1994). Information Technology and Brain Injury Rehabilitation. In MAJ Finlayson, SH Garner (eds), Brain Injury Rehabilitation: Clinical Considerations. Baltimore: Williams & Wilkins, 238.

Friedman MB (1993). A Wearable Computer that Gives Context-Sensitive Verbal Guidance to People with Memory or Attention Impairments. Proceedings of the Rehabilitation and Assistive Technology Society of North America 1993 Annual Conference. Washington, DC: Rehabilitation and Assistive Technology Society of North America, 199.

Gans BM, Mann NR, Ylvisaker M (1990). Rehabilitation Management Approaches. In M Rosenthal, MR Bond, ER Griffith, JD Miller (eds), Rehabilitation of the Adult and Child with Traumatic Brain Injury. Philadelphia: Davis, 593.

Gianutsos R (1992). The computer is cognitive rehabilitation: it's not just a tool anymore. J Head Trauma Rehabil 7(3);26.

Golinker L, Mistrett SG (1997). Funding. In J Angelo (ed), Assistive Technology for Rehabilitation Therapists. Philadelphia: Davis, 211.

Guerette P, Sumi E (1994). Integrating control of multiple assistive device: a retrospective review. Assist Technol 6(1);67.

Harris J (1984). Methods of Improving Memory. In BA Wilson, N Moffat (eds), Clinical Management of Memory Problems. Rockville, MD: Aspen, 46.

Henry K, Friedman M, Szekeres S, Stemmler D (1989). Clinical Evaluation of a Prototype Electronic Memory Aid. Proceedings of the Rehabilitation and Assistive Technology Society of North America Twelfth Annual Conference. Washington, DC: Rehabilitation and Assistive Technology Society of North America, 254.

Jaffe MB, Mastrilli JP, Molitor CP, Valko AS (1985). Intervention for Motor Disorders. In M Ylvisaker (ed), Head Injury Rehabilitation: Children and Adolescents. San Diego: College Hill, 167.

Kanyer B (1992). Meeting the seating and mobility needs of the client with traumatic brain injury. J Head Trauma Rehabil 7(3);81.

Kirsch NL, Levine SP, Lajiness R, et al. (1988). Improving Functional Performance with Computerized Task Guidance Systems. Proceedings of the International Conference of the Association for the Advancement of Rehabilitation Technology. Washington, DC: Rehabilitation and Assistive Technology Society of North America, 564.

Ladtkow M (1993). Traumatic brain injury and severe expressive communication impairment: the role of augmentative communication. Semin Speech Lang 14(1);61.

Levine SP, Horstmann HM, Kirsch NL (1992). Performance considerations for people with cognitive impairment in accessing assistive technologies. J Head Trauma Rehabil 7(3);46.

Levine SP, Kirsch NL (1985). Cogorth: A Programming Language for Computerized Cognition Orthoses. Proceedings of the Eighth Annual Conference on Rehabilitation Technology. Washington, DC: Rehabilitation and Assistive Technology Society of North America, 359.

Male M (1994). Technology for Inclusion: Meeting the Special Needs of All Students. Needham Heights, MA: Allyn and Bacon.

Molnar GE, Perrin JCS (1983). Rehabilitation of the Child with Head Injury. In K Shapiro (ed), Pediatric Head Trauma. Mount Kisco, NY: Futura, 241.

Napper SA, Narayan S (1994). Cognitive Orthotic Shell. Proceedings of the Rehabilitation and Assistive Technology Society of North America 1994 Annual Conference. Washington, DC: Rehabilitation and Assistive Technology Society of North America, 423.

Reid S, Strong G, Wright L, et al. (1995). Computers, assistive devices, and augmentative communication aids: technology for social inclusion. J Head Trauma Rehabil 10(5);80.

Scherer MJ (1993). Living in the State of Stuck. Cambridge, MA: Brookline Books.

Scherer MJ, McKee BG (1989). But Will the Assistive Technology Device be Used? Proceedings of the Rehabilitation and Assistive Technology Society of North America Twelfth Annual Conference. Washington, DC: Rehabilitation and Assistive Technology Society of North America, 356.

Shaw CG, Monahan LC (1989). Survey of Seating Providers for Patients with Traumatic Brain Injury. Proceedings of the Rehabilitation and Assistive Technology Society of North America Twelfth Annual Conference. Washington, DC: Rehabilitation and Assistive Technology Society of North America, 272.

Trefler E, Hobson DA, Taylor SJ, et al. (1993). Seating and Mobility for Persons with Physical Disabilities. Tucson, AZ: Therapy Skill Builders.

Turnbull AP, Turnbull HR III, Shank M, Leal D (1995). Exceptional Lives: Special Education in Today's Schools. Englewood Cliffs, NJ: Prentice Hall.

Vanderheiden GC, Cress CJ (1992). Applications of Artificial Intelligence to the Needs of Persons with Cognitive Impairments: The companion aid. Proceedings of the Rehabilitation and Assistive Technology Society of North America Twelfth Annual Conference. Washington, DC: Rehabilitation and Assistive Technology Society of North America, 388.

Ylvisaker M, Szekeres SF, Hartwick P, Tworek P (1994). Cognitive Intervention. In R Savage, GF Wolcott (eds), Educational Dimensions of Acquired Brain Injury. Austin, TX: PRO-ED, 165.

Appendix 8-1
Assistive Technology: Organizations and Information Sources

Organizations

Closing the Gap, Inc.
P.O. Box 68
Henderson, MN 56044
Tel: 507-248-3294
Web site: http://www.closingthegap.com

International Society for Augmentative and Alternative Communication (ISAAC)
P.O. Box 1762
Station R
Toronto, ON M4G 4A3
Canada

National Easter Seal Society
230 West Monroe Street
Suite 1800
Chicago, IL 60606
Tel: 800-221-6827
Web site: http://www.seals.com

National Rehabilitation Information Center (NARIC)
8455 Colesville Road, Suite 935
Silver Spring, MD 20910-3319
Tel: 800-346-2742
Web site: http://www.naric.com/naric

Rehabilitation and Assistive Technology Society of North America (RESNA)
1700 North Moore Street, Suite 1540
Arlington, VA 22209-1903
Tel: 703-524-6686
Web site: http://www.resna.org/resna/reshome.htm

Team Rehab Report
Miramar Communications Inc.
23815 Stuart Road
P.O. Box 8987
Malibu, CA 90265-8987
Tel: 800-543-4116
Web site: http://www.teamrehab.com

Trace Research and Development Center
S-151 Waisman Center
1500 Highland Avenue
University of Wisconsin
Madison, WI 53705-2280
Tel: 608-262-6966
Web site: http://www.trace.wisc.edu

Web Sites of Interest

The following list suggests World Wide Web sites for assistive technology, TBI, special education, and related topics:

http://www.icdi.wvu.edu/others.htm
West Virginia Rehabilitation Research and Training Center. A comprehensive list of disability-related sites.

http://www.asel.udel.edu
Applied Science and Engineering Laboratories at the University of Delaware–A.I. DuPont Institute, a resource for assistive technology research, development, and information dissemination.

http://www.cec.sped.org
Home page of the Council for Exceptional Children.

http://www.sped.ukans.edu
Home page for the Department of Special Education at the University of Kansas.

http://www.callamer.com/~cns/rehab/refs.html
Use to gain access to research articles in the field TBI from this site. Updated weekly.

http://www.familyvillage.wisc.edu
The Family Village is a virtual community of disability-related resources on the World Wide Web.

Appendix 8-2
Assistive Technology: Manufacturers and Distributors

Category key:
AAC = alternative and augmentative communication
CA = computer access
EC = environmental control
ID = input devices and switches
SM = seating-positioning and mobility
SW = software (educational, cognitive, etc.)
VS = vision-sensory devices or software

AbleNet, Inc. (AAC, ID)
1081 10th Avenue SE
Minneapolis, MN 55414-1312
Tel: 612-379-0956; 800-322-0956

ADAMLAB (AAC)
33500 Van Born Road
P.O. Box 807
Wayne, MI 48184
Tel: 313-467-1415

Adaptivation (ID)
224 SE 16th Street, Suite 2
Ames, Iowa 50010
Tel: 515-233-9185

Ai Squared (CA)
P.O. Box 669
Manchester Center, VT 05255-0669
Tel: 802-362-3612

American Printing House for the Blind (VS)
P.O. Box 6085
1839 Frankfort Avenue
Louisville, KY 40206-0085
Tel: 502-895-2405; 800-223-1839

Apt Technology, Inc. (CA, EC, ID)
DU-IT Control Systems Group, Inc.
8765 Township Road 513
Shreve, OH 44676-9421
Tel: 216-567-2001

Arkenstone, Inc. (VS)
555 Oakmead Parkway
Sunnyvale, CA 94086-4023
Tel: 408-245-5900; 800-444-4443

Artic Technologies (VS)
55 Park Street
Troy, MI 48083
Tel: 810-588-7370

Berkeley Access (VS)
Division of Berkeley Systems, Inc.
2095 Rose Street
Berkeley, CA 94709
Tel: 510-883-6270

Blazie Engineering (VS)
105 E. Jarrettsville Road
Forest Hill, MD 21050
Tel: 410-893-9333

BrainTrain, Inc. (SW)
727 Twin Ridge Lane
Richmond, VA 23235
Tel: 804-320-0105

Broderbund Software, Inc. (SW)
500 Redwood Boulevard
P.O. Box 6121
Novato, CA 94948-6121
Tel: 415-382-4400; 800-521-6263

Cascade Designs/Varilite (SM)
4000 1st Avenue
Seattle, WA 98134
Tel: 206-583-0583

Davidson and Associates, Inc. (SW)
19840 Pioneer Avenue
Torrance, CA 90503
Tel: 310-793-0600; 800-545-7677

Don Johnston Incorporated (AAC, CA, ID, SW)
1000 North Rand Road
Building 115
P.O. Box 639
Wauconda, IL 60084
Tel: 847-526-2682; 800-999-4660

Dragon Systems, Inc. (CA)
320 Nevada Street
Newton, MA 02160
Tel: 617-965-5200

Dunamis, Inc. (CA, SW)
3423 Fowler Boulevard
Lawrenceville, GA 30244
Tel: 770-279-1144; 800-828-2443

Edmark Corporation (CA, SW)
P.O. Box 97021
Redmond, WA 98073-9721
Tel: 206-556-8427; 800-426-0856

Everest and Jennings (SM)
4203 Earth City Expressway
Earth City, MO 63045
Tel: 800-235-4661

Freedom Designs, Inc. (SM)
2241 Madera Road
Simi City, CA 93065
Tel: 800-331-8551

Gus Communications, Inc. (AAC, CA, EC)
1006 Lonetree Court
Bellingham, WA 98226
Tel: 360-715-9633

Hartley (SW)
9920 Pacific Heights Boulevard
San Diego, CA 92121-4330
Tel: 619-587-0087; 800-247-1380

Imaginart (AAC)
307 Arizona Street
Bisbee, AZ 85603
Tel: 800-737-1376

Innocomp (AAC, ID)
26210 Emery Road
Suite 302
Warrensville Heights, OH 44128
Tel: 216-464-3636; 800-382-8622

IntelliTools (AAC, CA, SW)
55 Leveroni Court
Suite 9
Novato, CA 94949
Tel: 415-382-5959; 800-899-6687

Invacare Corporation (SM)
899 Cleveland Street
Elyria, OH 44035
Tel: 216-329-6000

Jay Medical (SM)
Sunrise Medical
4745 Walnut Street
Boulder, CO 80301
Tel: 303-422-5539

LaBac Systems, Inc. (SM)
8955 South Ridgeline Boulevard
Highlands Ranch, CO 80126
Tel: 303-791-6000

Laureate Learning Systems, Inc. (SW)
110 East Spring Street
Winooski, VT 05404
Tel: 802-655-4755; 800-562-6801

Learning Company (SW)
6493 Kaiser Drive
Fremont, CA 94555
Tel: 510-713-6011; 800-227-5609

Life Sciences Associates (SW)
1 Fenimore Road
Bayport, NY 11705-2115
Tel: 516-472-2111

Madenta Communications. Inc. (CA, ED, ID)
9411A-20 Avenue
Edmonton, AB T6N 1E5
Canada
Tel: 403-450-8926; 800-661-8406

MarbleSoft (SW)
12301 Central Avenue NE, 205
Blaine, MN 55434
Tel: 612-755-1402

Mayer-Johnson Company (AAC)
P.O. Box 1579
Solana Beach, CA 92075-1579
Tel: 619-550-0084

MECC (SW)
6160 Summit Drive N
St. Paul, MN 55430-4003
Tel: 612-569-1500, ext. 529; 800-685-6322, ext. 529

Microsystems Software, Inc. (CA, VS)
600 Worchester Road
Framingham, MA 01701
Tel: 508-879-9000; 800-828-2600

MindPlay (SW)
160 West Fort Lowell
Tucson, AZ 85705
Tel: 520-888-1800; 800-221-7911

Origin Instruments (CA, ID)
854 Greenview Drive
Grand Prairie, TX 75050
Tel: 972-606-8740

Otto Bock Reha (SM)
3000 Xenium Lane North
Minneapolis, MN 55441
Tel: 612-553-9464

Parrot Software (SW)
6505 Pleasant Lake Court
West Bloomfield, MI 48322
Tel: 800-727-7681

Permobil, Inc. (SM)
6B Gill Street
Woburn, MA 01801
Tel: 800-736-0925

Prentke Romich Company (AAC, CA, EC, ID)
1022 Heyl Road
Wooster, OH 44691
Tel: 330-262-1984; 800-262-1984

Psychological Software Services, Inc. (SW)
6555 Carrollton Avenue
Indianapolis, IN 46220
Tel: 317-257-9672

Quickie Designs (SM)
Sunrise Medical
2842 Business Park Avenue
Fresno, CA 93727
Tel: 209-292-2171

RJ Cooper and Associates (CA, ID, SW)
24843 Del Prado
Suite 283
Dana Point, CA 92629
Tel: 714-240-4853; 800-RJ-COOPER

Sentient Systems Technology, Inc. (AAC)
2100 Wharton Street
Suite 630
Pittsburgh, PA 15203
Tel: 412-381-4883; 800-344-1778

Snug Seat, Inc. (SM)
10810 Independence Pointe Parkway
Matthews, NC 28105
Tel: 704-847-0772

Sunburst Communications (SW)
101 Castleton Street
Pleasantville, NY 10570
Tel: 914-747-3310; 800-321-7511

TASH Inc. (CA, EC, ID)
Unit 1, 91 Station Street
Ajax, ON L1S 3H2
Canada
Tel: 905-686-4129; 800-463-5685

TeleSensory (VS)
455 North Bernardo Avenue
Mountain View, CA 94039-7455
Tel: 415-960-0920

Tumble Forms/Sammons Preston (SM)
4 Sammons Court
Bolingbrook, IL 60440
Tel: 708-226-1300

UCLA Intervention Program for Children with Disabilities (SW)
1000 Veteran Avenue
Room 23-10
Los Angeles, CA 90095
Tel: 310-825-4821

Whitmyer Biomechanix, Inc. (SM)
1833 Junwin Court
Tallahassee, FL 32308
Tel: 904-656-9448

Words+, Inc. (AAC, CA, ID)
40015 Sierra Highway, B-145
Palmdale, CA 93550-2117
Tel: 800-869-8521

World Communications (CA)
245 Tonopah Drive
Fremont, CA 94539
Tel: 510-656-0911

Zygo Industries, Inc. (AAC, EC, ID)
P.O. Box 1008
Portland, OR 97207
Tel: 503-684-6006; 800-234-6011

Chapter 9

A Framework for Cognitive Rehabilitation

Mark Ylvisaker and Shirley F. Szekeres

Clinicians and investigators alike have long observed that cognitive and related behavioral and psychosocial themes tend to dominate the long-term outcome after traumatic brain injury (TBI). In addition, cognitive profiles of children whose injuries occur after they have established a solid base of knowledge and skill often differ greatly from the common profiles of children with congenital cognitive impairment. The issues associated with cognitive disability after TBI can be exceedingly complex, justifying considerable effort on the part of those charged with helping children with TBI in their pursuit of cognitive improvement and success in daily tasks. Knowledgeable intervention requires a thorough understanding of cognition, its development, its disruption after TBI, and its potential for rehabilitation. This chapter, which is designed to facilitate such understanding, lays the foundation for subsequent chapters that address cognitive assessment and intervention.

Rationale for a Conceptual Framework

Clinical activity without a conceptual framework is blind; models and theories uninformed by clinical experience, therapeutic skill, and personal commitment are hollow. In this chapter, we offer a set of descriptive categories and intervention principles to guide cognitive rehabilitation for children and adolescents in medical and educational settings. The framework is derived from current cognitive research and theory filtered through many years of clinical experience with several hundred children and adolescents with TBI.

A framework of categories for understanding cognition and of principles for directing cognitive rehabilitation enables clinicians to achieve the following goals:

- To organize observations and descriptions of individuals' cognitive strengths and weaknesses, thereby enabling comprehensive assessment and effective communication among the many professionals interested in the cognitive dimensions of behavior
- To design intervention at two levels: (1) general, or concerned with overall program development, and (2) specific, or concerned with goals, objectives, and activities for specific individuals
- To define criteria for measuring progress and making judgments about placement, services, and supports
- To generate novel intervention procedures

A rehabilitation program for individuals with cognitive disability inevitably involves assumptions about normal cognitive functioning and about the nature of and interrelationships among cognitive deficits after brain injury. In the absence of a considered theoretical framework for cognitive intervention, clinicians may use a haphazard workbook-exercise approach, assuming that components of cognitive dysfunction can be isolated and treated separately and that aspects of cognition respond most effectively to decontextualized strengthening exercises. Both of these assumptions are very likely mistaken with regard to most aspects of cognition. In contrast, rehabilitative efforts that are consistent with current theories in cognitive science are sensitive to important interrelationships among aspects of cognitive functioning and to the need to embed intervention in meaningful context and content. Furthermore, when underlying theoretical hypotheses are stated and examined within an explicit intervention framework, principles of intervention are more readily derived, and the framework itself can be more easily evaluated in relation to the progress of the individuals served.

The selection of a framework for cognitive rehabilitation for children and adolescents is particularly challenging. In addition to differing conceptions of cognition (Flavell et al., 1993), there are varied explanations of cognitive development (e.g., piagetian versus vygotskyan

Table 9-1. Framework of Categories for Describing Cognitive Functions

Component systems
    Working memory
    Long-term memory (knowledge base)
    Executive system
    Response system
Component processes
    Attentional processes
    Perceptual processes
    Memory and learning processes
    Organizational processes
    Reasoning and problem-solving processes
Functional-integrative performance
    Efficiency
    Level
    Scope
    Manner

versus information-processing perspectives [Flavell et al., 1993; Siegler, 1991]), emerging but incomplete information about brain-behavior relationships (e.g., Pennington, 1991), sketchy information about the long-term evolution of symptoms over the years after an acquired brain injury in children (see Chapter 2; also Koskiniemi et al., 1995), and inadequately validated measures of cognitive functioning in children with specific types of brain injury, especially prefrontal injury (although work in this area is progressing rapidly; see Chapter 10).

A framework that is capable of guiding cognitive rehabilitation for children and adolescents must at least provide working answers to the following questions:

- What is the nature of the cognitive system that has been disrupted by brain injury?
- What are the dominant features of cognitive development in childhood?
- What are the typical patterns of cognitive disability after brain injury and of natural cognitive recovery?
- What are the general goals of cognitive rehabilitation?
- What are the most defensible approaches to cognitive rehabilitation at different ages and stages of recovery?
- What is the best system within which to deliver needed services and provide appropriate supports?

These questions form the outline for this chapter, which closes with a list of cardinal rules for cognitive rehabilitation.

Aspects of Cognition

Cognition, understood in appropriately broad terms, encompasses all of the mental processes, operations, and

systems that are posited to explain the acquisition and use of knowledge and, more precisely, to explain organized, goal-directed behavior (Flavell et al., 1993). For more than three decades, cognitive functioning has commonly been described in broad information-processing terms. We have followed this tradition because its general categories support comprehensive descriptions of cognitive disability and are clinically fruitful. Detailed theories within this tradition are presented in a number of published texts (e.g., Ashcraft, 1994; Baddeley, 1990; Parkin, 1993). We emphasize that the descriptive framework of categories of cognitive components presented here is intended to be nothing more than a proposal for talking about complex cognitive phenomena and organizing cognitive intervention. The framework certainly is *not* an explanatory model of the sort that abound in textbooks on cognitive science.

For clinicians in the field of cognitive rehabilitation to embrace a specific model of cognition is hazardous and certainly unnecessary. Among other dangers, defining intervention efforts around specific boxes and arrows hypothesized in a particular model of cognitive activity runs the risk of targeting purported psychological realities that may well be absent from subsequent models. More than 100 years ago, William James (1890) explained the heuristic value of models that included connected circles, squares, and lines to represent hypothesized aspects of cognition, but he cautioned against assuming that a given model might present an accurate picture of real structures and events in the human brain. More generally, careless talk of cognitive processes and systems in cognitive rehabilitation easily transports practitioners back a century to faculty psychology (i.e., the mind as composed of separate faculties) and the doctrine of formal discipline associated with faculty psychology (i.e., that it is possible to "discipline" or train the forms or faculties of the mind, in a way that has enduring and generalized effects, with exercises such as studying Latin and geometry) (Mann, 1979; Singley and Anderson, 1989). We do not wish to promote such retrograde intellectual motion.

Dodd and White (1980) noted that much of the research in cognitive psychology has been dominated by three approaches: (1) studying the *structure* of cognition (i.e., components such as working memory, long-term memory, and the executive system and their interrelationships); (2) studying the *processes* or *operations* or *activities* that are believed to be involved in taking in, interpreting, considering, and retrieving information and formulating a response; and (3) studying *functional behavior in context*, including the purposes and goals of individuals dealing with available or potential information as they act within and interact with an environment. Thus, cognition encompasses the processing of information, which occurs within certain mental systems or structures and for purposes of achieving meaningful goals in natural contexts.

Table 9-1 summarizes one of many ways to categorize the components hypothesized to explain complex cognitive behavior. The three main headings in this descriptive category system—cognitive systems, cognitive processes, and functional-integrative performance—capture the three primary dimensions of cognition reviewed by Dodd and White (1980).

Cognitive training for individuals with no identified cognitive impairment and for those with developmental cognitive problems (e.g., a learning disability) has been attempted for centuries. Many reviews of the effectiveness of this intervention (e.g., Herrmann et al., 1992; Mann, 1979), as well as some reviews of more recent attempts to retrain cognition after brain injury (e.g., Butler and Namerow, 1988; Ponsford, 1990; Ylvisaker and Urbanczyk, 1990), have cautioned clinicians to avoid conceiving of cognition as a set of separate components that can be understood as operating independently of one another and as yielding to training efforts that are insensitive to the complex interrelationships among aspects of cognition and between cognition and other dimensions of human function. Indeed, the word *interrelationships* might itself imply a greater degree of independence than can be legitimately assumed.

Consistent with this wise counsel, we do not apply categorical terms such as *attention, memory, organization,* or subcategorical terms such as *selective attention, episodic memory,* or *sequencing processes,* to refer to separate boxes in a mechanistic model of cognitive activity or to geographically distinct regions of the brain. Indeed, our discussions of assessment and intervention (Chapters 10–12) emphasize the difficulties and dangers inherent in attempting to separate enmeshed functions such as memory, organization, and the executive system and to understand them as existing independently of the individuals in whom they are studied, people who are pursuing meaningful goals in their real worlds. The value of the somewhat arbitrary category scheme proposed in this chapter is simply that it (1) gives diverse professionals a vocabulary with which they might communicate clearly with one another about complex cognitive issues, (2) supports comprehensive exploration and description of individuals' cognitive strengths and weaknesses, (3) creates a basis for exploring interrelationships among aspects of cognition, and (4) proffers an invitation to intervene creatively on the basis of that exploration.

The inclusion of aspects of functional-integrative performance in our category scheme (which serves as our operational definition of cognition) highlights the functional and real-world approach to cognitive rehabilitation we wish to promote. Research neuropsychologists and clinicians alike have noted the frequency with which individuals with frontal lobe injury or immaturity exhibit evidence of content knowledge and cognitive skill in response to highly structured and decontextualized tests yet do not make use of that knowledge and skill in real-world tasks (Lezak, 1982; Stuss and Buckle, 1992; Varney and Menefee, 1993). Teuber (1964) described this "riddle of the frontal lobes" as "the curious dissociation between knowing and doing." This situation parallels that documented for decades by developmental language specialists, who have frequently observed individuals' acquisition of linguistic knowledge and skills in training contexts with no application of these skills in natural settings.

In other cases, the relationship is reversed, such that high-level cognitive performance is evident in real-world tasks but not in response to formal tests. This latter situation is parallel to that of infants and toddlers who often interact effectively in natural contexts with caregivers but who doggedly refuse to reveal their knowledge and skill under formal testing conditions. These and related observations have led us to include functional-integrative performance variables in our operational definition of cognition, perhaps increasing the likelihood that these important dimensions of human cognition will be included in functional assessment and intervention plans.

Component Systems of Cognition

Working Memory

Working memory has traditionally been characterized as the *short-term storage* or *holding space* in which organizing and coding occur (Deutsch and Deutsch, 1975). Its primary characteristics are limited storage capacity and rapid loss of information. Although the *structural* capacity of working memory is limited (seven plus or minus two units in normal adults [Miller, 1956]), its *functional* capacity can be increased by grouping or "chunking" elements into meaningful units and by making these organizing systems automatic (Chi, 1978). Information is lost easily from working memory unless deliberate action is taken to preserve it (e.g., rehearsing information or coding it for storage). What is done with information in working memory depends in part on an individual's goals. As characterized, working memory is closely tied to the traditional concept of short-term memory, associated with transient electrochemical events in the brain, and is contrasted with long-term storage, which entails structural nervous system change.

The concept of working memory has grown richer and more interesting in recent years as a result of the work of Baddeley and his colleagues. These investigators approached the study of working memory from an evolutionary perspective (i.e., "What is the purpose of working memory?") and used a series of clever experiments (Baddeley, 1986, 1989). To explain their interesting findings, Baddeley and colleagues developed a model that "assumes a controlling central executive of limited capacity that is aided by a number of subsidiary slave systems" (Baddeley, 1989, p. 111).

The two working memory subsystems that have been explored are the visuospatial sketchpad and the articulatory loop. The *visuospatial sketchpad*, involved in the setting up and temporary maintenance of visuospatial images, is said to underlie the effect of imagery in verbal learning and is possibly associated with performance of spatial problem-solving and other tasks. The *articulatory loop* is hypothesized to be a short-term phonologic store, and impairment in this system might be associated with language comprehension deficits, difficulty learning to read and speak a second language, and difficulty with mental arithmetic.

Although structural capacity of working memory (as measured by digit span) is not among the memory functions most commonly impaired by closed head injury (Brooks, 1983), its capacity *is* reduced by the injury in some cases, whereas in others its capacity is limited pretraumatically, and in yet others the *functional* capacity of working memory is dramatically reduced by virtue of impaired organizing processes. Because effective processing of information that exceeds an individual's working memory capacity is difficult, organizational processes that expand functional working memory are essential to effective processing. If the capacity of an individual's working memory has been reduced or if his or her organizational skills are weak, information must be presented in graphic form for permanence (e.g., written words, symbols, pictures) or in small quantities, with cues, that enable the individual to chunk the information.

Long-Term Memory (Knowledge Base)

Long-term memory, sometimes referred to as the *knowledge base*, is the permanent memory record or store of knowledge. It contains memories of personal experiences (episodes); general information; social information, rules, and roles; learned skills and routines; knowledge of organizational frameworks; abstracted life scripts; goals; and self-concept. The system is believed to be highly organized, with multiple connections among related concepts, words, events, and other stored information. A variety of models have been proposed to explain how information is stored and organized in semantic memory (e.g., in networks and systems of networks of semantic relations or in feature hierarchies, propositions, and schemes) (Anderson, 1976; Rummelhart, 1984; Smith, 1978).

Rehabilitation professionals' interest in the integrity of long-term memory is often restricted to retrograde amnesia, the inability to recall events experienced during a period before the injury. However, the intactness of long-term retention and organization of all types of knowledge, not just autobiographical knowledge, has great functional significance for cognitive recovery because this knowledge and its organization are involved in virtually every human activity. It is commonly reported that pretraumatically acquired knowledge and skills return quite completely in all but the most severe cases of TBI (Kinsbourne and Wood, 1982). In our experience with large numbers of children and adolescents with moderate or severe injury, however, in-depth academic

and language testing reveals, in most cases, some reduction in semantic memory or major gaps in the system or decreased organization of the information. Many individuals continue to evidence a reduction in their pretraumatically acquired knowledge base after resolution of posttraumatic amnesia (PTA) and the return of functional episodic memory.

More importantly, young people with severe TBI typically evidence reduced learning capacity, resulting in a failure to add to their knowledge base at an age-appropriate rate. Because the effect of this new learning impairment is cumulative, the student may fall progressively further behind in school over the years after the injury. This is one of several explanations for the common phenomenon of delayed consequences of TBI in children (see Chapter 2). Locating gaps in the knowledge base, promoting recovery of preinjury knowledge, and identifying the most effective ways to teach new content are primary areas of cognitive concern in working with young people with TBI.

The following descriptions of types (or divisions) of memory (Ashcraft, 1994) do not imply a commitment to the view that each type represents a cognitively and anatomically distinct memory system that operates differently from the others. Our discussion is consistent with the view that, from a neuropsychological perspective, distinct types of memory can be understood as different only in that they involve different networks and systems of networks of stored units of information. Thus, for example, episodic memories are stored in a way that involves binding of information with awareness of the context of learning. This understanding of types of memory is consistent with Neisser's (1989) characterization of domains of memory as categories of "memoria," or things we remember. Using this definition, one can be sensitive to the variety of possible memory disturbances but remain focused on the questions that are most critical for intervention:

1. How do people get information into storage so that the units are as strongly represented as possible?
2. How do people store information (including facts, meanings, rules, episodes, movement patterns, and much more) in organized networks and systems of networks for ease of retrieval?
3. How do people most efficiently get information out of organized storage when they need it?

Episodic and Semantic Memory.   *Episodic memory* includes the encoding, storage, and retrieval of personally experienced events or episodes and associated information about when and where the events were experienced (e.g., remembering that I saw the Yankees play the Red Sox yesterday at Fenway Park) (Tulving, 1972, 1989). It has been described as a sort of autobiographical memory in that the memory traces include contextual information, such as the time, place, and conditions of an episode. There is some evidence that episodic memory develops over the preschool years partly as a result of caregivers' elaborative interactions with children about their past experiences (Nelson, 1992; Reese et al., 1993).

In contrast, *semantic* memory is free of context. That is, information is stored independently of when, where, and how it was acquired (e.g., knowledge that baseball games have nine innings). A large quantity of general information as well as abstracted and organized knowledge about words, meanings, relations, concepts, rules, scripts, and strategies is stored in semantic memory (Brown, 1975, 1979; Kinsbourne and Wood, 1982; Tulving, 1972).

Episodic and semantic memory interrelate in many ways. For example, some researchers presume that many items currently in semantic memory may first have been represented as specific episodes (Baddeley, 1982). Furthermore, not uncommonly, episodic elements are combined with abstracted knowledge. The distinction may not be neat, but it is clinically useful nonetheless. Amnesia is associated most closely with severe episodic memory disorders, consistent with an individual's residual ability to learn information and skills but with no awareness of having had the learning experience (see the section on Explicit and Implicit Memory).

Measures of PTA are commonly used to chart recovery and predict outcome after TBI (Brooks, 1984). By standard definition, PTA includes elements of episodic memory loss and of disorientation to person, place, and time (Levin et al., 1982). In very severe cases, confusion, disorientation, and severe memory problems can last months after an injury or continue indefinitely. Furthermore, the return of adequate orientation does not necessarily coincide with the return of continuous memory for ongoing events, and both may recover so gradually that assigning a termination date to PTA is virtually impossible.

Declarative and Procedural Memory.   The distinction between declarative memory and procedural memory corresponds roughly to the distinction between *knowing that* (i.e., memory for facts) and *knowing how* (i.e., memory for rules, motor patterns, mechanical procedures, and similar sequences). This distinction overlaps with other memory types listed in this section (e.g., both episodic and semantic memory have been characterized as types of declarative memory [Squire, 1987]) and is not completely unambiguous. Some investigators emphasize the conscious awareness and explicitness of declarative memory, aligning this distinction from procedural memory more closely with the distinction between explicit and implicit memory. Nonetheless, the classification of declarative versus procedural memory serves to remind clinicians that individuals with apparently severe learning difficulties and difficulty consciously recalling facts may nevertheless be successful at learning rules and procedures (Parkin, 1993; Schacter, 1987). This is notably true of people with selective hippocampal damage, which

is common in TBI. Procedural learning may be relatively more critical in vocational and independent living contexts than in school, where the focus is on learning facts.

Explicit and Implicit Memory.   Over the last 10 years, increasing attention has been paid to the distinction between explicit and implicit memory to explain the observed capacity of people with dense amnesia to learn new information and skills (Graf and Masson, 1993). The distinction is between different ways in which the effects of earlier experiences can be revealed (Schacter and Church, 1992). Explicit memory includes deliberate recollection of information and conscious recognition of having learned the information. By contrast, implicit memory occurs when an individual's performance is influenced by previous exposure to information, even though that person may not intend to recall the information and has no recollection of having been exposed to the information. Implicit memory experiments often involve verbal learning paradigms in which the individual may fail to recall any of the previously presented words or the experience of exposure to the words but nevertheless will recognize previously presented words more readily than nonpresented words or will recall previously presented words with phonetic priming. A vivid illustration of this distinction is the teenager with brain injury subsequent to a gunshot wound, who learned algebra in math class at a normal rate and scored well on tests without recalling that he had been taught the material or had been present in the classes.

This distinction is sufficiently new that there continues to be controversy about the phenomena and associated definitions (e.g., Jacoby, 1994). From an intervention perspective, however, the introduction of the categories of explicit and implicit memory is fruitful because they acknowledge that people with severe amnesia might nonetheless be able to learn and that assessment of that learning must be creative and circumvent the manifest impairment of these people—namely, that affected individuals do not consciously recall either the information or the experience of learning it.

Recent developments in the understanding of implicit memory have also yielded a caution that "errorless learning" must be promoted for people with severe explicit memory impairment (Wilson and Evans, 1996): That is, for the person who does not consciously recall learning experiences, avoidance of rehearsing errors is particularly important; otherwise, those errors might become part of the individual's repertoire. This important principle is distinct, however, from the notion that errors may contribute significantly to self-awareness in the case of people with less severe memory impairment.

Executive System

The executive system comprises those mental functions "necessary for formulating goals, planning how to achieve them, and carrying out the plans effectively" (Lezak, 1982). Discussions of cognitive psychology, developmental cognitive psychology (e.g., Bjorklund, 1990; Flavell et al., 1993; Siegler, 1991), cognitive neuropsychology (e.g., Shallice, 1988), and cognitive rehabilitation (see Chapter 12) have increasingly emphasized the critical role of the executive system in the development of cognition, effective use of cognitive functions in everyday life, and long-term outcome after TBI in both children and adults. Broadly associated with the large prefrontal areas of the brain (the most vulnerable part of the brain in closed head injury [Levin et al., 1991b]), executive functions are believed to be involved in the control of cognitive activity, including conscious and deliberate activity (e.g., actively creating mnemonic schemes in studying for an examination) as well as more routine cognitive activity (e.g., filtering out distractions so that one can remain focused in conversation). In relation to cognition, *executive functions* might be synonymous with *metacognitive functions*, assuming that the latter term encompasses both a static aspect (i.e., possessing knowledge about one's cognitive system) and a dynamic aspect (i.e., controlling cognitive behavior) (Ylvisaker and Szekeres, 1989). Understood more generally, the concept of executive functions is closely related to the more familiar concepts of self-control, self-management, and self-regulation.

As we use this term, *executive functions* include awareness of one's cognitive strengths and needs and, on the basis of that awareness, the ability to set reasonable goals, plan and organize behavior in pursuit of those goals, initiate behavior toward achievement of the goals, inhibit behavior incompatible with achievement of the goals, monitor and evaluate behavior in relation to the goals, and think strategically and solve problems flexibly in the event of obstacles to achievement of the goals. In relation to language and communication, executive functions are presupposed in controlled and organized conversation, in noninteractive discourse, in controlled searches for words, in directing oneself to interact with others in a socially appropriate manner, in the ability to use language flexibly and abstractly (e.g., decipher ambiguity, understand indirect or abstract language), and, generally, in the effective use of linguistic knowledge and skill in the pursuit of real-world goals. In relation to social behavior, development of executive functions enables one to perceive and appreciate other people's intentions and needs and to guide one's behavior actively by knowledge of social rules, roles, and routines.

Understanding the consequences of frontal lobe injury and possible executive system dysfunction is particularly difficult in children. Standardized measures of executive function development in children are emerging (Levin et al., 1991a, 1996), and the integration of developmental psychology and developmental neuropsychology has yielded considerable insight in this domain (e.g., Roberts and Pennington, 1996; Welsh and Pennington, 1988).

However, variability in individual development, the interaction of organic issues with personality and cultural issues, and the relatively small quantity of long-term outcome data combine to make any predictions of long-term outcome after frontal lobe injury hazardous. Most importantly, the protracted period of normal development of prefrontal areas of the brain and of associated executive functions (from infancy through the adolescent years [Welsh et al., 1991]) creates the possibility—or likelihood—of delayed consequences of the injury, as evidenced by a child's failure to mature in a developmental area that is supported by a part of the brain injured earlier in life (Eslinger et al., 1992; Feeney and Ylvisaker, 1995; Grattan and Eslinger, 1991, 1992; Marlowe, 1992; Mateer and Williams, 1991; Price et al., 1990; Williams and Mateer, 1992; Ylvisaker and Feeney, 1995, 1996).

Response System

The response system, which controls output (including gross- and fine-motor activity, speech, and facial expression), is an element of a broad description of cognition within an information-processing perspective. Response system disability includes neuromuscular disorders (e.g., weakness, spasticity, tremors) and motor-planning problems (incoordination). In addition, many individuals with TBI continue indefinitely to perform motor tasks slowly and to fatigue easily, even with otherwise excellent recovery of motor ability. Thorough cognitive assessment should include an investigation of the relationships between the response system and other cognitive processes and systems. For example, generally slow processing and responding can easily be misunderstood and result in academic failure in school in the absence of appropriate accommodations (e.g., extra time for tests).

Furthermore, if a child has even mildly severe motor problems, a portion of "space" in working memory might be occupied by deliberate attempts to control motor functioning, which is automatically controlled in healthy individuals; the result of such deliberate control attempts is reduced cognitive efficiency. For example, a child may be able to respond effectively in class if his or her body is supported but not if he or she has to fight gravity to remain upright; or a child may be able to converse adequately when seated comfortably but unable to do so when walking or standing in a way that requires effort. Conversely, cognitive impairment can negatively affect motor output. For example, slow cognitive processing or disorganized perception can create the appearance of an impaired motor system.

Component Processes of Cognition

Attention

Attention is the complex process of admitting and holding information in consciousness. Its components include basic *arousal*, *directing* attention, *maintaining* attention, *selecting* particular objects of attention and *filtering* out irrelevant information, *shifting* attention from object to object, and *dividing* attention among two or more objects. (The word *concentration* is often used to refer to the selecting and maintaining aspects of attention.) What one attends to is determined by the characteristics of the impinging stimuli (external or internal) and by the level of arousal or alertness of the individual and by momentary intentions and long-term goals (i.e., motivation). On the one hand, attention may be captured by strong, novel, or significant environmental stimuli (e.g., a loud noise or noxious odor) and is thus a phenomenon of considerable survival value. On the other hand, a person may deliberately direct attention to stimuli if doing so serves a particular purpose (e.g., studying a text or mentally reviewing information in preparation for an examination). Deliberate control over attention is necessary for effective and efficient information processing in less-than-ideal contexts.

Attentional problems resulting from TBI in adults have been emphasized as an important focus of cognitive remediation programs (Ben-Yishay and Diller, 1983; Mateer and Mapou, 1996; Ponsford, 1990; Sohlberg and Mateer, 1989; Wood, 1984, 1992), particularly those programs grounded in a hierarchical approach to cognition and restoration of cognitive function. A certain level of arousal and external focus is assumed by all cognitive activity and, in this sense, attention is basic and should be targeted early in recovery by means of a combination of planned stimulation and environmental and pharmacologic efforts. However, it is possible that attentional problems occur secondary to other cognitive disabilities (e.g., difficulty attending because of a lack of comprehension or organizing skill) or are part of a larger syndrome of impaired executive functions. In these cases, exercises that specifically target attention may be less efficient than interventions that focus on the primary disability. In recent years, a number of clinicians and investigators have come to view a large class of children with congenital attention deficit disorder as having attentional problems secondary to broader executive system dysfunction (e.g., Pennington, 1991) and have promoted an approach to intervention that targets broader organizational and self-regulatory deficits rather than specific attentional symptoms (Hallowell and Ratey, 1994).

In this book, we have chosen to emphasize the purportedly higher-level cognitive functions—organization, executive functions, and social cognition—in part as a response to the disproportionate emphasis on attention and perception in traditional cognitive rehabilitation programs after brain injury. In the real world of clinical decision making, however, decisions must be made carefully and on an individual basis. If a thorough investigation of a child's performance suggests that difficulty focusing, attending selectively, maintaining focus, and shifting and dividing focus are specific to attentional functions, then remedial

exercises, compensatory procedures, or pharmacologic intervention specific to attention may be warranted. Even in this case, however, attentional exercises probably should be structured around meaningful content—for example, practice in selecting, shifting, or dividing using educational software (e.g., math or reading programs)—because of the well-known difficulty of transferring cognitive skills (Singley and Anderson, 1989). In other cases, apparent attentional problems (e.g., wandering conversation, inattention in class) may be more intelligently addressed by a focus on comprehension, organization, or general executive self-regulation of cognitive functions. In every case, the individual's goals and motivation must be considered.

Perception

Perception is the process of detecting distinctive features, invariant relationships, and patterns in stimuli (Gibson, 1969). With experience, it is possible to differentiate more and more features and patterns within stimuli, and recognition may become automatic (e.g., as a football coach sees players running helter-skelter, yet perceives a simple, well-executed fullback-counter-off-tackle-right). In contrast, if an array of stimuli is both complex and unfamiliar, one attempting to understand the stimuli must attend to the array in detail until distinctive features and patterns emerge (e.g., as a novice learning to follow a fast-paced hockey game) (Flavell et al., 1993).

Preexisting knowledge, attentional bias, and preferences make some features of stimuli more noticeable than others (Gibson, 1969). Developmental studies of perception in children 3 years of age and older indicate that as attentional control and knowledge develop, the isolation of perception from other aspects of cognition (e.g., memory, organization, and executive functions) becomes increasingly inappropriate and misleading (Flavell et al., 1993). Mature perceivers process specific kinds of information as circumstances require and, if necessary, search through stimuli for relevant information, directed by their knowledge of the subject and goals. Features also become perceptually salient when an environment is externally structured to highlight them.

The visual-perceptual problems of children and adolescents with TBI may be specific to perception (e.g., the neglect of a visual field or visuospatial disorientation). Alternatively, perceptual problems can result from more general cognitive deficits (e.g., inefficient perception relative to rate, amount, and complexity of the stimuli; difficulty shifting perceptual focus in a flexible manner; and ineffective simultaneous processing of the object of perception and contextual cues). Perceptual symptoms may also be the consequence of impairments of so-called higher cognitive processes or symptoms. For example, perceptual inefficiency may result from generally weak organizing processes, from a shallow knowledge base, or from impaired executive control over attentional or perceptual processes.

Even in those cases in which perceptual problems are primary, if higher functions are relatively intact, effective treatment might involve engaging the child in meaningful higher-level tasks. For example, using meaningful reading texts, rather than conceptually simpler, nonmeaningful materials, as treatment materials may most effectively promote systematic scanning to the left for a student with left visual-field neglect or scanning problems. Construing the meaning of sentences (a purportedly higher-level cognitive activity) often facilitates the task of systematic visual scanning (a purportedly lower-level cognitive activity) for those whose language systems are relatively intact. Of course, improved scanning in reading might not transfer to other perceptual tasks; however, improved reading of meaningful texts would benefit the student substantially in a way in which improved scanning of nonmeaningful materials would not.

Learning and Memory

At the core of cognitive psychology in recent years has been investigation into the nature of memory and learning, types of memory, disorders of memory, and factors that promote improved memory (Baddeley, 1990; Baddeley et al., 1995; Parkin, 1993). The issues are so complex that to summarize a perspective on memory in a chapter such as this is indeed difficult. However, because memory impairment is so common after TBI, attempts to understand cognitive functioning and promote improvement in function require familiarity with basic distinctions in this domain.

Within the general domain of memory, a large number of memory systems and processes have been proposed to explain neuropsychologically distinct types of memory disorders as well as distinct memory phenomena that have emerged in studies of normal subjects. In some cases, the proposed systems and processes have resulted from opposing theoretical perspectives and are intended to cover much the same territory. The net result of reading the current literature is a picture of multiple maps, each bearing the same outline of a large and bewildering territory but crisscrossed by many lines, some indistinct and many appearing in different positions depending on the map-maker (i.e., the theoretical foundation). We have chosen to highlight some of the aspects of memory of particular importance from the perspective of intervention.

The process of learning or remembering involves three stages: encoding, storage, and retrieval of information, each of which applies to varied types of information or *memoria*. The *encoding* or acquisition stage includes the construction of an internal representation of a perceived event. The representation might include a nearly accurate replica (e.g., remembering a speaker's exact words) or an interpretation of the event, contextual information, concurrent internal experiences, and knowledge integrated with the event at the time of encoding. Several interacting factors determine which events are encoded and how much of a given event is encoded, such as the

attentional focus and orientation of the individual (Postman and Kruesi, 1977); the social, emotional, and intellectual significance of the event (Smirnov, 1973); the depth of understanding or degree to which information is integrated into existing knowledge (Brown, 1975, 1979; Moely, 1977; Piaget and Inhelder, 1973); and the type and extent of deliberate elaboration that an individual performs at the time of encoding (Craik and Tulving, 1975; Pressley and El-Dinary, 1992). Therefore, different people may encode the same event quite differently, some forming a shallow or incomplete representation of the event (possibly making the event less memorable) and others forming a deeper and more complete representation that is well integrated with other knowledge (possibly making the event more memorable).

The *storage* stage of memory involves holding information over time in what is believed to be a highly organized long-term memory system (Smith, 1978). At the *retrieval* stage of memory, information is transferred from long-term memory to consciousness. Retrieval can be deliberate and effortful, involving a strategic searching of memory and creative problem solving to reconstruct an event from the bits of information that have been retrieved (Norman, 1976). Retrieval can also be automatic and effortless (e.g., retrieving words during relaxed conversation). Retrieval can even be out of control as, for example, when one finds it impossible to exclude distressing events and ideas from consciousness.

Retrieval is referred to as *recognition* when the stimulus is present and one must merely identify it (e.g., responding to yes-no or multiple-choice questions, or identifying objects or pictures as having been seen before); as *cued recall* when specific cues are given to prompt retrieval (e.g., *wh-* questions or category label); and as *free recall* when the stimulus is not present and must be recalled without cues (e.g., "Tell me what you remember about . . .") (Hintzman, 1978).

Involuntary and Deliberate Memory.   A critical distinction in working with young children and individuals with significant cognitive impairment is that between involuntary (i.e., incidental) memory and deliberate (i.e., effortful, strategic) memory. Here the distinction is not between types of memory content (e.g., episodic and semantic; visual and auditory), but rather between significantly different orientations of the learner at the time of exposure to the information to be learned.

If, by means of the task design, instructions, or incentives, an individual is oriented to the goal of learning or remembering, the task is said to be a *deliberate* or *strategic* learning task (e.g., studying for a test). To be efficient, deliberate learning or memory requires some degree of metacognitive awareness and planning. Means selected to achieve the goal of learning or remembering are generally referred to as *learning* or *memory strategies*, ranging in sophistication from simply looking at information a little longer to rehearsing it mentally to associating it with other knowledge to creating an elaborate organizational framework that ensures retrieval. Although motivation and initiation are prerequisites for efficient deliberate learning, these demands are reduced when the context of learning is a meaningful activity (Brown, 1975).

Deliberate memory is often ineffective in individuals with TBI because of deficits in executive functions, particularly if there is frontal lobe involvement. In extreme cases, turning learning tasks into deliberate memory tasks by suggesting strategies or simply calling attention to the goal of learning ("John, you've got to learn this for the test on Friday" or "Please remember to bring your memory book") may actually *reduce* the individual's ability to learn or remember. Similarly, asking a preschooler to work at remembering or learning interferes with the youngster's natural learning ability. In the case of very young children, one cannot assume the ability to relate to the abstract cognitive goal of learning, the possession of strategic procedures to achieve that goal, or the control over cognitive processes implicit in using strategic procedures to achieve the goal.

In the case of children who, because of immaturity or impairment, are not strategic learners, teaching must focus on the design of the learning activity so that involuntary memory is enhanced. *Involuntary memory* (or *incidental learning type 1* [Postman, 1964]) refers to a condition in which an individual learns and remembers information despite not having been oriented to the task of learning or remembering. That is, the individual does not specifically intend to learn or remember the information but rather is simply engaged in an interesting or personally meaningful activity that has its own internal goal and of which learning is a by-product (Brown, 1979; Smirnov and Zinchenko, 1969). Preschool teachers are masters of creating incidental learning experiences, and preschool students tend to be masters of learning under these circumstances.

It is sometimes mistakenly said that individuals with memory and learning problems must learn under deliberate learning conditions because, by definition, their ability to pick up information "incidentally" is not as efficient as that of their nonimpaired peers. Unfortunately, this recommendation misses the point of involuntary or incidental learning. Great effort can and should go into designing learning tasks so that the learner is actively engaged, wants to achieve the concrete goal of the task, and is clearly oriented to the to-be-learned information as critical to process in order to complete the task. Furthermore, repetition can be as extensive in involuntary learning paradigms as in deliberate learning. Often, individuals with TBI who have become less strategic learners profit from teaching that uses the involuntary learning paradigm, even though their age and knowledge base seem to suggest that they should profit from mature deliberate learn-

ing tasks. These aspects of intervention are discussed further in Chapter 11.

Verbal and Nonverbal Memory.   Because any combination of strengths and deficits is possible after TBI, one might observe relatively severe impairment of *verbal memory* (e.g., memory for language units or information presented with language) or of *nonverbal memory* (e.g., memory for designs, melodies, faces, routes). Certainly, if language comprehension is impaired, one would expect verbal memory to be relatively strongly affected. Within nonverbal memory, the impact on memory for events, routes, faces, and newly taught procedures may vary considerably. The areas of verbal and nonverbal memory should be explored separately during comprehensive cognitive assessment. Discussions of discrete verbal or nonverbal memory impairment have historically been based on studies of individuals with focal and clearly lateralized temporal lobe lesions (Milner, 1970). Closed head injury is generally associated with injury that is bilateral and less likely to produce clearly distinguishable verbal or nonverbal memory disturbance.

Sensory Modality–Specific Memory.   Discussions of congenital learning disability often highlight profound asymmetries between auditory and visual information-processing skills. Indeed, neurologic impairment, whether congenital or acquired, can disrupt auditory and visual information processing and storage systems differently. Therefore, exploration of differential effects is recommended (Lezak, 1983). However, two of the most common sites of injury associated with memory problems in TBI—bilateral prefrontal areas and the hippocampus—are not associated with differential auditory versus visual system effects. Often, memory and learning problems after TBI cut across auditory and visual boundaries.

Retrospective and Prospective Memory.   *Retrospective memory* refers to the usual memory paradigm—that is, the presentation of material to be remembered and subsequent request for recall of that material. Prospective memory is memory for appointments or other events scheduled in the future. Memory for planned future events for children is rarely a major problem because the children's parents and others play the role of a prosthetic prospective memory system. However, prospective memory problems can be manifested in children who routinely forget to do homework or other assigned tasks. (There are, of course, alternative explanations for this forgetfulness, including motivational and cultural variables.) Prospective memory problems in adults can be debilitating, rendering otherwise adequately functional people unable to work or live independently because they routinely "forget to remember" to do what needs to be done. Standard compensatory procedures, such as writing appointments on calendars or in appointment books, may be unsuccessful because the individual forgets to look at the calendar or appointment book. Recently, sophisticated electronic paging and cueing systems (e.g., NeuroPage, discussed in Chapter 11) have been developed for adolescents and adults with severe prospective memory problems.

Implications. Memory and learning problems are among the most commonly reported deficits after TBI. Among these deficits, inefficiency in new learning is the most common and most debilitating for children and adolescents who return to school, as school demands learning efficiency. In this brief discussion of various aspects of memory, we have emphasized its complexity and the variety of possible memory disorders. This complexity and variety call out for comprehensive assessment and careful differential diagnosis of memory and related cognitive problems (discussed in Chapter 10). However, separating memory into components is not necessarily an invitation to address those components separately during intervention. Indeed, the rich literature in educational psychology that deals with students with severe learning problems has increasingly moved toward a holistic approach to intervention, simultaneously addressing many cognitive and noncognitive areas that influence efficiency of information processing and learning (Borkowski et al., 1990; Deshler and Schumaker, 1988; Pressley et al., 1990; Pressley and El-Dinary, 1992). This research has influenced our discussions of cognitive intervention in Chapters 11 and 12.

Organization

An argument could be made for grouping cognitive organization under the heading Executive System. Planning and organizing are often uttered in the same breath when theorists attempt to characterize executive functions. Furthermore, there is considerable evidence that prefrontal injury, associated with executive system dysfunction, commonly results in organizational impairment (Grafman et al., 1993; Levin and Goldstein, 1986; Schwartz et al., 1993; Szekeres, 1992).

An equally strong argument could be made for the inclusion of cognitive organization under the heading Long-Term Memory (Knowledge Base). It is the organization of the knowledge base into networks of information units and systems of networks that supports efficient processing of complex information and organization of complex behavior (Ashcraft, 1994; Bjorklund et al., 1990).

Despite the validity of these points, there remains a rationale for including organizing processes within the category of cognitive processes rather than cognitive systems. Organizing processes are the means by which people relate and group stimuli (ideas, objects, events, people) with reference to information and organizing schemes that are already stored in permanent memory. These processes include analyzing information, identifying relevant perceptual and conceptual features, compar-

ing features and concepts, identifying similarities and differences, classifying and categorizing, sequencing, and integrating information into larger units (e.g., main ideas, themes, scripts). Organizing at the most basic level of processing involves "chunking" or grouping perceptual units (e.g., perceiving visual stimuli as a specific object or recognizing a sequence of sounds as a word). Most organizing at this basic level is automatic. At more complex levels, organizing engages reasoning and problem solving as well as the executive system in complex activities, such as organizing complex content for presentation in a textbook.

Organizing processes are not skills that exist independently of any domain of content. Therefore, it is not necessarily true that an individual who is skilled at organizing things or information in one domain will be skilled at organizing things or information in another domain. For example, a stock boy who is great at organizing products on shelves of a supermarket may be incompetent at organizing books on the shelves of a library. Organizing skill, like other cognitive skills, is tied to more or less specific domains of content. Although it does occur, transfer of cognitive skills across tasks and domains of content is far from automatic, even in the case of bright adults. In children with brain injury, it is important to make no assumptions about transfer and therefore to be sensitive to the importance of contextualizing intervention in meaningful ways.

Organizational disability after closed head injury is common (Levin and Goldstein, 1986) and includes difficulty analyzing a task into its components, sequencing steps in activities of daily living or other complex tasks, arranging task materials and work space, understanding main ideas or central themes in a text, presenting information or telling stories in an organized manner, and remaining on topic in a conversation. Information about the development of organized thinking, acting, and talking is presented in Chapter 11, along with three neuropsychological explanations for breakdowns in the performance of organizationally demanding tasks. We devote a chapter to cognitive organization because it is so frequently impaired after TBI and because of its importance in relation to effective thinking, acting, and talking and its intimate relation to other cognitive functions, notably memory.

Reasoning

Reasoning is the process of considering evidence and making inferences or drawing conclusions. The types of reasoning most commonly analyzed in logic texts and rehearsed using logic and reasoning skills workbooks—namely, deductive and inductive reasoning—are also the types of reasoning least commonly used in everyday life, at least in an explicit manner.

In *deductive reasoning*, inferences are drawn on the basis of formal relations among propositions: That is, if the premises are true, the conclusion *must* be true. Students who acknowledge that passing grades necessitate regular class attendance and admit that they routinely cut class but insist that they will nevertheless receive passing grades are guilty of faulty deductive reasoning. Because reasoning in daily life rarely takes the form of explicitly deductive arguments, training in this type of reasoning (e.g., exercises in syllogistic reasoning common to cognitive rehabilitation workbooks) is of negligible clinical value. The reasoning of even normally bright college students in political science or physics class—or daily life— rarely improves after the students have mastered syllogistic thinking in logic class.

Inductive reasoning involves *direct* inferences from experience, ranging from scientific generalizations to everyday reasoning: For example, "My first two therapies were a waste of time, so they are all probably a waste if time." Induction is distinguished from deduction in that a good inductive argument may have true premises yet a false conclusion. True premises simply increase the probability that the conclusion is true. Errors of induction often take the form of faulty generalizations: For example, "Sarah said she won't go to the prom with me so I'm sure nobody will go with me; nobody likes me."

Analogical reasoning, sometimes considered a type of inductive reasoning, allows us to draw inferences *indirectly* from experience when known relationships are used to explain or predict different but related phenomena. Analogical reasoning is perhaps the most useful form of reasoning in everyday problem solving and decision making. As with most aspects of cognition, it originates in one's preschool years, and there is great variability in development and in adult performance (Gholson et al., 1990). One common example of analogical reasoning is saying to oneself, "In situations such as this in the past, I have tried such and such a solution and it has generally worked, so it's probably a good idea to try that again now."

Problem solving is often based on tacit analogies, which can be dangerous if one sees too many parallels and draws too few distinctions (see next section also). Judging the acceptability of analogical reasoning usually means weighing the *relevance* of the analogy. For example, is the situation in former Yugoslavia more like Vietnam or Iraq or Europe before World War II or none of these? The value of reasoning by analogy depends entirely on the relevance and strength of the analogy. Therefore, although analogy is a powerful and common form of reasoning in both children and adults, evaluation of and training in analogical reasoning are difficult because there are no firm rules, and effective analogical reasoning depends heavily on knowledge of the content. This is one of many reasons to promote acquisition of content knowledge as a critical component of cognitive rehabilitation rather than as an alternative to "rehabilitating cognition."

Evaluative reasoning involves considering the merits of ideas, courses of action, things, or people in relation to explicit or assumed criteria and making judgments of value on the basis of these considerations (e.g., "That's a good idea" or "What he did was wrong" or "It's a great car" or "Tom is a terrific person"). As in induction, mistakes in evaluative reasoning often result from a failure to gather sufficient information before making a value judgment.

From a different perspective, some clinicians have found it useful to classify reasoning or abstract thinking as either convergent or divergent. *Convergent thinking* involves the search for main ideas, central themes, or single conclusions. It includes all the types of reasoning just defined. *Divergent* (lateral or flexible) *thinking* includes identifying a number of exemplars of a concept, listing items that fall under categories, and creatively exploring possible courses of action, information that may be relevant to a given topic, and alternative interpretations of behavior and events.

In young children, reasoning with ideas (versus concrete trial-and-error problem solving with objects) develops slowly, probably as an internalization of "reasoning" interactions with adults and with objects (Vygotsky, 1978). If the latter is true, it provides some support for a conversational and everyday approach to improving reasoning skills after TBI, using everyday communication partners to model and coach increasingly careful thinking in real-world contexts. This approach is in sharp contrast to the standard cognitive rehabilitation practice of rehearsing reasoning skills, in much the same way that logic is taught to undergraduates. In older children with TBI, reasoning impairments can range from a near-total inability to think abstractly and inferentially, to a failure to use reasoning ability when appropriate (impulsive thinking), to a weak exploration of alternative possibilities, to a failure to relate known information to new problems. Stress often contributes to failures in reasoning, including disorganization and impulsiveness. In the years after the injury, young children with TBI may experience difficulty developing abstract thinking and reasoning skills in an age-appropriate manner.

Problem Solving and Judgment

The categories of problem solving and judgment are included in our list of cognitive processes largely because of their significance after TBI. A case could be made for including them under the heading Reasoning or for grouping them with cognitive systems under the heading Executive System. In the final analysis, placement in a descriptive category scheme is less important than appropriate attention to the realities identified by the categories.

Problem solving is a complex form of cognitive activity designed to achieve a goal in the presence of obstacles. Organized, deliberate problem solving includes (1) identifying the goal and clarifying the problem; (2) gathering and considering information that may be relevant to solving the problem; (3) exploring possible solutions, weighing their relative merits, and choosing the best; (4) formulating a plan of action; (5) executing the plan; and (6) monitoring and evaluating the plan's effectiveness. As such, problem solving includes as components most other types of thinking and reasoning. If a procedure exists that can generate a single correct solution (e.g., problem solving in mathematics), the problem-solving process is regarded as closed-ended. Real-life problem solving (or decision making) is most often open-ended in that no rule or set of rules determines exactly what information is relevant in thinking about the problem or which of the possible solutions is best. *Judgment* is a decision to act based on available information, which includes the prediction of consequences.

As with other aspects of cognition, there is a domain specificity to skill in problem solving. It is a common observation that individuals who are masters of problem solving in one domain, such as chess, may be incompetent in other domains, such as marriage counseling. One of the obvious reasons for this domain specificity is that problem solving is not simply a cognitive skill; it also presupposes solid content knowledge in the domain in which problems are to be solved.

For this and other reasons, formal tests of problem solving often yield ecologically unsatisfactory results. First, test tasks generally present problems in explicit terms and request problem-solving behavior; thus, individuals who fail to recognize problems or to initiate problem-solving behavior in the real world may score well relative to their real-world disability. Second, many tests request a verbal answer to the question, "What would you do if . . . ?," thereby neglecting the requirement to act and to evaluate one's action, two critical dimensions of mature problem solving. Tests of this sort may yield useful information about the individual's procedural or social knowledge without giving insight into his or her problem-solving skill. Ideal tasks for evaluating problem solving have the following characteristics: (1) The individual has a goal, (2) there is an obstacle to achieving the goal, (3) there are real-world distractions and stressors, and (4) there are available solutions.

Because the cognitive processes and systems that support effective problem solving and sound safety and social judgment are numerous, a wide variety of cognitive deficits can depress real-world problem solving and judgment. At least at some stages of recovery, many people with TBI appear confused, impulsive, childish (relative to age expectations), and socially inappropriate as a likely consequence of a combination of cognitive deficits. Intervention in this area is discussed in Chapter 12. Children and adolescents whose intervention programs are designed to make them more reflective and strategic in their problem solving and decision making often protest that they are being asked to be more deliberate and careful in their thinking and acting than are their peers and than they were before the injury. The meaningful response to this protest is that, although the situation appears unfair, these children have and will have more problems to solve than will their peers and therefore must be as good as they can be at solving problems. Strategic problem-solving behavior is required only when automatic behavior is insufficient to overcome obstacles to achieving goals. Because of the injury and consequent impairment, individuals with TBI have more physical, cognitive, and social obstacles to overcome and therefore must be better at strategic thinking than those whose automatic behavior serves them well.

Functional-Integrative Performance

By *functional-integrative performance,* we mean performance of real-life activities (e.g., dressing, playing, conversing, reading, participating in sports or job-related activities) in a real-world setting (e.g., classroom) with real-world stressors (e.g., limited time frame, peer pressure, the perceived need to receive a good grade). Such performance entails integration of many cognitive processes and systems as well as noncognitive contributors to performance (e.g., motivation, self-concept, interpersonal relations, environmental support, physical ability). From a cognitive perspective, identification of the effects of performance variables (e.g., efficiency, level, scope, and manner) on real-world task performance is critical. Clinical observations commonly reveal that performance in sanitized test situations and improvements in performance in isolated cognitive processes and systems do not automatically transfer to more functional tasks in real-world contexts. Certainly, the measure of success of intervention must be improved performance in functional academic, social, vocational, or recreational activities. Systematically tracking real-world performance with the variables *efficiency*, *level*, *scope*, and *manner* enables clinicians to maintain a focus on the functional outcome of intervention and to document real progress for family members, third-party payers, and the individuals themselves.

Efficiency refers to the *amount* that is accomplished in a *given period*, holding quality of performance constant. For example, many students with TBI can read short texts and comprehend them adequately, given a reasonable amount of time. However, often a precipitous deterioration in comprehension occurs with increases in the amount of reading or the speed required. This deterioration may be due to inefficient organizing processes or generally slow processing and may be consistent with adequate performance under less stressful conditions (Ylvisaker, 1993).

Level refers to the developmental, academic, linguistic, or vocational level of a task as it is measured on scales such as early to late grade level and simple to complex, concrete to abstract, or low to high language level. *Scope* refers to the variety of situations in which a level of performance can be maintained (e.g., familiar or unfamiliar, structured or unstructured, quiet or noisy). Because individuals with TBI are often concrete thinkers and learners, clinicians must be even more alert than normal to problems of transfer of learning or performance from one context to another.

Manner refers to the characteristic style or way a task is performed, such as impulsive or reflective, flexible or rigid, dependent (needing cues) or independent, or active or passive. The manner of performance has an effect on the other performance variables. For example, if children are highly dependent or inflexible in the way they perform, then their scope of activity will be restricted. Furthermore, the manner of performance profoundly affects cooperative activity.

The inclusion, in our operational definition of cognition, of the executive system and factors that influence functional-integrative performance of real-world tasks transports cognitive rehabilitation far beyond remedial exercises designed to improve separate components of cognition, an approach that dominated the early decades of special education (Mann, 1979) and the early years of cognitive intervention efforts for individuals with TBI. In the latter case, cognitive restoration workbooks and computer programs—often focusing exclusively on basic-level cognitive processes (e.g., attention, perception, rote memory, simple organizing processes, and speed of processing)—once dominated clinical activity. Movement toward a broader, more functional, contextualized, and integrative approach to cognitive rehabilitation followed the recognition of predictable difficulties with transfer of learning and the recognition that effective cognitive processing in context is more than the sum of cognitive components.

Although including executive functions, defined broadly, in the definition of cognition creates substantial overlap between cognitive rehabilitation and psychosocial counseling, cognitive functioning in context cannot be understood without some explanation of the executive direction of the mechanism. Similarly, including functional-integrative performance in the definition of cognition creates substantial overlap between cognitive rehabilitation and academic instruction, vocational training, and other areas of intervention. We believe that clinicians should embrace this inevitable overlap and its obvious implication—that professionals involved in intervention with a cognitive focus should work collaboratively to achieve goals rather than attempt to artificially split humans into components that exist separately only within the scope of practice statements of professional organizations.

Domains of Cognitive Functioning Not Explicitly Recognized in the Proposed Classification System

Language

We intend the information in this and subsequent chapters to be of special interest to professionals, such as speech-language pathologists and educators, who have an interest in the comprehension and production of language (including reading and writing). These professionals are accustomed to seeing their special content—oral and written language—addressed under its own heading rather than distributed under a combination of more general cognitive headings. Indeed, this is the most reasonable practice when specific oral language disorders or reading and writing disorders are the focus of the discussion. However, after TBI, it is common for language and reading and writing problems to be associated with more general cognitive or self-regulatory deficits (reviewed by Ylvisaker, 1992, 1993). For example, researchers and clinicians alike have highlighted the following language-processing disorders as being strongly associated with TBI:

- Disorganized discourse (spoken and written) and difficulty comprehending extended text (auditory and reading comprehension), likely associated with generally impaired organizational functioning
- Difficulty processing rapidly spoken language and reading quickly, likely associated with generally depressed rate of information processing
- Difficulty retrieving words, especially under stress, likely associated with more general retrieval difficulties or with disorganization of the semantic representation of word meaning in semantic memory
- Difficulty learning new words or other forms of language, likely associated with general new learning problems
- Difficulty processing linguistic abstractions, likely associated with generally impaired abstract thinking
- Difficulty using language in a socially appropriate manner, likely associated with difficulty maintaining socially appropriate behavior in general

Because these symptoms are not specific to the language system, we believe it is reasonable to follow the practice reflected in many cognitive psychology texts and discuss language-related issues under a variety of cognitive headings. Chapters 10–13 include assessment and intervention discussions directly related to the work of speech-language pathologists and educators.

Academic Knowledge and Skill

For reasons exactly parallel to those presented in the preceding section, academic knowledge and skill could be discussed under its own heading in a cognitive framework or could be included in a discussion of a variety of cognitive processes and systems. As in the case of language, we have chosen the latter route. However, we hope that educators will recognize the direct relevance to their work of our chapters on cognitive assessment, organization and memory, executive functions, and social cognition.

Social Cognition

Chapter 13 includes a discussion of intervention for deficits in the area of social cognition, deficits that result in the impairment of both social interaction and general social skills. The types of knowledge, insight, perceptual skill, and reasoning that characterize a socially competent individual are often brought together into an integrated discussion of social cognition, as we have done in Chapter 13. However, for reasons similar to those elucidated in the preceding two sections, we have presented in this chapter an approach to understanding cognition in which social cognitive processing and knowledge are subsumed into more general categories (e.g., perception, organization, reasoning, knowledge base, executive system) that also include nonsocial knowledge and processing.

In an important sense, social information processing is more demanding than nonsocial processing. The "objects" of social thinking (e.g., people's feelings, intentions, motives, attitudes, relationships) are typically hidden and can be identified only be inference. Furthermore, these objects are fluid; that is, they change with changing circumstances, as do other objects of social thought, such as topics of conversation and the meaning of words and expressions. These features of social processing make it especially vulnerable to processing deficits, thereby necessitating careful attention to social cognition in rehabilitation after TBI.

Cognitive Development

With appropriate qualifications, normal sequences of cognitive development can serve as a useful guide in selecting goals and objectives for intervention and in identifying effective intervention procedures for children with TBI. With respect to sequences of objectives, it is reasonable to believe that normal development reveals not only a natural sequence of acquisitions but also natural and important interrelationships within component cognitive processes and systems. For example, children become competent in attacking academic problems strategically only after they have acquired a reasonable amount of content knowledge and the ability to discriminate between easy and difficult tasks, to monitor their performance, to engage in problem-solving behavior with concrete objects, to understand abstract language, and to control impulsive responses. There is not only a temporal sequence here, there is also every reason to believe that these acquisitions make strategic academic behavior possible. Normal developmental sequences can thus be used to plan a broad and long-term approach to cognitive rehabilitation, in this case rehabilitation that focuses on strategic thinking (see Chapter 12).

Observation of normally developing children reveals potentially fruitful procedures for promoting cognitive growth after TBI. For several decades, specialists in child language disorders have carefully observed normally developing children and their caregivers for clues regarding procedures most effective in promoting language and communication development. Similarly, students of cognitive development in children (e.g., Flavell et al., 1993; Schneider and Pressley, 1989; Vygotsky, 1978) have used the study of normal cognitive development to identify experiences and interventions that may promote cognitive growth in children whose development is delayed. Although few concrete solutions to these questions are available, there is at least a *prima facie* reason to keep intervention procedures as consistent as possible with procedures that have evolved within our species as means of promoting cognitive development. For example, many developmental cognitive psychologists believe that both efficiency and depth of episodic memory, as well as organization and elaboration of narrative discourse, are facilitated in preschoolers by ensuring, first, that preschool children have meaningful routines in their lives that serve as the basis for internalization of script representations and, second, that parents or others provide conversational scaffolding that promotes progressively more complete and better-organized narrative accounts of real routines or scripts in children's lives (Nelson, 1992; Reese et al., 1993). These and other developmental insights serve as the basis for some of the intervention procedures we present in Chapters 11, 12, and 14.

Detailed descriptions of cognitive development, and theories designed to explain that development, are presented in a number of excellent texts (Bjorklund, 1990; Flavell et al., 1993; Schneider and Pressley, 1989; Siegler, 1991; Sternberg and Berg, 1992). Flavell and colleagues (1993) suggested that the four leading theories of cognitive development—piagetian, neo-piagetian, information processing, and contextual (vygotskyan)—are compatible in many ways, and all contribute to a full understanding of child development. The most we can hope for here is to highlight broad trends in cognitive development and to identify intervention principles in these trends. A developmental template is obviously critical in working with children who are injured at an early age and who have yet to move through subsequent stages of development. Such a template is also important in working with older children and adolescents because, although brain injury does not necessarily cause systematic developmental regression, there are often important ways in which TBI is associated with developmentally early stages of cognitive functioning (e.g., concrete thinking, egocentric thinking, impulsive and poorly controlled thinking and acting, nonstrategic approaches to problems, poorly organized thinking and acting, reduced self-awareness). Therefore, intervention procedures useful in promoting early cognitive development are at least strong candidates for promoting cognitive recovery after brain injury.

Interrelated Patterns of Normal Cognitive Development

Major interrelated patterns of normal cognitive development include (1) progression from surface to depth, (2) progression from concrete to abstract and hypothetical, (3) progression from context dependence to context independence, (4) growth in metacognition (progression from thinking that is not deliberately strategic to strategic thinking and problem solving), (5) progression from egocentric to nonegocentric thinking and acting, (6) progression from cognitive centration to decentration, (7) growth in the knowledge base, and (8) increased efficiency or capacity of information processing. Many of these areas of development, particularly strategic thinking, nonegocentric thinking, abstract thinking, decentration, and efficient use of organizing schemes, are associated with the slow and protracted neuroanatomic and neurophysiologic development of the prefrontal areas of the brain. One way of supporting a developmental perspective in cognitive rehabilitation is to note the frequency with which the frontal lobes are injured in closed head injury, resulting in a cognitive profile that, in many respects, can strongly resemble that of a younger child.

Progression from Surface to Depth

Children's awareness develops from attention to superficial characteristics of objects, persons, and events (perceived appearances) to a focus on underlying causes and inferred meanings and realities. Their thinking develops from gross qualitative judgments about things and people (e.g., big, good) to more precise quantitative judgments that evidence an understanding of measurement, proportions, degrees of feeling, and balanced interactions (e.g., 6 feet tall; "straight A" student).

Progression from Concrete to Abstract and Hypothetical

Children's thinking begins as an ability to think only about concrete physical things and people, to solve problems only by trial and error with real objects, and to apply learned skills only in contexts that closely resemble the context of learning. It develops into an ability to think about possibilities; reflect on past experience; reason hypothetically; experiment strategically; comprehend abstract attributes, relationships, and principles; and to transfer learned skills and knowledge to an increasingly broad domain of comparable problems and experiences. For example, preferred modes of organizing things and information progress from the organization inherent in familiar, concrete routines and scripts to more abstract categories and associations. Similarly, memory progresses from an early ability to remember concrete things and places to an increasingly wide domain of types of memories.

Progression from Context Dependence to Context Independence

The ability of young children to learn, comprehend, and express meaningful language and maintain adaptive behavior is dependent on context cues. In this sense, young children are relatively stimulus bound. As children mature, their thinking and behavior become increasingly independent of specific context cues. To some degree, context dependence in learning continues into adulthood, evidenced by apprenticeship programs and internships in many fields of study. Sensitivity to context in rehabilitation, promoted in the chapters of this book devoted to cognition rehabilitation, is supported by this developmental principle.

Growth in Metacognition: Progression from Thinking That Is Not Deliberately Strategic to Strategic Thinking and Problem Solving

Associated broadly with the development of metacognition and executive functions, children's thinking and problem-solving abilities progress from generally unplanned and uncontrolled to potentially very strategic. Associated with this broad domain of development are several related components, including (1) growth in distinguishing between easy and difficult tasks (in relation to the child's abilities) and therefore understanding which tasks require special effort; (2) the ability to inhibit initial impulses to act or to think and to engage in increasingly goal-directed, persistent, and reflective behavior; (3) the ability to represent and to direct oneself toward abstract goals, such as learning; (4) growth of knowledge of procedures or strategies that may be effective in overcoming obstacles; (5) understanding of oneself as a potential problem solver; and (6) the ability to monitor and evaluate performance and cognitive activity to determine the need for strategic behavior. This development corresponds to progression from learning in only involuntary learning tasks (young preschoolers) to learning deliberately as well as involuntarily. Ultimately, the outcome of this developmental progression is that children use strategies automatically without necessarily devoting space in working memory to strategic thinking (Bjorklund, 1990; Schneider and Pressley, 1989).

It is important not to underestimate the strategic abilities of preschoolers. Investigators (e.g., Istominia, 1977) have found that 4- and 5-year-old children can be deliberately strategic in natural contexts and with memory tasks that are important for them. Our focus on the development of strategic behavior in young children is based in part on these and related findings (see Chapter 14).

Progression from Egocentric to Nonegocentric Thinking and Acting

Whereas very young children are unable to represent other minds with their own points of view, intentions, and desires, cognitive development includes progress toward such representational ability and a corresponding ability to adjust one's behavior to meet the needs of others as well as oneself. For example, preschoolers find it difficult to describe objects and events from another person's perspective and to adjust their language to meet the informational needs of their communication partner.

Recently, the progression from egocentric to nonegocentric thinking and acting has been discussed as the child's evolving *theory of mind.* It has been proposed that the same developmental acquisitions that enable a child to appreciate another's perspective also enable the child to understand lies, jokes, metaphors, and false presentations of self (Flavell et al., 1993). These are often major issues in rehabilitation after TBI in young children (see Chapter 13).

Progression from Cognitive Centration to Decentration

Related to a child's development from egocentric to non-egocentric thinking is a progression from thinking that is focused on one's immediate situation and needs and on only one aspect of a situation to an ability to represent events that are spread widely in space and time, to assume other people's perspectives, to guide one's behavior in part by the representations of other perspectives, and generally to consider varied aspects of a problem situation.

Growth in the Knowledge Base

One of the most critical aspects of cognitive development, highlighted in recent discussions of cognitive development but often overlooked in rehabilitation programs, is growth in content knowledge and its organization. Deep and well-organized knowledge about people, objects, events, and ideas enables an individual to comprehend and assimilate new information in an efficient manner, to retrieve information efficiently, to express organized thoughts, and to solve problems in an informed manner. The knowledge base also includes knowledge of strategies, rules, and other abstract entities that facilitate efficient performance of cognitively demanding tasks. This relationship of stored knowledge to processing explains the domain specificity of cognitive efficiency: That is, a person may process information efficiently and solve problems strategically in one domain but not in others. This important developmental fact supports a contextualized approach to cognitive intervention.

Increased Efficiency or Capacity of Information Processing

The speed of processing, functional capacity of working memory, and flexibility of the retrieval system have all been found to increase with age, while reaction time decreases. These age-related improvements may result from increases in the amount and organization of stored knowledge: That is, as domain-specific knowledge and strategies become automated, both processing efficiency and the functional capacity of working memory increase (Flavell et al., 1993; Kail, 1990).

Limitations of a Developmental Model for Cognitive Rehabilitation

For two important reasons, it would be a mistake to commit oneself without qualification to a developmental model in cognitive rehabilitation for children and ado-

lescents with TBI. First, TBI is often associated with a long-term profile of strengths and weaknesses that includes preserved high-level strengths and major losses in lower-level knowledge and skill. This may even be true within a hierarchically arranged domain of content. For example, it is possible for an individual injured in ninth grade to recover some knowledge of algebra acquired shortly before the injury despite having lost much of the knowledge of basic arithmetic (e.g., multiplication tables) acquired much earlier. Individuals exhibiting profiles of this sort need creative teachers and clinicians who can capitalize on preserved knowledge and skill (and respect the individual's sense of self) while helping the individual to recover lost knowledge and skill. This critical orientation may be lost in a purely developmental approach to intervention.

Second, for certain individuals, it may be possible and desirable to accelerate developmental schedules in important areas of cognitive development. For example, it is generally believed that preschoolers are incapable of understanding the difficulty level of cognitive tasks. However, because of the importance of strategic thinking and behavior for people with disability, identification of task difficulty might be an important objective for a child functioning generally at a preschool level. Although this intervention may not bear fruit for many months or years, its importance in relation to the goal of fostering a more strategically thinking and acting person may necessitate an early start to this process.

What Cognitive Development Is Not

Serial Progression

Cognitive development is *not a serial progression from acquisition of one component of cognition to another*: That is, young children do not master sophisticated attentional skills before acquiring perceptual skills, followed by organizational skills, followed by problem-solving skills, followed by development of executive control over cognitive function, and so on (Bjorklund and Harnishfeger, 1990; Flavell et al., 1993). Furthermore, within a given cognitive component, children do not, for example, master selective attention before maintained attention before shifting attention, or divided attention.

In contrast, at every age and level of cognitive development, evidence exists of at least simple and developmentally early forms of all cognitive processes and systems, each developing in ways that are intimately linked with development of the others. For example, 2-year-old children have a level of attentional, perceptual, learning, organizational, problem-solving, and executive skill superior to that of 1-year-old children but inferior to that of 3-year-old children, and so on for the entire period of development. Furthermore, development in each area facilitates development in the others throughout the developmental years. For example, as the knowledge base grows and as organizational skills improve, so does a child's ability to maintain attention, to filter out distractions, to divide attention, and to assimilate and encode new information efficiently. In a reciprocal fashion, as attentional skills mature, the ability to acquire and organize knowledge likewise matures.

This interactive perspective on the development of components of cognition is supported not only by studies of cognitive development but also by developmental neurophysiologic studies. Cortical surface in all parts of the brain matures simultaneously (Dennis, 1991), supporting simultaneous and interactive development of all aspects of cognition. These observations are inconsistent with a rigid distinction between "lower" and "higher" cognitive processes. For example, it is common for professionals to refer to *higher-level executive functions* and *higher-order reasoning skills,* thereby encouraging an unwelcome neglect of very early development (as early as in infancy) of executive control (Goldman, 1971) and of simple, concrete planning, problem-solving, and reasoning skills (Willatts, 1990).

Stage-Wise Development

Cognitive development is also *not stage-wise development*. Recent discussions of cognitive development favor a perspective that describes development in continuous and quantitative terms (as opposed to qualitatively different stages) and that acknowledges domain and context variability of cognitive functioning (Bjorklund and Harnishfeger, 1990; Flavell et al., 1993; Siegler, 1991). These are two of the ways in which the powerful and still important views of Piaget have been transcended. Thus, for example, it is incorrect to describe preschoolers as being completely nonstrategic; rather, they are strategic in simple ways in relation to important and concrete problems. Similarly, it is incorrect to say that children cannot engage in hypothetico-deductive reasoning prior to entering the stage of formal operations (at age 10 or 11); rather, observers of children acknowledge that reasoning of this type can occur earlier in connection with significant and concrete problems and with adult encouragement.

Furthermore, adolescents and adults with generally mature cognitive function are known to think in immature ways in connection with certain domains of thought or under stress. For example, adults may use mature hypothetico-deductive reasoning in relation to familiar problems in domains of content in which they have been trained to think and reason critically but might revert to immature trial-and-error reasoning in unfamiliar domains. Similarly, an adult's social reasoning may be mature under ideal circumstances, taking into account the perspectives of varied interested parties, but might become fiercely concrete and egocentric under stress. This domain specificity of cognitive skill has been emphasized in studies of transfer of cognitive skill (Singley and Anderson, 1989).

Learning the Lessons from Other Intervention Fields

These are not merely academic points. Tacit or explicit acceptance of a serial-order approach to cognitive development easily leads to a hierarchical approach to cognitive rehabilitation that encourages an exclusive focus on attention, perception, and basic organization before introducing any intervention focus on components of executive functions, strategic behavior, reasoning, problem solving, and the like. Similarly, tacit or explicit acceptance of a stage model of cognitive development easily leads to a rehabilitation perspective in which certain types of cognitive interventions (e.g., executive system intervention) are postponed entirely until the individual demonstrates recovery to a predetermined stage. Finally, failure to recognize the domain specificity of cognitive skill encourages the use of cognitive exercises that are insensitive to the person-relative meaningfulness of the exercise's content, on the assumption that a cognitive skill, once acquired, will transfer readily to other domains of content or cognitive problems. The approach to cognitive rehabilitation presented in this book follows findings in cognitive science and cognitive development in rejecting all three of these assumptions. Chapters 11, 12, and 14 present intervention strategies that integrate a developmentally appropriate focus on all aspects of cognition at each stage of recovery beyond emergence from coma, within the context of appropriately selected, meaningful activities.

Hierarchical thinking of the sort questioned here is known to have deleterious effects in intervention fields having a longer history than does cognitive rehabilitation. For example, until recently, programs for very young children with developmental disabilities commonly focused primarily on basic-level content and cognitive and language processes, neglecting executive functions and decision making. The unwanted long-term result of such neglect too often was an adult who may have possessed a variety of basic skills but who lacked judgment and independence in decision making. This is one definition of the often accurate and always ominous term, *learned helplessness*. Professionals in the field of TBI rehabilitation would be well served by attending to this and other lessons learned in related areas of intervention.

Cognitive Disability and Improvement After Traumatic Brain Injury

It has been customary in the TBI literature to describe cognitive improvement in terms of qualitatively distinct stages. (The word *improvement* may be preferable to the more customary word *recovery* in that the latter term carries a suggestion, at least to family members and other lay people, of return to normal, which is rarely a realistic expectation after severe TBI.) Just as descriptions of cognitive development in children have evolved from stages to continuity, so also we would propose that improvement after TBI, although often characterized by bursts of progress, nevertheless be seen more as a continuum than as a sequence of a small number of abruptly changing, qualitatively distinct stages. Similarly, just as one can separate continuous normal development into roughly distinguishable phases (e.g., the preschool phase, the grade-school phase, and the high-school phase), so one can divide cognitive improvement after TBI into roughly distinguishable phases, as is done in Table 9-2. Establishing this rather arbitrary division allows us to highlight three roughly distinguishable phases of rehabilitation, which are not associated with specific lengths of time.

Early Phase of Improvement

The early phase of improvement includes the period from early medical stabilization to consistent responsiveness to environmental events. This phase generally occurs in a hospital setting and may last for hours, days, weeks, or, in some cases, persist indefinitely. The transition to the middle phase occurs when the individual gives evidence of consistent comprehension of simple language and appropriate use of everyday objects.

From a cognitive rehabilitation perspective, the focus of intervention during the early phase is to control sensory stimulation so as to prevent the negative effects of sensory deprivation and sensory overload, to channel recovery by providing specific sensory and sensorimotor stimulation that is consistent with the individual's ability to process stimulation and to respond, to create as much familiarity in the environment as possible so that the processing burden is made as light as possible, and to ensure that everyday people in the environment attempt to engage the individual in as many familiar sensorimotor routines as possible. Physically prompting familiar sensorimotor activities (e.g., self-care) serves to stimulate neural networks that cannot be stimulated by passive sensory stimulation alone and also ensures that the individual with TBI "wakes up" in a world in which he or she is an agent engaged in familiar activities, not just a passive recipient of care and stimulation.

Middle Phase of Improvement

The middle phase is the period during which the individual is alert and generally responsive but to some degree confused, disoriented (relative to age expectations), unable to process information in depth, unable to remember information effectively from day to day, and generally unable to maintain effective and appropriate social interaction (again, relative to age expectations). General cognitive disruption may be exacerbated by deficits in specific domains of processing (e.g., language, visual perception) associated with focal lesions. Children

are often in an inpatient setting during this phase of recovery but, with the trend toward decreasing lengths of stay in medical facilities, children may be discharged to home and attempt to return to school. Cognitive rehabilitation during this phase focuses on reducing confusion and disorientation through careful environmental structuring, gradually and systematically improving general information-processing abilities by controlled use of activities of daily living and familiar academic and recreational activities, helping individuals to reaccess their knowledge base acquired before the trauma, and supportively improving decision-making and problem-solving ability. There is also a preventive emphasis during this phase. Specialists in cognition must ensure that people present in the child's everyday life understand his or her cognitive strengths and limitations so that they provide needed supports and adjust their expectations accordingly so as to prevent the behavioral and emotional problems that are otherwise predictable.

Late Phase of Improvement

In the late phase, many children and adolescents recover to the point at which they are generally oriented, goal directed, and purposeful (relative to age expectations). Learning new information and skills may still be difficult and processing efficiency may deteriorate precipitously with increases in cognitive demands or psychosocial stress. Furthermore, individuals may have specific cognitive deficits related to specific focal injuries (e.g., language impairment, perceptual impairment, difficulty with specific academic content). Cognitive rehabilitation during this phase focuses on increasing independence and adaptability to varied environments, refining skills, enhancing individuals' strategic behavior so that they can compensate for ongoing cognitive deficits, generalizing treatment gains to functional settings, and identifying the teaching procedures that will result in the most effective academic instruction possible.

Critical Considerations in Assessing Improvement by Phases or Stages

This talk of phases must not obscure the following five critical points:

1. *Variability in improvement:* At any point in general cognitive recovery, individuals may have quite dissimilar profiles, depending on the ways in which specific focal injuries compound the effects of diffuse injury.

2. *Continuity in improvement:* See earlier discussion under What Cognitive Development Is Not.

3. *Limited recovery in some cases:* Some individuals with very severe injuries remain severely compromised indefinitely. In other cases, long-term improvement may be generally good, but the individual may continue to

Table 9-2. Aspects of Cognition and Phases of Improvement after TBI

Aspects of Cognition	Early Phase	Middle Phase	Late Phase*
Component processes			
Attention: holding objects, events, words, or thoughts in consciousness *Components:* span, selectivity, filtering, maintaining, shifting, dividing	Severely decreased arousal or alertness Minimal selective attention, focusing, shifting Possibly, attention primarily to internal stimuli	Attention generally focused on external events Short attention span Poor control of attention: highly distractible, inflexible	Attention span possibly reduced Relatively weak concentration, selective attention, and fluid attentional shifts Possibly, weak organizational processes, absence of goals, or both reflected by attending problems
Perception: recognition of features and relationships among features; affected by context (figure-ground) and intensity, duration, significance, and familiarity of stimuli	Begins to recognize (and perhaps use) familiar objects when they are highlighted May perceive only one feature or aspect of stimulus Adaptation to continuous stimulation	Clear recognition of familiar objects and events Inefficient perception in context Sharp deterioration with increases in rate, amount, and complexity of stimuli Difficulty in distinguishing whole from part	Possibly subtle versions of perceptual problems related to rate, amount, and complexity Possibly specific deficits (e.g., field neglect) Possibly inefficient shifting of perceptual set Possibly weak perception of relevant features
Memory and learning: *Encoding:* recognition, interpretation, and formulation of information, including language, into an internal code; coding affected by knowledge base, personal interests, and goals *Storage:* retention over time *Retrieval:* transfer from long-term memory to consciousness	Progression in comprehension from minimal responses to vocal intonation and stress to recognition of simple, context-bound instructions No evidence of encoding or storage of new information	Weak encoding due to poor access to knowledge base, poor integration of new with old information, or inefficient attention or perception Inefficiently encoded information often lost after short delay Recognition stronger than recall; receptive vocabulary superior to expressive vocabulary Disorganized search of storage system	Possibly subtle versions of earlier problems, particularly with increases in cognitive stress Memory problems—any combination of comprehension, encoding, storage, or retrieval deficits Memory problems—problems recalling information related to personal experience (episodic memory) or abstracted knowledge (semantic memory)
Organizing: analyzing, classifying, integrating, sequencing; identifying relevant features of objects and events; comparing for similarities or differences; integrating into organized descriptions, higher-level categories, and sequenced events; these processes presupposed by higher-level reasoning and efficient learning	No evidence of these processes	Weak or bizarre associations Weak analysis of objects into features Disorganized sequencing of events Weak identification of similarities and differences in comparisons and classifications Can integrate concepts into propositions; difficulty integrating propositions into main ideas Major difficulty imposing organization on unstructured stimuli	Possibly subtle versions of earlier problems Difficulty maintaining goal-directed thinking Ongoing difficulty discerning main ideas and integrating main ideas into broader themes Possibly gets lost easily in details Can impose organization on unstructured stimuli with prompting

Table 9-2. *Continued*

Aspects of Cognition	Early Phase	Middle Phase	Late Phase*
Reasoning: considering evidence and drawing inferences and conclusions, involving flexible exploration of possibilities (divergent thinking) and use of past experience *Deductive:* strict logical formal inference *Inductive:* direct inference from experience *Analogical:* indirect inference from experience	No evidence of these processes	Minimal inferential thinking; may deal with concrete cause-effect relationships, particularly if overlearned General inefficiency with abstract ideas and relationships	Fair to good concrete reasoning in controlled settings; disorganized thinking in stressful or uncontrolled settings Abstract thinking deficient
Problem solving and judgment: *Problem solving:* occurs when a goal cannot be reached directly; ideally involves goal identification, consideration of relevant information, exploration of possible solutions, and selection of the best *Judgment:* decision to act, based on consideration of relevant factors, including prediction of consequences	No evidence of these processes	Inability to see relationships among problems, goals, and relevant information Inflexibility in generating or evaluating possible solutions; impulsive; trial-and-error approach Inability to assess a situation and predict consequences Severely impaired safety and social judgment	Possibly subtle versions of earlier problems Impulsive; disorganized problem solving Inflexible thinking and shallow reasoning Primary residual deficits possibly poor safety and social judgment; manifested in academic and social situations
Component systems			
Working memory (attentional focus): storage or holding "space" where coding and organizing occur; limited information capacity; *functional* capacity increased by making processes automatic or by "chunking" information	Severely limited capacity Progression from single-modality to multimodality processing of simple stimuli Attentional space possibly exhausted by attention to internal stimuli	Gradual increase in attention span to near normal, as measured by digit span Possibly maintained severe restriction of *functional* capacity due to lack of automatic organizing processes Rapid deterioration of processing with increases in the information load	Often normal digit span Possibly, continual reduction of *functional* capacity, due to inefficient organizing processes, as information load increases, and to generally inefficient executive functions
Long-term memory: contains knowledge of concepts and words; rules, strategies, and procedures; organizational principles and knowledge frames; goals, experience and self-concept	Emerging evidence of remote memory; recognition of familiar objects and persons May assume that other contents are present but inaccessible	Growing access to pre-trauma contents Recognition of strong associations (e.g., hammer-nail), basic semantic relations, and common two- or three-event sequences	Stabilization of recovery of access to pretraumatically acquired knowledge base Variable growth of long-term memory, depending on type and severity of residual cognitive deficits
Response system: controls all output, including speech,	Severely limited; often perseverative responses	Speaks or begins augmentative system	Generally functional communication system—

Aspects of Cognition	Early Phase	Middle Phase	Late Phase*
facial expression, and fine- and gross-motor activity; includes motor planning	May use some gestures and speech toward end of this stage, but with motor planning problems or delayed responses	Possible motor-planning problems or general slowness Impulsiveness and possible perseveration Variable motor function depending on site and extent of injury	usually speech Possible motor-planning problems or slowness Possible rapid fatigue
Executive system ("central processor"): sets goals; plans and monitors activity; directs processing and operations according to goals, current input, and perceptual-affective set	Minimal awareness of self and current condition No apparent self-direction of behavior or cognitive processes	Growing awareness of self; poor awareness of deficits Weak metacognitive awareness of self as thinker Minimal goal setting, self-initiation or self-inhibition, self-monitoring or self-evaluation	Shallow awareness of residual deficits Mild to severe deficits in executive functions, related in part to anterior frontolimbic damage Strategy training possible, depending on meta-cognitive level

Functional-integrative performance

Functional behavior: performance of real-life tasks and activities (e.g., reading a book or conversing) *Efficiency:* rate of performance and amount accomplished *Level:* developmental or academic level of performance *Scope:* variety of situations in which child can maintain performance *Manner:* dependence or independence (need for prompts and cues; impulsive or reflective style)	Cannot adapt to environment; activity level ranges from inactive to hyperactive; activity marginally purposeful (e.g., pulling at tubes, restraints, clothes; attempting to get out of bed); gives little or no assistance to daily care May perform a limited range of routine tasks when prompted (e.g., brushing hair) Profound confusion or disorientation to person, place, time, and condition Communication severely limited, inconsistent, and prefunctional; may begin to comprehend simple context-bound instructions Minimal social interaction; little variation in facial expression; reflexive crying; may reflexively hold or shake hands Agitated behavior at the end of this stage more pronounced in adolescents	Performs many overlearned routines (e.g., self-care, games) in structured settings with prompts; poor retention of information from day to day; severely impaired learning of new skills Performs simple sequential tasks (e.g., dressing) in structured setting if stimuli are controlled for rate, amount, and complexity; rapid deterioration of organization of behavior in uncontrolled setting Continued confusion but growing orientation to person, place, and time in structured settings and with orientation cues; gross awareness of the structure of the day Communication: *Expressive:* Usually verbal and functional (barring motor speech disorder), but often characterized by confabulation, word retrieval problems, excessive and often inappropriate output *Receptive:* Control of rate amount and complexity of verbal interaction necessary to assure comprehension Social interaction strained and often unsuccessful, due to	Performance of pretraumatically acquired skills related to type and extent of residual deficits and ability to compensate; possibly continued sharp deterioration of performance with increasing processing load; reduced-rate learning of new skills and strategies Deficient performance of complex tasks requiring organization, persistence, and self-monitoring; low efficiency, with slow rate and low productivity Solid orientation to person, place, and time, but possible recurrence of disorientation with sudden changes in routine Communication usually conventional in form, with possible word-finding problems, expressive disorganization, and comprehension limited in efficiency; social use of language possibly strained or inappropriate Social interaction and

Table 9-2. *Continued*

Aspects of Cognition	Early Phase	Middle Phase	Late Phase*
		disinhibition, inappropriateness, impaired social perception Possibly minimal adaptation to the environment due to impulsiveness, agitation, and inability to set goals	judgment possible dominant residual symptoms, related to weak awareness of social conventions and rules, persistent impulsiveness, and poorly defined self-concept (with shallow awareness of residual deficits) Generally goal-directed behavior, but goals possibly unrealistic and social and safety judgment significantly impaired; prompts needed to set goals and subgoals

*Functioning also related to age and pretrauma developmental and educational level.
Source: SF Szekeres, M Ylvisaker, AL Holland (1985). Cognitive Rehabilitation Therapy: A Framework for Intervention. In M Ylvisaker (ed), Head Injury Rehabilitation: Children and Adolescents. Austin, TX: PRO-ED, 230. Copyright 1997, Butterworth–Heinemann.

require support for effective cognitive functioning in academic, vocational, and social tasks.

4. *Possible delayed consequences:* It is well established that frontal lobe injury, very common in closed head injury, is often associated with delayed consequences in children and adolescents (Eslinger et al., 1992; Feeney and Ylvisaker, 1995; Grattan and Eslinger, 1991, 1992; Marlowe, 1992; Mateer and Williams, 1991; Price et al., 1990; Williams and Mateer, 1992; Ylvisaker and Feeney, 1995). For example, a toddler who incurred a brain injury may appear quite well recovered at age 3 but, because the injured frontal lobes fail to mature, the child may be unable to negotiate the cognitive and behavioral demands of school at age 6. Similarly, an adolescent injured at age 12 may appear quite well recovered at age 12 but years later think in ways that are relatively concrete and act in ways that are socially immature because of delayed effects of the earlier injury. (This theme is elaborated in Chapter 2.)

5. *Impact of preinjury functioning:* One must remember that outcome after TBI is a function of the individual who was injured as well as of the injury itself: That is, children with outstanding intellectual resources and solid family and social support before the injury may fare better than comparably injured children who were impaired or had less solid support before the injury.

Goals of Cognitive Rehabilitation

To rehabilitate is to re-enable people to do what they want to do after an injury or other cause of acquired disability. The target of rehabilitation is people and their real-world pursuits. It is sometimes said that the goal of rehabilitation is to improve the functioning of arms and legs or to improve eating and talking or language and social skills or cognition. This way of speaking is potentially dangerous in that it leads to a framework within which the only truly legitimate goal of rehabilitation is remediation or cure—that is, elimination of the disability. In an ideal world, people who had completed their rehabilitative course would be able to achieve success in their social, academic, and vocational lives with no special effort or accommodations. Unfortunately, after severe brain injury, this is seldom a realistic goal. Therefore, rehabilitation efforts generally require a flexible mix of stimulation and retraining, personal and environmental strategies and accommodations, and procedures to promote adjustment to disability.

In other fields of habilitation and rehabilitation for individuals with chronic disability, including special education and vocational rehabilitation for individuals with developmental disability, progress in the last 30 years has resulted largely from a shift away from the medical model of services, with its emphasis on eliminating or reducing the underlying impairment through technical intervention delivered by specialists in clinical settings. Instead, meaningful real-world goals have been achieved by providing services and supports in natural settings and by including a variety of people who interact regularly with the child (so-called everyday people) as important members of the collaborative team of service providers.

The general goal of cognitive rehabilitation is to enable people to do what they would like and need to do to be successful but what they find difficult because of their cognitive disability. This very broad goal gives way to many combinations of subgoals, depending on a variety of factors. These subgoals include assisting the individual in achieving the following objectives:

- Processing information more effectively because of improved cognitive processes and systems
- Processing information more effectively by deliberately using special strategic procedures
- Performing everyday tasks at a higher level because of external supports, including environmental accommodations for ongoing cognitive disability
- Learning new information and skills despite significant disability, by means of teaching procedures consistent with the individual's profile of cognitive ability and disability
- Acquiring content knowledge, which by itself facilitates improved information processing
- Understanding his or her cognitive abilities and disabilities and adjusting to ongoing disability

Approaches to Cognitive Rehabilitation

Controversies in the field of cognitive rehabilitation during the last 20 years have included competing approaches to intervention and competing views of the goals of intervention (i.e., improved cognition versus improved performance of functional tasks in natural contexts). During the first decade of active program development for individuals with cognitive impairment after TBI (roughly 1975–1985), most efforts focused on improving performance either by retraining discrete aspects of cognition using process-specific retraining exercises organized within a hierarchical curriculum or by promoting compensation for specific cognitive impairment by teaching specific strategic procedures outside of the context of functional application. Like many interventions for other populations, these efforts were greeted initially with enthusiasm because of measurable improvement on training tasks or neuropsychological tests when pretreatment and post-treatment performance or experimental and control groups were compared. Again, as with many other interventions, initial enthusiasm gradually gave way to skepticism and searches for more functional approaches

to cognitive rehabilitation, as the historical nemesis of treatment effects—generalization and maintenance—inevitably raised its ugly head. An appreciation of several decades—even centuries—of clinical experience and empirical research in educational psychology and in cognitive training for people with disabilities other than TBI (e.g., Mann, 1979) may have accelerated this maturation within the field.

Restorative Versus Compensatory Approaches: A False Dichotomy

Disagreements in the field of cognitive rehabilitation after brain injury are often discussed as differences in relative emphasis either on restoration of cognitive process and skill by means of targeted exercises or on compensation for permanently impaired functions by means of strategic procedures or environmental modifications. This is an unfortunate dichotomy for several reasons.

First, this dichotomy between restoration and compensation is inconsistent with the important fact that normal cognitive functioning involves strategic use of cognitive processes and systems. Indeed, development of metacognitive awareness and strategic cognitive behavior are among the most critical aspects of cognitive development in childhood. Therefore, "restoration" of cognitive functioning must focus, at least in part, on strategic or compensatory behavior, as it is part of normal cognitive behavior.

Second, this dichotomy does not provide a comfortable home for a variety of goals and activities vital to cognitive rehabilitation. For example, helping children to acquire and use organizing schemes to process information more efficiently, to remember more effectively, and to express themselves successfully, all of which are central to cognitive rehabilitation (see Chapter 11), does not fit neatly into either of these schemes. Similarly, acquisition of content knowledge, identification of the best teaching procedures, and adjustment counseling are central to cognitive rehabilitation for children and adolescents, but do not find a natural home in the restoration-compensation dichotomy.

Finally, in young children, cognitive rehabilitation includes attempts to accelerate acquisition of new developmental skills. For example, knowing that a child will need to be more strategic than other people because of some degree of cognitive weakness, it is wise for the rehabilitation team to begin working early—even in the preschool years—on the prerequisites for strategic behavior. If the people in that child's everyday environment are appropriately trained, the child might receive hundreds of coached experiences in natural contexts that focus on the child's ability to (1) identify how difficult a task might be, given what the child is capable of doing; (2) recognize that there might be a special way to accomplish the task; and (3) pay attention to the degree of the child's success and to attempt another approach if the first failed. Having spent 2 or 3 years in an environment rich in these coached experiences, the child may be in a better position to apply strategic behaviors and thinking in relation to the cognitive challenges that emerge during the school years.

The significance of these issues is more than academic. The restoration-versus-compensation dichotomy is associated with at least two unfortunate tendencies in cognitive rehabilitation that are rejected in our framework: The first is the notion that rehabilitation is initially restorative and moves into a strategic or compensatory mode only if it becomes clear that restorative exercises combined with spontaneous recovery are incapable of achieving satisfactory goals. The second is that a compensatory approach is restricted to teaching very specific strategies to compensate for specific deficits; it does not promote a broad-based and long-term focus on the development of strategic thinking and strategic behavior generally.

Process-Specific Versus Integrated Approaches

Process-specific retraining approaches to cognitive rehabilitation have an advantage over loosely organized workbook exercises in that there is a rationale for the selection of training tasks and intervention is organized around specific treatment goals and objectives, with a theoretical rationale (Sohlberg and Mateer, 1989). However, the targeting of specific, discrete cognitive processes (e.g., selective attention, visual memory, prospective memory) assumes something about the discreteness and independence of these processes that is not supported by recent developments in cognitive science. For example, *memory* processes do not operate independently of *organizing* processes, whether the focus is organizing information for encoding, storing information in organized (cognitive-neural) networks, or retrieving information based on organized searches of organized networks of information. More generally, remembering a text that one has read is a consequence of many interacting cognitive and noncognitive processes and activities, including selective attention, perception, language comprehension, content knowledge, organization of information, retrieval processes, reasoning, strategic behavior, interest, attribution, motivation, and physical state. Indeed, a recent summary of research in memory improvement (Herrmann et al., 1992) had as its central theme this "multimodal" nature of memory.

These same types of interactions can be described between and among other aspects of cognition also. Thus, so-called memory tasks are not merely memory tasks, nor are attention tasks merely attention tasks, and so on for all aspects of cognition. The practical consequences of embracing the essential interdependence of cognitive functions are several:

- Breakdowns in performance of cognitively demanding tasks must be analyzed from a variety of per-

spectives to identify the primary contributors to the breakdown (see Chapter 10).

- Efforts to improve cognitive functioning must, in most cases, be broad-based, focusing not just on the manifest problem (e.g., inattention) but also on the many possible contributors to the problem (e.g., shallow knowledge of the topic, difficulty organizing information, impaired executive control over cognitive processes generally, belief that one cannot succeed, disinterest).

- Careful decisions must be made about how best to approach a specific cognitive breakdown in individual cases (see Chapter 10).

Improved Cognition Versus Improved Performance of Functional Activities

It is unfair to construe improved cognition and improved performance of functional activities as mutually exclusive goals of cognitive rehabilitation. Proponents of retraining exercise approaches to improvement of cognition would certainly counter that the point of these exercises is to improve performance of functional activities and that probes of generalization should be a component of all retraining programs (e.g., Sohlberg and Mateer, 1989). If there were solid evidence that cognitive training or retraining exercises not embedded in functional activities or content had a generalized effect on performance of any task requiring that aspect of cognition, then this issue would be easily resolved. Furthermore, responsible proponents of decontextualized retraining exercises conscientiously advocate a generalization phase of intervention during which transfer to functional activities is targeted explicitly (Sohlberg and Raskin, 1996).

Unfortunately, historical evidence for broad transfer of cognitive skills is weak (see Contextualized Versus Decontextualized Approaches). Furthermore, for many types of interventions in which generalization is considered the final phase, generalization is allotted insufficient time, effort, and energy after the hard work of reducing the underlying impairment has been completed. Practical constraints in health care facilities and decreasing funding for rehabilitation contribute to the difficulty of ensuring adequate attention to generalization to real-world settings and tasks.

In addition to these practical considerations, it makes theoretical sense to embed the child's training in a functional application task from the outset. If improvement of the process or skill in question is not broadly transferable, then at least the training time will have been well spent on functional tasks (e.g., academic tasks, activities of daily living, vocational tasks) that require specific improvement. If transfer does occur, it should occur when functional activities comprise the training and transfer tasks as readily as it occurs when specially designed drill-and-practice cognitive retraining tasks are the context of training (e.g., computerized cognitive retraining programs). Therefore, within our perspective, even if the goal of training is improvement of pervasive aspects of cognition (e.g., selective attention, speed of processing, strategic remembering, organized thinking), it is wise to use training tasks that have meaningful, useful content for the child. For example, for school-age children, computerized math or reading exercises can be used to target selective attention or speed or processing. Similarly, organization exercises can be structured around meaningful text comprehension or production of organized narratives versus the decontextualized categorizing and sequencing exercises frequently found in cognitive retraining programs. (See Chapters 11 and 12 for additional examples.)

In promoting a more functional approach to cognitive rehabilitation than is traditional, we certainly do not mean to suggest that cognitive exercises are irrelevant to recovery and improvement in cognitive functioning after TBI or that rehabilitation is entirely a matter of compensating for disability that persists after spontaneous neurologic recovery has achieved its ultimate benefit. It is important to exercise cognitive processes and systems as intensively as possible after TBI. Even in the absence of brain injury, failure to exercise domains of knowledge and skill, such as foreign languages or math, easily results in progressively deteriorating efficiency of processing in those domains. Our point is that the history of cognitive training combines with current theory in cognitive science to support an approach to retraining that is functional in its selection of training tasks, that is respectful of the limits of mental muscle-building exercises, and that recognizes that, in many cases, improved cognitive functioning is a consequence of increased knowledge, skill, and strategic behavior *in specific domains of content* as opposed to generally improved cognition.

Hierarchical Versus Nonhierarchical Approaches

The tradition in cognitive rehabilitation has been to promote restoration of function using tasks and objectives that are arranged hierarchically. In some senses of the term *hierarchy*, this approach is unobjectionable, although in others it is questionable and perhaps misleading. If by *hierarchy of exercises* one means exercises that progress from simple to more difficult for the individual, then there can be little dispute with a hierarchical approach. However, this meaning of the term is insufficient to support a curricular approach to cognitive intervention. Many factors contribute to the difficulty of a task and therefore difficulty levels can be ranked very differently for different individuals. Furthermore, a given task can be made easy or difficult depending on the amount of support that is offered.

A more substantive sense of *hierarchy* has been part of Western psychology for 2,500 years or more, and it is presumably involved in the recommendation that cognitive

rehabilitation be hierarchical. For example, Aristotle proposed that there are five major human faculties, arranged hierarchically from lowest to highest: vegetative, locomotive, perceptual, intellectual, and volitional. In the nineteenth century, a number of educational theorists described hierarchies of cognitive faculties and promoted exercises that began with the lowest faculties and proceeded sequentially to the highest. Many discussions of cognitive rehabilitation in the 1980s similarly suggested that detailed hierarchies of cognitive process could be identified, such that cognitive rehabilitation comprised the organized presentation of tasks to exercise and improve cognitive processes from lowest to highest in the hierarchy.

Certainly, some aspects of cognition are more pervasive than others. For example, all cognitive activity presupposes some degree of alertness and attentiveness, but not all cognitive activity presupposes reasoning or executive control. Based on these considerations, it is tempting to focus sequentially in cognitive rehabilitation on "lower" processes such as attention and perception and to move to "higher" processes and systems only after a high level of success has been achieved at the lower levels. Unfortunately, this approach is strikingly inconsistent with normal cognitive development in children (described earlier under Cognitive Development). For example, between the ages of 6 and 12 months, there is active development of reasoning and problem-solving skill (Willatts, 1990) and of executive control over cognitive processes (Diamond and Goldman-Rakic, 1989), developmental facts that are inconsistent with purported hierarchies underlying many cognitive retraining programs. The important point here is that just as aspects of cognition are not discrete in normal adult cognition, aspects of cognition develop in a mutually interactive manner throughout childhood. This developmental model suggests that in rehabilitation, there should be an appropriate focus on all aspects of cognition at all stages of recovery and intervention. It is in part because of our opposition to the hierarchical approach to cognitive rehabilitation that we have selected organization and memory, executive functions, and social skills as our topics for the three cognitive intervention chapters in this book.

Contextualized Versus Decontextualized Approaches

Context of training includes the *content* of training activities as well as the *setting* where training occurs and the *people* in that setting. In this sense, a retraining activity can be contextualized if it contains meaningful content, even though it occurs in a clinical setting. The primary rationale for engaging individuals in cognitive exercises not embedded in personally meaningful content is that the opposite approach may run the risk of yielding stimulus-bound cognitive improvements that do not extend beyond the concrete, meaningful content that is the training context

(Sohlberg and Raskin, 1996). For example, if attention training is administered to a child using only current classroom materials, improved ability to attend may be restricted to these materials, and no generalized improvement of attentional functions may result. Therefore, within this framework, cognitive exercises are promoted that may have varied content but content that is as nonspecific as possible so as to promote the most general development of cognitive skills.

Nineteenth-century educational practices provided an interesting experiment related to transferability of cognitive skill in people with no cognitive disability. One of the linchpins of the doctrine of formal discipline, the prevailing philosophy of education at the time, was that thorough training in Latin and geometry, along with other formal training, would result in organized thinking and careful reasoning that would transfer broadly to any task that required organization and reasoning. When Thorndike put this theory to the test near the turn of the century, little evidence was adduced to support the predicted general transfer (Singley and Anderson, 1989). These experiments helped to discredit faculty psychology, the theoretical support for the doctrine of formal discipline. Faculty psychologists of the nineteenth century maintained that the mind was composed of highly general cognitive faculties (e.g., faculties of attention, discrimination, and reasoning) that could be separately strengthened with exercise, the result of which would be improvement of performance in all activities that engage that faculty. The assumptions underlying the process-specific approach to cognitive training in special education in the nineteenth century and into the 1950s and 1960s and to cognitive rehabilitation in the 1970s and 1980s closely resemble those made by nineteenth-century faculty psychologists.

The fallacy of cognitive training based on the principles of faculty psychology can be expressed as follows:

1. Task *T* engages cognitive process *P*.
2. Repetitive performance of *T* results in improved performance of *T* and, by inference, improvement in *P*.
3. Therefore, performance should improve in all tasks that engage process *P*.

This line of reasoning would predict that As in geometry and logic classes will result in improved reasoning in political science class and everyday life; that faster reaction times in response to meaningless signals on a computer screen will result in faster reading and writing; that improved problem-solving skill playing video games will result in improved problem solving in everyday life; that a person who is a master of strategic thinking in baseball will be a fine strategist in chess or on a military battlefield; that increased flexibility in attentional shifts using computerized cognitive retraining tasks will result in a child with greater flexibility in shifting from reading class to math class or from recess back to the classroom; and that improvements in cognitive rehabilitation workbook exercises will result in improved cognition in everyday life. Unfortunately, such predictions are rarely met when put to the test (Singley and Anderson, 1989).

The natural rebuttal to this argument in support of meaningful content for cognitive rehabilitation tasks is that transfer or generalization from training task to application task is not expected without systematic efforts to promote such generalization. This is certainly a giant step in the right direction. Furthermore, there is no question that it is desirable to equip individuals with the most generally applicable knowledge and skill possible. However, it makes greater sense to us to follow the normal and gradual developmental progression from successful performance in concrete and personally meaningful tasks to acquisition of more abstract and more readily transferable knowledge and skill. Not only is this a sage developmental principle; it is also a safer plan in that, if generalization does *not* occur, the child's practice at least occurred in a context and with activities in which improved performance is important for the child.

Improving Cognitive Functioning: Intervention Procedures

Chapters 11, 12, and 14 present a variety of procedures designed to promote improvement in cognitive functioning or improvement in performance of tasks when that performance is impeded by chronic cognitive disability. Those procedures have their rationale and historical origin in several theories of cognitive change and development in children. Understanding relationships between brain structure and behavior, between brain injury and impairment, and among aspects of cognition does not yet answer the question, "What should I do to help improve the functioning of a child with cognitive impairment?" The earlier discussion of approaches to cognitive rehabilitation begins to answer this question by answering others: For example, should the targets be components of cognition or functional-integrative performance? Should the focus be restorative or compensatory? Should the progression be based on a hierarchical view of cognition? Should the activities be meaningfully contextualized? These questions, however, do not squarely address the critical issue of effective intervention procedures.

In this brief discussion of cognitive development and ways of promoting cognitive change, we wish to recommend an eclectic and experimental approach. Although we emphasize the special contribution of Vygotsky's social interactionist approach, each theory contributes to a functional approach to cognitive rehabilitation.

Alternative schemes exist that could be used to organize a discussion of theories regarding the "how" of cognitive development. Here we highlight theories that yield specific and interestingly different intervention procedures. The responsible clinician's goal is not to commit to one theory and reject the others but rather to glean from each whatever it might contribute to an approach to intervention that works for the individual child.

Applied Behavior Analysis

Applied behavior analysis, with its emphasis on contingencies of reinforcement—including social, emotional, and informative feedback as well as tangible rewards—has evolved a set of procedures for changing behavior and maintaining motivation, the effectiveness of which has been documented in a wide variety of treatment areas (Bandura, 1977; Harter, 1978; Miller and Dollard, 1971; Skinner, 1969). In its broadest terms, change in performance is a result of breaking complex behaviors into components, modeling and otherwise eliciting targeted responses, differentially reinforcing desired responses, chaining component behaviors into desired complexes, and systematically varying stimuli, responses, and reinforcement contingencies so that behaviors can generalize to many real-world tasks and contexts. The literature that addresses procedural technology within a behavioral framework is enormous. In Chapter 13, Ylvisaker and Feeney recommend some deviations from the tradition of behavior modification in working with children with TBI who have behavior problems. In particular, the approach they recommend focuses more on setting events and other antecedents than on consequences.

Traditional procedures of applied behavior analysis may be appropriate in cognitive intervention (Sohlberg and Raskin, 1996), particularly for individuals whose motivation and cognitive levels are relatively low. The contributions of behavioral learning theory that are particularly critical include (1) a focus on behavior or skill generalization, (2) an understanding of behavior as evolving out of and being shaped by everyday routine interactions, (3) an appreciation of modeling and cueing procedures, and (4) a recognition of the importance of automating cognitive processes (through practice) to reduce the burden on working memory. These contributions have occasionally been neglected in cognitive rehabilitation. Furthermore, because development of the knowledge base is an important contributor to improved cognitive functioning, Direct-Instruction procedures (based on an applied behavior analytic theory of instruction) may be useful in teaching children with TBI (Glang et al., 1992), especially in the case of material that must be immediately accessible (e.g., math facts) and skills that must be automatic (e.g., reading). Ideally, these procedures are applied in the context of everyday routines (vs. a service restricted to relatively infrequent specialized treatment sessions), in which everyday teachers and others model and encourage cognitive targets in meaningful activities, using natural rewards.

Cognitive Behavior Modification

Cognitive behavior modification (CBM; Meichenbaum, 1977) adds to traditional learning theory a useful emphasis on self-instruction as a means of controlling and mediating one's behavior (for older children and adolescents with reasonable cognitive recovery). In work with other disability groups, CBM procedures have received mixed experimental support, the criticism often focusing on failures of generalization and maintenance. However, it is possible that published reports have been based on specific studies in which CBM procedures were isolated (i.e., used in a highly controlled manner and divorced from other interventions). Our view is that CBM, probably like all cognitive intervention procedures, is unlikely to have a powerful effect unless infused into a wide domain of everyday activities, integrated with other interventions appropriate for individual children, and actively promoted for years (vs. the few weeks characteristic of research designs). Recent investigations by educational psychologists suggest that intervention to improve strategic learning and controlled processing must be long term to be effective (Pressley, 1993).

Feuerstein's (1980) techniques of mediated learning have a similar focus on understanding and controlling one's cognitive behavior. A critical element of Feuerstein's approach is that the cognitive mediation is designed to occur throughout the instructional day, infused into the normal academic curriculum.

Feuerstein's approach and Meichenbaum's recent application of CBM principles to TBI rehabilitation (Meichenbaum, 1993) are both explicitly linked to Vygotsky's theory of cognitive growth, discussed next.

Social Interactionist (Vygotskyan) Approaches

Understanding cognitive development and intervention as social interaction (Vygotsky, 1978) recently has experienced a lively revival among developmental cognitive psychologists (e.g., Nelson, 1992; Rogoff, 1990; Rogoff and Misty, 1990), educational psychologists (e.g., Brown et al., 1992; Campione and Brown, 1990), early childhood educators (e.g., Bodrova and Leong, 1996), special educators (e.g., Evans, 1993), speech-language pathologists (e.g., Schneider and Watkins, 1996; Westby, 1994), and others. According to Vygotsky (1981), "[H]igher mental functions evolve through social interactions with adults; they are gradually internalized as the child becomes more and more proficient and needs less and less cueing and other support from the adult." This principle has been used to explain the origin of language and conversational interaction (Bruner, 1975), of episodic (or autobiographical) memory and discourse organization (Nelson, 1992; Reese et al., 1993), of deliberate self-regulation (Leont'ev, 1978), and of other mental functions.

Within the vygotskyan framework, psychological processes such as problem solving, organizing, planning, remembering, social reflection, and self-regulation exist initially as interactions between the child and an adult or another child. Gradually these conversations are internalized, and the child is ultimately able to carry out the same cognitive activity but now as an internal mental process. Despite their demonstrated usefulness in many domains of education and intervention for children, and despite the close historical connection between vygotskyan psychology and Luria's popular neuropsychological framework, Vygotsky's principles have received surprisingly little attention in discussions of neuropsychological rehabilitation after brain injury.

Vygotskyan theory is a major component of the theoretical basis for our recommendation (in Chapters 11, 12, 14, and 20) that cognitive intervention use as primary agents of cognitive growth appropriately trained communication partners (e.g., parents, aides, siblings, teachers) who function in the child's everyday environment. This approach applies throughout the developmental spectrum, from the interaction between parents and infants (e.g., designed to facilitate simple problem solving and interactive competence) to that between teachers and adolescents (e.g., designed to improve reading comprehension, writing skill, metacognitive awareness, and general strategic behavior). In Chapter 14, our description of the use of everyday conversations about the past as a means for improving memory and thought and language organization illustrates this approach.

The developmental theories of Vygotsky and their recent implementation in the intervention literature support the increasingly popular concepts of *cognitive coaching* and *apprenticeship,* in which adults who interact with the child on an everyday basis (e.g., teachers, therapists, parents, nurses) interact in a way that is natural and conversational but that also provides scaffolding (i.e., various forms of support, including joint activity, modeling, cueing, and elaboration) for incremental growth in cognitive performance in specifically targeted areas, using as the context everyday activities and interaction: That is, the adult's role is to engage children in interesting activities and interaction associated with those activities, ensuring that the cognitive activity (e.g., problem solving, reading for comprehension, remembering, organizing) is apparent and effective in the interaction, and taking responsibility for as much of the cognitive activity as is necessary while turning over to the child increasing responsibility for cognitive dimensions of the task.

Throughout the interaction, adults try to engage children within their "zone of proximal development," which is "the distance between the actual developmental level

as determined by independent problem solving and the level of potential development as determined through problem solving under adult guidance or in collaboration with more capable peers" (Vygotsky, 1978). This aspect of Vygotsky's theory of instruction connects his work directly with the dynamic assessment movement in educational psychology. Dynamic assessment is a set of procedures designed to determine what a child is capable of doing if aided and what kind of help (e.g., instructions, modeling, cueing, task modification) is most effective at raising the child's level of performance (Feuerstein, 1979; Lidz, 1987; Minick, 1987). In Chapter 10, Ylvisaker and Gioia expand this concept of dynamic assessment to include collaborative, contextualized, hypothesis-testing assessment as the primary form of intervention-relevant evaluation.

Working within a vygotskyan perspective requires professionals to modify their implicit understanding of their role, moving from a combined animal trainer–pedagogue–surgeon metaphor to a combined master craftsperson–coach–consultant metaphor. Like a master craftsperson working with an apprentice, the adult ensures that the jointly produced "product" (e.g., a well-organized narrative about the past, a solution to a problem, a plan, a resolution of a conflict) is a good one, that the child has a role to play in its creation (i.e., the child and adult are collaborators), and that the child increasingly appreciates the cognitive activity that goes into creating the product. Like a coach, the adult models cognitive processes, encourages exploration and development, and praises accomplishment, both on the practice field (e.g., therapy sessions) and in real games (i.e., activities and contexts that are meaningful and important for the child). These metaphors are explored further by Ylvisaker and Feeney in Chapter 20.

One of the benefits of a vygotskyan theoretical foundation for cognitive rehabilitation is the promise it holds for creating a bridge between the worlds of behaviorally and cognitively oriented clinicians. In both cases, the core of intervention is facilitation of positive *routines.* In the case of behavioral intervention, the routines are behavior chains in which each behavior is a discriminative stimulus for the next behavior. A goal of behavioral intervention is to create positive routines and then to make them sufficiently flexible to fit a variety of real-world contexts by systematically varying eliciting stimuli and consequent responses. In the case of cognitive intervention, the goal is to create, by systematically varying the experiences to which they apply and the mediation that the adult supplies, routines of interaction that gradually are internalized as cognitive processes or scripts and that become sufficiently flexible to fit a variety of real-world contexts.

Another interesting benefit of vygotskyan instructional theory is that it challenges the distinction between compensatory and restorative approaches to intervention. *Scaffolding* within this framework can be understood as a set of environmental *compensations* (including modifications in the behavior of others) that enable the child to complete a task effectively. However, providing such scaffolding and then either systematically reducing the support structure or increasing the difficulty of the task as the child improves is also the recommended approach to *restoration* after TBI and ongoing cognitive development. Thus, it becomes possible to avoid disputes between restoration-focused and compensation-focused approaches to cognitive rehabilitation, because a single intervention can be at the same time restorative and compensatory.

Structuralist (Piagetian) Approaches

Despite serious concerns about basic aspects of the structuralist theory of cognitive development devised by Piaget (e.g., Siegler, 1991; Willatts, 1990), including his commitment to discrete, qualitatively distinct stages of cognitive development and to the existence of cognitive structures that are fully independent of specific domains of content, elements of Piaget's perspective remain valid, including the focus on balancing assimilation and accommodation and on promoting cognitive growth with concrete problem-solving experiences. According to Piaget (1970), individuals add to their knowledge and restructure their conceptual framework through interaction with the environment. As they interpret events and objects in terms of what is already known (assimilation), they simultaneously take into account unknown properties and relations (accommodation). Balancing these two adaptive mechanisms gradually modifies schemata of interaction and results in cognitive growth. Therefore, improvement can be promoted when presented tasks offer some components that can be easily understood in terms of existing knowledge structures and other components that require some schematic modification before the task can be completed. Because learning occurs primarily through discovery, the key to effective intervention is designing tasks that create optimal conditions for discovering targeted information or cognitive schemata.

The High/Scope Curriculum, discussed in Chapter 14, is a good example of Piaget's views applied to the education of children at risk for academic failure. Children with significant cognitive disability after brain injury clearly need more direction, focusing, highlighting, motivating, coaching, and cueing than do children with no disability. For this reason, vygotskyan interactionist principles, with their emphasis on the guiding and mediating activity of adults and more accomplished peers, are a useful antidote to the shortcomings of Piaget's view. Nevertheless, these core themes (assimilation, accommodation, and task design) in Piaget's theory are useful in cognitive rehabilitation. Furthermore, a large number of piagetian tasks (e.g., object permanence [*A*-not-*B*], means-end [i.e., early problem solving–strategic behav-

ior]), and conservation tasks have recently been reinterpreted within the framework of modern theories of cognitive development, with a particular emphasis on development of executive functions (Roberts and Pennington, 1996; Willatts, 1990).

Service Delivery Systems

Perhaps because cognitive rehabilitation after TBI evolved as a specialized service within the medical rehabilitation system, published descriptions of the service have emphasized components of the medical model. Cognitive rehabilitation is often described as a discrete service, delivered by cognitive rehabilitation specialists in a clinical setting using specialized activities that target specific aspects of cognition. Indeed, during the 1980s, many people came to associate computerized exercises with cognitive rehabilitation. Although we do not intend to argue that this picture is completely mistaken, our discussion of cognition, cognitive development, and cognitive growth in children leads inevitably to a system that emphasizes the infusion of cognitive intervention throughout the child's day and program, with all people who are active in the child's everyday life playing a role in the service.

In the case of rehabilitation hospitals, the everyday people who need to know how to use everyday activities and interaction to facilitate cognitive recovery include parents, nursing staff (including nursing assistants), all rehabilitation therapists, and others who spend time with the child. Chapters 11, 12, 14, and 20 include suggestions for implementing such a contextualized cognitive rehabilitation program. Professionals who specialize in cognitive rehabilitation (whatever their specific training) must acquire considerable competence as consultants because much of their professional time and energy is devoted to equipping other people with competencies in this area of intervention.

As lengths of hospital stay decrease dramatically, most professional services designed to improve children's cognitive functioning are being provided by outpatient or school-based clinicians and teachers. In a managed-care environment, a service explicitly referred to as *cognitive rehabilitation* is often not reimbursed. Under these circumstances, it is critical that a professional culture be developed that values and facilitates role sharing within teams of professionals and everyday people. Most of the intervention activities described in our chapters on application can be part of physical, occupational, or speech-language therapy; tutoring sessions; or recreational and daily living activities supervised by parents. It is not the title but rather the knowledge, skill, energy, and commitment of the person delivering the intervention that makes a difference. Specialists in cognition may find themselves working in the background, consulting with others who, because of the frequency of their interaction with the child or because of the reimbursable nature of their service, are in a better position to help the child.

Cardinal Rules of Cognitive Rehabilitation

The discussions in this chapter lead to an approach to cognitive rehabilitation that is driven by the following rules and is illustrated in subsequent chapters:

1. *Meaningful developmental hierarchies:* In designing cognitive rehabilitation tasks, follow normal developmental progressions in these areas: surface to depth; concrete to abstract; context dependent to context independent; real-event routines and scripts to more abstract categories and other organizing schemes; involuntary, nonstrategic to controlled and strategic information processing.

2. *Knowledge base:* Help children to recover pretraumatically acquired content knowledge and to acquire and organize new content knowledge. Because efficient processing of information is, in part, a function of the depth and organization of the knowledge base, it is misguided to attempt to promote development of cognitive processes without regard to meaningful and relevant content.

3. *Efficiency of processing:* Help children to process information more quickly and efficiently, recognizing that both speed of processing and amount of information that can be processed are, in part, a function of existing knowledge and its organization.

4. *Organization and habituation:* Help children to increase the functional capacity of working memory by equipping them with functional organizing schemes that they practice in meaningful tasks to the point of habituation.

5. *Balance in approaches:* Within every phase of intervention, ensure that there is an appropriate balance of restorative exercises, compensation training, and environmental support, based on functional short-term and long-term goals and on available evidence regarding the effectiveness of the interventions being considered. These three approaches can be integrated with a vygotskyan-supported cognition approach to facilitating cognitive growth.

6. *Functional outcome:* Ensure that the child not only possesses a cognitive skill or capacity in artificial training tasks but also uses it in real-world activities. The standard of success must be improved performance of meaningful tasks in real-world contexts, maintained and strengthened over the long term.

7. *Functional context:* Unless there is good reason to do otherwise, provide cognitive rehabilitation services within the context of the child's meaningful daily living, academic, social, vocational, or recreational

activities. If the initial stages of training use decontextualized exercises, expand to meaningful activities and real-world settings as quickly as possible.

8. *Motivation and executive function focus:* Ensure that children are as engaged as possible in identifying their own problems and goals, choosing activities, planning and organizing their activities, identifying the difficulty level of tasks, monitoring and evaluating their performance, and solving problems that arise. Recognizing that children with TBI will probably face a large number of obstacles in life, help them to become as strategic a thinker as possible in order to overcome those obstacles.

9. *Integration and organization:* Ensure that the child's activities are clearly integrated within a treatment or instructional session, between sessions, and from day to day. Try to avoid contributing to fragmentation by addressing too many goals and objectives at one time (across the entire program) and by proceeding through too many unrelated activities over the course of a day or treatment session. Provide external support that the child may need to remain organized.

10. *Everyday people as cognitive coaches:* Ensure that all adults who regularly interact with the child know how to provide cognitive coaching in their arena of interaction with the child. Increase both intensity and functionality of cognitive intervention by infusing it throughout the child's day.

11. *Cognitive support and success:* Ensure that all adults who regularly interact with the child understand how much support is needed by the child to succeed in everyday tasks and that they provide neither too little nor too much support. Ensure that support is reduced as the child demonstrates capacity to succeed independently.

12. *Cognition and behavior:* Ensure that all adults who regularly interact with the child understand that appropriate and frequently adjusted levels of cognitive support are often the key to preventing the evolution of behavior problems after TBI.

Concluding Comments

In this chapter, we have attempted to articulate a framework for cognitive rehabilitation for children and adolescents with TBI. Clinicians who wish to deliver a service knowledgeably must have an understanding of the components of mature cognition and their interrelationships; of the general patterns and driving forces of cognitive development; of likely consequences of TBI and their evolution over time in various age groups; and of the basis and empirical support for intervention options with this and other disability groups. This is a tall order. Although TBI rehabilitation for children is in the early stages of development, we believe that a framework for intervention can be derived from research in cognitive functioning and cognitive development, investigations of cognitive intervention with other disability groups, and experience "in the trenches." We hope that this framework will provide a helpful structure within which to place the assessment and intervention practices described in Chapters 10–14.

References

Anderson JR (1976). Cognitive Psychology and Its Implications. San Francisco: Freeman.

Ashcraft M (1994). Human Memory and Cognition. New York: HarperCollins.

Baddeley A (1982). Amnesia: A Minimal Model and Interpretation. In L Cermak (ed), Human Memory and Amnesia. Hillsdale, NJ: Lawrence Erlbaum, 305.

Baddeley A (1986). Working Memory. Oxford: Clarendon.

Baddeley A (1989). The Uses of Working Memory. In P Solomon, G Goethals, C Kelley, B Stephens (eds), Memory: Interdisciplinary Approaches. New York: Springer, 107.

Baddeley A (1990). Human Memory. Boston: Allyn & Bacon.

Baddeley A, Wilson BA, Watts FN (1995). Handbook of Memory Disorders. New York: Wiley.

Bandura A (1977). Social Learning Theory. Englewood Cliffs, NJ: Prentice Hall.

Ben-Yishay Y, Diller L (1983). Cognitive Deficits. In M Rosenthal, M Bond, E Griffith, JD Miller (eds), Rehabilitation of the Head Injured Adult. Philadelphia: Davis.

Bjorklund DF, Harnishfeger KK (1990). Children's Strategies: Their Definition and Origins. In DF Bjorklund (ed), Children's Strategies: Contemporary Views of Cognitive Development. Hillsdale, NJ: Lawrence Erlbaum, 309.

Bjorklund DF (1990). Children's Strategies: Contemporary Views of Cognitive Development. Hillsdale, NJ: Lawrence Erlbaum.

Bjorklund DF, Muir-Broaddus J, Schneider W (1990). The Role of Knowledge in the Development of Strategies. In DF Bjorklund (ed), Children's Strategies: Contemporary Views of Cognitive Development. Hillsdale, NJ: Lawrence Erlbaum, 93.

Bodrova E, Leong DJ (1996). Tools of the Mind: The Vygotskyan Approach to Early Childhood Education. Englewood Cliffs, NJ: Prentice Hall.

Borkowski JG, Carr M, Rellinger E, Pressley M (1990). Self-Regulated Cognition: Interdependence of Metacognition, Attributions, and Self-Esteem. In BF Jones, L Idol (eds), Dimensions of Thinking and Cognitive Development. Hillsdale, NJ: Lawrence Erlbaum, 53.

Brooks DN (1983). Disorders of Memory. In M Rosenthal, E Griffith, M Bond, JD Miller (eds), Rehabilitation of the Head Injured Adult. Philadelphia: Davis, 185.

Brooks DN (1984). Closed Head Injury: Psychological, Social, and Family Consequences. New York: Oxford University.

Brown AL (1975). The Development of Memory: Knowing, Knowing About Knowing, and Knowing How to Know. In HW Reese (ed), Advances in Child Development and Behavior, vol 10. New York: Academic, 103.

Brown AL (1979). Theories of Memory and Problems of Development, Activity, Growth, and Knowledge. In FIM Craik, L Cermak (eds), Levels of Processing and Memory. Hillsdale, NJ: Lawrence Erlbaum, 225.

Brown AL, Campione JC, Weber LS, McGilly K (1992). Interactive Learning Environments: A New Look at Assessment and Instruction. Berkeley, CA: University of California, Commission on Testing and Public Policy.

Bruner J (1975). The ontogenesis of speech acts. J Child Lang 2;1.

Butler RW, Namerow MD (1988). Cognitive retraining in brain-injury rehabilitation: a critical review. J Neurol Rehabil 2;97.

Campione JC, Brown AL (1990). Guided Learning and Transfer. In N Fredrickson, R Glaser, A Lesgold, M Shafto (eds), Diagnostic Monitoring of Skill and Knowledge Acquisition. Hillsdale, NJ: Lawrence Erlbaum, 141.

Chi MTH (1978). Knowledge Structures and Memory Development. In R Siegler (ed), Children's Thinking: What Develops? Hillsdale, NJ: Lawrence Erlbaum, 73.

Craik FIM, Tulving E (1975). Depth of processing and the retention of words in episodic memory. J Exp Psychol 104;268.

Dennis M (1991). Frontal lobe function in childhood and adolescence: a heuristic for assessing attention regulation, executive control and the intentional states important for social discourse. Dev Neuropsychol 7(3);327.

Deshler DD, Schumaker JB (1988). An Instructional Model for Teaching Students How to Learn. In JL Graden, JE Zins, MJ Curtis (eds), Alternative Educational Delivery Systems: Enhancing Instructional Options for All Students. Washington, DC: National Association of School Psychologists, 391.

Deutsch D, Deutsch JA (1975). Short-Term Memory. New York: Academic.

Diamond A, Goldman-Rakic PS (1989). Comparison of human infants and rhesus monkeys on Piaget's AB task: evidence for dependence on dorsolateral prefrontal cortex. Exp Brain Res 74;24.

Dodd D, White RM (1980). Cognition, Mental Structures and Processes. Boston: Allyn & Bacon.

Eslinger PJ, Grattan LM, Damasio H, Damasio AR (1992). Developmental consequences of childhood frontal lobe damage. Arch Neurol 49;764.

Evans P (1993). Some Implications of Vygotsky's Work for Special Education. In H Daniels (ed), Charting the Agenda: Education Activity After Vygotsky. London: Routledge.

Feeney TJ, Ylvisaker M (1995). Choice and routine: antecedent behavioral interventions for adolescents with severe traumatic brain injury. J Head Trauma Rehabil 10(3);67.

Feuerstein R (1979). The Dynamic Assessment of Retarded Performers: The Learning Potential Assessment Device,

Theory, Instruments, and Techniques. Baltimore: University Park.

Feuerstein R (1980). Instrumental Enrichment: An Intervention Program for Cognitive Modifiability. Baltimore: University Park.

Flavell J, Miller P, Miller S (1993). Cognitive Development. Englewood Cliffs, NJ: Prentice Hall.

Gholson B, Morgan D, Dattel AR, Pierce KA (1990). The Development of Analogical Problem Solving: Strategic Processes in Schema Acquisition and Transfer. In DF Bjorklund (ed), Children's Strategies: Contemporary Views of Cognitive Development. Hillsdale, NJ: Lawrence Erlbaum, 269.

Gibson EJ (1969). Principles of Perceptual Learning and Development. New York: Appleton-Century-Crofts.

Glang A, Singer G, Coole E, Tish N (1992). Tailoring direct instruction techniques for use with elementary students with brain injury. J Head Trauma Rehabil 1;93.

Goldman PS (1971). Functional development of the prefrontal cortex in early life and the problem of neuronal plasticity. Exp Neurol 32;366.

Graf P, Masson M (1993). Implicit Memory: New Directions in Cognition, Development, and Neuropsychology. Hillsdale, NJ: Lawrence Erlbaum.

Grafman J, Sirigu A, Spector L, Hendler J (1993). Damage to the prefrontal cortex leads to decomposition of structured event complexes. J Head Trauma Rehabil 8;73.

Grattan LM, Eslinger PJ (1991). Frontal lobe damage in children and adults: a comparative review. Dev Neuropsychol 7;283.

Grattan LM, Eslinger PJ (1992). Long-term psychological consequences of childhood frontal lobe lesion in patient DT. Brain Cogn 20;185.

Hallowell EM, Ratey JJ (1994). Driven to Distraction. New York: Pantheon Books.

Harter S (1978). Effective motivation reconsidered: toward a developmental model. Hum Dev 21;34.

Herrmann DJ, Weingartner H, Searleman A, McEvoy C (1992). Memory improvement: implications for memory theory. New York: Springer.

Hintzman DL (1978). The Psychology of Learning and Memory. New York: Freeman.

Istominia ZM (1977). The development of voluntary memory in preschool age children. Soviet Psychol 13(4);5.

Jacoby LA (1994). A process disassociation framework: separating automatic from intentional uses of memory. J Mem Lang 30;513.

James W (1890). The Principles of Psychology. New York: Holt.

Kail R (1990). The Development of Memory in Children (3rd ed). New York: Freeman.

Kinsbourne M, Wood F (1982). Theoretical Considerations Regarding the Episodic-Semantic Memory Distinction. In L Cermak (ed), Human Memory and Amnesia. Hillsdale, NJ: Lawrence Erlbaum, 195.

Koskiniemi M, Kyykka T, Nybo T, Jarho L (1995). Long term outcome after severe brain injury in preschoolers is worse than expected. Arch Pediatr Adolesc Med 149;249.

Leont'ev A (1978). Activity, Consciousness, and Personality. Englewood Cliffs, NJ: Prentice Hall.

Levin H, Benton A, Grossman R (1982). Neurobehavioral Consequences of Closed Head Injury. New York: Oxford University.

Levin HS, Culhane KA, Hartman J, et al. (1991a). Developmental changes in performance on tests of purported frontal lobe functioning. Dev Neuropsychol 7;377.

Levin HS, Fletcher JM, Kufera JA, et al. (1996). Dimensions of cognition measured by the Tower of London and other cognitive tasks in head-injured children and adolescents. Dev Neuropsychol 12;17.

Levin HS, Goldstein FC (1986). Organization of verbal memory after severe head injury. J Clin Exp Neuropsychol 8;643.

Levin HS, Goldstein FC, Williams DH, Eisenberg HM (1991b). The Contribution of Frontal Lobe Lesions to the Neurobehavioral Outcome of Closed Head Injury. In HS Levin, HM Eisenberg, AI Benton (eds), Frontal Lobe Function and Dysfunction. New York: Oxford University, 318.

Lezak MD (1982). The problem of assessing executive functions. Int J Psychol 17;281.

Lezak MD (1983). Neuropsychological Assessment. New York: Oxford University.

Lidz CS (1987). Dynamic Assessment: An Interactional Approach to Evaluating Learning Potential. New York: Guilford.

Mann L (1979). On the Trail of Process: A Historical Perspective on Cognitive Processes and Their Training. New York: Grune & Stratton.

Marlowe WB (1992). The impact of a right prefrontal lesion on the developing brain. Brain Cogn 20;205.

Mateer CA, Mapou RL (1996). Understanding, evaluating, and managing attention disorders following traumatic brain injury. J Head Trauma Rehabil 11;1.

Mateer CA, Williams D (1991). Effects of frontal lobe injury in childhood. Dev Neuropsychol 7;359.

Meichenbaum D (1977). Cognitive Behavior Modification: An Integrative Approach. New York: Plenum Press.

Meichenbaum D (1993). The "potential" contributions of cognitive behavior modification to the rehabilitation of individuals with traumatic brain injury. Semin Speech Lang 14;18.

Miller G (1956). The magical number seven, plus or minus two: some limits on our capacity for processing information. Psychol Rev 63;81.

Miller NE, Dollard J (1971). Social Learning and Imitation. New Haven: Yale University.

Milner B (1970). Memory and the Medial Temporal Regions of the Brain. In KH Pribram, DE Broadbent (eds), Biological Bases of Memory. New York: Academic, 29.

Minick N (1987). Implications of Vygotsky's Theories for Dynamic Assessment. In CS Lidz (ed), Dynamic Assessment: An Interactional Approach to Evaluating Learning Potential. New York: Guilford, 116.

Moely B (1977). Organization of Memory. In R Kail, J Hagen (eds), Perspectives on the Development of Memory and Cognition. Hillsdale, NJ: Lawrence Erlbaum, 203.

Neisser E (1989). Domains of Memory. In P Solomon, G Goethals, C Kelley, B Stephens (eds), Memory: Interdisciplinary Approaches. New York: Springer, 84.

Nelson K (1992). Emergence of autobiographical memory at age 4. Hum Dev 35(3);172.

Norman DA (1976). Memory and Attention: An Introduction to Human Information Processing (2nd ed). New York: Wiley.

Parkin AJ (1993). Memory Phenomena, Experiments, and Theory. Oxford, UK: Blackwell.

Pennington BF (1991). Diagnosing Learning Disorders: A Neuropsychological Framework. New York: Guilford.

Piaget J (1970). Piaget's Theory. In PH Mussen (ed), Carmichael's Manual of Child Psychology, vol 1. New York: Wiley.

Piaget J, Inhelder B (1973). Memory and Intelligence. New York: Basic Books.

Ponsford J. (1990). The Use of Computers in the Rehabilitation of Attention Disorders. In RL Wood, I Fussey (eds), Cognitive Rehabilitation in Perspective. London: Taylor & Francis, 48.

Postman L (1964). Short-Term Memory and Incidental Learning. In AW Nelson (ed), Categories of Human Learning. New York: Academic, 145.

Postman L, Kruesi E (1977). The influence of orienting tasks on the encoding and recall of words. J Verbal Learn Verbal Behav 2;353.

Pressley M (1993). Teaching cognitive strategies to brain-injured clients: the good information processing perspective. Semin Speech Lang 14;1.

Pressley M and Associates (1990). Cognitive Strategy Instruction That Really Improves Children's Academic Performance. Cambridge, MA: Brookline Books.

Pressley M, El-Dinary PB (1992). Memory Strategy Instruction That Promotes Good Information Processing. In DJ Herrmann, H Weingartner, A Searleman, C McEvoy (eds), Memory Improvement: Implications for Memory Theory. New York: Springer, 79.

Price B, Doffnre K, Stowe R, Mesulam M (1990). The compartmental learning disabilities of early frontal lobe damage. Brain 113;1383.

Reese E, Haden CA, Fivush R (1993). Mother-child conversations about the past: relationships of style and memory over time. Cogn Dev 8;403.

Roberts RJ, Pennington BF (1996). An interactive framework for examining prefrontal cognitive processes. Dev Neuropsychol 12;105.

Rogoff B (1990). Apprenticeship in Thinking: Cognitive Development in Social Context. New York: Oxford University.

Rogoff B, Misty J (1990). The Social and Function Context of Children's Remembering. In R Fivush, JD Hudson (eds), Knowing and Remembering in Young Children. New York: Cambridge University.

Rummelhart D (1984). Schemata and the Cognitive System. In R Wyer, T Srull (eds), Handbook of Social Cognition, vol 1. Hillsdale, NJ: Lawrence Erlbaum, 161.

Schacter D (1987). Memory, amnesia, and frontal lobe dysfunction. Psychobiology 15;21.

Schacter D, Church B (1992). Auditory priming: implicit and explicit memory for words and voices. J Exp Psychol 18;915.

Schneider P, Watkins RV (1996). Applying Vygotskyan developmental theory to language intervention. Lang Speech Hear Services Schools 27;157.

Schneider W, Pressley M (1989). Memory Development Between 2 and 20. New York: Springer.

Schwartz MF, Mayer NH, Fitzpatrick DeSalme EJ, Montgomery MW (1993). Cognitive theory and the study of everyday action disorders after brain damage. J Head Trauma Rehabil 8(1);59.

Shallice T (1988). From Neuropsychology to Mental Structure. Cambridge, UK: Cambridge University.

Siegler R (1991). Children's Thinking (2nd ed). Englewood Cliffs, NJ: Prentice Hall.

Singley MK, Anderson JR (1989). Transfer of Cognitive Skill. Cambridge, MA: Harvard University.

Skinner BF (1969). Contingencies of Reinforcement. New York: Appleton-Century-Crofts.

Smirnov A (1973). Problems in the Psychology of Memory. New York: Plenum.

Smirnov A, Zinchenko P (1969). Problems in the Psychology of Memory. In M Cole, I Maltzman (eds), A Handbook of Contemporary Soviet Psychology. New York: Basic Books, 45.

Smith EE (1978). Theories of Semantic Memory. In WK Estes (ed), Handbook of Learning and Cognitive Processes, vol 6. Hillsdale, NJ: Lawrence Erlbaum.

Sohlberg M, Mateer C (1989). Introduction to Cognitive Rehabilitation: Theory and Practice. New York: Guilford.

Sohlberg MM, Raskin SA (1996). Principles of generalization applied to attention and memory interventions. J Head Trauma Rehabil 11;65.

Squire L (1987). Memory and the Brain. New York: Oxford University.

Sternberg R, Berg C (1990). Intellectual Development. Cambridge, UK: Cambridge University.

Stuss DT, Buckle L (1992). Traumatic brain injury: neuropsychological deficits and evaluation at different stages of recovery and in different pathologic subtypes. J Head Trauma Rehabil 7;40.

Szekeres S (1992). Organization as an intervention target after traumatic brain injury. Semin Speech Lang 13;293.

Teuber HL (1964). The Riddle of Frontal Lobe Function in Man. In JM Warren, K Akert (eds), The Frontal Granular Cortex and Behavior. New York: McGraw-Hill.

Tulving E (1972). Episodic and Semantic Memory. In E Tulving, W Donaldson (eds), Organization of Memory. New York: Academic, 382.

Tulving E (1989). Remembering and knowing the past. Am Scientist 77;361.

Varney NR, Menefee L (1993). Psychosocial and executive deficits following closed head injury: implications for orbital frontal cortex. J Head Trauma Rehabil 8;32.

Vygotsky LS (1978). Mind in Society: The Development of Higher Psychological Processes. Edited and translated by M Cole, V John-Steiner, S Scribner, E Souberman. Cambridge, MA: Harvard University.

Vygotsky LS (1981). The Genesis of Higher Mental Functions. In JV Wertsch (ed), The Concept of Activity in Soviet Psychology. Armonk, NY: ME Sharps, 144.

Welsh MC, Pennington BF (1988). Assessing frontal lobe functioning in children: views from developmental psychology. Dev Neuropsychol 4;199.

Welsh MC, Pennington BF, Groisser DB (1991). A normative-developmental study of executive function: a window on prefrontal function in children. Dev Neuropsychol 7(2);131.

Westby CE (1994). The Effects of Culture on Genre, Structure, and Style of Oral and Written Texts. In GP Wallach, KG Butler (eds), Language Learning Disabilities in School-Age Children and Adolescents. New York: Merrill, 180.

Willatts P (1990). Development of Problem-Solving Strategies in Infancy. In DF Bjorklund (ed), Children's Strategies: Contemporary Views of Cognitive Development. Hillsdale, NJ: Lawrence Erlbaum, 23.

Williams D, Mateer CA (1992). Developmental impact of frontal lobe injury in middle childhood. Brain Cogn 20;196.

Wilson B, Evans J (1996). Error-free learning in the rehabilitation of people with memory impairments. J Head Trauma Rehabil 11;54.

Wood RL (1984). Management of Attention Disorders Following Brain Injury. In BA Wilson, N Moffatt (eds), Clinical Management of Memory Problems. London: Croom Helm.

Wood RL (1992). Disorders of Attention: Their Effect on Behavior, Cognition, and Rehabilitation. In B Wilson, N Moffatt (eds), Clinical Management of Memory Problems. San Diego: Singular Publishing, 216.

Ylvisaker M (1992). Communication outcome following traumatic brain injury. Semin Speech Lang 13;239.

Ylvisaker M (1993). Communication outcome in children and adolescents with traumatic brain injury. Neuropsychol Rehabil 3;367.

Ylvisaker M, Feeney T (1995). Traumatic brain injury in adolescence: assessment and reintegration. Semin Speech Lang 16;32.

Ylvisaker M, Feeney T (1996). Executive functions after traumatic brain injury: supported cognition and self-advocacy. Semin Speech Lang 17;217.

Ylvisaker M, Szekeres S (1989). Metacognitive and executive impairments in head-injured children and adults. Top Lang Dis 9(2);34.

Ylvisaker M, Urbanczyk B (1990). The efficacy of speech-language pathology intervention: traumatic brain injury. Semin Speech Lang 11;215.

Chapter 10
Cognitive Assessment

Mark Ylvisaker and Gerard A. Gioia

Cognitive assessment can serve a variety of purposes. In this chapter, we restrict our focus to assessment designed primarily to contribute to rehabilitative and educational intervention. With this as our goal, we focus less on tests and more on ongoing assessment activities that are collaborative, contextualized, and structured around the testing of hypotheses that relate directly to decisions about how to teach, interact with, and otherwise support the child. To that end, we present a broad and functional framework for collaborative cognitive assessment and describe in some detail the process of ongoing, collaborative, contextualized hypothesis-testing assessment. We close the chapter with a discussion of specialized assessment challenges in a variety of domains. The discussions in this chapter are relevant to the assessment activities of neuropsychologists, school psychologists, educators, speech-language pathologists (SLPs), occupational therapists, vocational specialists, social workers, and others involved in evaluating cognitive functions (broadly construed) or behavior that has a cognitive dimension.

Cognitive assessment occupies a central place in rehabilitation and special education for children with traumatic brain injury (TBI) because of the frequency of cognitive impairment after TBI (see Chapters 2 and 9), the unusual cognitive profiles encountered in this group, the often unpredictable cognitive changes over time in children with TBI (both improvement and delayed onset of symptoms), and the importance of cognitive integrity for success in school and in social and vocational life. Furthermore, even sophisticated neuroimaging procedures often fail to detect neurologic disruption capable of affecting cognitive function. For all these reasons, professionals who serve these children must commit themselves to acquiring information that is not only reliable and valid, but also useful in serving the children effectively.

Scope of Cognitive Assessment

There is a cognitive dimension to everything that human beings do. Therefore, all professionals and others working with children with TBI need to understand their cognitive strengths and weaknesses. Because general cognitive and executive system weaknesses (see Chapter 2) are often more pronounced in children with TBI than are specific academic, linguistic, perceptual, or motor deficits, professionals in rehabilitation and school settings must become comfortable with general cognitive descriptors in addition to the discipline-specific descriptors with which they may be more familiar. For example, SLPs must be comfortable evaluating and describing cognitive-communicative functions (e.g., general organizational impairment in relation to language comprehension and expression), not just speech and language in a narrow sense. Similarly, educators must be comfortable in evaluating and describing academic performance as it is affected by organizational problems, various types of memory disorders, and executive system weakness. The same point can be made about other professionals. Later in this chapter, we explore in greater detail the implications of common cognitive impairment after TBI for educational and communication assessment.

As we use the term in this chapter, *cognition* is a broad category that plots out an expansive territory that can be mapped in a variety of ways, depending on one's purposes (Flavell et al., 1993; Krasnegor et al., 1994). In Chapter 9, Ylvisaker and Szekeres break the category of cognition into component systems (i.e., working memory, the executive system, the knowledge base, and the response system), component processes (i.e., attention, perception, memory and learning, organization, and reasoning), and variables that characterize functional-integrative performance (i.e., scope, level, manner, and

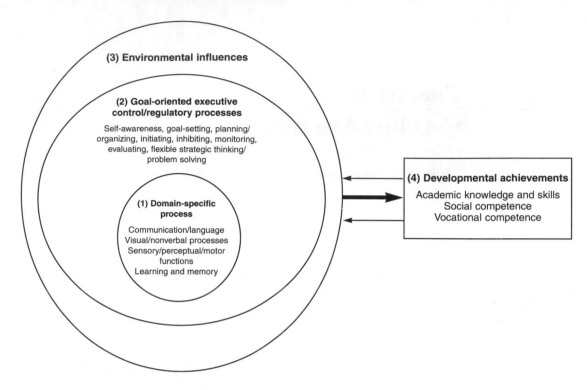

Figure 10-1. A neuropsychological classification system for cognitive functions in children.

efficiency) and delineate subcomponents within each of these. (See Chapter 9 for a definition of these categories.) Ylvisaker and Szekeres emphasize the arbitrariness in this and all other classification systems but stress that a shared understanding of cognitive categories helps team members to understand one another and plan coherent assessment and intervention.

An alternative classification system (Figure 10-1), illustrating the grouping of psychological processes and skills and the influences on the use of those processes and skills, sheds light on assessment practices in many rehabilitation and special education settings. Most tests administered by psychologists, SLPs, occupational therapists, and others are designed to identify strengths and weaknesses in specific processing domains (see Figure 10-1). These are the "worker bee" functions that enable people to take in and process within specific modalities information received from the world. These functions are at the core of the cognitive system and are relatively amenable to traditional testing methods.

Executive control processes (see Figure 10-1) include interrelated regulatory functions responsible for the production, regulation, and management of all cognitive activity and behavior. Executive functions are dynamic and are not wedded to specific content or sensory modalities; instead, they serve to direct appropriate goal-oriented processing in all domains. Because these functions are associated with the frontal lobes—most vulnerable in TBI—they must be considered a high priority in the assessment of children with TBI. Assessment of executive functions is notoriously problematic (Crépean et al., 1997; Lezak, 1982; Stuss and Buckle, 1992), and attempts to validate standardized pediatric assessments in this area are in their infancy (Levin et al., 1991a, 1996).

Academic, vocational, and social knowledge and skills (see Figure 10-1), stored in long-term memory, are the achievements of interaction between executive control processes and specific cognitive processes. In Figure 10-1, bidirectional arrows indicate the complementary relationship between the cognitive system and developmental achievements: That is, cognitive processing contributes to developmental achievements, just as stored knowledge that is organized well contributes to effective and efficient cognitive processing.

Assessment of cognition must take into account not only specific cognitive processes, executive control functions, and stored knowledge, but environmental influences on the development and expression of the cognitive system (see Figure 10-1). Negative effects of environmental stressors and positive effects of environmental supports are particularly important in acquired brain injury, given the potential for stimulus overload and the consequent need for active control of environmental input. All four of these domains are the legitimate focus of comprehensive cognitive assessment.

It is critical for a hospital or school staff to adopt some set of commonly understood descriptive categories with which to discuss cognitive realities. A shared conceptual framework helps team members to communicate effectively with one another. Furthermore, the absence of such a shared framework and collaborative teamwork can result simultaneously in both overassessment (several professionals using similar tests to assess the same aspects of cognition) and underassessment (some aspects of cognition remaining insufficiently explored). In an ideal world, diverse staff organize and integrate their assessment perspectives and activities within the context of collaborative hypothesis testing, described later in this chapter.

Goals of Cognitive Assessment and Assessment Procedures: Form Follows Function

Cognitive assessment can serve a variety of purposes, including diagnosis of brain injury, diagnosis of specific disability within a disability classification system, prognosis for recovery, establishment of eligibility for services, establishment of baseline levels and measurement of progress, preparation for legal testimony, epidemiologic investigation of the population of children with TBI, and planning of rehabilitative and educational intervention. Each of these purposes is associated with specific and often distinct constraints and assessment tools. For example, the use of a test to help to diagnose a type of brain injury presupposes thorough validation of the test for that purpose and with that population. The use of a test to measure progress assumes that the test is a valid indicator of the type of real-world progress that the intervention is designed to facilitate. The use of a test to establish eligibility for services assumes that the test has predictive validity for that child (i.e., that adequate performance on the test predicts success without special services, whereas poor performance predicts lack of success without special services).

The research base for making any of these claims for standardized tests of cognitive function when used with children and adolescents with TBI is weak. More importantly, there is growing evidence that many children with TBI perform in misleading ways on standardized tests, which we discuss in the section on executive system impairment (associated with frontal lobe injury) and assessment. The important point is that clinicians using standardized tests to achieve any of the purposes of cognitive assessment must be familiar with the special characteristics of children with TBI and interpret test results flexibly in light of these characteristics.

Because our focus is restricted to one purpose of cognitive assessment—planning intervention—most of this chap-

ter is devoted to assessment activities that are collaborative, that exploit everyday contexts of intervention and interaction, and that are designed specifically to help the intervention team members to do their jobs most effectively. Many excellent textbooks may be helpful to clinicians seeking guidance in relation to the other goals of assessment (e.g., Rourke et al., 1986; Sattler, 1990; Simeonsson, 1986).

General Considerations in Frontal Lobe Injury, Executive Function Impairment, and Cognitive Assessment

Many of the tests and related assessment procedures developed for other disability groups or for general cognitive, educational, and language assessment are appropriate for many children with cognitive disability after TBI. However, for four important reasons, cognitive assessment of children and adolescents with TBI is complex and often requires some customized assessment procedures and flexibility in interpreting the results of traditional assessments.

1. Most children with severe TBI improve neurologically, in ways that are not predicted easily for several weeks or months or possibly even years after the injury. Therefore, an assessment completed in the early weeks or months may quickly lose its validity as an accurate description of the child's profile of strengths and weaknesses.

2. Executive function deficits (associated with prefrontal lobe injury) are notoriously resistant to identification and classification with standardized office tests alone.

3. Recovered knowledge and skills acquired before the injury can combine with new disability, including severe difficulty acquiring new knowledge and skills, to create misleading profiles of ability.

4. Pronounced inconsistency in the child's performance, related to neurologic, emotional, and contextual factors, adds to the difficulty of straightforward interpretation of test results.

Damage to prefrontal lobes, the most common site of brain damage in closed head injury (Levin et al., 1991b, 1993), is associated with several outcome characteristics that affect decisions about and interpretation of cognitive assessment. For example, many children and adults with prefrontal injury maintain relatively good performance on standardized tests, including those specifically designed to detect the effects of prefrontal injury, while demonstrating great difficulty in performing effectively on real-world tasks in stressful contexts, such as school (Benton, 1991; Bigler, 1988; Crépean et al., 1997; Dennis, 1991; Eslinger and Damasio, 1985; Grattan and Eslinger, 1991; Mateer and Williams, 1991; Stelling et al., 1986; Stuss and Benson, 1986; Welsh et al., 1991). This well-documented phenomenon was articulated more than three decades ago by the neurologist Teuber (1964) when he described the "riddle of the frontal lobes" as "the curious dissociation between knowing and doing."

In discussing the rationale for contextualized assessment (see later), we suggest reasons for the frequently observed inaccuracy of the results of standardized tests. The general theme underlying this inaccuracy is the paradox inherent in presenting brief and highly structured tasks in a highly controlled environment to determine how effectively individuals (1) set goals for themselves (based on their insight into their abilities), (2) plan and organize behavior in pursuit of those goals, (3) monitor and evaluate their performance, (4) shift strategies flexibly in the event of failure, and (5) remain focused over time, with unstructured and challenging tasks in complex real-world contexts (Lezak, 1982). In other words, the evaluator and standard evaluation context easily become the "prosthetic frontal lobes" for the student with frontal lobe injury, in effect masking the difficulties that are manifest in unstructured contexts (Stuss and Benson, 1986). This feature of prefrontal injury often necessitates creative deviation from traditional school assessment policies to ensure that needed services and supports are provided to students with TBI (e.g., going beyond standardized tests and fixed performance criteria to determine eligibility for services).

Furthermore, prefrontal injury is associated with delayed onset of certain types of symptoms (Eslinger et al., 1992; Goldman and Alexander, 1977; Grattan and Eslinger, 1991; Kolb, 1995; Mateer and Williams, 1991). Because physical development of prefrontal parts of the brain is slow and continues through adolescence (Yakovlev and Lecours, 1967), it is possible to incur an injury that has few functional consequences for the child until the function associated with maturation of that part of the brain is expected to emerge. For example, a 3-year-old child who has TBI and is impulsive, disinhibited, concrete in thinking, egocentric, nonreflective, disorganized, and socially immature is like most other 3-year-old children. However, if over the next 3 years the child fails to mature in these areas, he or she will be a first grader with a substantial and possibly growing disability. The same pattern of growing disability may characterize the future development of a child injured during the grade-school years or even early in adolescence (Ylvisaker and Feeney, 1995). This feature of frontal lobe injury necessitates a long-term plan for careful monitoring of development through the developmental years, even in the event of relatively good early recovery.

Finally, prefrontal injury is associated with primary social disability, including disinhibited, overly familiar, and otherwise socially inappropriate behavior; lack of social initiation; difficulty in reading social cues and in interpreting social situations; difficulty in organizing complex social responses; rigid social behavior; awkward behavior in novel situations; failure to respond to feedback from communication partners in social situations;

and others (Brown et al., 1981; Fletcher et al., 1990; Marlowe, 1992; Mateer and Williams, 1991; Perrott et al., 1991; Petterson, 1991; Price et al., 1990; Thomsen, 1989). In children, social disability may grow over time, an ominous finding emphasized in two studies that followed young children with prefrontal lesions into adulthood (Ackerly, 1964; Eslinger et al., 1992) and in two that described the evolution of negative social-behavioral consequences of frontal lobe injury over the adolescent years (Feeney and Ylvisaker, 1995; Williams and Mateer, 1992). Because this type of disability can coexist with adequate cognitive functioning in structured situations, it is difficult to identify or predict with formal tests alone (Grattan and Eslinger, 1992; Williams and Mateer, 1992), thus necessitating the use of contextualized measures.

Ongoing, Contextualized, Collaborative Hypothesis-Testing Assessment

Rationale

Ongoing, contextualized, collaborative hypothesis-testing assessment of cognitive and related functions occupies a clinical dimension far removed from the more customary practice of comprehensive cognitive assessment that (1) occurs at a discrete time (and may or may not be repeated later), (2) consists largely of standardized tests, and (3) is completed by diverse professionals working in relative isolation. For several reasons, we offer a departure from this traditional model of cognitive assessment, a departure that has its clinical roots in process assessment (Kaplan, 1988) and dynamic assessment (Feuerstein, 1979; Lidz, 1987; Vygotsky, 1986). The primary purpose of process assessment as described by Kaplan is to identify—more precisely than is possible with standardized scores alone—the processing breakdowns that contribute to weak performance of a test item or real-world task. The primary purpose of dynamic assessment, increasingly promoted by educational psychologists (Palincsar et al., 1994), is to identify the variables (task variables, situational variables, motivational variables, cues, or other supports) that could be modified to improve weak performance, thereby identifying aspects of the child's potential ("zone of proximal development," Vygotsky, 1978) and what can be done to help the child realize that potential. Although these two approaches emphasize slightly different elements, the flexible hypothesis-testing procedures are very similar. To these procedures, we add an emphasis on collaboration and contextualized experimentation.

This approach to assessment can also be thought of as a cognitive application of assessment procedures commonly used in behavioral psychology. Within the framework of applied behavior analysis, clinicians sometimes explore variables and test hypotheses in systematically controlled environments ("analogue assessment"; e.g.,

Iwata et al., 1982). Alternatively, clinicians can measure the relative influence of environmental conditions on behavior in natural environments by means of questionnaires distributed to individuals familiar with the child (e.g., Durand, 1990) or by means of a functional analysis interview (e.g., O'Neill et al., 1990). Recently, Kern and colleagues described classroom and curriculum-based hypothesis testing (similar to that advocated in this chapter) to identify the factors that were related to on-task behavior of a student with challenging behaviors (Kern et al., 1994). Whatever the details, these assessments are designed to identify the factors that elicit and maintain challenging behavior as well as the factors that can be manipulated to reduce challenging behavior and increase appropriate behavior. The goal is to provide a solid experimental basis for a behavioral intervention plan, which is also the goal of functional cognitive assessment.

Why Ongoing?

Following severe TBI, neurologic change may continue for months and often longer. Because this change can be rapid in the early months after the injury, the results of formal assessment may be invalid (for purposes of planning instruction or intervention) by the time the testing is completed and interpreted and the reports written and disseminated. In addition, even in the absence of neurologic change, students with TBI often have very complex profiles of ability and need, necessitating frequent modification and refinement of their rehabilitation and educational programs. Ongoing cognitive assessment, as we use the term, contributes to this process. Finally, it is well known that TBI in children and adolescents, especially prefrontal injury, is associated with delayed consequences that affect educational decisions. For all of these reasons, a system for ongoing dynamic assessment is preferable to (or at least supplements) an assessment that captures only one or a small number of discrete points in the student's life after the injury.

Why Contextualized?

Hospital personnel, educators, parents, and others often observe that the behavior of many children with TBI is inconsistent, varying from day to day and from situation to situation. The contributors to this inconsistency are often elusive. However, factors that are relatively predictable in their negative effect on performance include fatigue, cognitive or social stress, anxiety, complexity and novelty of the task, organizational demands of the task, environmental interference, and lack of motivation. It is in part for this complex of reasons that many students with frontal lobe injury perform better on standardized tests in a controlled testing environment than in stressful real-world contexts (Benton, 1991; Bigler, 1988; Dennis, 1991; Eslinger and Damasio, 1985; Grattan and Eslinger, 1991; Mateer and Williams, 1991; Stuss and Benson, 1986; Welsh et al., 1991). The supportive interactive man-

ner of the examiner, clear orientation to the tasks, elimination of environmental distractions, use of relatively short tasks, and use of tasks that do not require integration of multiple sources of information or retention from day to day combine to elevate performance in a student who may have difficulty performing effectively on real-world tasks in a busy classroom or in a stressful or novel social situation. Furthermore, formal testing situations rarely require that students initiate behavior on their own (they are told when to start and stop), inhibit irrelevant behavior (the examiner generally keeps the student on task), monitor and evaluate performance (the examiner evaluates the results), or think of clever ways to succeed that may be outside the limits of the test (e.g., asking to take notes when listening to a paragraph during a test of auditory comprehension). It is for these reasons that many clinicians have characterized examiners as "prosthetic frontal lobes" and have questioned the validity of test results for children and adults with frontal lobe injury.

Alternatively, children with TBI may perform poorly on test tasks that are unfamiliar or unmotivating, and proceed to surprise everybody by their solid performance in real-world settings, given the support provided by familiar routines and motivating tasks. To be sure, these challenges to ecological validity of standardized tests could be raised in connection with all children. However, for the reasons given, frontal lobe injury requires particularly serious consideration of the ecological validity of tests.

Therefore, it is critical that cognitive assessment include procedures designed to carefully identify strengths and weaknesses of the student's performance in relation to a variety of contextual variables, including setting, people, time of day, activity, and materials. It is especially important for hospital staff to simulate an educational setting, including a classroom-like space, the student's own school books and materials, and activities that resemble classroom instruction. In the absence of such contextual exploration, hospital staff will find it difficult to offer recommendations that are both tested and relevant to educational planning. Procedures that enhance sensitivity to context can include the primary evaluator's (e.g., a neuropsychologist's) making structured and unstructured observations in varied settings and also obtaining reports from others through standardized questionnaires or informal interviews. It is most useful, however, to engage those people who are active in the student's everyday life (so-called everyday people; e.g., parents, therapists, teachers, assistants) in the process of collaborative hypothesis testing. In addition to ensuring that the assessment is relevant to planning intervention, this practice has the other advantages associated with collaboration and hypothesis testing (listed later).

Why Collaborative?

Ideally, cognitive assessment includes contributions from all of the members of the professional team as well as parents, paraprofessionals (e.g., nurses aides, teacher aides), and others. The most obvious reason to promote collaboration in cognitive assessment is that it increases the number of people available to interact with and observe the child in varied contexts, to brainstorm about hypotheses that need to be tested, to test those hypotheses, and to apply the results of the experiments to planning and implementing intervention. Related to this advantage, collaborative assessment in this shared professional territory helps to promote collegiality and cohesion within teams of professionals.

In addition, if staff and family members who interact with the child on a daily basis are active collaborators in identifying what causes breakdowns in functioning and what can be done to improve performance, the likelihood of their compliance with the recommendations that emerge from this assessment is increased. In contrast, when staff and family members are simply told what to do by a specialist in cognitive functioning who has unilaterally completed an assessment (which may appear mysterious to other staff and family members), they often understandably resist these instructions and follow their own instincts. This may be due to a genuine difference of opinion, a lack of understanding, or old-fashioned oppositional behavior. Collaborative assessments hold the promise of diminishing all of these sources of noncompliance, much as they do in the field of applied behavior analysis.

Furthermore, active participation in assessment is an efficient learning process for staff and others who are not specialists in cognition or cognitive consequences of TBI. Having participated in assessments of this sort under the guidance of a specialist in cognition, these participants are positioned to make better observations and improved judgments about cognitive intervention in the future. When a neuropsychologist or other cognitive specialist consults with a rehabilitation program or school, the goal should not simply be to help create the best program for the student or patient in question, but also to leave expertise behind so that future students will be served effectively.

Finally, inviting a wide variety of professionals, paraprofessionals, and family members to participate in the assessment is a powerful statement of respect. This statement is always worth making but particularly so in the presence of potentially adversarial relationships. In both rehabilitation hospitals and schools, it is common for sharply different opinions to exist among staff and between staff and family. An ideal way to respond to such differences is to say, in effect, "We seem to disagree about this. What do you suppose we can do to test our views and come to agreement?" Differences of opinion should be invitations to collaborative testing of competing hypotheses rather than occasions for argument and potentially growing conflict. Seizing occasions for collaboration with family members has increasingly been seen as a mandate in all areas of health care.

Similarly, students, especially adolescents, can be active participants in this assessment process. For example, it is common for adolescents who are hospitalized after TBI to insist prematurely that they are ready to return to school with no special supports. An appropriate response may be to say, in effect, "You may be right and we certainly hope you are right. But we suspect that you would have a very hard time returning to school right now and might be happier being a little better prepared when you go back to school. Let's try to think of something that you could do to prove that you are right and we are wrong about this—or at least identify the supports that you might need in school." This invitation would then be followed by negotiation that might result in simulating school tasks (e.g., lectures, projects, tests), varying the supports provided, in an attempt to test the conflicting hypotheses. It is important for staff and student to make general predictions regarding the student's performance and to agree in advance to interpretations of possible outcomes of these experiments: That is, the student (and possibly family) would agree that a certain level of performance would mean that returning to school now would not be a good idea; staff would agree that a higher level of performance would indicate greater readiness to return to school than they had anticipated.

Why Hypothesis Testing?

Because all human activities are supported by a variety of abilities and functions (i.e., they are multiply determined), they can be disrupted by a variety of deficits. Failure to perform any given real-world task effectively (e.g., reading a chapter and answering questions; maintaining a social conversation; getting ready for school in the morning; walking from homeroom to art class) can be explained by reference to a wide variety of possible cognitive and noncognitive breakdowns. As a corollary, a variety of modifications and supports holds the potential to improve performance. In the case of students with TBI, this variety is exaggerated by the potentially bewildering pattern of damaged and preserved parts of the brain, often accompanied by complex emotional and behavioral reactions after the injury. Therefore, without experimentation it is never possible to know with certainty how to interpret failure on a test or other task, or what recommendation would be most effective in improving performance.

For example, failure of a student to read a paragraph and correctly answer the questions that follow could be explained by any combination of the following:

1. *Physical problems:* The student may be fatigued, hungry, overmedicated, undermedicated, in pain, sick, or experiencing subclinical seizures.
2. *Sensory or perceptual problems:* The student may be unable to see the print, maintain one clear image, track from left to right, or scan back to the left.

3. *Cognitive problems*
   - *Attention:* The student may be unable to sustain attention sufficiently, filter out internal or external distractions, divide attention between the information and the questions, or shift attention from the previous task to the current task.
   - *Orientation:* The student may be unclear about what is expected of him or her.
   - *Memory:* The student may have difficulty encoding the information for subsequent storage and retrieval, storing information long enough to answer the questions, or retrieving information from storage to answer the questions.
   - *Organization and integration:* The student may have difficulty organizing information to comprehend the text, to understand how details relate to each other, to understand how the questions relate to the text, or to formulate an organized answer.
   - *General speed of information processing:* The student may simply be very slow at all tasks.
4. *Language problems:* The student may be unable to comprehend the vocabulary or syntax of the text or questions, or may have difficulty retrieving words to answer the questions.
5. *Academic problems:* The student may unable to decode printed language efficiently.
6. *Emotional, motivational, and behavioral problems:* The student may be depressed, anxious, fearful, angry, unmotivated, oppositional, or euphoric.

Clearly a teacher or therapist would not know how to proceed in rehabilitation or classroom instruction without understanding which combination of variables is significant in explaining the student's impaired performance. Everyday assessments conducted by psychologists, psychoeducational evaluators, SLPs, and others commonly begin the process of testing those hypotheses that can be explored in a testing context. For example, if there is reason to suspect that a 15-year-old adolescent may have scored at a first-grade level on a reading test because of visual-perceptual problems, most evaluators would repeat the test with modifications (e.g., enlarged print, a line marker, or other support). If performance improved dramatically with this support, one could conclude safely that visual-perceptual problems are the exclusive or primary cause of impaired reading and could recommend some combination of compensations and exercises to improve performance in this area.

Figure 10-2 outlines the structure of collaborative, contextualized hypothesis-testing assessment. Although it may not be obvious in some cases, all the cognitive variables that can impair or support effective performance can be explored systematically in this manner. In Table 10-1, we list several common assessment questions that arise in planning rehabilitation and educational services for students with TBI and outline a variety of contextualized probes or experiments that can be used to answer the questions.

Selection of Hypotheses for Testing

Exploring all these variables and testing all possible hypotheses for a specific child would be an enormous undertaking, as well as unnecessary and exhausting. Generally, collaborative brainstorming reduces the domain of active hypotheses to a manageable number. Hypotheses are selected for testing on the basis of some combination of the following considerations: (1) the plausibility of the hypothesis relative to what is known about the child, (2) the ease with which the hypothesis could be tested, and (3) the importance of the implications of this hypothesis for intervention planning.

We refer to this process as *experimentation* in a rather loose sense. Clearly, these so-called experiments are not exactly like experiments in chemistry. For example, multiple factors often negatively influence performance, and it may not be possible to isolate their relative contributions. Indeed, sometimes it is appropriate to design experiments that test combinations of factors at once. For example, Feeney and Ylvisaker (1995) tested a four-component hypothesis regarding the aggressive behavior of three adolescents with TBI (i.e., that the students needed intensive organizational support, increased control over their program, positive behavioral momentum before attacking difficult tasks, and respect from others for their communication style). These authors tested the hypotheses together rather than separately because of the seriousness of the behavior and the consequent need to implement effective intervention procedures quickly.

Despite this looseness, promoting a generally experimental approach to assessment has great value. Experimental assessment sets the stage for flexible and experimentally based intervention (i.e., it gets teachers, therapists, and others in the habit of identifying issues clearly, experimenting with intervention options, and determining systematically what works and what does not work). This focus on thoughtful experimentation increases the likelihood that staff will navigate successfully between the "rock" of inflexible test batteries tied to inflexible intervention programs and the "hard place" of unplanned and unsystematic trial-and-error intervention.

Implementing Ongoing, Contextualized, Collaborative Hypothesis-Testing Assessment in a Hospital or School

The minimum requirements to ensure that the system for assessment is organized and implemented effectively are (1) a facility-wide commitment to principles of collaborative assessment and intervention, including mutual respect among staff and between staff and family members; (2) a designated cognitive specialist who takes responsibility for organizing ongoing collaborative assessment; (3) meetings that are sufficiently frequent and are structured to facilitate collaborative problem identifi-

To answer the question: _____

_____

staff (and family) will systematically collect and compare information about the child's performance, gathered under the following conditions:

1. _____

   versus

2. _____

Results of these miniexperiments will be evaluated by the team on <u>(date)</u>, leading to decisions about the educational program.

Illustration: Deliberate versus incidental learning

Question: Does John perform better and learn more efficiently when the task is organized
1. So that his explicit goal is to learn (deliberate learning)?
   or
2. So that he is pursuing concrete meaningful goals and learning is a by-product (incidental learning)?

If John's learning is systematically more efficient under one or the other condition, staff members will attempt to structure their teaching in a way that is consistent with this finding.

Experiment: Staff and family systematically will observe and compare John's performance (especially his learning rate) on equally demanding tasks but with a different task orientation for John:
1. Deliberate learning: The task is preceded with a statement such as "John, today we will work on _____
   _____."; "John, let's see whether you can remember _____."; "John, I bet you can learn this if you try hard." With these orienting instructions, John's goal becomes the goal of learning.
   versus
2. Incidental learning: John is engaged in a play activity or in a practical activity designed in such a way that mastering the concept or learning the information is a by-product of completing the meaningful activity. His goal is not to learn but rather to play, to complete the practical task, or to produce a concrete product. For example, John is asked to write a story for the class newspaper. The teacher introduces an outline format that John is to learn. However, John's goal is not to learn the format (the teacher's goal for John) but to produce the story.

Figure 10-2. Structure of collaborative, contextualized hypothesis-testing assessment for developing an educational program. (Adapted from M Ylvisaker, T Feeney, N Maher-Maxwell, et al. [1995] . School reentry following severe traumatic brain injury: guidelines for educational planning. J Head Trauma Rehabil 10[6];25–41. Copyright 1995, Aspen Publishers, Inc.)

Table 10-1. Illustrations of Common Assessment Questions, Hypotheses, and Tests of Hypotheses for Students with TBI

Assessment question 1

Why does John try the same approach to a problem over and over even when it clearly does not work? What should we do about this?

Collaborative hypothesis generation

John's problem could be a consequence of many cognitive or executive-system breakdowns or combinations of them. For example, (1) John may not have any other ideas about what to try; (2) he may perseverate; (3) he may have difficulty in registering and processing feedback; (4) the behavior may be self-stimulatory or attention seeking; (5) the behavior may be oppositional; (6) he may have forgotten the previous failed attempt; (7) he may fear success; (8) he may lack motivation to succeed; or (9) he may simply be convinced he is correct.

Collaborative hypothesis testing

Hypothesis 1: John simply does not know of other possibilities.

Test: When John begins to repeat a failed approach, offer an alternative. If he regularly agrees to try the alternative and is pleased with the result, his response presents some reason to believe that the problem lies in his knowledge base (stock of possible solutions) and that it must be the focus of intervention (e.g., providing varied experiences with problem-solving situations and cataloging successful solutions for later review).

Hypothesis 2: John perseverates.

Test: When John begins to repeat a failed approach, redirect him in a way that does not offer a solution but simply breaks his set. If, after redirection, he routinely tries another possibility or gives up and does something else, his response provides some reason to believe that the problem lies in perseveration and that it must be the focus of intervention (e.g., self-cues or cues from others to try something new).

Hypothesis 3: John may have difficulty registering and processing feedback.

Test: When John begins to repeat a failed approach, engage him in clear, objective demonstration of the failure. If he routinely moves on to an alternative and is pleased with the result, the results offer some reason to believe that the problem lies in self-monitoring and that it must be the focus of intervention (e.g., a system for recording attempts and their success).

Hypothesis 4: The behavior is oppositional.

Test: Observe John's behavior to determine whether the frequency of repetitive behavior increases when he has been instructed to get on with other possibilities or when, for other reasons, some adult obviously is invested in John's solving problems in a flexible manner. If he is observed to be more flexible when nobody opposes him, the situation provides some reason to believe that the problem is found in oppositional behavior and that it must be the focus of intervention (e.g., increasing his opportunities to choose his therapeutic or instructional tasks).

Hypothesis 5: John may have forgotten the previous failed attempt.

Test: When John is engaged in problem solving, ensure that he has access to an objective record of his attempts (video tape, log book, photograph, or other). If perseverative behavior decreases in the presence of this prosthetic memory, the change gives some reason to believe that the problem lies in memory and that it must be the focus of intervention (e.g., ongoing use of memory aids).

Hypothesis 6: John may lack motivation to succeed.

Test: When John is engaged in problem solving, offer him $10 for a successful solution. If flexible problem solving increases in the presence of such motivation, the gain offers some reason to believe that the problem is rooted in motivation and that it must be the focus of intervention (e.g., structuring teaching around motivating tasks, routinely reviewing the purpose of therapy and educational tasks).

Assessment question 2

Why does John seem to understand information when I present it to him but rarely can state the next day what he had learned? What should we do about this?

Collaborative hypothesis generation

John's problem could be a consequence of many cognitive or executive-system breakdowns or combinations of them: (1) retrieval, whereby John processes, encodes, and stores the information but has difficulty retrieving it the next day; (2) storage, whereby he encodes the information but simply does not retain it; (3) organization and encoding, whereby his initial processing of the information is superficial, making it possible for him to answer questions immediately but not to retain the information; (4) attention, whereby he can remember information but only when he is not distracted at the time of encoding and at the time of retrieval; or (5) repetition, whereby he can remember information but only if it is repeated many times.

Collaborative hypothesis testing

Hypothesis 1: John processes, encodes, and stores the information but has difficulty in retrieving it the next day.

Test: Systematically compare John's performance on *free-recall* tasks (e.g., "Tell me about the story we read yesterday") versus *recognition-memory* tasks (e.g., true-or-false questions). If John does much better on recognition memory tasks, teachers and others will need to use such tasks in assessing his retention of information.

Hypothesis 2: John encodes the information but simply does not retain it.

Test: Systematically compare John's performance on immediate-recall tasks versus delayed-recall tasks. Vary the time delay. If storage is impaired specifically, John will need memory prostheses.

Hypothesis 3: John's initial processing of the information is superficial, making it possible for him to answer questions immediately but not to retain the information.

Test: Systematically compare John's performance on memory tasks both with advance organizers and without advance organizers. If organizers make a substantial difference, he may benefit from a rich assortment of advance organizers for tasks throughout the day.

Hypothesis 4: John can remember information but only when he is not distracted at the time of encoding and at the time of retrieval.

Test: Systematically compare John's performance in both the presence and the absence of distractions. If distractions substantially impair performance, he may need to receive instruction in a nondistracting environment.

Hypothesis 5: John can remember information but only if it is repeated many times.

Test: Systematically compare John's performance both when given only one or two repetitions and when given many repetitions. If repetition makes a substantial difference, staff and family will need to find a way to encourage large amounts of repetition.

cation, brainstorming, and hypothesis testing; and (4) a system for tracking assessment activity and the child's responses to intervention.

1. *Commitment to collaborative assessment and intervention:* The approach to assessment described in this chapter cannot be implemented successfully in a professional environment in which staff work in relative isolation and jealously guard their assessment and intervention territory. In contrast, truly collaborative teams embrace the reality of shared professional territory and value the professional growth facilitated by ongoing collaboration with other professionals. Additionally, they welcome participation of family members and other everyday people.

2. *Cognitive specialist:* Some facilities have one professional play the role of cognitive specialist (e.g., a hospital neuropsychologist or school psychologist) for all patients or students; others assign separate children to different members of the team. In addition to possessing a thorough grounding in cognitive functioning and cognitive assessment, the individual must be well organized, an effective communicator, and a person with genuine respect for the contributions of all staff and family members. The cognitive specialist facilitates discussion of cognitive assessment questions that must be answered, of reasonable hypotheses, of ways to test the hypotheses, and of implications of the results for intervention.

3. *Meetings:* Meetings designed to facilitate ongoing, collaborative, contextualized hypothesis-testing assessment begin with identification of assessment questions that must be answered (for purposes of ensuring the most effective intervention) and are not yet answered. Then, hypotheses are generated, followed by brainstorming about ways to test the hypotheses and assignments to staff and family to use their special contexts to test the hypotheses. At the next meeting, data are shared and intervention plans are discussed. In the real worlds of busy rehabilitation centers and schools, these discussions may occur over lunch, in teacher lounges, and the like. Ideally, time is set aside during daily rounds or at staff conferences for this important collaborative activity.

Hypothesis Testing: Recommendations from Hospital to School

Recommendations associated with this approach to assessment are quite different from the recommendations typically found in traditional reports written by neuropsychologists, psychoeducational evaluators, SLPs, occupational therapists, and others. For example, a traditional recommendation regarding attention might read: "Testing revealed weak attentional control. Therefore, John should receive one-to-one instruction in a quiet environment when he returns to school." A comparable recommendation from a facility committed to hypothesis testing might read (or, better, be presented in person as):

"Exploration of attentional functioning in our facility revealed that new or particularly difficult information is presented to John best through one-to-one instruction in a familiar setting, even if it includes distractions. More routine teaching or interaction is accomplished best in a small group (e.g., four to six children) with well-established group routines. In an unusual teaching environment (e.g., a quiet alcove), internal distraction becomes a major problem for John. It is recommended that school staff begin with these teaching arrangements but continue to compare John's behavior and academic performance systematically under varied teaching conditions. We would be happy to discuss possibilities at any time with school staff." Ylvisaker and colleagues (1994) described cognitive assessment as, in part, a dialectical process among varied professionals.

A traditional recommendation regarding memory might read: "At the present time, John's ability to process and remember information presented in class is limited severely. Therefore, it is critical for him to use a tape recorder in class for later review and to have his teachers write assignments in an assignment book." A comparable recommendation from a facility committed to hypothesis testing might read (or, better, be presented in person as): "John's ability to process and remember information presented in class is limited severely at this time. We tested the following compensations: a tape recorder, a peer note taker, an assignment book in which he records assignments, and an assignment book in which the teacher records assignments. At present, a tape recorder is too complicated and frustrating for John. He profits from peer note taking, but he must participate in choosing the peer. He profits from an assignment book, which must be organized by the teacher, or assignments will be lost. School staff should continue to explore compensations for impaired memory, as new possibilities will emerge as John recovers. We would be happy to discuss possibilities at any time with school staff."

In summary, rehabilitation staff members, having rich experience with the child, communicate to school staff (1) that they systematically have explored issues directly relevant to educational planning and teaching; (2) their exploration results as they might effect educational decision making; (3) the instructional methodologies, supports, and arrangements that probably will be a good starting point in school; (4) encouragement for the school staff to continue this active exploration; and (5) a willingness on the part of hospital staff to help school staff, if appropriate, in this exploration.

Recommendations on Video

In Chapter 12, Ylvisaker, Feeney, and Szekeres discuss transitional videos that can be used to train and orient staff as the student moves from one level of care or education to another. For children who require prolonged inpatient rehabilitation, the results of collaborative hypothesis testing can be captured on a video illustrating what have been identified as the best teaching practices, behavior management practices, communication routines, and the like. Engaging family members and the student in planning and producing this training video can also be a useful procedure for helping them to understand the cognitive issues that will figure prominently in school reentry. Engaging the child and family in the process of creating the video may help all participants to understand the child's strengths and weaknesses in a more functional way and is a component of the critical empowerment process. Bringing rehabilitation staff together to produce these transitional videos is a useful contributor to team building.

Obstacles to Ongoing, Contextualized, Collaborative Hypothesis-Testing Assessment

Despite its solid grounding in scientific methodology, clinical experience, and common sense, in our experience as consultants to a large number of hospitals and schools, the approach to cognitive assessment (for planning intervention) described in this chapter is practiced infrequently. This state of professional affairs can be explained best by reference to some combination of the following obstacles.

Inadequate Training in the Use of These Assessment Procedures

Most professionals—neuropsychologists, school psychologists, psychoeducational evaluators, SLPs, occupational therapists, and others with an important stake in cognitive assessment—receive thorough training in the use of standardized, norm-referenced tests and (possibly) in questionnaires and informal observation techniques. Rarely is contextualized, collaborative hypothesis-testing assessment featured in preservice training programs. The all-too-pervasive unfamiliarity with these assessment procedures is illustrated by an event that occurred at the end of a recent workshop dealing exclusively with this type of assessment. One of the participants (a special education teacher with considerable experience) commented that the workshop was interesting but that she wished that the stated topic (functional cognitive assessment) had been addressed. After 3 hours of presentation, discussion, and group exercises, she did not think that the topic of functional cognitive assessment had come up. In our judgment, the approach to assessment presented in this chapter (and in that workshop) is as functional as cognitive assessment can become. Changing old habits may require persistent and patient leadership from those professionals who appreciate the positive impact that this approach can have in developing effective rehabilitation and education plans and in creating collaborative relationships.

Administrative Requirements

Commonly, in both hospitals and schools, an administrative requirement mandates that the assessment be completed within a specified and limited period and that it result in some sort of diagnosis, prognosis, and judgment about the need for specialized services and supports. These requirements can be met without illegitimately restricting the meaning of the word *assessment* to those procedures designed to meet such administrative requirements. In an important sense, the difficult but critically important part of assessment *begins* when assessment in an administrative sense has ended. Leaders within rehabilitation and special education programs must take responsibility for ensuring that staff understand that assessment for intervention planning is a different process and has standards different from those of assessment designed to meet administrative requirements.

Confusion Regarding Varied Purposes Served by Cognitive Assessment

Assessments designed to yield a diagnosis or prognosis, to establish candidacy for services, to prepare for legal testimony, or to yield epidemiologic data about a population must meet psychometric standards that the procedures described in this chapter are not intended to meet. Many tests have been developed to meet these standards and to achieve these assessment goals. However, it is a fatal error to assume that an assessment procedure designed to serve one purpose will meet others as effectively or that one type of assessment must meet standards established for another. Our focus in this chapter has been on ecologically valid assessment for purposes of intervention planning. The ultimate standard to which this type of assessment must be held is that it results in intervention that is as effective as it can be for the individual being served. The best way to meet this important standard is to experiment thoughtfully and systematically with intervention approaches in real-world contexts.

Desire to Retain Special Expertise

On the surface, the assessment procedures described in this chapter appear to dull the professional luster associated with highly technical and discipline-specific assessment procedures. A highly trained professional needs considerable maturity and self-confidence to say to family members or paraprofessionals—or even to professional colleagues—that they are critical contributors to his or her assessment and that it is necessary to experiment with intervention procedures before confidently recommending them. Certainly it is easier and, in a superficial way, more gratifying to foster the misconception that tests of cognitive functioning are like laboratory tests that yield a diagnosis, prognosis, and prescription for cure. However, beneath the surface lies a satisfying and challenging professional life associated with a commitment to collaboration and to concretely helping people with disability to be successful in their specific, real-world contexts.

Territorialism

Many facilities have achieved an admirable level of collegiality and interdisciplinary collaboration. The type of assessment described in this chapter tends to emerge naturally and to develop effectively in these settings. However, it is common for staff both in hospitals and in schools to be in conflict about the choice of person to take responsibility for various areas of cognitive assessment and intervention. For example, psychologists may find themselves in conflict with educators about the choice of person to evaluate academic skills, in conflict with SLPs about assessment of language and language-related functions, and in conflict with occupational therapists about perceptual and perceptual-motor assessment. Collaborative assessment is unlikely to occur in a professional setting dominated by such adversarial relationships among professionals. In a healthy environment, the primary concern is not the choice of professional who should be responsible for this area of assessment but rather the questions that must be answered about John and how all involved can contribute to addressing these questions. Territorial instincts must be put aside for this type of assessment to flourish.

Special Considerations in Frontal Lobe Injury, Executive System Impairment, and Cognitive Assessment

Neuropsychological Assessment

Neuropsychologists contribute to the collaborative cognitive assessment team in several important ways, on the basis of their comprehensive training in understanding cognition and behavior as related to brain development, injury, and recovery. Critical information about a child's strengths and weaknesses comes from a variety of sources. Often, the neuropsychologist is in a position to organize this information in relation to a comprehensive model (like that depicted in Figure 10-1), to work with staff in formulating contextualized experiments to answer outstanding questions, and to formulate intervention plans that cross disciplinary boundaries and are influenced by current information about recovery after brain injury. The neuropsychologist must ensure that all the areas outlined in Figure 10-1 are explored adequately, although specific disciplinary responsibilities for testing may vary from program to program. The neuropsychologist must also ensure that functions known to be vulnerable to a specific type of brain injury are explored thoroughly, including

executive functions and new learning in the case of closed head injury.

In recent years, child neuropsychologists have devoted considerable energy to (1) modifying adult executive-function ("prefrontal") tests and providing norms for children (e.g., Levin et al., 1991); (2) interpreting traditional developmental measures from a neuropsychological perspective as measures of executive-function development (e.g., Roberts and Pennington, 1996; Welsh et al., 1991; Welsh and Pennington, 1988); (3) creating measures to capture deficits believed on clinical or theoretical grounds to be associated with executive-function development and impairment (e.g., Dennis, 1991); (4) applying factor-analytic procedures to the results of children's performance on purported executive-function measures to derive models of executive functioning applicable to child development and disability (e.g., Levin et al., 1996; Taylor et al., 1996; Welsh et al., 1991); and (5) developing procedures for experimentally using paired tests to detect executive-system weakness (e.g., Denckla, 1996).

Adapting Existing Neuropsychological Procedures for Use with Children

Many of the neuropsychological tasks currently used to explore functioning of children with brain injury are downward extensions of tests originally developed to explore brain-behavior relationships in adults. Used cautiously and with a thorough understanding of cognitive and neurologic development in children, many of these procedures can be helpful. However, for reasons that we reviewed earlier in promoting the use of contextualized assessment procedures, results of such tests must be interpreted with great caution, especially in the cases of children with executive-system impairment associated with frontal lobe injury.

Traditional Developmental Tasks as Measures of Executive Functions

Roberts and Pennington (1996) argued that many of the insights and developmental measures associated with traditional developmental cognitive psychology (e.g., Piaget's theories) can be incorporated readily into a view of early child development that highlights the maturation of executive functions (in particular, working memory and its inhibitory functions; see Case, 1992). For example, within this framework, success on the traditional piagetian multiple hiding task for infants (A-not-B) is seen as evidence for development of inhibitory control over prepotent responses (i.e., development of executive self-regulation) versus development of qualitatively distinct cognitive structures during the sensorimotor period of cognitive development. Similarly, later in development, success on piagetian conservation tasks can be given a parallel explanation: Children learn to inhibit a prepotent response based on perceptually salient features and, in contrast, base their judgment on mature logical considerations.

In a similar fashion, Willatts (1990) recast Piaget's discussion of early sensorimotor means-ends coordination in terms of the infant's gradual development of strategic behavior and executive control over planning. Understanding intentional or goal-directed behavior as (1) selecting an action appropriate for obtaining a goal, (2) persisting in efforts to achieve a goal, (3) making corrections for errors, and (4) stopping when the goal is achieved, researchers have documented goal-directed, problem-solving behavior in infant development much earlier than that proposed by Piaget. According to Willatts (1990), the rapid development of children's strategic behavior over the first 2 years of life is not explained by changes in the structure of intelligence but rather by improvements in executive control (e.g., monitoring, task analysis, error detection, inhibition) and growth in the knowledge base (e.g., recall of successful solutions, transfer between tasks).

Reframing traditional cognitive psychology in terms of development of executive functions has two critical advantages for pediatric rehabilitation professionals. First, it invites creative use of qualitative measures and ordinal scales of development (e.g., Uzgiris and Hunt, 1978) that have a long history in developmental cognitive psychology and, with the change in theoretical perspective, can be used in evaluating executive-function impairment and recovery after brain injury. Second, it alerts rehabilitation specialists to the potential usefulness of the traditional apprenticeship model of cognitive growth (championed by Vygotsky, 1978) as a framework for cognitive rehabilitation of children. This suggestion is developed in Chapters 11, 12, 14, and 20.

Creating Executive-Function Assessment Tasks

Since the 1970s, Maureen Dennis and her colleagues have developed a variety of tasks designed to capture specific aspects of executive functioning in children and adolescents, with an emphasis on executive control of language functions. For example, the Premise and Transitive Inference Test (Lovett and Dennis, 1977) assesses a child's ability to draw inferences about objects on the basis of a mental model. The Anomalies Test (Dennis and Whitaker, 1976) assesses semantic monitoring by asking a child to detect and correct lexical and grammatical anomalies. The Presupposition Test (Dennis, 1980) evaluates a child's ability to identify presuppositions of epistemic verbs (*know, remember,* and *pretend*) within various types of sentences. The Beliefs and Intentions Test (Dennis and Winner, 1990) evaluates a child's ability to distinguish falsehood from irony from deception. Studies using these measures have enabled Dennis to conclude that head injury with significant frontal lobe involvement causes impairment in children's metacognitive and metalinguistic skills, with the understanding that metacognition and metalanguage are components of more general executive functions.

Factor Analysis and Models of Executive Functions

Recently, developmental neuropsychologists have sought to characterize executive functions in children by administering batteries of tests to various clinical populations, including children with TBI, and by identifying relatively independent components of the executive system by means of factor analysis. Using this methodology, Levin and colleagues (1996) examined children and adolescents with TBI and proposed five factors: conceptual/productivity (e.g., word fluency), planning/execution (e.g., number of broken rules on the Tower of London task), schema (e.g., number of constraint-seeking questions on a 20-questions task), cluster (e.g., use of organizational strategies in memory tasks), and inhibition (e.g., false-alarm errors on a Go–No Go task). In contrast, Taylor and colleagues (1996) derived a three-factor analysis of executive functions in children: response speed, planning/sequencing, and response inhibition. These studies have contributed to our understanding of disability groups and the executive-function tasks used to test them.

However, because these characterizations of executive functions in children are based on administration of available tests, it is not surprising that they omit critical components of the executive system, including self-awareness and awareness of task difficulty (as few tests require the individual to predict performance accurately), initiation (because, in testing situations, the examiner takes responsibility for initiation), inhibition under conditions of social stress (as testing environments do not include social stressors problematic for many children with TBI), and self-evaluation (because the individual being tested rarely is responsible for evaluating personal performance). A more meaningful methodology for examining executive functions as they are relevant to success in rehabilitation and school is that preferred by many investigators in the field of attention deficit–hyperactivity disorder (another executive-system impairment): characterizing the disability as it manifests itself in real-world activities and then creating assessment procedures tested for validity against that real-world standard.

Experimental Use of Paired Tests to Evaluate Executive Functions

Denckla (1996) proposed creative use of paired tests to explore executive-function development or impairment. Because all tasks involve both specific content (e.g., language, visual-perceptual material, academic content) and general executive-control dimensions, single tasks cannot be used to unambiguously demonstrate impairment in executive functions. However, if it is possible to create or discover two tasks that are similar in their content except that one has executive-function demands that the other lacks, it might be possible to isolate the executive-system contribution to impaired performance by comparing results on the two tasks. For example, adequate performance on a vocabulary test combined with poor performance on a letter-word fluency test would suggest that the content domain (language, in this case) is intact but that executive control over searches within the lexicon is impaired. Similarly, adequate recall performance on the California Verbal Learning Test (Delis et al., 1983) combined with poor performance on the clustering measure from the same test suggests adequate nonstrategic verbal memory but weak executive control over verbal learning. Ongoing, contextualized, collaborative hypothesis-testing assessment, as we described it earlier in the chapter, involves a similar experimental use of paired tasks to isolate executive-function breakdowns but within the context of more natural tasks and settings.

Cautions in Interpreting Results of Executive-System Assessment

For many reasons, clinicians should exercise great caution in interpreting the results of executive-function testing in children with TBI. First, no sufficiently solid data base exists to support confident interpretation of test results, particularly for children with prefrontal injury. In addition, functions included under the heading *executive functions* are subject to substantial normal developmental, cultural, and personality variability, especially during early childhood. Third, for reasons described earlier in this chapter, the ecological validity of tests administered in a sanitized and supportive environment must be routinely questioned, particularly in the case of children with known or suspected prefrontal injury.

Collaborative, Contextualized Assessment

If the primary goal of neuropsychological assessment is to help therapists and educators deliver the most effective educational and therapeutic services, neuropsychologists should participate with other staff in ongoing, collaborative, contextualized hypothesis-testing assessment. In many settings in which children with brain injury are served, the child neuropsychologist may be the most comprehensively trained member of the team that addresses cognitive disability and intervention, creating for that person a natural leadership role. Collaboration in assessment not only increases the likelihood of compliance with recommendations (as discussed earlier) but presents the neuropsychologist with an ideal opportunity to teach staff and family members about practical implications of brain injury and the best methods to explore the child's strengths and needs.

Role of Neuropsychological Assessment in Planning Special Education

Neuropsychological assessment has become a staple in pediatric rehabilitation programs. However, questions about its usefulness in educational settings remain. To be sure, if the goal of assessment is to help school staff plan

the child's educational program, little value is gained from assessment that results in nothing more than a technical report written in language unfamiliar to educators and insensitive to the child's real-world issues in school. In contrast, a child neuropsychologist knowledgeable about brain-child-school interactions (versus brain-behavior relations alone)—and *willing to work with the school team*—can be very helpful (Bernstein and Waber, 1990). Referral for comprehensive neuropsychological assessment for a student who has TBI and has returned to school should be based on the following criteria:

- Important questions related to educational programming must be answered.
- The questions are in some way related to brain injury.
- The neuropsychologist has extensive experience with children and with children with acquired brain injury.
- The neuropsychologist is willing to collaborate with educational staff both before the evaluation to identify the questions that must be explored and after the evaluation to explore educational implications of the findings.

Routine Informal Assessment of Executive Functions

Whatever specific measures are used, some general assessment practices can be used routinely by all staff to add incrementally to an understanding of children's executive functions and to contribute over time to improvement of those functions. These practices are listed in Table 10-2. If all staff and family members can make these interviews part of their everyday interaction with the child, assessment data accumulate quickly and such interaction creates an environment in which adults routinely engage the child in nonthreatening conversations that have the effect of facilitating development of executive functions.

Language and Communication Assessment

Children with TBI can exhibit any combination of language and communication strengths and weaknesses (Ylvisaker, 1993). Some children have injuries that include damage to the parts of the brain associated specifically with speech and language processing. For this group and for those children with preinjury delays, tests developed for children with congenital speech and language disorders are useful. However, many children with TBI, including many with severe injuries, escape this type of injury and enjoy an apparently excellent recovery of speech and language. The most common types of language and communication disability after TBI are those resulting from executive-system problems (associated with commonly occurring prefrontal injury); from slow

Table 10-2. Procedures That Contribute to Assessment and Improvement of Executive Functions

Before beginning a task
  1. Self-awareness of ability; goal setting: Ask the child whether the task will be easy or difficult and to explain the choice of answer. If relevant, ask for a prediction of performance.
  2. Strategic behavior and problem solving: Ask the child to explain plans for achieving his or her goal.
During the task
  1. Initiation: If appropriate, create opportunities for initiation (e.g., insufficient materials, requiring the child to initiate a request).
  2. Inhibition: If appropriate, create some distractions that would require active inhibition from the child.
  3. Self-monitoring: Ask the child how he or she is doing.
  4. Strategic behavior and problem solving: If appropriate, create obstacles that require active problem solving from the child.
After completion of the task
  1. Self-evaluation: Ask the child how he or she did and how results compare to expectations.
  2. Strategic behavior and problem solving: Ask what the child did to succeed; list relevant strategic procedures; ask the child whether he or she used them or whether they might be useful.

and inefficient processing of information, including language (associated with commonly occurring diffuse injury); and from general problems in learning new information (associated with commonly occurring medial temporal lobe damage and prefrontal injury) (Ylvisaker, 1993). These types of communication disability are consistent with average or above-average performance on most language tests.

From the perspective of language and communication, executive-system dysfunction (prefrontal injury) is associated with six main types of language and communication disability:

1. *Disorganized language or impaired discourse:* This disability is observed most easily in expressive tasks that require an individual to organize a substantial amount of language, either in speaking (e.g., extended conversation, narratives, or descriptions) or in writing. Organizational impairment also depresses comprehension of extended language, including reading comprehension. Therefore, language evaluation of a person with known or suspected prefrontal injury must include tasks that stress the student's ability to organize language (both receptively and expressively). This may include having the student (a) listen to a story and repeat it in an organized manner; (b) at a higher-functioning level, listen to a real or simulated classroom lecture and answer questions or summarize the information; (c) read a chapter of a classroom text, write an organized summary, and answer questions; (d) write an essay; (e) maintain an extended conversation on a single topic; and (f) engage in other tasks designed to identify possible breakdowns when organizational demands are at realistic levels relative to the child's age and grade level. Analysis of expressive discourse should include measures of the amount of information expressed, the coherence or logical organization of the information, and the cohesiveness of the discourse (i.e., the use of linguistic markers of organization) (Chapman et al., 1997).

Analysis of receptive discourse should include identification of the effects of increasing length on reading comprehension and the relative success in comprehending factual information versus themes, main ideas, and inferences. To contribute to planning intervention, assessment in this area should also explore the effects of organizational strategies on language organization (e.g., giving varied advance organizers to identify their effect on receptive or expressive discourse tasks).

2. *Inflexibility:* Many children and adults with prefrontal injury are inflexible in their thinking and acting. Linguistically, this disability may manifest itself in difficulty in interpreting ambiguous words or sentences, difficulty in finding alternate ways to express a thought, and difficulty in maintaining a fluid, ever-changing conversation. Tests that probe the child's facility with multiple meaning, such as the Test of Language Competence (Wiig and Secord, 1988), are useful and should be supplemented by informal probes of multiple interpretation of stories or events, of the child's ability to express thoughts in more than one way, and of the ability to manage topic shifts in conversation.

3. *Concrete thinking:* Children with prefrontal injury also tend to have difficulty with abstract thinking, abstract language, and indirect meaning (e.g., metaphor, figures of speech, irony) (Dennis and Barnes, 1990). Tests of metaphor or figure-of-speech comprehension may be useful. It is also important to interview parents and other everyday communication partners to determine the child's ability to detect humor, irony, and other subtleties of language. Exploration of metalinguistic and metacognitive skills is particularly important for school-age children whose learning environment is filled with metalanguage (Dennis et al., 1996).

4. *Inefficient word retrieval:* Children with prefrontal injury also tend to have word retrieval problems, more pronounced in word fluency tasks (e.g., in 1 minute, naming as many members of a semantic category as possible

Table 10-3. Informal Assessment of Reading and Writing for Generally Well-Recovered Middle-School and High-School Students with TBI

Reading

Ask the student to read a previously unread chapter of a school textbook. Give the student a form that requests the following information:

1. How long did it take you to read the chapter?
2. How many times did you read the chapter so as to write a summary?
3. How well did you understand the information after one reading?
4. How well did you understand the information after the final reading?
5. What did you do to help yourself to understand the chapter (vocabulary; main ideas)?

Writing

Ask the student to write a clear and well-organized summary of the chapter. Give the student a form that requests the following information:

1. How long did it take you to write the summary (total time)?
2. What did you do to organize the summary?
3. What did you do to ensure that the summary was adequately complete?
4. What did you do to ensure that you used correct grammar, spelling, punctuation?
5. What did you do to ensure that the writing was clear?
6. How many drafts did you write? Please bring in all drafts.

---

or reciting as many words as possible that start with a certain letter) than in confrontation naming tasks (i.e., naming objects or pictures, the usual procedure for identifying word retrieval abilities). Therefore, assessment should include a word fluency test, such as the SFA task (Gaddes and Crocket, 1975) or the category-naming task from the Clinical Evaluation of Language Fundamentals (Semel et al., 1987) or a more comprehensive word-finding test, such as the Test of Word Finding (German, 1989), the Test of Word Finding in Discourse (German, 1991), or the Test of Adolescent and Adult Word Finding (German, 1990). Equally important is documentation and analysis of word retrieval breakdowns in conversation and classroom recitation. Various types of stress (e.g., social stress, time pressure, stress associated with the level of the required language) should be explored systematically to determine what types of supports may be needed to help the child with word retrieval problems to succeed.

5. *Impaired social communication (pragmatics of language):* As stated in the last section, the most pronounced consequence of prefrontal injury may be impaired social communication (Alexander et al., 1989; Ylvisaker and Feeney, 1994), or what SLPs refer to as pragmatics of language. Assessment should include some functional measure of conversational competence, such as the Pragmatic Protocol of Prutting and Kirchner (1987), based on observation of the child with a variety of conversation partners and in a variety of settings. Social skills inventories, associated with social skills curricula, may also be helpful.

6. *Inefficient new learning of language:* Damage to medial temporal lobe memory centers (e.g., the hippocampus) may impair learning of new verbal information despite adequate recovery of semantic information acquired before the injury, associated with normal scores on vocabulary tests. Prefrontal injury may also reduce

learning efficiency by rendering a child relatively nonstrategic in language-learning tasks. Efficiency of learning and age-appropriate use of language-learning strategies can be explored with tests of verbal memory and learning, such as the California Verbal Learning Test—Children's Version (Delis et al., 1994) or the Test of Memory and Learning (Reynolds and Bigler, 1993). An attempt can be made to estimate the child's ease of new learning by using standardized tests that mimic a teaching situation, teaching verbal information that is new to the child, using multiple learning trials with feedback (e.g., the Visual-Auditory Learning Subtest of the Woodcock-Johnson Psychoeducational Battery, Cognitive Tests by Woodcock and Johnson, 1989). Most revealing, however, is real, contextualized teaching of concepts and associated language not in the child's preinjury knowledge base. Teachers and clinicians can document (a) the child's rate and style of learning, (b) the child's spontaneous use of learning strategies and response to strategy suggestions, and (c) teaching procedures that seem to be most effective.

Depressed *speed of language processing* is not necessarily associated with prefrontal injury but should be targeted in a thorough language assessment of children with TBI. Speed of language processing can be assessed by systematically comparing performance under time constraints with performance with no time constraints. Some reading and writing tests are designed to yield these results in a standardized manner. In other cases, clinicians can compare language performance informally (listening, talking, reading, writing) under varying time constraints, being careful to interpret differences as diagnostic only if they are substantial. Table 10-3 suggests a procedure for assessing real-world reading and writing performance, including speed.

Educational Assessment

One of the purposes of educational assessment is to determine a student's levels of performance, relative to age and grade levels, in areas of academic interest, including reading, writing, spelling, and mathematics and (for older students) specific content areas. This information is critical for those planning the student's educational program in school. Educational diagnosticians have many standardized, norm-referenced tests available for this purpose. In selecting tests or other procedures for evaluating reading and writing, evaluators should be particularly sensitive to the factors discussed in the previous section regarding language assessment for children with TBI:

- Reading and writing tasks must be long enough to capture possible breakdowns in organizational ability. For students who are relatively well recovered, it is important to assign reading and writing tasks comparable in length and difficulty to those encountered in their school programs. If a student is required to read and write no more than short paragraphs, the consequences of organizational impairment may not be revealed.
- The evaluator must document the effects of time pressure on academic performance. If a test does not have provisions for timed versus untimed scoring, the evaluator should use double-scoring procedures (i.e., first administer the test according to the manual, then readminister it, varying critical parameters, including but not limited to time pressure). A large difference in performance may indicate that the variable being manipulated may play a critical role in educational planning.
- The evaluator should include some abstract or indirect language in the reading material. (See section on language assessment, Concrete Thinking.)

Table 10-3 contains the outline of an informal reading and writing assessment task for middle- and high-school students who are relatively well recovered. The task engages students in observing and describing their performance, thereby beginning the process of helping them to understand the consequences of their injury.

The written product can be evaluated for all aspects of writing: mechanics, organization, style, and content. If the evaluator is not familiar with typical performance at various grade levels, a control student of the same age can be used to serve as a reference point. As with all assessment procedures that are not standardized or norm referenced, only large deviations from normal expectations have interpretable significance. Reading performance, including speed and comprehension, can be evaluated in much the same way. Because students do not always recognize that they are using strategies, the evaluator should interview them to get a complete list of strategic maneuvers used.

If a student performs poorly, a second assignment can be given, accompanied by recommendations for compensatory procedures that may improve reading performance: using an advance organizer, highlighting and self-questioning while reading, using a dictionary, surveying before reading, and others. Similarly, the second writing assignment can include recommendations for compensatory writing procedures: semantic mapping, outlining, following an editing guide, using a peer or adult editor, and others. Comparing reading and writing performance under these two conditions may reveal useful instructional strategies and also begin to engage the student in identifying strategic behaviors that will be necessary for success in school.

Performance on tests of educational functioning can be misleading for the aforementioned reasons (see under Why Contextualized). Students with executive-system problems may score misleadingly well because the conditions of formal testing compensate for many of that student's most debilitating deficits. In addition, information and skills mastered before an injury may be recovered despite substantial difficulty with new learning and effective classroom behavior. Therefore, decisions about services and supports for the student in school must be made on the basis of considerations that go far beyond test performance.

In addition to identifying levels of academic performance, educational assessment aims to determine how the student processes information and learns new information and skills. This assessment includes identifying the student's best processing strategies and manner of handling materials, activities, and social demands in an educational setting. Close observation of the student during testing can contribute to this assessment but must be complemented by contextualized assessment, including situational observation, curriculum-based probes, and contextualized hypothesis testing. To accomplish this type of assessment in a rehabilitation hospital, it is critical to create a classroom-like environment complete with teachers (or other rehabilitation staff functioning as teachers), educational materials from the child's school, and educational activities similar to those of a regular classroom (Ylvisaker et al., 1995). In such a setting, the variables that affect academic success can be explored systematically (see also Chapters 17 and 18).

Introduction of Cognitive Assessments Over the Term of Recovery

Early in recovery, systematic observation of a child's level of alertness and responsiveness in relation to varied environmental stimuli, people, and activities can be useful in providing stimulation recommendations to nursing staff and family members. Systematic tracking of alertness, responsiveness, goal-directed behavior, and orientation continues as the child emerges from the very early phase of cognitive recovery and enters the phase characterized by general alertness combined with some degree of confusion and disorientation. Many programs use the Children's Orientation and Amnesia Test to track general aspects of cognitive functioning during this period (Ewing-Cobbs et al., 1989; Iverson et al., 1994). If these phases of recovery are prolonged, hypothesis testing (as described earlier) is useful in identifying factors that influence alertness, external focus, and orientation to task. From the perspective of cognitive recovery, a primary goal during this period is to have children spend maximum time processing information at their highest level and minimum time in a confused, agitated, or withdrawn state. Well-designed tracking systems, used by professionals and everyday people alike, can contribute to this goal by enabling staff to organize and disseminate information about factors that increase the likelihood of focused information processing and organized behavior.

When the child is rested, adequately oriented (and able to be oriented to new tasks), out of pain, and able to maintain attention for 15 minutes or more, standardized testing becomes possible. At this time, it is generally not appropriate to administer a battery of tests. The child's rate of change will likely render the results meaningless not long after the tests are scored and the results are organized and disseminated. During the period of relatively rapid recovery, standardized tests may be helpful but only if they contribute to decisions about how best to serve the child. For example, a receptive vocabulary test may help staff identify the appropriate level at which to converse with the child; a test of visual perception may help staff identify appropriate materials to use in therapy; a test of memory may help staff understand how best to teach the child. As always, the gold standard for selecting rehabilitation-relevant assessment procedures is identifying which information is needed to serve the child most effectively at this stage of recovery and how to acquire that information. For example, standardized tests are an unnecessary and relatively inefficient method for marking progress; during this phase, progress can be documented easily with daily observations of behavior in natural contexts.

Cognitive Assessment of Infants and Preschoolers

Whereas models of brain-behavior relationships have been articulated for use with older children and adolescents (Rourke, 1985; Rourke et al., 1983, 1986; Rudel et al., 1988; Tramontana and Hooper, 1988), such is not the case for children younger than 5 years old. Assessment challenges are compounded by the great variability in normal infant and preschooler development, the limited availability of validated and reliable formal measures of cognitive functioning, and the lack of objective preinjury baseline data.

For infants, clinicians have available the large domain of developmental checklists and scales, such as the sec-

ond edition of the Bayley Infant Scales of Development (Bayley, 1993), and ordinal scales of development, such as the Uzgiris-Hunt Scale (Uzgiris and Hunt, 1978), which are useful global indicators of recovery and which can also be used as screening tools to identify areas of development that may require close monitoring. Early childhood specialists have access to a large number of scales and tests for use in cognitive assessment of preschoolers. Piagetian tasks are particularly useful because of the importance of the functions identified by these tasks from both traditional structuralist and current information-processing perspectives (Willatts, 1990).

However, assessment tools designed to track maturation of early developmental achievements may be insensitive to subtle changes in areas of executive functioning such as initiation and flexibility in shifting sets, both common areas of concern after TBI. For this reason, combined with the well-documented context variability in infant and preschooler behavior, the procedures described earlier (ongoing, contextualized hypothesis-testing assessment) are especially important for this age group. Fortunately, an efficient way to orient parents to their critical role in stimulation and intervention is to engage them in this contextualized assessment, thereby simultaneously meeting assessment and intervention objectives. Clinicians can ask parents to observe a child's responses to various types of interaction, activities (including play activities), and environments. If the clinician's requests are sufficiently clear and ongoing encouragement and support are provided, the parents are likely to learn for themselves about the experiences, activities, and interaction that are most important for their child. Some parents require more concrete instruction than do others.

Infants and preschoolers with good early recovery after apparently severe TBI must be monitored at least into the early grades. The phenomenon of delayed developmental consequences after early brain injury is sufficiently common to justify this concern. In their chapter on preschoolers with TBI (Chapter 14), Ylvisaker and colleagues explore these and other issues related to preschool TBI in greater depth.

Cognitive Assessment After Mild Traumatic Brain Injury in Children

Most children with concussions (defined generally as a blow to the head resulting in minimal to no immediate loss of consciousness and no secondary neurologic sequelae, such as subdural hematoma or seizures) experience excellent outcome (Bijur et al., 1990; Fay et al., 1994; Rutter et al., 1980; Winogren et al., 1984). However, some investigators have documented persistent morbidity in some cases of mild TBI (Casey et al., 1986, 1987; Gulbrandsen, 1984). Others have suggested that mild TBI might interact with environmental disadvantages and preinjury vulnerability to create a need for special supports when the child returns to school (Greenspan and MacKenzie, 1994).

Concerns about the ability of psychological or neuropsychological tests to detect potentially troubling consequences of relatively severe, isolated prefrontal injury also apply to mild injuries and suggest that a valid method for identifying potential needs after such injuries should rather use careful observation of the child's real-world performance in school and social settings as the identification procedure of choice. In Chapter 17, Ylvisaker and Feeney outline such a "red-flag" system of contextualized assessment associated with a safety-net system of temporary supports for students with cognitive weakness after mild TBI (Ylvisaker et al., 1995).

Summary

In this chapter, we present and defend an approach to comprehensive cognitive assessment that highlights ongoing, contextualized, collaborative hypothesis testing. Besides creating a solid foundation for planning intervention, the procedures associated with this approach can help to solidify collaborative teams of professionals and facilitate competence and participation among everyday people, including family members and direct-care staff. We also offer important cautions regarding the use of standardized tests and address selected issues in cognitive assessment that are important for children with TBI.

References

Ackerly SS (1964). A Case of Paranatal Frontal Lobe Defect Observed for Thirty Years. In JM Warren, K Ackert (eds), The Frontal Granular Cortex and Behavior. New York: McGraw-Hill, 192.

Alexander MP, Benson DF, Stuss DT (1989). Frontal lobes and language. Brain Lang 37;656.

Bayley N (1969). Bayley Scales of Infant Development: Birth to Two Years (rev ed). New York: Psychological Corporation.

Benton A (1991). Prefrontal injury and behavior in children. Dev Neuropsychol 7;275.

Bernstein JH, Waber DP (1990). Developmental Neuropsychological Assessment: The Systematic Approach. In AA Boulton, GB Baker, M Hiscock (eds), Neuromethods: Vol 17, Neuropsychology. Clifton, NJ: Humana Press.

Bigler ED (1988). Frontal lobe damage and neuropsychological assessment. Arch Clin Neuropsychol 3;279.

Bijur PE, Haslum M, Golding J (1990). Cognitive and behavioral sequelae of mild head injury in children. Pediatrics 86;269.

Brown G, Chadwick O, Shaffer D, et al. (1981). A prospective study of children with head injuries: III. Psychiatric sequelae. Psychol Med 11;63.

Case R (1992). The role of the frontal lobes in the regulation of cognitive development. Brain Cogn 20;51.

Casey R, Ludwig S, McCormick MC (1986). Morbidity following mild head trauma in children. Pediatrics 78;497.

Casey R, Ludwig S, McCormick MC (1987). Minor head trauma in children: an intervention to decrease functional morbidity. Pediatrics 80;159.

Chapman SB (1997). Cognitive-communication abilities in children with closed head injury. Am J Speech Lang Pathol 6;50.

Chapman SB, Watkins R, Gustafson C, et al. (1997). Narrative discourse in children with closed head injury, children with language impairment, and typically developing children. Am J Speech Lang Pathol 6;66.

Crépean F, Scherzer BP, Belleville S, et al. (1997). A qualitative analysis of central executive disorders in a real-life work situation. Neuropsych Rehabil 7;147.

Delis M, Kramer J, Kaplan E, Ober B (1994). California Verbal Learning Test—Children's Version. San Antonio, TX: Psychological Corporation.

Denckla MB (1996). Research on executive function in a neurodevelopmental context: application of clinical measures. Dev Neuropsychol 12;5.

Dennis M (1980). Capacity and strategy for syntactic comprehension after left and right hemidecortication. Brain Lang 10;287.

Dennis M (1991). Frontal lobe function in childhood and adolescence: a heuristic for assessing attention regulation, executive control, and the intentional states important for social discourse. Dev Neuropsychol 7;327.

Dennis M, Barnes M (1990). Knowing the meaning, getting the point, bridging the gap, and carrying the message: aspects of discourse following closed head injury in childhood and adolescence. Brain Lang 39;428.

Dennis M, Barnes MA, Donnelly RE, et al. (1996). Appraising and managing knowledge: metacognitive skills after childhood head injury. Dev Neuropsychol 12;77.

Dennis M, Whitaker HA (1976). Language acquisition after hemidecortication: linguistic superiority of the left over the right hemisphere. Brain Lang 3;404.

Dennis M, Winner E (1990). The Beliefs and Intentions Test [unpublished test]. Toronto: The Hospital for Sick Children.

Durand VM (1990). Severe Behavior Problems: A Functional Communication Training Approach. New York: Guilford.

Eslinger PJ, Damasio AR (1985). Severe disturbance of higher cognition following bilateral frontal lobe oblation: patient EVR. Neurology 35;1731.

Eslinger PJ, Grattan LM, Damasio H, Damasio AR (1992). Developmental consequences of childhood frontal lobe damage. Arch Neurol 49;764.

Ewing-Cobbs L, Levin HS, Fletcher JM, et al. (1989). Post-Traumatic Amnesia in Children: Assessment and Outcome. Paper presented at the International Neuropsychological Society annual meeting, February 1989, Vancouver, BC.

Fay GC, Jaffe KM, Polissar NL, et al. (1994). Outcome of pediatric traumatic brain injury at three years: a cohort study. Arch Phys Med Rehabil 75;733.

Feeney TJ, Ylvisaker M (1995). Choice and routine:

antecedent behavioral interventions for adolescents with severe traumatic brain injury. J Head Trauma Rehabil 10(3);67.

Feuerstein R (1979). The dynamic Assessment of Retarded Performers: The Learning Potential Assessment Device, Theory, Instruments, and Techniques. Baltimore: University Park Press.

Flavell J, Miller P, Miller S (1993). Cognitive Development (3rd ed). Englewood Cliffs, NJ: Prentice Hall.

Fletcher JM, Ewing-Cobbs L, Miner M, Levin HS (1990). Behavioral changes after closed head injury in children. J Consult Clin Psychol 58;93.

Gaddes WH, Crocket DJ (1975). The Spreen-Benton Aphasia Tests: normative data as a measure of normal language development. Brain Lang 2;257.

German DJ (1989). Test of Word Finding. Allen, TX: DLM Teaching Resources.

German DJ (1990). Test of Adolescent/Adult Word Finding. Allen, TX: DLM Teaching Resources.

German DJ (1991). Test of Word Finding in Discourse. Allen, TX: DLM Teaching Resources.

Goldman PS (1971). Functional development of the prefrontal cortex in early life and the problem of neuronal plasticity. Exp Neurol 32;366.

Goldman PS, Alexander GE (1977). Maturation of prefrontal cortex in the monkey revealed by local reversible cryogenic depression. Nature 267;613.

Grattan LM, Eslinger PJ (1991). Frontal lobe damage in children and adults: a comparative review. Dev Neuropsychol 7;283.

Grattan LM, Eslinger PJ (1992). Long-term psychological consequences of childhood frontal lobe lesion in patient DT. Brain Cogn 20;85.

Greenspan AI, MacKenzie EJ (1994). Functional outcome after pediatric head injury. Pediatrics 94;425.

Gulbrandsen GB (1984). Neuropsychological sequelae of light head injuries in older children 6 months after trauma. J Clin Neuropsychol 6;257.

Iverson GL, Iverson AM, Barton EA (1994). The Children's Orientation and Amnesia Test: educational status is a moderator variable in tracking recovery from TBI. Brain Inj 8;685.

Iwata BA, Dorsey MF, Slifer KJ, et al. (1982). Toward a functional analysis of self-injury. Anal Interv Dev Disabil 2;3.

Kaplan E (1988). A Process Approach to Neuropsychological Assessment. In T Boll, BK Bryant (eds), Clinical Neuropsychology and Brain Function: Research, Measurement, and Practice. Washington, DC: American Psychological Association, 129.

Kern L, Childs KE, Dunlap G, et al. (1994). Using assessment-based curricular intervention to improve the classroom behavior of a student with emotional and behavioral challenges. J Appl Behav Anal 27;7.

Kolb B (1995). Brain Plasticity and Behavior. Hillsdale, NJ: Lawrence Erlbaum.

Krasnegor NA, Otto DA, Bernstein JH, et al. (1994). Neurobehavioral test strategies for environmental exposures in pediatric populations. Neurotoxicol Teratol 16;499.

Levin HS, Culhane KA, Hartman J, et al. (1991a). Developmental changes in performance on tests of purported frontal lobe functioning. Dev Neuropsychol 7;377.

Levin HS, Culhane KA, Mendelsohn D, et al. (1993). Cognition in relation to magnetic resonance imaging in head-injured children and adolescents. Arch Neurol 50;897.

Levin HS, Fletcher JM, Kufera JA, et al. (1996). Dimensions of cognition measured by the Tower of London and other cognitive tasks in head-injured children and adolescents. Dev Neuropsychol 12;17.

Levin HS, Goldstein FC, Williams DH, Eisenberg HM (1991b). The Contribution of Frontal Lobe Lesions to the Neurobehavioral Outcome of Closed Head Injury. In HS Levin, HM Eisenberg, AI Benton (eds), Frontal Lobe Function and Dysfunction. New York: Oxford University, 318.

Lezak MD (1982). The problem of assessing executive functions. Int J Psychol 17;281.

Lidz CS (1987). Dynamic Assessment: An Interactionist Approach to Evaluating Learning Potential. New York: Guilford.

Lovett MW, Dennis M (1977). The Premise and Transitive Inference Test [unpublished test]. Toronto: Hospital for Sick Children.

Marlowe WB (1992). The impact of a right prefrontal lesion on the developing brain. Brain Cogn 20;205.

Mateer CA, Williams D (1991). Effects of frontal lobe injury in childhood. Dev Neuropsychol 7;359.

O'Neill RE, Horner RH, Albin RW, et al. (1990). Functional Analysis of Problem Behavior. Sycamore, IL: Sycamore Publishing.

Palincsar AS, Brown AL, Campione JC (1994). Models and Practices of Dynamic Assessment. In GP Wallach, KG Butler (eds), Language Learning Disabilities in School-Age Children and Adolescents. New York: Macmillan, 132.

Perrott SB, Taylor HG, Montes JL (1991). Neuropsychological sequelae, familial stress, and environmental adaptation following pediatric head injury. Dev Neuropsychol 7;69.

Petterson L (1991). Sensitivity to emotional cues and social behavior in children and adolescents after head injury. Percept Mot Skills 73;1139.

Price B, Doffnre K, Stowe R, Mesulam M (1990). The compartmental learning disabilities of early frontal lobe damage. Brain 113;1383.

Prutting CA, Kirchner DM (1987). A clinical appraisal of the pragmatic aspects of language. J Speech Hear Dis 52;105.

Reynolds CR, Bigler ED (1993). Test of Memory and Learning. Austin, TX: PRO-ED.

Roberts RJ, Pennington BF (1996). An interactive framework for examining prefrontal cognitive processes. Dev Neuropsychol 12;105.

Rourke BP (ed) (1985). Neuropsychology of Learning Disabilities: Essentials of Subtype Analysis. New York: Guilford.

Rourke BP, Bakker DJ, Fisk JL, Strang JD (1983). Child Neuropsychology: An Introduction to Theory, Research and Clinical Practice. New York: Guilford.

Rourke BP, Fisk JL, Strang JD (1986). Neuropsychological Assessment of Children: A Team-Oriented Approach. New York: Guilford.

Rudel RG, Holmes JM, Pardel JR (1988). Assessment of Developmental Learning Disorders: A Neuropsychological Approach. New York: Basic Books.

Rutter M, Chadwick O, Shaffer D, Brown G (1980). A prospective study of children with head injuries: I. Design and methods. Psychol Med 10;633.

Sattler JM (1990). Assessment of Children (3rd ed). San Diego: JM Sattler.

Semel E, Wiig E, Secord W (1987). Clinical Evaluation of Language Fundamentals (rev ed). San Antonio, TX: Psychological Corporation.

Simeonsson R (1986). Psychological and Developmental Assessment of Special Children. Newton, MA: Allyn and Bacon.

Stelling MW, McKay SE, Carr WA, et al. (1986). Frontal lobe lesions and cognitive function in craniopharyngioma survivors. Am J Dis Child 140;710.

Stuss DT, Benson DF (1986). The Frontal Lobes. New York: Raven.

Stuss DT, Buckle L (1992). Traumatic brain injury: neuropsychological deficits and evaluation at different stages of recovery and in different pathologic subtypes. J Head Trauma Rehabil 7;40.

Taylor HG, Schatschneider C, Petrill S, et al. (1996). Executive dysfunction in children with early brain disease: outcomes post *Haemophilus influenzae* meningitis. Dev Neuropsychol 12;35.

Teuber HL (1964). The Riddle of Frontal Lobe Function in Man. In JM Warren, K Ackert (eds), The Frontal Granular Cortex and Behavior. New York: McGraw-Hill.

Thomsen IV (1989). Do young patients have worse outcomes after severe blunt head trauma? Brain Inj 3(2);157.

Tramontana MG, Hooper SR (1988). Assessment Issues in Child Neuropsychology. New York: Plenum.

Uzgiris I, Hunt J (1978). Assessment In Infancy: Ordinal Scales of Psychological Development. Urbana, IL: University of Illinois.

Vygotsky LS (1978). Mind in Society: The Development of Higher Psychological Processes. Edited and translated by M Cole, V John-Steiner, S Scribner, E Souberman. Cambridge, MA: Harvard University, 79. (Original work published 1935.)

Vygotsky LS (1986). Collected Works: Problems of General Psychology, vol 1. Translated by N Minick. New York: Plenum. (Original work published in 1934.)

Welsh MC, Pennington BF (1988). Assessing frontal lobe functioning in children: views from developmental psychology. Dev Neuropsychol 4;199.

Welsh MC, Pennington BF, Groisser DB (1991). A normative-developmental study of executive function: a window on prefrontal function in children. Dev Neuropsychol 7;131.

Wiig EH, Secord W (1988). Test of Language Competence (expanded edition). San Antonio: Psychological Corporation.

Willatts P (1990). Development of Problem-Solving Strategies in Infancy. In DF Bjorklund (ed), Children's Strategies: Contemporary Views of Cognitive Development. Hillsdale, NJ: Lawrence Erlbaum, 23.

Williams D, Mateer CA (1992). Developmental impact of frontal lobe injury in middle childhood. Brain Cogn 20;196.

Winogren HW, Knights RM, Bawden HN (1984). Neuropsychological deficits following head injury in children. J Clin Neuropsychol 6;269.

Woodcock R, Johnson M (1989). Woodcock-Johnson Psycho-Educational Test Battery (rev ed). Allen Park, TX: Teaching Resources.

Yakovlev PI, Lecours A-R (1967). The Myelogenetic Cycles of Regional Maturation of the Brain. In A Minkowski (ed), Regional Development of the Brain in Early Life. Oxford: Blackwell.

Ylvisaker M (1993). Communication outcome in children and adolescents with traumatic brain injury. Neuropsychol Rehabil 3;367.

Ylvisaker M, Feeney T (1994). Communication and behavior: collaboration between speech-language pathologists and behavioral psychologists. Top Lang Dis 15;37.

Ylvisaker M, Feeney T (1995). Traumatic brain injury in adolescence: assessment and reintegration. Semin Speech Lang 16;32.

Ylvisaker M, Feeney T, Maher-Maxwell N, et al. (1995). School reentry following severe traumatic brain injury: guidelines for educational planning. J Head Trauma Rehabil 10(6);25.

Ylvisaker M, Feeney T, Mullins K (1995). School reentry following mild traumatic brain injury: a proposed hospital-to-school protocol. J Head Trauma Rehabil 10(6);42.

Ylvisaker M, Hartwick P, Ross B, Nussbaum N (1994). Cognitive Assessment. In R Savage, G Wolcott (eds), Educational Dimensions of Acquired Brain Injury. Austin, TX: PRO-ED, 69.

Chapter 11

Cognitive Rehabilitation: Organization, Memory, and Language

Mark Ylvisaker, Shirley F. Szekeres, and Juliet Haarbauer-Krupa

In this chapter, we discuss themes in cognitive intervention that are often presented separately for cognitive rehabilitation specialists, educators or special educators, speech-language pathologists, psychologists, occupational therapists, recreation therapists, and vocational specialists. These professionals are the primary intended audience for this chapter. However, we have elected to address the themes in an integrated rather than a discipline-specific manner for two important reasons. First, in children and adolescents with traumatic brain injury (TBI), typically the same underlying cognitive weakness results in difficulty in organizing thoughts and behavior for effective learning and performance of activities of daily living (ADLs), complex play activities, expressive discourse tasks (speaking and writing), extended-text comprehension, and other complex social, academic, or vocational tasks that require organization. Second, presenting these themes in separate chapters for different groups of professionals runs the risk of suggesting that a fragmented intervention program can meet the needs of children and adolescents whose internal fragmentation requires intensely integrative and collaborative rehabilitation and special education programs. Although they are not the primary audience for this chapter, members of the physical restoration team, nursing staff, and family members are most certainly primary deliverers of cognitive rehabilitative services, necessitating a fierce commitment to collaboration among those with special expertise in the cognitive dimensions of behavior and between specialists and people who interact daily with the child or adolescent (so-called everyday people).

We recommend that this chapter be read in conjunction with Chapters 9, 10, 12, and 14. At several points in this chapter, we make the assumption that the reader either is familiar with material in those chapters or will read them to pursue those themes in greater depth. We especially hope that the reader will study Chapter 9, because many of the practical recommendations made in this chapter are based on theoretical and empirical supports discussed there. Chapter 12 is in some respects a continuation of this chapter, including discussions of intervention for disorders of organization and memory from a compensatory or strategic perspective.

Because of dramatically decreasing lengths of stay in pediatric rehabilitation centers, some of the issues discussed in this chapter may not be relevant for children and adolescents during their period of inpatient rehabilitation. Rehabilitation activities that once took place in inpatient settings—when lengths of stay after severe brain injury were counted in months—now take place, if at all, in homes or schools because lengths of stay for children with comparable injuries are now typically counted in days or weeks. Nevertheless, it is critical that inpatient staff have solid expertise in these areas of intervention, because it is their job to ensure that family members and staff at the next level of rehabilitation or education are as well oriented and trained as possible to carry on the rehabilitative efforts begun in a medical setting. Indeed, from a cognitive perspective, orienting and training people who will later be involved with the child, and collaborating with them in developing effective reintegration programs, are often the most important contributions of cognitive specialists in inpatient rehabilitation facilities (see Chapter 20): That is, in today's health care climate, inpatient staff typically play a more important role as consultants to and educators of family members, school personnel, and other professionals than as direct providers of cognitive rehabilitation services.

First in this chapter, we plot out the territory and clarify our general orientation to cognitive rehabilitation. We believe that this background information merits careful study, because it provides the theoretical support for the practical intervention suggestions that follow. In the intervention sections, we present practical procedures, heuristics, and recommendations we hope will guide clinicians and teachers in their search for effective interventions and supports for children and adolescents with TBI. Included in this chapter is an organization checklist that clinicians and teachers can use to develop and evaluate their interventions from the perspective of cognitive organization.

Foundations: Intervention Premises

The selection of themes to be discussed in this chapter and the intervention activities and procedures that we recommend are based on a small set of premises. These premises are derived from our clinical experience with several hundred children and adolescents with TBI and from the small but growing outcome and intervention literature in this area as well as from the large body of theoretical and experimental work in developmental cognitive psychology, educational psychology, and developmental neuropsychology. The theoretical and practical issues raised in these premises are elaborated, with concrete examples, later in the chapter. Several of these premises are discussed at greater length in Chapter 9.

Premise I

The first premise is that problems with organization and memory are common after TBI in children and adolescents and have far-reaching effects. Among the vulnerable areas of the brain in closed head injury (as well as in other causes of acquired brain injury) are those associated with cognitive organization and memory or new learning (Grafman et al., 1993; Schwartz et al., 1993; Szekeres, 1992; Tranel and Damasio, 1995). For example, medial temporal lobe structures (e.g., the hippocampus) are critical to memory and learning and are vulnerable to anoxic brain injury. Prefrontal structures, the most vulnerable parts of the brain in closed head injury (Levin et al., 1991), are associated with strategic organizing and learning.

Therefore, it is very common for children who may have been good students before incurring a brain injury to experience generally good recovery after TBI but nevertheless to have difficulty with any complex task and to learn slowly in school, which often results in failing grades. Impaired new learning has serious negative implications for children and adolescents who face years of formal education, social learning, and vocational training in order to succeed as adults. Difficulty organizing information and behavior interferes with ADLs, academic and vocational performance, social interaction, and all other complex tasks that cannot be completed automatically. In the absence of careful attention to these cognitive consequences of TBI, children are likely to fail academically and socially, and behavioral and emotional deterioration are likely to be secondary results.

Premise II

The second premise is that different types of TBI can differentially impair organization and memory. With respect to cognitive organization, prefrontal injury (which is very common in head injury) reduces executive control over cognitive processes (e.g., remaining focused on the task at hand and choosing the correct organizing scheme to complete the task) (Schwartz et al., 1993). Posterior injury, in contrast, may disrupt stored knowledge and the organizing networks or schemes within which knowledge is stored, thereby interfering with organized behavior as well as retrieval of old information and efficient encoding of new information (Patterson and Hodges, 1995). With respect to memory, prefrontal injury might reduce an individual's control over memory processes, including the use of strategic procedures (e.g., organizational strategies) to learn new information or retrieve stored information (Shimamura, 1995; Stuss and Benson, 1986). In contrast, medial temporal lobe injury (e.g., injury to the hippocampus) reduces the individual's ability to consolidate new (declarative) memory traces for subsequent storage (Markowitsch, 1995; Tranel and Damasio, 1995).

Premise III

The third premise is that organization and memory are intimately related. Many distinct types of memory processes and systems exist and are affected by a variety of factors outside of and within the learner (Tulving, 1995). However, for most types of memory, the four keys to effective encoding, storage, and subsequent retrieval are (1) the frequency of presentation of the information to be remembered (repetition), (2) its personal meaningfulness, (3) knowledge of the topic already possessed by the learner, and (4) the degree to which the information to be learned is organized in a way that is meaningful to the learner. One of the most thoroughly established principles of memory and learning is that the better organized information to be learned is, the easier it is to attend to, comprehend, encode, store, and subsequently retrieve that information—assuming that the learner appreciates that organization (Brown, 1979). Because of this intimate connection between organization and memory, we have chosen to address them together, focusing primarily on cognitive organization. In the next chapter, we discuss memory and learning from the perspective of learning strategies.

Premise IV

The fourth premise is that normal development of organization and memory yields insights for intervention. As a general rule, sequences of normal cognitive and linguistic development provide clues to hierarchies of difficulty that can be used in planning rehabilitation. For example, important guidance in the selection of rehabilitation goals and activities for children and adolescents with cognitive impairment results from knowing (1) that young children learn more efficiently when oriented to concrete, meaningful goals in a natural context rather than to the abstract goal of learning; (2) that they are more comfortable with organization based on their own everyday routines and life experiences than on more abstract categories and associations (commonly found in cognitive rehabilitation workbooks); and (3) that their learning is facilitated when adults impose meaningful organization on the to-be-learned information (Schneider and Pressley, 1989; Ylvisaker et al., 1992).

Premise V

The fifth premise is that there are many approaches to cognitive rehabilitation (including intervention for deficits in organization and memory), all of which are appropriate for some individuals at certain stages of recovery in relation to specific goals. In Chapter 9, goals for and approaches to cognitive rehabilitation are discussed in detail. The general goal of cognitive rehabilitation is to help individuals achieve real-world objectives that may be difficult to master because of cognitive impairment. Approaches to achieving this goal include general cognitive stimulation early in recovery, direct retraining of weak areas (when possible), teaching of strategic behavior to compensate for ongoing disability, provision of cognitive supports, modification of the environment, and adjustment of interaction with the child and teaching procedures to fit the child's profile of abilities. A need for the latter types of cognitive support, and the continuous problem solving and creative adapting that accompany them, often continues throughout the child's school career and vocational development. In addition, acquisition of academic knowledge and other content should be considered a component of cognitive rehabilitation in that stored knowledge itself facilitates cognitive processing of new information.

Premise VI

The sixth premise is that everyday functional activities are the best context for cognitive intervention. Studies in cognitive science (e.g., Singley and Anderson, 1989), developmental cognitive psychology (e.g., Flavell et al., 1993; Light and Butterworth, 1993), and educational psychology (e.g., Schneider and Pressley, 1989) yield the important conclusion that cognitive skills are acquired in a way that ties them to more or less specific domains of content. This domain specificity of cognitive skill is particularly true of young children and individuals with frontal lobe injury or immaturity. This important reality argues for a rehabilitation approach that attempts to facilitate improved processing of information and effective

compensatory behavior within the contexts (content, place, person, activity) in which improvements are needed. Appropriate contexts for children can include play with peers, classroom academic activities with teachers, social interaction at mealtimes or during other social activities, ADLs on the nursing unit or at home, and prevocational activities. Exercising cognitive processes in a wholly decontextualized manner (e.g., using cognitive training workbooks and software in isolated cognitive retraining therapy sessions with the general goal of improving cognition in a way that will positively influence all practical applications of the trained skill) is of questionable value from the perspectives of transfer of cognitive skill and motivation. Although drill and repetition may be important for people with impaired learning, special attention must be paid to *what is being drilled* and to *the context in relation to promoting transfer of learning.*

Premise VII

The seventh premise is that cognitive rehabilitation is a collaborative enterprise: Everyday people are the ideal providers of cognitive intervention services and supports. If context (person, place, activity, content) is critical in improving cognitive processes and systems (Premise VI), it follows that the people in those meaningful contexts are the primary facilitators of improved cognitive functioning. The inescapable conclusion is that family members, nursing staff, teachers, aides, and other people who function regularly in the child's everyday life must be thought of as primary deliverers of the service (i.e., everyday cognitive "coaches"; see Chapter 20). Specialists in cognitive rehabilitation, regardless of their disciplinary background, play a critical role in thoroughly understanding the child's profile of cognitive strengths and weaknesses (typically through diagnostic intervention, including systematic testing of hypotheses, discussed in Chapter 10) and using that understanding to orient and train everyday people and to help develop appropriate educational programs.

Premise VIII

The eighth premise is that problems with organization and memory are often misdiagnosed, resulting in inappropriate intervention. Children with organizational problems find it difficult to focus and remain on task. These difficulties might be diagnosed as an attentional problem, possibly resulting in a decision to focus intervention on attention and thereby missing the primary issue. Similarly, many children with undiagnosed organizational problems fail to perform as expected, and a misdiagnosis of oppositional behavior results, initiating a downward behavioral spiral (see Chapter 13). Sorting through these complex issues is not easy and necessitates collaborative, contextualized hypothesis testing (described in Chapter 10).

Cognitive Organization and Memory and Their Relationship

Memory processes as well as distinct types of memories that are retained in long-term storage are discussed in Chapter 9.

Cognitive Organization

Organizational activity (i.e., arranging objects, people, events, language, or ideas into a structured whole) takes many forms. For example, preschoolers tend to have highly organized behavioral routines around bedtime; they typically start a story by saying something about characters, place, and time; and they may group items in play by function (e.g., placing the plate, cup, fork, and spoon together), by perceptual characteristics (e.g., sorting out all the dowels, blocks, and wheels before playing with construction toys), and by categories (e.g., grouping all the animals together). In each case, they are engaged in organizational activity, which can be understood as having three dimensions: the product, the process, and the underlying conceptual structure (Pellegrino and Ingram, 1978).

Dimensions of Organizational Activity

Organization as *product* is the set of stable and identifiable relationships among the organized items (Mandler, 1967). For example, a table set for dinner has predictable relationships between and among the table and chairs, and the plates, glasses, utensils, napkins, serving bowls, and the like. Similarly, a story has a predictable order and relationships among its components (characters, settings, actions, reactions, plans, resolution), as does a day at school.

Organizing as a *process* or *activity* (i.e., the act of arranging objects, people, events, language, or ideas) is what people do to create the relationships that are identified as an organized product. Setting the table and telling a coherent story are among the many organizing activities in which people engage daily. Much of an individual's organized behavior is routine or habitual. However, when organizing activity is deliberate, it typically involves a goal, a plan, arrangement of the items or ideas to be organized, and an evaluation of the product in relation to the goal. Effective organizing of behavior and ideas enables people to function efficiently in complex and novel environments and to deal with amounts of information that exceed processing capacity.

Organization as a *conceptual structure* is the mental representation of organizational relationships and principles, which is hypothesized to explain an individual's organizing of objects, people, events, and ideas into predictable patterns. For example, when a child creates a truck from Tinkertoys, it can be inferred that he or she has a mental representation of a truck, which also plays a role in perception and verbal descriptions of trucks. Likewise, when a child pretends to feed a baby and put it to bed, it is inferred that he or she has a mental representation of an event schema or script. Similarly, when an older child tells an organized story, it is inferred that there exists a mental schema for storytelling, a schema that also guides efficient listening to, comprehension of, and memory for stories. More generally, cognitive activity, including learning, is guided by these conceptual structures or *knowledge structures*. These organizing schemes enable people to make sense of complex experiences, comprehend new material, store information in an organized and readily retrievable manner, express themselves clearly, and negotiate demanding or novel tasks and environments without becoming confused and anxious (Bartlett, 1958). From a neuropsychological perspective, organization as conceptual structure is understood to include networks and systems of networks of neural connections, spanning multiple cortical areas, damage to any part of which can result in inefficient and disorganized behavior, language, thinking, and learning.

Acquisition and Use of Knowledge Structures

A primary goal of cognitive rehabilitation is to help children (re)acquire important knowledge structures and use them to guide behavior and thinking. Recognizing that organized behavior and thinking have their basis in these knowledge structures (organized mental representations of things and events) helps teachers and clinicians focus on meaningful domains of content in their attempts to facilitate improved organizational functioning in children and adolescents with TBI. This recognition also helps discourage clinicians from "exercising" children's organizing processes in the absence of meaningful content that is to be organized (e.g., "contentless" categorizing, sequencing, associating, and problem-solving exercises), as though those processes were merely tools that could be sharpened with exercise, thereby improving the child's ability to organize *any* kind of content with that tool. Cognitive (re)training workbooks and software are filled with exactly this type of highly abstract exercise, which at best is useful in helping a child to understand the concept of organization.

Unfortunately, more than a century of studies of the transfer of cognitive skill has revealed that exercises of this sort (i.e., cognitive exercises outside of the context of any meaningful content) rarely yield transferable, functional improvements in general cognitive functioning (Singley and Anderson, 1989). Indeed, it is misleading to refer to cognitive processes as *skills* because of this term's implicit suggestion that improvement comes with practicing or rehearsing the skill without regard to the content to be attended to, perceived, organized, comprehended, learned, and used.

Table 11-1. Illustrations of Organizing Schemes Important to Children

Familiar event scripts	Grouping people, things, events, and associated dialogue according to sequences of events that are common in life. For children, familiar event scripts typically include daily routines (e.g., getting up and getting ready for school, going to school, after-school activities) as well as events that occur less frequently (e.g., going to a birthday party, visiting the doctor, eating out, going camping).
Common task scripts	Grouping things and events that constitute common activities of daily living (e.g., bathing, eating) and household, school, or vocational tasks (e.g., cleaning one's room, writing a term paper, delivering papers).
Function (use)	Grouping items that have a similar function (e.g., cup, glass) or that are used together to accomplish a goal (e.g., brush, rag, soap, pail, and sponge for washing a car).
Main idea and detail	Grouping related facts under the main idea that holds those facts together.
Story schema	Grouping people and events in a story under headings such as setting, characters, initiating event, psychological reaction, plan, action, resolution.
Perceptual similarity	Arranging items according to color, shape, size, sound, texture, taste, and the like.
Semantic relations	Arranging items according to features such as superordinate categories (e.g., dogs and cats are animals), part-whole relations, opposites, analogic relations, and the like.
General life scripts	Organizing biographical events according to a general representation of passages through life: People are born, go to school, establish friendships and partnerships, get jobs, and so on.

Let us illustrate this point with two brief exercises. First, quickly place the following events and documents in chronological order: Articles of Confederation, Boston Tea Party, Bill of Rights, Stamp Act, Declaration of Independence. Difficulty in sequencing these items (as is experienced by most people) is *not* evidence of a weak general faculty or skill of sequencing, a weakness that necessitates decontextualized sequencing exercises to strengthen the skill. Rather, difficulty suggests that you lack adequate knowledge of the events surrounding the American Revolution and how they are related to one another (i.e., organized). Similarly, a child who cannot sequence morning ADLs needs help learning the morning routine (as well as other routines and schemas), not abstract practice with sequencing. Similarly, a child who has difficulty sequencing material in a narrative needs to practice narrating using relevant supports, such as a narrative guide.

Next, quickly determine which of the following famous historical figures does not belong in the group: Aristotle, Duns Scotus, Saint Augustine, Plato, Thomas Aquinas. Difficulty in identifying which does not belong with the others (as is experienced by most people) is *not* evidence of a weak general faculty or skill of categorizing, a weakness that necessitates decontextualized categorizing exercises to strengthen the skill. Rather, this difficulty would suggest that you lack adequate knowledge of ancient and medieval philosophy, including how philosophies are grouped (i.e., organized). Similarly, a child who is unable to categorize common objects in the environment requires experiences that will result in an enriched knowledge base, including knowledge of the relationships among common objects (i.e., how they are or can be organized), and needs to practice using that knowledge in practical ways. Appreciation of this simple,

commonsense point has powerful implications for cognitive rehabilitation, including intense skepticism regarding decontextualized cognitive retraining exercises.

Our point is not that drill and exercise associated with cognitive domains are inappropriate. It is rather that clinicians and teachers must clearly understand the goal of the practice. Practice in the area of cognitive organization must be focused on organizing schemes that are particularly important for the child in question and at the correct level of concreteness for that child. A problem with decontextualized workbook exercises is that they are characteristically at a level of abstractness too high for most cognitively impaired children and adolescents.

Common Organizational Schemas

There are many ways in which people, objects, events, and ideas can be related to one another. Table 11-1 presents common organizational schemes that figure prominently in the daily life and academic functioning of children. Preferred modes of organization, as well as the level of abstractness that can be appreciated within each mode, depend on age, education, and culture.

The recognition of organization in things and events can exist on a continuum from concrete to abstract. For example, a preschooler who frequently eats at a specific McDonald's may be aware of a sequence of events common to all visits (e.g., arrive, stand in line, give the order, wait for the food, find a table, eat, throw away refuse, leave) but might not recognize the connection between this pattern and the sequence of events at other restaurants. Because of its concreteness, this type of organization sometimes is referred to as a *routine*.

At a more general or abstract level, a child who has visited many types of restaurants may become aware of abstract patterns common to them all (e.g., arrive, examine a menu, interact with a waiter or waitress, eat, pay). This more abstract representation of organization—which is important for guiding behavior in novel contexts—is sometimes referred to as a *script* and can include knowledge of people, places, event sequences, props, and dialogue common to a variety of similar experiences.

At an extremely abstract level, an individual may acquire a general representation (or general schema) of the components of a visit to any place of business. Similarly, function categories may begin with a concrete recognition that knives and spoons go together, then proceed to a more general and abstract representation of utensils, and end at an extremely general and abstract category of tools. Likewise, problem solving may begin with an infant's concrete understanding of specific relations between specific means and ends (e.g., if I cry, I'll get food) and then progress to the very abstract general understanding of problem solving possessed by logicians, mathematicians, and cognitive psychologists. This concrete-to-abstract continuum in the mental representation of organization is a useful guide in planning a sequence of cognitive rehabilitation goals and activities. Often clinicians make the mistake of beginning at a level that is too abstract and general for a child or adolescent with TBI and who is a concrete thinker (e.g., general practice in determining which items belong together in decontextualized categorizing drills; general practice in decontextualized problem-solving drills without meaningful engagement in solving real problems).

Relation Between Cognitive Organization and Memory

The ability to think and act in an organized manner serves many purposes. One important consequence of improved organization is more efficient learning and memory. During the 1960s and 1970s, the intimate relationship between organization and memory/learning was a major theme in the study of memory (e.g., Mandler, 1967). Indeed, to this day, cognitive and educational psychologists of differing theoretical orientations agree that information that is well organized and organized in a way that "fits the head of the learner" is easier to attend to, comprehend, encode, store, and retrieve (Bower, 1972; Brown, 1975, 1979; Flavell et al., 1993; Hagen et al., 1975). That is, the way information is organized must be congruent with the organizational structures available in the learner's knowledge base (i.e., semantic memory). Thus, organization cuts across all three basic dimensions of memory. Information that is encoded in an organized way leads to "a well-integrated trace that stores the information in more than one dimension, hence making it resistant to forgetting. Furthermore, the presence of several dimensions will increase the number of retrieval routes" (Baddeley, 1995, p. 9).

Young children, including preschoolers, similarly profit from organization in information that is to be learned. However, unlike older children and adults who can actively organize information in a way that makes sense to them, young children profit most from organization that is imposed and highlighted by adults, assuming that the organization is congruent with the children's internal organization (Baumeister and Smith, 1979; Ceci, 1980; Horowitz et al., 1969; Moely, 1977). This places an obligation on teachers of young children (and of older children and adolescents recovering from brain injury) to present information that is to be learned in the most meaningful and concrete terms, emphasizing relationships with the child's real-life knowledge of and interest in things as well as real-world routines and scripts. In contrast, when teachers highlight forms of organization that are too abstract for the child (e.g., categories like fruits and vegetables for young children), the effect on the child may be confusion rather than facilitation of learning.

Relation Between Organization and Other Cognitive Processes

In addition to its association with memory and learning problems, organizational impairment can easily masquerade as some other type of cognitive or behavioral problem. For example, people who are generally disorganized—that is, people who lack organizing schemas or who fail to use them when needed to guide behavior or thinking—often appear to be unable to pay attention or to concentrate.

Case Illustration: Organization and Attention

Early in life, TK had a brain tumor removed, followed by intracranial radiation and chemotherapy. His cognitive disability, which appeared to be moderate initially, grew over the course of his grade-school years as the curricular demands increased. His fourth-grade teacher stated that he was incapable of learning in a regular educational setting, regardless of the support available to him. However, at his mother's urging, he remained in a regular education class for fifth grade (with considerable special education and therapeutic support). By January of that year, his regular education teacher claimed that he was getting little out of her instruction, largely because he appeared unable to focus his attention on his work or her classroom discussions. His inattention was so extreme that she proposed that he may be having ongoing seizures. At that point, an intervention began that included easy-to-follow written or pictured organizational guides for all of TK's lessons and independent work in the classroom. With that organizational support, his apparently severe attentional problem was virtually eliminated.

Clearly, TK's primary problem was not an inability to attend but rather a severe inability to organize his thinking and behavior, a consequence of which was severe inattention. It is interesting to note that intervention recommendations for children and adults with attention deficit disorder often emphasize the importance of organizational support and training more than procedures that directly target attention and concentration (e.g., Hallowell and Ratey, 1994).

Normal Development of Organization and Memory

Normal sequences of cognitive development can serve as a useful guide in selecting goals and objectives for cognitive rehabilitation and in identifying effective intervention procedures. In Chapter 9, Ylvisaker and Szekeres discuss important principles and patterns of cognitive development and their implications for intervention after TBI. They caution against understanding development (and rehabilitation after TBI) as a serial-order progression from so-called lower-order (e.g., attention, perception) to so-called higher-order (e.g., reasoning, executive control) processes and systems. They also caution against understanding development (and rehabilitation) as a series of qualitatively distinct stages at which new types of cognitive behavior emerge in the absence of functional predecessors at earlier stages. In addition, they offer two reasons for flexibility in using a developmental template as a basis for rehabilitation planning: First, after TBI, knowledge and skill at relatively high levels of development are often preserved, whereas gaps are commonly found at relatively low levels. Second, in some areas (e.g., self-awareness and executive-control functions), it is important in working with children with disability to try to accelerate development beyond normal developmental expectations. Table 11-2 lists patterns of normal cognitive development, which are discussed in Chapter 9.

Development of Cognitive Organization

Important themes in the development of conceptual organization include (1) progression from concrete and context dependent to abstract and free of context, (2) changes in preferred modes of organization, (3) progression from organizational behavior that does not involve the deliberate use of organizational strategies to that which does, and (4) growth in the number and variety of organizing schemes.

Concrete to Abstract

The knowledge structures, or mental representations of organized objects and events, possessed by preschoolers tend to be concrete—that is, elicited by and applicable to

Table 11-2. Major Interrelated Patterns of Normal Cognitive Development

Progression in perception and thought from surface to depth
Progression from concrete to abstract and hypothetical thinking
Progression from context-dependent learning and behavior to increasingly context-independent learning and behavior
Progression from behavior that is not deliberately strategic to deliberately strategic thinking and problem solving
Progression from egocentric to nonegocentric thinking and acting
Progression from cognitive centration to decentration
Growth in the knowledge base
Increased efficiency of or capacity for information processing

specific circumstances (Flavell et al., 1993). For example, a 3 year old might be very clear about his or her bedtime routine at home but become confused and disorganized at bedtime when visiting another home. Adults, in contrast, possess bedtime scripts that are general, flexible, and applicable in widely varied circumstances. Similarly, preschoolers can effectively organize concrete physical objects, but they have difficulty organizing ideas and language to describe their experiences. After TBI (especially frontal lobe injury), older children and adolescents may return to a state of extremely concrete thinking, necessitating an initial focus on the (re)acquisition of concrete and contextualized organizational routines and scripts before children with TBI can progress to more abstract types of organization. The normal progression in the development of narrative ability (described later) is one example of a concrete-to-abstract progression that can be applied to brain injury rehabilitation.

Preferred Modes of Organization

Preschoolers are able to organize objects in a variety of ways (e.g., by function, perceptual characteristics, part-whole relations). However, they appear to *prefer* thematic or episodic organization based on the themes or routines of their own lives. For example, a preschooler's strongest association with the word *pie* may be *Grandma* (versus *bake* or *eat*, which are syntagmatic associations, or *cherry* or *cake,* which are paradigmatic associations and preferred associations for older children), because Grandma is the person in the preschooler's experience who has the most to do with pies. For young people, information presented in the context of real-life routines or scripts is more readily processed and remembered than information organized in any other way (Ceci and Howe, 1978; Szekeres, 1988).

By the late grade-school years (or earlier, if category organization is highlighted in school), children seem to be equally comfortable with more abstract forms of organization (e.g., superordinate-subordinate categories). After TBI, the initial therapeutic focus should be on the concrete organization of personally meaningful routines and scripts, including play routines, ADLs, common social and academic routines, and concrete categories (e.g., sorting clothes) before attempts are made to facilitate the use of more abstract organizing schemes.

Nondeliberate to Deliberate Strategic Organization

Although often very organized in their behavior, preschoolers rarely formulate explicit intentions to organize their thinking or behavior in order to accomplish a difficult task. Formulated intentions to use strategies generally start with physical activity. Take, for example, a 3 year old pondering how to walk on a balance beam: "Maybe I'll try it sideways." Another starting point for formulating intentions to use strategies is highly motivating cognitive activity that has a physical component and is in a natural context: Consider a 4 year old who is wondering where to put a present that he or she must remember to take home from school: "I think I'll put it in my cubby." The rate at which children develop is, in part, a function of the expectations for independent functioning placed on them by parents and teachers (e.g., "Make sure you have all of your soccer things together and ready to go.").

In contrast, middle- and high-school students, particularly those whose parents and teachers have highlighted the importance of independently strategic and organized behavior, have sufficient metacognitive understanding of organization and of their own organizational limitations that they can write outlines for papers; make a plan for how to get everything done on a particularly busy day; write assignments in an assignment book; with peers, talk through difficult material in preparing for examinations; and the like. A peer culture supportive of this type of strategic behavior facilitates such development. Furthermore, middle-school and older students may be aware of a variety of organizational schemas from which to choose. For example, many middle-school students can describe the general organization of a fictional story and how that organization differs from the organization of language in explaining a complex game. After TBI, there is reason to focus initially on organized behavior without metacognitive reflection on the nature of the organizing schemes used; subsequently, metacognitive reflection and deliberate strategic use of organizing schemes can be taught (see Chapter 12).

Development of Narrative Ability

Development of the ability to organize language into coherent descriptions, narratives, and other types of discourse has, for a variety of reasons, received considerable attention in recent years. First, the organization of language is a useful indicator of a child's ability to organize thoughts. Second, the development of narrative ability may be causally related to the development of memory and thought organization (Fivush and Reese, 1992; McCabe and Peterson, 1991; Nelson, 1992; Reese et al., 1993; Reese and Fivush, 1993). Third, difficulty in organizing narratives at ages 4 and 5 years is associated with difficulty in learning to read and write in the early grades (Paul and Smith, 1993) and may be an important indicator of ongoing language impairment. Finally, it is possible to understand early language disability generally as a manifestation of organizational weakness, with language-delayed toddlers having difficulty organizing sounds into words, 2–4 year olds having difficulty organizing words into semantically and syntactically appropriate utterances, 4–6 year olds having specific difficulty organizing their thoughts and language to produce coherent connected discourse, and older children with language disability having difficulty comprehending longer texts and producing organized written and spoken language consistent with age expectations. Unfortunately, the richness of this child development literature has not been adequately reflected in the development of intervention procedures for children with congenital or acquired organizational impairment. We return to this point later, in the section on Organization and Language.

Most descriptions of the normal developmental sequence of narrative skill are based on observations of white, middle-class children attempting to recount an event or tell a story without help. Studies of other cultures have revealed different patterns of development and varied organizational structures underlying narration (Westby, 1994). Therefore, clinicians should be cautious in their application of normative information to cultures other than mainstream American culture. In addition, most children do not develop their narrative skill by independently producing narratives (i.e., narratives as *performances*) and then receiving feedback. Rather, most children's narratives are co-constructed with a caregiver within the context of a conversation, with the adult providing the support (the so-called scaffolding) needed to generate an adequately elaborated and coherent narrative. The skill and communication style of that partner has much to do with the development of preschoolers' episodic memory, thought organization, and narrative competence. (See Chapter 14 for further discussion of this point.)

Acknowledging these qualifications as background, the developmental literature suggests the following outline of normal development of narratives that the child produces without external support (McCabe and Rollins, 1994):

1. *Approximately age 2:* The child may produce a *single-event narrative* (e.g., "me fall") or a *miscellaneous narrative* (sometimes called a *heap*), which is an apparently unrelated set of words and word combinations about

an event or theme. An adult who is familiar with the event described can recognize the utterances as a narrative. Generally, adults ask questions and add content to turn the single-event description or miscellaneous narrative into a more elaborate and coherent conversational or chained narrative.

2. *Approximately age 4:* Between the ages of 3 and 4, the child progresses to *leap frog narratives*. The events may still be somewhat out of order, but it is clearer that the descriptions all relate to a single event. By age 4, most children produce occasional chronological narratives— that is, appropriately sequenced descriptions of events but with no clear theme or end point (e.g., "I had a Pocahontas cake for my birthday. It has four candles. I got presents and we played games."). In general, preschoolers are better at organizing descriptions of their own routines or scripts, or singular experiences from their own life, than at organizing fictional stories.

3. *Approximately age 5:* Most 5 year olds can produce an appropriately sequenced set of events that culminates in a particularly important or climactic event (*end-at-high-point narrative*). Furthermore, the narratives tend to include causal relationships, including causal explanations of internal states (e.g., "I was scared 'cause . . ."').

4. *Approximately age 6 or 7:* Most 6- or 7-year-old children are capable of producing a simple story with all the basic elements: characters and setting, initiating event, reaction, plan, sequence of events leading to a high point, and resolution. Referred to as *classical* narrative organization (or basic *story grammar*), this organizational scheme is important for both understanding and producing stories in first grade. By this age, most children can impose narrative structure on fictional narratives as well as stories about their own experiences.

5. *Early adolescence:* By early adolescence, many children, though certainly not all, have acquired sufficient metacognitive awareness of discourse structure that they can describe the general outline of a story, indicate how that organization differs from the organization needed to explain how to play a game (for example), and deliberately choose an organizational framework that is useful in communicating a specific kind of information to a specific audience. Furthermore, older children are better at meeting the needs of the listener (e.g., giving clearer introductions and changes of settings and characters; providing fewer unrelated details and unresolved problems) and at creating more complex episodic structure (Johnston, 1982). The ability to choose an organizing scheme that will be helpful for a specific task is a theme to which we return later in this chapter, in the section on Organization and Deliberate (Strategic) Learning.

McCabe and Rollins (1994) described procedures for using this developmental information in assessing preschoolers' narrative development. It should be noted, however, that *independent* narration, useful in assessing

the child's development of thought and discourse organization, is not as useful as are *socially co-constructed* narratives in helping children to improve their ability to organize their thoughts and their language and to remember more past experiences. We return to this important vygotskyan theme in the section on Organization and Narrative Discourse. Log- or memory-book reviews with parents or other adults are an ideal context for facilitating development of event, thought, and discourse organization and episodic memory in children (including older children) with TBI, owing to the relative ease with which young children are able to narrate real events or real routines from their lives, as compared to constructing fictional stories.

Development of Memory

In this section, our goal is simply to highlight aspects of development critical to planning rehabilitation goals and activities. The development of memory is a central theme in current developmental cognitive psychology and has been comprehensively addressed in a number of excellent texts (e.g., Kail, 1990; Schneider and Pressley, 1989). Indeed, in post-piagetian developmental cognitive psychology using information-processing categories, memory may be *the* central theme in cognitive development.

Schneider and Pressley (1989) classified the development of memory and learning into four interconnected categories: memory strategies, metamemory, the knowledge base, and short-term or working memory. From an information-processing perspective, these are the critical areas of memory development and must be understood in planning cognitive rehabilitation after brain injury. Related to these four areas of memory development is the distinction between incidental and deliberate learning, which also is critical to teaching people with TBI.

Memory Strategies

In a narrow sense, strategies are *deliberately* applied procedures designed to achieve some goal. By this definition, then, memory strategies, which could be used at the time of encoding (i.e., placing information into memory) or retrieval (i.e., pulling information out of memory), are procedures used deliberately to achieve the cognitive goal of remembering. Used in a fully conscious manner, strategies presuppose substantial cognitive and metacognitive sophistication and are typically not attributed to children younger than school age. However, like intentional communication, which evolves gradually over several months in infancy, strategic behavior also evolves gradually. Preschoolers can function strategically in relation to memory tasks (e.g., placing skates in front of the door in response to "Remember to take your skates"; Flavell et al., 1993), but only if they have a concrete, practical, meaningful goal and access to a familiar concrete strategy. Preschoolers also benefit from modeling of concrete strategies and practice designed to make concrete strategic behavior part of their everyday routines. We emphasize this point, because in the next chapter we promote an early focus on strategic behavior and executive functions generally, a focus that would seem ill advised if one assumed that strategic behavior was simply out of the question for people with less mature cognitive functioning than that of mature 6 or 7 year olds.

Metamemory

Metamemory (i.e., understanding one's own memory, factors that affect it, and strategies that facilitate it) is a component of metacognition. The development of metamemory is the context within which memory strategies develop, making this a critical area of concern after TBI because (1) memory is often weak, necessitating greater reliance on memory strategies, (2) frontal lobe injury often weakens metacognitive and executive functions, and (3) organizational impairment heightens the need to control cognitive functions deliberately.

Preschoolers appear to have little understanding of their memory, particularly when the assessment tasks rely on understanding words such as *remember* (Brown, 1978; Flavell, 1979; Kail, 1990). For young children, remembering is more like finding something even if one does not know it is there. However, 3 and 4 year olds may shy away from difficult memory tasks, revealing some understanding of task difficulty, and they are capable of maintaining a higher level of use of memory terms when supported by conversations with their parents about shared experiences (e.g., "Do you 'member when we . . ."), which suggests greater metacognitive maturity than is traditionally attributed to preschoolers. Similarly, although preschoolers are notoriously poor at predicting their ability to remember (they generally overestimate their ability), they are capable of becoming progressively better at identifying cognitively difficult tasks if they receive intense coaching and practical feedback. This potential is analogous to deaf preschoolers who have a greater understanding than their age-matched peers of communication breakdowns, the difficulty of communicating effectively, and strategies to use when breakdowns occur. Their precociousness in this area is a likely result of the frequency with which breakdowns occur for them and the coaching these children receive in strategically overcoming communication barriers.

As in our discussion of strategies, we emphasize the early forms of development of metacognitive awareness as a basis for our call for an early but developmentally appropriate focus on metacognition in rehabilitation (see Chapters 12 and 14). Approaches to cognitive rehabilitation are often based on stage-wise, hierarchically organized theories of development and recovery after TBI, yielding the unfortunate recommendation that metacognitive and strategic approaches to memory impairment be postponed entirely until some advanced stage of recov-

ery or substantial cognitive criterion is reached. This theme is addressed under Teaching the Functional Use of Organization Schemes and in Chapters 12 and 14.

Knowledge Base

The knowledge base includes information, autobiographical episodes, concepts, words, strategies, principles, and values and their interrelations or connections. Obviously, children progressively acquire more and more knowledge from life experiences and school instruction. Of direct relevance to cognitive rehabilitation is the important point that stored knowledge (and its organization or networks of interconnections) increases the efficiency of information processing and the ability to process information deeply by making connections with that previously stored knowledge: That is, as knowledge increases, information is more easily organized, integrated, and elaborated (Bjorklund, 1985; Chi, 1978). Based in part on this thesis, we resist the recommendation, common in cognitive training and retraining manuals, to focus intervention on cognitive processes *rather than* on academic or other content. We argue, in contrast, that intervention should focus on cognitive processes and systems *in the context of* academic and other content. Acquisition and reacquisition of knowledge are critical components of cognitive rehabilitation after TBI. Furthermore, as organizational, memory, problem-solving, and other types of strategies are rehearsed and become routine, they are stored as procedures in the knowledge base and can be used automatically, thereby increasing the efficiency of information processing and creating "space" for other kinds of mental operations (Case, 1985).

Working Memory

The traditional concept of working (or short-term) memory is that of a limited-capacity, rapid-loss storage space in which organizing, filtering, and coding of information occur prior to transfer of that knowledge to long-term storage (Deutsch and Deutsch, 1975). Its structural capacity (i.e., the number of units of information that can be held in mind at one time) in older children and adults has been established at seven plus or minus two. More recent concepts of working memory emphasize subsystems such as the visuospatial sketchpad (wherein visuospatial information can be held temporarily) and the phonologic loop (wherein verbal information can be held temporarily) and executive-control functions assumed to be responsible for the selection and operation of strategies and for maintaining and switching attention as needed (Baddeley, 1995).

The *structural* capacity of working memory may be fixed and may not change with age (Case, 1985), but its *functional* capacity increases with increasingly effective and automatic use of organizing schemes and strategies: That is, growth in organization and strategic behavior improves the functioning of working memory. This phenomenon explains much in the development of children's cognition (Case, 1978). Similarly, impairment of working memory after TBI is more often associated with loss of organizing schemes or (more likely) ineffective executive control over organizing behavior (associated with frontal lobe injury) than with loss of structural capacity. Therefore, brute exercises designed to "stretch" working memory (e.g., practice repeating sequences of numbers or words) are generally ill advised. Rather, as with other aspects of memory, the focus should be on helping the child to acquire and habituate organizing schemes and on increasing the child's executive control over cognitive behavior.

Involuntary and Deliberate Memory and Learning

Involuntary memory (sometimes referred to as *incidental learning*, although this term is ambiguous) occurs as a by-product of an individual's engagement in personally meaningful activities, in which the learned information is processed to accomplish the goals of the activity. In other words, there is no explicit goal to learn anything. Deliberate (voluntary or effortful) learning, on the other hand, is characterized by the intent to learn or remember some information: That is, the goal of the activity is the abstract cognitive goal of learning, as when college students study for an exam (Brown, 1975, 1979; Smirnov, 1973).

Young children (and adults) are masters of involuntary learning. Information that they must process to accomplish a concrete, meaningful goal often "sticks." In contrast, when young children are instructed to try hard to remember, their success rate often deteriorates badly (Schneider and Pressley, 1989). Presumably, this is because the children are not clear about the abstract goal of remembering, because they are not particularly motivated to try and, more importantly, because effort toward achieving that abstract goal assumes voluntary access to means to achieve the goal (i.e., memory strategies). Preschoolers simply do not have easy, voluntary access to memory strategies. Thus, it is *not* a good idea to tell a preschooler—or an older child with significant cognitive impairment as a result of TBI—to try to remember. Rather, tasks must be designed so that the learner processes the information to be learned in the context of concrete, personally meaningful activity. We provide illustrations of such task design in the section on Cognitive Organization and Involuntary (Incidental) Learning.

Unfortunately, when children have specific memory impairment, which is common after TBI, professionals and parents alike are often inclined to increase rather than decrease the frequency with which they orient the child to the abstract task of remembering. For example: "John, you have to try hard to remember this." "Mary, please try to remember to lock the wheels of your wheelchair." "Jim, how many times have I told you? You must remember to bring your memory book to memory group!" These may be the worst possible instructions for very young or cognitively impaired children.

Rather, these children need to process information such as "lock my breaks" and "write it in a memory book" because this is *necessary to achieve a meaningful, concrete goal*; therefore, the information to be learned must be practiced sufficiently to be stored as a procedure. Adults must structure meaningful learning tasks to encourage this type of processing. However, as with all aspects of development, the ability to orient to the abstract task of learning or remembering develops gradually (DeLoache, 1985; Ornstein and Baker-Ward, 1983; Schneider and Pressley, 1989; Wellman et al., 1975, 1985). Therefore, in our intervention recommendations, we suggest tasks that gradually shift focus from completely involuntary learning to the abstract, metacognitive activity of deliberately using learning strategies to learn new information.

TBI and Impairment of Organization and Memory

Any combination of cognitive strengths and weaknesses is possible after TBI, depending on many factors, including the individual's age and preinjury profile of abilities, the nature and severity of the injury, services and supports (including family and friends) available after the injury, and the individual's personality, mode of adjustment, motivation, and related affective variables. However, TBI has come to be considered a useful disability category, in part because some parts of the brain—and therefore some domains of function—are more vulnerable than others, including parts critical to organization and memory (see Chapter 2).

Disorders of Organization

Schwartz and colleagues (1993), taking a neuropsychological perspective, identified three different types of organizational impairment. The subject of their analysis was breakdowns in organization of ADLs (e.g., grooming, dressing, eating). Action errors in daily activities can take the form of faulty sequencing (e.g., putting on shoes before socks), omission (e.g., brushing teeth without the toothpaste), perseveration (e.g., continuing to brush one's hair long after the job is satisfactorily completed), and object substitution or misuse (e.g., buttering bread with a fork). However, their three neuropsychological categories of organization impairment appear to apply also to other types of organizational breakdown (e.g., disorganized narration, tangential conversation, difficulty organizing materials and steps for an academic or vocational task) and are useful for planning intervention.

Ideational apraxia is the label these investigators use for a disability characterized by disorganized action and verbal behavior in real-world contexts, combined with poor performance on structured tests specifically designed to reveal organized knowledge. In this sense, individuals with ideational apraxia not only would have difficulty getting dressed but also would fail structured tests designed to reveal knowledge of dressing (e.g., sequencing pictures that illustrate the steps of an organized dressing routine). Similarly, they not only would have difficulty finding words and remaining organized in conversation but also would perform poorly on tests of word knowledge (e.g., identifying which among a group of four words did not belong with the others) and underlying world knowledge (e.g., demonstrating how to use an egg beater), despite adequate perceptual abilities and knowledge of the referential meaning of words (e.g., ability to point to the correct picture) (Ochipa et al., 1989). People with ideational apraxia cannot think, speak, or behave in an organized manner because they have lost some or all of the organizing schemes (or knowledge structures) that hold together connected units of knowledge. This loss of organizational ties in the knowledge base (which is partial, in most cases) sometimes is referred to as a *disorder of semantic memory* (Patterson and Hodges, 1995) and is presumably associated with damage to multiple neural networks distributed over broad areas of bilateral cerebral cortex, possibly including bilateral temporal lobe cortex in the case of disrupted declarative knowledge (Patterson and Hodges, 1995) and occipitoparietal cortex in the case of disrupted action routines (Schwartz et al., 1993). Using our earlier analysis of organization as a process, product, and conceptual structure, ideational apraxia is an impairment of organization as a conceptual structure. Of course, young children may lack organizational knowledge not as a result of brain injury but rather because they have not yet acquired the knowledge.

The other two types of cognitive disorganization described by Schwartz and colleagues (1993)—frontal apraxia and supervisory attentional system distractibility syndrome—are associated with frontal lobe lesions, and both are consistent with adequate performance on structured tasks, including tests designed to assess organizational knowledge. *Frontal apraxia* refers to a condition that includes a weakened connection between an intention (e.g., I want to get dressed; I want to tell a story) and the organized action schemas needed to accomplish the intention: That is, the organizational scheme, which may be stored in the knowledge base, is not selected and activated for the job at hand. Alternatively, the components of a complex action scheme may be only weakly related and therefore lead to incoherent action or talk. People with frontal apraxia may behave in a disorganized manner in the absence of environmental stressors, even though they possess the requisite knowledge and organizing schemes. Frontal apraxia is an impairment of organization as a process.

Individuals with weakened control over their attentional system (supervisory attentional system distractibility syndrome), another possible result of prefrontal injury

(Norman and Shallice, 1986), generally perform well-rehearsed action routines in an organized manner, revealing intact knowledge of organizing schemes and activation of those schemes in familiar contexts with minimal distractions. However, in novel or stressful contexts or in the presence of distractions, the organization of behavior may deteriorate into rigid or perseverative patterns of routine behavior or total dependence on environmental cues (i.e., the child becomes stimulus bound) (Lhermitte, 1986). This pattern of behavior is familiar to parents whose young children may appear organized and independent in moving through familiar routines at home but who act and converse in ways that may appear completely incoherent or inflexible in novel settings or in the presence of distractions and other stressors.

Frontal apraxia and supervisory attentional system distractibility syndrome are types of executive-system impairment (discussed in the Chapter 12). They are both concerned with *control over* cognitive activity, not possession of the requisite knowledge or cognitive structures. Because these serious organizational disabilities are compatible with adequate performance on tests of organizational knowledge, their identification and description require planned observation in naturalistic contexts (see Chapter 10).

The organizational activities and graphic advance organizers discussed in the intervention sections of this chapter can be used for individuals with all three types of organizational breakdown or any combination of them. For children and adolescents with ideational apraxia (lack of stored organizing schemes), the activities are designed to teach the organizing schemes (e.g., how to get dressed, how to make lunch, how to tell a story, how to write an organized term paper) as well as to help the children or adolescents to guide their behavior deliberately by using the scheme. For those with either of the frontal lobe syndromes, the activities and organizers are designed to help the individuals stay organized, stay on task, and generate an organized product (e.g., a story, an art project, completion of dressing, eating, or bathing) without relying on the ongoing guidance of another person (which is often interpreted as nagging).

Disorders of Memory

Much of the literature on memory processes is based on differentiation of memory disorders. The working assumption has been that if one type of learning or remembering can be disrupted by brain injury while other types are left intact, then the disrupted type must represent a neuropsychologically distinct memory process or system. Various classification systems have evolved, which are explored in Chapter 9. From a rehabilitation perspective, it is useful to distinguish the following five types of memory disorder (see Tulving, 1995): anterograde versus retrograde amnesia, semantic versus episodic memory problems, declarative versus procedural memory problems, visual versus auditory and verbal versus nonverbal memory problems, and somatic markers and impaired learning from consequences. It is, however, unnecessary to make the controversial assumption that each disorder corresponds to a neuropsychologically distinct memory process or system.

Anterograde Versus Retrograde Amnesia

Retrograde amnesia refers to inability to remember events that occurred and information that was acquired before the injury. *Anterograde amnesia* refers to difficulty in learning new information and remembering day-to-day events after the injury. When recovery of preinjury information is good (resulting in good test performance on academic tests) and recovery of day-to-day episodic memory is adequate, identification and appreciation of the extent of new learning problems may be difficult. New learning problems can result from damage to frontal lobes (e.g., inefficient use of memory strategies) and to medial temporal lobes (inefficient consolidation of new memory traces), both very commonly damaged areas in closed head injury. Loss of stored preinjury knowledge and skill is more likely a result of posterior cortical damage.

Declarative Versus Procedural Memory Problems

Procedural memory includes memory for action patterns (e.g., riding a bike, brushing teeth), skilled action (e.g., reading), rules of games, and other procedures, whereas *declarative memory* refers to memory for propositional information (including both semantic and episodic information). Schwartz and colleagues (1993) suggested that posterior (parietal or occipital) damage is involved in loss of daily action schemas, whereas Patterson and Hodges (1995) identified cortical temporal lobe damage as the most important in disrupting semantic or declarative memory (e.g., word knowledge).

It is important to remember that individuals can learn procedures, routines, skills, and the like without remembering the context of learning and without being explicitly aware that they have learned the procedures. This neuropsychological possibility serves as the foundation for teaching and training during the period of posttraumatic amnesia (Slifer et al., 1996). *Implicit memory* refers to the change in future behavior that results from a learning trial even though the child does not *explicitly* remember the event or information or the context of learning (i.e., there is no conscious experience of recalling the information or event). The knowledge that even people who appear to remember nothing from one minute to the next may be able to learn skills and other information with very systematic teaching or behavioral conditioning is a source of considerable optimism.

Semantic Versus Episodic Memory Problems

Semantic and episodic memory systems are subcategories of declarative memory. Many children with TBI recover their ability to recall episodes in their own life from both before and after the injury (i.e., episodic memory) but continue to experience relatively marked difficulty in learning new academic information that needs to be stored as something other than a biographical episode (i.e., semantic memory). This difficulty may be related to attentional problems, organizational problems, motivational problems, or some other problem that does not necessarily implicate memory processes, strictly speaking. This pattern of recovery establishes the need for a much more thorough exploration of memory after TBI than is accomplished by the usual interview about recent events in the person's life (episodic memory). With both semantic and episodic memory problems, it is important to distinguish anterograde and retrograde dimensions of the problem, because one may have difficulty remembering autobiographical information from before the injury (retrograde episodic memory disorder) or from recent events (anterograde episodic memory disorder).

Visual Versus Auditory and Verbal Versus Nonverbal Memory Problems

Because the neural pathways that underlie distinct types of processing diverge, memory problems specific to certain kinds of information are possible. However, this possibility does not imply that these systems are different *memory* systems or that intervention for these disorders should necessarily be different in kind. Obviously, people with specific visual-processing problems may profit from learning tasks that exploit preserved auditory-processing abilities, and people with specific language-processing weakness profit from learning tasks that exploit nonverbal strengths. The same principle applies to the other combinations of processing strengths and weaknesses. Closed head injury can, but often does not, pick out specific sensory modalities of information processing for specific impairment.

Somatic Markers and Impaired Learning from Consequences

Finally, a dimension of memory and memory disorders has been described in recent years that has important implications for behavioral intervention after brain injury. The ventromedial prefrontal region of the brain (also vulnerable in closed head injury) has been said to help link factual knowledge (e.g., "When I leave my desk without permission, the teacher makes me stay after school") with emotions and feelings (e.g., "I hate staying after school") (Damasio et al., 1991). These so-called somatic markers help people to profit from personal experiences that include either positive or negative consequences or feedback.

Because most intervention programs for children with behavioral problems are based on the imposition of consequences (rewards or punishments) for behavior, damage to the ventromedial prefrontal cortex may seriously interfere with the effectiveness of these programs. Indeed, in extreme cases, damage to this area has been linked to sociopathic behavior that may be influenced in the *short term* by serious consequences, though such consequences have no *enduring* effects on behavior (Tranel and Damasio, 1995). Children and adolescents who are suspected of having this type of disorder are candidates for behavioral intervention that emphasizes control over the *antecedents* of behavior (and other setting events) versus strict contingency management (see Chapter 13).

Goals of Cognitive Rehabilitation

The overarching goals of cognitive rehabilitation or cognitive intervention for a child or adolescent are the individual's achievement of important real-world goals, which may be difficult to achieve because of cognitive weakness, and prevention of academic and behavioral deterioration that might result from failure associated with cognitive weakness. These two important and expansive goals, which extend far beyond the limited goal of retraining cognition, can be achieved through a combination of approaches, some of which are directed at improving the child's cognitive resources and capacities, others are directed at modifying the demands placed on those resources and capacities. Changes in the child can include (1) improved cognitive processes (e.g., better-focused attention; more efficient habitual use of organizing schemes); (2) an improved ability to process information effectively by deliberately using compensatory strategic procedures (e.g., organizational strategies, learning strategies, problem-solving strategies); and (3) growth in the knowledge base, which alone facilitates improved information processing. Helpful changes outside of the child can include (1) external supports (e.g., posted reminders, removal of distractions, ongoing coaching in cognitive skills), (2) improved teaching procedures sensitive to the child's profile of cognitive abilities, and (3) understanding of the child's cognitive strengths and weaknesses.

Achieving the goals of cognitive rehabilitation and intervention generally involves some combination of directly (re)training the child (e.g., having the child practice cognitive skills such as organized perception, coherent narration, systematic planning), teaching the child strategic procedures to compensate for ongoing difficulties, putting the best system of external supports in place, and ensuring that all teachers, therapists, and others know how best to teach, interact with, and support the child. The varied goals of cognitive rehabilitation and intervention approaches are discussed more thoroughly in Chapter 9.

Case Study: Supported Cognition

For most children and adolescents, a combination of cognitive rehabilitation goals and approaches may be appropriate at any given time, and this combination changes over time. The ultimate goal for most individuals is to achieve independence in relation to the cognitive demands of academic, vocational, social, and daily-living activities. For many people, however, independence may be an unrealistic goal, and supported cognition is an acceptable alternative. The case of MS illustrates this principle (Ylvisaker and Feeney, 1996).

MS was severely injured in an automobile accident at age 14. Early in her recovery, as she emerged from coma, the focus of her cognitive program was twofold: (1) to provide whatever support she needed to remain oriented and focused on external realities and goal-directed activities, and (2) to engage her in activities, including ADLs and therapy-based activities, that stimulated her cognitive functions at the limit of her processing ability without overwhelming her.

Her cognitive profile at 6 months after injury was characterized by adequate attention, perception, basic academic skills (e.g., decoding words, calculating), and episodic memory but severe new academic learning impairment, disorganized thinking and acting, severely depressed self-awareness, and minimal strategic thinking and acting (related, in part, to frontal lobe injury). MS responded positively to a program of compensatory strategy intervention (for organizational impairment) that enabled her to improve functional levels in reading comprehension, writing, and memory (Ylvisaker et al., 1994). This was a primary focus of her extended inpatient cognitive rehabilitation.

At the time of discharge from inpatient rehabilitation, MS scored at normal levels on a test of reading comprehension using her outlining strategies but continued to score at least two standard deviations below the mean on standardized tests of verbal memory, indicating that her improvement in reading comprehension and functional memory was indeed a compensatory effect. However, because she had very weak insight into her deficits and needs, staff and family members had to continue to cue her to use her special procedures. Staff at the rehabilitation hospital worked closely with school staff to ensure that the reading, writing, study, and other strategies acquired in the rehabilitation hospital setting would continue to be encouraged when MS returned to school and would evolve as she improved neurologically and academically.

Ten years later, MS graduated from college, a remarkable accomplishment in light of the severity of her injury. An interview with her at that time revealed that she continued to have shallow insight into her cognitive strengths and weaknesses and was not yet an independent strategic thinker. However, she had been enrolled throughout her college career in a special program for students with learning problems. This program mandated 8 hours per week of coached study time. Although MS was not yet independent in using her cognitive strengths, she was supported effectively by this system and consequently achieved a level of academic success that no one had predicted for her.

In retrospect, the most important contribution made by MS's cognitive rehabilitation therapist at the rehabilitation program was to learn enough about her cognitive functioning (and strategic procedures that improved that functioning) to permit an appropriate set of cognitive strategies and supports to be transferred from rehabilitation to school. A major contribution of her high school staff was to learn enough about her cognitive functioning so that an appropriate set of cognitive strategies and supports could be transferred from high school to college. Ideally, a major contribution of her college staff would have been to transfer an appropriate set of cognitive strategies and supports to her work site. MS was capable of behaving in an effectively strategic manner to compensate for her serious cognitive weakness. However, she required ongoing knowledgeable support and coaching to do so. Unfortunately, this support was not available to her at her first job (as a telemarketer), and she lost the job within the first month because on two occasions she failed to control her anger in conversations with customers.

MS presents us with one illustration of the important concept of supported cognition, which is analogous to supported employment and supported living and which, for many people with chronic cognitive weakness after TBI, is a noble alternative to the goal of complete independence.

Intervention: Functional Everyday Approaches to Cognitive Rehabilitation

In the remaining sections of this chapter, we present intervention procedures designed to help children and adolescents with organizational impairment and associated memory and language disability after TBI. For reasons described earlier in this chapter, we emphasize the use of settings, people, activities, and content that are as natural, meaningful, and functional for the child as possible. Chapter 12 extends these themes into the territory of compensatory strategies and executive control over cognitive behavior.

In many ways, the cognitive rehabilitation procedures espoused in this chapter could be called a *conversational approach*, based on the developmental cognitive psychology of Vygotsky (1978). A fundamental principle of Vygotsky's view of development is that mature, covert, abstract cognitive processes have their basis in concrete

everyday interactive routines between young children and their parents, teachers, and others. This deceptively simple principle has had, and continues to have, a powerful impact on educational psychology and intervention in many domains. The principle, which was discussed in Chapter 9, should be kept in mind as the reader considers the intervention procedures discussed in the following sections, many of which are based on everyday interaction between the child and adults.

Figure 11-1 uses an organic metaphor to illustrate this vygotskyan theme. The key idea is that abstract and esoteric-appearing cognitive and executive system functions gradually emerge out of simple, everyday social-behavioral routines, in an environment in which these components of development are *valued* (i.e., given large numbers of learning trials, with successful performance meaningfully reinforced [for those who prefer behavioral language]), in which there is plenty of opportunity for *practice*, and in which adults or older peers are good at *coaching* (including concrete feedback) and at incrementally encouraging development.

This developmental phenomenon of gradually internalizing interactive routines is familiar to students of language development. For example, on the basis of Vygotsky's popular theory, Bruner (1975) proposed that conversational rules and competence emerge from frequently repeated communication games played by infants and their caregivers. These views have led to some of the most productive approaches to early language intervention, designed primarily to equip caregivers with the knowledge and skill needed to facilitate the developmental process in their everyday interaction with a child (e.g., MacDonald, 1989). Our approach to cognitive rehabilitation similarly emphasizes participation of everyday communication partners. Therefore, this chapter should be read in conjunction with Chapter 20, in which Ylvisaker and Feeney discuss procedures for supporting everyday people in their attempt to play the role of coach and facilitator for children with TBI.

Cognitive Organization and Activities of Daily Living

For children and adults alike, probably the best contexts in which to begin cognitive rehabilitation after TBI, from an organizational perspective, are ADLs, including dressing, bathing, eating, and the like. In all but the youngest children, these are well-rehearsed routines and therefore can capitalize on recovery of preinjury learning. In addition, there are many occasions over the course of a day to engage the child in these familiar, functional, organized routines. We emphasize two guidelines for using ADLs to promote improved cognitive organization: First, provide the child with as much, and only as much, external support as is needed to complete the task in an organized manner, systematically reducing the support as the child becomes increasingly competent and

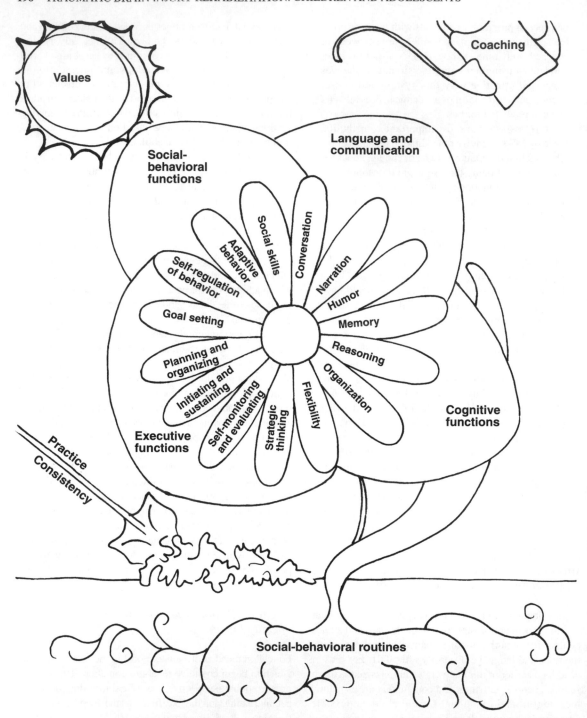

Figure 11-1. Development of cognitive and related executive and communication functions out of everyday interactive routines. In environments in which the functions are valued, coaching and supported practice are liberally provided. This is a graphic representation of Vygotsky's interactionist view of cognitive and communication development. (Copyright, Mark Ylvisaker, Ph.D.)

independent. Second, increasingly use language that highlights the organizational components of the activity (e.g., "This comes first, this next, this last"; "It's important to do these in order"). Young children can also practice "ADL scripts" in play, to reinforce the organized patterns of behavior targeted during functional ADLs.

Cognitive Support

Children and adolescents emerging from coma typically require a great deal of support to become oriented and to remember their organized routines and scripts. A similar level of support may again be necessary when environmental cues change with the transition to home and school. Specialists in cognition (possibly an occupational therapist, psychologist, speech-language pathologist, or special educator) may be needed to analyze daily activities from the perspective of their organizational demands and to advise everyday people (e.g., nursing staff, family members) about the child's current need for organizational support. These recommendations should be updated frequently and clearly posted in the child's environment. Supports can include some combination of those listed in Table 11-3, all designed to improve organizational functioning and enable the child to succeed with daily living activities as independently and with as little nagging as possible. Parents and staff must always remember that for an older child or adolescent, language that we try to legitimize by calling it a *helpful verbal cue* is nagging, pure and simple, and should therefore be used with caution.

The language that adults use during the child's ADLs can vary from none to highly pedagogical language. With children who are aphasic, highly distractible, or oppositional, it may be preferable for adults not to talk. Rather, such children might simply be oriented to the task, be given a model or shown photographs of how to proceed, be physically prompted if necessary, and be physically reassured and rewarded for successful performance (e.g., with a hug). In the case of children who comprehend language but who are still very disorganized, adults can similarly orient such a child to the task but can also provide simple running commentary that highlights the organizational components of the task (e.g., "You'll need toothpaste and toothbrush . . . good . . . now, first you take the cap off . . . great . . . next—take a look at the picture and see what comes next . . ."). At a somewhat higher level of functioning, a child might be asked to make a plan physically (e.g., by sequencing the photographs on a planning board before beginning the activity) or verbally (e.g., responding to a request for such information with a stated sequence of actions in the form of "First I will . . ."). At the highest level, children who are well oriented to the organization of ADLs can be asked to serve as helpers for children who still are quite disorganized (e.g., explaining the morning routine to a new child on the nursing unit or in the classroom). Understanding the organization of tasks well enough to help others represents a higher level of organiza-

Table 11-3. Possible Cognitive Supports for Independent Performance of Activities of Daily Living

Create consistent daily routines, in the hospital and at home.

Ensure consistent location of needed items (e.g., clothes, bathroom items, eating utensils).

Label closets, drawers, containers, and the like with helpful photographs, symbols, or words, so the child knows where to look for needed items.

Provide useful external advance organizers (e.g., sequenced photographs of children engaged in their own specific routines, drawings, charts with words), so the child can guide himself or herself through the activity. For the very disorganized child, frequent rehearsal of the child's script with customized photographs and coaching may be useful. (See also J Groden, P LeVasseur [1995]. Cognitive Picture Rehearsal: A System to Teach Self-Control. In KA Quill [ed], Teaching Children with Autism: Strategies to Enhance Communication and Socialization. Albany, NY: Delmar Publishers, 287.)

If unfamiliar people are involved in the child's routine, have photographs available to orient the child to the unfamiliar people.

Encourage the child to observe peer models who are competent with the task. Use peers as coaches if this is helpful for the child.

Reduce support as the child's competence improves.

tional functioning (i.e., *meta-organization*) than simply being able to stay organized (Meichenbaum, 1993).

The level of difficulty of a given task can be increased by systematically reducing the support provided, increasing the complexity of the task, or increasing other forms of stress (e.g., time pressure, novelty of the context). A cognitive specialist can help nursing staff and family members decide when to reduce levels of support, when to add complexity or stress, and how to mix these progressions, ensuring that the child remains successful throughout. Too much support, in the long run, results in learned helplessness, whereas too little support generates frustration and growing behavior problems. The goal is to find the appropriate middle ground, which shifts frequently over the course of improvement after TBI, and to collaborate with others so that all adults in the child's life provide the appropriate amount and type of support.

Daily Routines and an Organized Life

Children and adolescents with significant organizational and memory impairment after TBI may have profound difficulty understanding how any one thing or event is related to any other thing or event in their lives. For infants and toddlers, this is a normal state and therefore not cause for great concern. However, older children and adolescents are accustomed to being able to integrate and

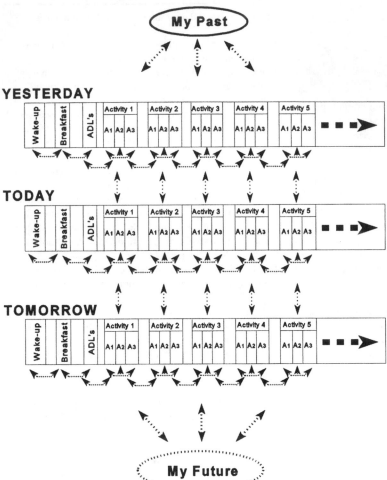

Figure 11-2. In lives that are organized, activities are meaningful because they are connected in clear ways to other activities in life and to one's past and future. These connections are represented by the arrows. Children in confused stages of recovery after brain injury require considerable support to re-establish the connections that promote orientation.

make sense of their experiences over the course of a day or week or lifetime. Moving beyond the here and now of infancy is a gradual process of decentration that renders a normally developing school-aged child able to perceive connections between the present and the past and future. Tragically, rehabilitation programs—including those that manage to maintain fairly consistent staff and schedules—often contribute to their patients' sense of fragmentation rather than to their sense of integration and orientation, because they do not sufficiently attend to the organization of life *from the perspective of the individual.*

A consistent schedule does not help a disorganized person unless that person is somehow made aware of the organization of the day and of the ways in which the episodes of the day are related to one another and to that individual's life: That is, what appears very organized to a staff person may lack coherence from the child's perspective. Most therapists and teachers are trained to design activities to meet specific physical, cognitive, communicative, academic, or psychosocial goals that they have set for the child. Each 30-minute therapy or instructional session may include three or four such activities. Adding to this number the 10 or 20 activities in which the child or adolescent may engage on the nursing unit or at home, potentially 20, 30, or more episodes occur per day—in many places and with many people—all of which the disorganized individual must try to integrate and understand. From the perspective of the individual, these episodes may appear completely unrelated, leaving him or her with a horrible sense of fragmentation and disorientation. Figure 11-2, in which arrows represent connections among events of the day, depicts the life of such a person. Endless recitation of "orientation information" (e.g., days and dates, names of strange people and places), common to brain injury rehabilitation programs, rarely helps to dispel this fragmentation. An important component of intervention for disorganized people is to aid them in making the connections and understanding

Table 11-4. Procedures to Help Disorganized Individuals Integrate Their Experiences

1. Ensure that the *daily schedule* is as *consistent* as possible (person, place, time) and is understood by the child. Consistency can never be total. However, consistent schedules are less critical than other procedures that follow.
2. Ensure that *daily routines* are as *consistent* and *orienting* as possible.
   a. Begin the day with a planning routine, in which the child creates a plan for the day, with concrete materials (e.g., photographs) to which he or she can refer back throughout the day to remember the plan.
   b. Transition routines may include a brief review of what was just done, with whom it was done, and why; a brief review of the entire day; a brief description of what is to come next and why it is important and meaningful to the child.
   c. This review should be accompanied by concrete support, including photographs of relevant people and places, written or pictured schedules, and the like.
3. Ensure that the child has *orienting materials*. These may all be combined in one log, memory, or orientation book, which should include
   a. Photographs of relevant staff, family members, peers, and visitors.
   b. Helpful maps and drawings for physical navigation and orientation.
   c. A schedule presented in a way that is helpful for the child, with photographs rather than words for the child who cannot read or who is easily confused.
   d. A log of recent events that can be reviewed frequently.
   e. Photographs and information about the child's life before the injury so unfamiliar staff can converse with the child about a meaningful life.
4. Ensure that *activities across the day and week are as connected as possible* and that the connections are understood by the child.
   a. If possible, each day or week should be assigned a theme that can be carried through all of the therapies and nursing unit activities.
   b. Connections among therapies, within each therapy, from one therapy to another, from day to day, and between therapies and real life should be reviewed frequently.
5. Ensure that the child or adolescent is as *actively engaged* and *independent* as possible in making plans and connections, including
   a. Making a plan for the day.
   b. Navigating from place to place.
   c. Following the plan.
   d. Making decisions about activities.
   e. Trying to see connections and relevance of activities.
   f. Narrating (with needed support, including photographs) his or her day for parents in the evening.
6. Systematically reduce organizational support as the child's condition improves.

how current activity is related to things that are important in their lives, past and future—in effect, adding the arrows in Figure 11-2. Table 11-4 presents procedures that contribute to that integrative process.

We have repeatedly recommended using photographs as support for various types of organizational thinking. A simple camera is perhaps the most important piece of equipment for a rehabilitation center or school that serves children and adolescents with organizational impairment. For example, to illustrate a sequence of events, it is far more meaningful, concrete, and interesting to have photographs of the child engaged in the activity than to use generic off-the-shelf therapy materials. Furthermore, for meaningful review of events that have passed or anticipation of events later in the day, it is important to have photographs of people and places that give meaning to these discussions. In the absence of this anchor in reality, talk about the past or future may be little more than a confusing heap of words. As children improve, photographs as a form of organizational support might give way to symbols or printed words, contributing to logistic ease in generating organizational materials and to the child's increasing ability to represent routines and scripts abstractly.

Cognitive Organization and Play

In Chapter 14, Ylvisaker, Sellars, and Edelman outline stages of play development in infants and preschoolers from the point of view of play with objects as well as social play with caregivers and peers. In both cases, development is in part a progression from minimal to substantial demands on organizational resources. For example, the sensorimotor play of 6 month olds (holding, looking, dropping, batting, mouthing) involves minimal organizational activity, whereas the complex object play of 5 year olds, integrating large numbers of toys and other props into complex scripts, requires high levels of organizational knowledge and skill. Similarly, the interactive vocal play of 6 month olds and their parents requires little organizing. In contrast, the sociodramatic play of 5 year olds, involving elaborate scripts, roles, dialogue, costumes, and props, is organizationally very demanding. Therefore, specialists in cognition can work with family members and other everyday people to help them to facilitate the child's gradual progression along these two important developmental continua. At the simplest level, improvement can be measured by the gradually increasing number of toys the child can organize in play, from one (e.g., a truck) to two (e.g., a truck with a driver) to three (e.g., a truck with a driver hauling logs) and so on (see Chapter 14).

Cognitive Organization and Visual Perception

In this section, we address only one of several possible visual-perceptual disorders associated with TBI, disorganized perception. Some children have specific visual disturbances that make organized searches difficult, possibly including visual-field cuts or neglect, figure-ground problems, and difficulty maintaining convergence. Other children simply are not systematic in their tracking and searching. For example, in reading, a child may not look systematically to the left and then track fluidly along the line of print from left to right. In searching for a math problem on a page, a child may not begin the search at the top and proceed systematically from top to bottom.

Intervention programs designed to improve organized visual-perceptual processing have been available for decades. In the field of special education, they became very popular in the 1950s and 1960s, consistent with what was at that time a popular bottom-up approach to academic disability. Subsequent analysis of the effectiveness of such programs showed them to be modestly effective in improving the specific skill being trained (e.g., left-to-right scanning) and ineffective in improving general cognitive or academic functioning (Kavale and Mattson, 1983).

Programs of this sort were also very popular in the early years of cognitive rehabilitation program development for people with TBI (e.g., Sohlberg and Mateer, 1989). For example, the century-old cancellation exercise (scanning rows of figures, letters, or numbers and canceling certain preidentified items) enjoyed renewed popularity as a way to train concentration and systematic visual searches. It has been documented repeatedly that, with practice, many people with TBI can improve their performance on tasks of this sort. However, the theoretical and empirical literature on transfer of training (discussed in Chapter 9 and referred to earlier in this chapter) suggests that the use of tasks having content that is meaningful to the individual is more effective. Therefore, we recommend that training in organized visual perception involve academic and other personally meaningful tasks that require efficient perception.

Early in recovery, communication boards and boards with photographs that are personally meaningful to the child using them are useful contexts for perceptual exercises. Even if a child does not communicate efficiently with such a board—and never initiates its use—many people over the course of a day can invite that child to point out specific words or pictures and thereby can encourage systematic searches as the child scans the board. Instructions regarding how to coach the child may have to be written on the board. Games that require finding pieces and places on a game board are also motivating and contextually meaningful. Motivating computer games meet the same standard, although it should not be expected that improvements in games will necessarily translate into improved reading or other unrelated tasks that require organized perception.

Schoolchildren can be given academic work (e.g., words or arithmetic problems on a page) that requires organized perception. Many inexpensive educational computer programs that present words and sentences or math problems as stimulus items can be used as part of the visual-perceptual retraining program. Difficulty can be systematically increased (e.g., number of words or problems on the screen, response time demand) as a child's skills improve. Perceptual skills that improve with this type of training are within the context of perceptual tasks important to the child, so transfer of training is a minimal problem. If perceptual skills do not improve, the time spent in training is nonetheless valuable from an academic perspective.

Adolescents may profit from word-processing exercises. Most adolescents today have experience keyboarding and can use this activity, as well as reading what they compose, as an exercise in organized perception. Familiarity with the keyboard and the meaning of what they have just composed can be considered cognitive supports, making the visual and reading tasks easier than they would be in the absence of familiarity and meaning. Ultimately, of course, an individual must be able to use efficient perceptual skills across a wide domain of familiar and unfamiliar tasks. Our point is simply that beginning this process with tasks that are as familiar and concrete as possible lends support to early success and transfer to other familiar tasks. Subsequently, transfer training in the context of other concrete tasks and, possibly, more abstract tasks may be necessary to promote broader generalization.

With visual-perceptual training, as with other types of training of children and adolescents with TBI, collaboration with everyday people in the child's life is essential. For example, if the child neglects the left side of the visual field, all everyday people should initially place items in the right visual field (to facilitate success) and later should systematically prompt the individual to scan the left side of space. Consistency requires collaboration.

Teaching the Functional Use of Organizational Schemes

Earlier in the chapter, we distinguished between ideational apraxia (loss or absence of relevant organizing schemes or conceptual structures) and frontal apraxia (failure to select and deploy organizing schemes when needed, i.e., impairment of organization as a process). For example, some children tell incoherent stories because they have no idea how stories are supposed to be organized, whereas others have an understanding of the organization of stories but simply do not guide their storytelling behavior with that knowledge. Although these possible consequences of TBI are distinct from a neuropsychological perspective, similar activities can be used in both situations to facilitate improvement in functioning. In both cases, the affected individuals need to practice the use of organizing schemes in the context of meaningful, goal-directed activity. Furthermore, children who reveal knowledge of pretraumatically acquired organizing schemes but fail to use them when needed (frontal apraxia) must continue to learn new organizing schemes as part of their ongoing development and, in this sense, are in the same position as children who have lost organizing schemes (ideational apraxia).

Broadly conceived, there are four components to teaching functional use of organizing schemes: (1) establishing or re-establishing an organized knowledge base— that is, knowledge of things and events and important ways in which they are related to one another; (2) facilitating use of these organizing schemes in functional activities; (3) developing awareness of the distinction between organized and disorganized behavior and awareness of the schemes that define organized behavior; and (4) developing organizational strategies that an individual can use deliberately to learn and retrieve new information or to accomplish any other task that is organizationally demanding. Young children and those who are still in the confused stages of improvement after TBI are candidates for the first and second components. In addition, facilitation of metacognitive awareness (i.e., component three) can be introduced as a long-term goal. Deliberately using organizing schemes as strategic procedures presupposes a higher level of cognitive development and recovery, the foundation for which is laid with earlier acquisitions.

Cognitive Organization and Involuntary (Incidental) Learning

Table 11-5 outlines the structure of intervention activities designed to teach organizing schemes to young children or to individuals with significant cognitive impairment. Virtually any interesting activity can be used (e.g., play with toys, daily activities such as snack time, art projects, household chores, academic or vocational projects). These activities can be used by cognitive specialists or educators in specialized therapy or instructional settings and by family members and other everyday people in everyday settings.

Table 11-6 includes a variety of activities that can be used with young children and children with significant cognitive impairment. The listed activities are grouped

Table 11-5. Teaching Organizing Schemes to Young Children and Older Children with Significant Cognitive Impairment

Goal: To help the child to acquire and to use organizing schemes, without necessarily understanding organizing as a cognitive process

Procedures:

1. Identify a personally meaningful task that (a) requires some type of organizing activity and (b) has an intrinsic, concrete goal that interests the individual.
2. Engage the individual in the task in such a way that he or she must process the organizing scheme in order to complete the task.
3. Highlight the organizing scheme as the activity progresses (if this is not confusing).
4. If possible, encourage the individual to reflect on the organizing scheme that enabled him or her to complete the task.
5. Repeat and gradually expand to other tasks, settings, organizing schemes, and activities.
6. Gradually reduce external control.

according to the type of organizing scheme that is the activity's focus. They are designed around an involuntary learning paradigm (i.e., in each case, the child's goal is concrete and internal to the activity), because it is not expected that children at this level can relate to the abstract goal of learning and using organizing schemes. However, the reflection questions, which can become increasingly prominent as the child matures or recovers cognitively, set the stage for more deliberate use of organizing schemes as compensatory strategic procedures.

Cognitive Organization and Deliberate (Strategic) Learning

Although teaching compensatory strategies is a central theme of the next chapter, here it is instructive to juxtapose these two levels of intervention (actually two points on a continuum)—involuntary and deliberate learning— for children and adolescents with organizational impairment. In the case of deliberate or strategic learning (versus involuntary learning), the individual is expected to participate in identifying why the task is difficult (e.g., much information must be included in the term paper; many components in the vocational task must be organized if the task is to be completed on schedule), in brainstorming about special procedures that might make it easier (e.g., an outline for the paper; a flowchart for the vocational task), in selecting a useful procedure, and in evaluating its effectiveness. Table 11-7 outlines the structure of these teaching tasks. In Chapter 12, we expand this discussion to include a number of other considerations critical to helping people adopt a strategic approach to difficult tasks across all domains of their lives.

Table 11-6. Procedures for Promoting Acquisition of Organizational Schemata in Children

Organizational Schemata (means for attaining goal)	Task and Goal	Activity	Reflection Questions*
Specific event scripts (e.g., going to a restaurant, going to the dentist)	"Let's play dentist." "Let's take turns being the dentist and the patient."	Select items from a large box of appropriate items and foils. Arrange items for dramatic play of the sequence. Play out the event assuming first the role of the patient, then the role of the dentist.	What things do we always see in the dentist's office? What different things (variations) might we see? What events always happen when we go to the dentist? How do they help us to remember? What events might happen only some of the time when we go to the dentist (e.g., dentist is late, get a shot)?
General life scripts (abstracted common life events)	"Let's do a 'This Is Your Life' for either Grandma or Grandpa." Talk about all the special things that happened to them.	Use pictures to represent each important category of event: birth, school, marriage, job, and special events. Using the pictures as a guide, make a storybook for the grandparents or older significant other person in the child's life. Then have each child tell the "life story" on the radio show.	How did the pictures help you to remember all the important events? How did we organize all the information about your grandma/grandpa? How did the "books" help you with your radio show?
Function (use)	"Let's clean the doll house and arrange all the furniture for the play family." "Now let's rearrange some of the furniture for a birthday party for one of the children."	Take all the furniture out of the doll house. Clean the rooms. Then place the furniture back into the house. Have the child rearrange furniture for a party.	How did we arrange all of the furniture and why did we do it that way? Is that the way that the store shows the furniture? How did we change things for the birthday party? Why did we change them?
Perceptual similarity (e.g., color, shape, size, texture, rhyme)	"The art teacher asked us to organize these crayons so that the children can easily and quickly find the ones they want. Let's find a good way to do this."	Label small boxes for different colors. Sort the pieces according to color and put them into the labeled boxes. Call out the colors and time how quickly the items can be found, compared with those in a container with a variety of colors.	How did we sort? Why this way? How did it help you find what you wanted? In what other situations might we sort by color? Would we ever want to sort by size (e.g., when we are deciding which crayons to throw away)?
Semantic similarity (e.g., superordinate category, opposites)	"We are going to set up a grocery store so that we can play store." "First, we will make our plan of where we want to put all the items." "Let's make it easy for people to find things."	Make a floor plan showing where the items will be placed. Place play items in the play store as indicated in the plan (e.g., all the fruits in one area).	How did we arrange the store? Why did we arrange it that way? When would this *not* be a helpful way to arrange the items? How could this arrangement help you to remember where to find things in the store?
Main idea and topic (discourse structure)	"Let's do a radio program (or write a letter to a special friend) about a	Let the child select a favorite or special person, place, or thing. Use pictures on a	How did the chart help you to think of details about the special person, place, or thing?

Organizational Schemata (means for attaining goal)	Task and Goal	Activity	Reflection Questions*
	favorite person, place, or thing."	chart to cue the child to focus on a main idea about the "topic" (e.g., focus on the main idea, "my dog is lots of fun"). Place representation (e.g., pictures) of main idea in the center of the chart, with boxes surrounding it for supporting details. Cue the child to add details to support the main idea (e.g., "he chases a stick; he plays with me," etc.). Use pictures as cues. Record the program (or write the letter).	How did the chart help you to stay organized when you were talking on the radio show or writing your letter? How did the chart help you to remember what you wanted to say?
Story schema	"Let's make a movie about ___ and show it to your classmates (or to another class)."	Give the child a set of props that are potential elements of a story: characters (dolls or animals); settings (e.g., house, barn, fence); potential problems or goals (e.g., container of water, mud); potential resolutions for problems (e.g., long stick or ladder, towels). Present a concrete story guide or cues to help the child create a story from the props (e.g., face to indicate who is in the story, a large blank square to indicate place, or ? to indicate a problem, a light bulb for solution, a happy face for reaction). Videotape the child's story. Watch the video. Use cues to help the child tell the story.	How did the story guide help you to think up your story? How did the story guide help you to tell your story so well (coherent and organized)? How did the story guide help to make your story more interesting? How could the story guide help you to remember the story?
Integration of scripts	"Let's play going grocery shopping; you be the checker and I'll be the shopper." Use check-out play set with small lunch bags. (Store items have been previously arranged according to semantic similarity.)	Play at going to the store and selecting items. Play at check-out, including scanning items, paying, and packing items into the bags. Pack items according to size, shape, and weight of items (perceptual) or functional categories (all refrigerated items together). Shift role of buyer and checker.	What different things could happen at the store (variations of the script)? How would your mom want you to pack the bags? How could this help you to remember what you bought?

*Possible probe question to develop metacognition, understanding, and awareness.

Source: Adapted with permission from M Ylvisaker, S Szekeres, K Henry, et al. (1987). Topics in Cognitive Rehabilitation Therapy. In M Ylvisaker, EMR Gobble (eds), Community Re-Entry for Head Injured Adults. San Diego: Singular Press, 165–168.

Table 11-7. Facilitating the Use of Organizational Strategies in Older Children and Adolescents with Mild to Moderate Cognitive Impairment

---

Goal: To help individuals to understand organizing as a cognitive activity so that they can become more deliberate in compensating for organizational weakness

Procedures:

1. Identify a meaningful task that the individual wants to accomplish and that requires some kind of organizing activity.
2. Identify why it would be difficult to complete the task successfully without special effort of some sort.
3. Discuss ways in which the task might be completed most easily and effectively (i.e., special procedures, forms, guides, outlines, and the like that might be used).
4. Out of this discussion, select an organizational strategy (e.g., a graphic organizer) that will enable the individual to complete the task effectively.
5. Complete the task, focusing on the importance of the organizational strategy.
6. Invite the individual to evaluate performance with and without the organizing procedure; encourage reflection about the reason for deliberate organizing activity.
7. Discuss other tasks for which this or related strategic procedures might be useful.
8. Encourage practice and generalization to other tasks and settings.

Cognitive Organization and Language

Helping children become better organized in their use of language (e.g., to describe objects or events, tell stories, explain, argue, persuade) is accomplished by the same procedures that are applied to any kind of organizational effort: That is, producing (or comprehending) a coherent piece of extended discourse is facilitated by internalized knowledge structures (organizing schemes) that enable the speaker (or writer, listener, or reader) to sift through large amounts of information and to identify what is central and what is peripheral, to place components in an order that is easy to follow, and to relate new information to old. However, because there is considerable literature on organization and language, and because this is an important area of competence for school-age people, we give it special attention.

Cognitive Organization and Narrative Discourse

Earlier in this chapter and in Chapter 14, we outline the stages in development of narrative ability in children and factors that influence that development. Of particular importance in that discussion are the following points:

1. The ability to organize language to produce coherent narratives is associated with the ability to orga-

nize thoughts and to remember events from one's past.
2. Children learn most effectively how to organize their thoughts and language by engaging frequently in socially co-constructed narratives about past experiences with parents or other caregivers who use an elaborative and collaborative style of interaction.
3. Specific competencies are associated with a positive, elaborative, collaborative, facilitative adult style of talking with children about the past.
4. Early narratives are most commonly descriptions of familiar routines or important singular events, with organized fictional narratives being a later developmental acquisition.
5. Children benefit from daily routines in which they are expected to organize a narrative with whatever support is necessary, including daily journal entries at school and discussion of the day over dinner at home.

Real-Event Narratives About the Recent Past.   These five themes combine to highlight the importance of reviewing the past with children with organizational impairment after TBI and in such a way that exploits the interactive competencies known to be part of a positive, *elaborative* and *collaborative* style of interaction. These important competencies are listed in Table 14-1. This style of interaction is far removed from the *inquisitorial* style frequently observed in rehabilitation hospitals (e.g., "Okay, what did you do after breakfast? And what did you do after physical therapy? No, you went to speech after physical therapy. Now, what . . . ?").

Particularly when children are in the confused stages of recovery, staff and family members must be helped to understand the value of reviewing the recent past and of the critical features of those reviews—namely, that this is a social activity, it should be fun, there should be considerable elaboration, the adult should develop the narrative collaboratively with the child, and the child should be supported in every way possible. Support can take the form of adult contributions of whatever information the child does not readily retrieve, photographs of the people and places that could help trigger the child's recollections and descriptions, and supportive language to encourage elaboration, organization, and effortful searches of memory.

To facilitate frequent reviews of daily events, rehabilitation hospitals—and schools that serve students with organizational impairment—must have in place an effective log- or memory-book system. Information that will be reviewed later must be recorded to ensure that the child does not confabulate as well as to provide the adult with information with which to elaborate on the child's narrative. In our experience, considerable effort is required to initiate and maintain the use of log or memory books in settings where professionals are very busy. However, this practice is sufficiently important to justify the effort and time, to ensure that children and adolescents have access to orienting information and that adults have access to relevant historical information. A simple, useful procedure in preschools and schools with self-contained classrooms is to complete form letters for each student during a group review at the end of each day and to send home a photocopy to the students' parents. In this way, parents know what transpired at school and can facilitate a narrative review at home.

As a child gains some facility with recalling routines or singular events from the recent past, some of this support can gradually be removed. For example, children can be given photographs to place on a planning board at the beginning of the day, generating a sort of narrative about the future, and they can be asked to review the day in a similar way in the evening. A photograph guide for simple chronological narratives is presented in Figure 11-3. When the photographs are no longer necessary, they can be removed as the child produces a coherent chronological narrative. An alternative strategy for a child who is improving is to expect more types of information and more elaboration from him or her (e.g., a recounting of problems that arose during the day and how these were reconciled).

Real-Event Narratives About Preinjury Scripts.   Concurrent with exercises in relating the recent past, it is useful to help children organize their thoughts about preinjury events, including important routines and scripts in their lives. To gain a common knowledge base, for purposes of socially co-constructing narratives about the child's preinjury routines, staff members need to ask parents to write or tape record detailed descriptions of very important singular events (e.g., a recent trip to Disney World) and, more importantly, of important routines (which are very concrete) and scripts (which are somewhat more general). The routines might have to do with household chores or other frequently repeated sequences of events, whereas the scripts might have to do with more general activities in school, family life, social and extracurricular activities, vocational experiences, or anything important to the child. Photographs again are helpful in triggering recollections that help to generate organized and elaborated narratives. Manipulative representational toys (e.g., to represent school scripts) or drawings may prove useful for formulating a visual representation of the routine or script and then dictating the narrative. The permanence of objects and pictures is useful for children with serious organizational and memory problems.

It is important that this co-construction of a narrative result in a written or printed story. First, this concrete product—an actual piece of paper with a story on it—makes the processing of the script (which is the information to be learned) meaningful in relation to a concrete goal: That is, the learning task becomes an involuntary or incidental learning task, which is important for children

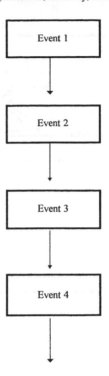

Figure 11-3. Photograph guide for a simple chronological narrative about past events.

and adolescents at this stage of recovery. Second, because the narrative is written, it can be reviewed many times over the course of a day by other staff and family members, providing needed repetition. Thus, the most critical factors in memory—personal significance, repetition, and organization—are all factored into the exercise. During the writing of the story, children may ask to look at the photographs, toys, or drawings to help them remember. After they have done this a few times, the adult can help by saying something such as, "I'm not sure you have to look at the pictures. Think about where we are in this story. I bet you'll be able to tell me what comes next." In this way, the adult invites the children to use the organizing scheme (script) in their head in the same way that they used the physical pictures or objects that represented the script. Thus, two of the important purposes of organizing schemes or scripts are stimulated: to guide the organization of thinking and talking and to facilitate retrieval of information.

Beyond the important cognitive rehabilitation goals and objectives that support this rehabilitation activity are hidden benefits. Having detailed information about a child's preinjury life helps staff know and appreciate a real human being who is more than a "head-injured patient." It also communicates respect to parents and gives them an important role in cognitive rehabilitation, that of providing the material for their children's narratives and of being

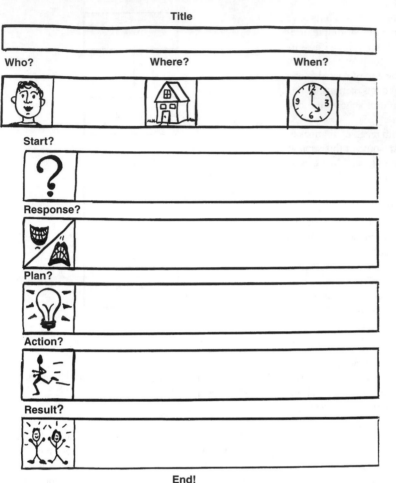

Figure 11-4. Simple graphic organizer for narrative information (story grammar).

effective narration partners for their child. Finally, it provides some integration of content across the rehabilitation program as all staff members review the day's story with the child. Research on the effectiveness of facilitating narrative development in preschoolers suggests that everyday people, including parents, must be involved in this long-term project (McCabe and Peterson, 1989; McCabe and Rollins, 1994).

Fictional Narratives.   Earlier, we observed that organized narratives about real events or routines generally precede organized fictional narratives in typical child development. Three and 4 year olds who are read to a great deal may begin stories in an organized and consistent way: For example, "Once upon a time there was a little girl who lived in the woods with her mother. One day as they were walking through the woods . . ." However, what follows is generally delightful but incoherent free association. For this reason, and because children with TBI need to become focused on real-world events, the process of organizing thoughts and language around the child's real events and routines is the initial best

approach. Ultimately, though, children need to internalize a variety of organizing schemes for discourse, including the organization of simple fictional stories.

Basic story grammar, or the organization of classical narratives, is illustrated in Figure 11-4. Internalizing this and related organizing schemes (knowledge structures) is important for telling and writing organized stories, which is a common task from first grade forward. The organizing scheme is also important for comprehending stories told by teachers or read in books. Without this guiding scheme (i.e., without knowing which information is important to listen for), a listener will likely find it difficult to pick out the most critical information and to follow a story without being overwhelmed by details. Children who lack these organizing schemes easily become inattentive and disruptive during story time because, from an organizational perspective, the task is beyond their ability.

Therefore, after they achieve an adequate level of independence with narrating familiar routines, children can be introduced to the organizational scheme underlying classical narratives. We do this by constructing stories with children—often in a group—using the outline in Figure 11-4. The outline can also be used to structure note taking as the group is reading a story. Parents are encouraged to use this same form to highlight information as they read children bedtime stories. Initially, children may contribute very little to the story construction process. However, as they become familiar with the form and the organization it represents, children will assume increasingly greater responsibility. In addition, the form can be used to help children listen to stories and summarize them, orally or in writing. As with real-event narration, upping the ante can take the form of systematically withdrawing supports (e.g., the printed forms, the assistance in constructing the narrative) or of requesting longer and more elaborate narratives.

Cognitive Organization and Other Types of Discourse

Varieties of Graphic Organizers. Not all organized language takes the form of a narrative. Figure 11-5 illustrates organizing schemes for discourse designed to *define concepts,* to *develop analogies*, to *analyze characters* in a text, and to *develop* a *perspective*. No particular magic resides in the boxes or connecting lines in Figure 11-5. Indeed, in working with children, adolescents, and young adults who are poor readers and writers because of organizational impairment, one will find it advantageous to collaborate with each individual to create a customized diagram (a type of graphic organizer) that fits the material that person needs to comprehend or express in writing. This creative process helps to emphasize the points that organizing is an activity in which we engage and that we can perform complex activities well with a little advance organizing. The illustrations of graphic advance organizers in Figures 11-3 through 11-6 and 11-8 may be of some assistance to teachers and clinicians in this creative process.

Some discourse tasks do not fit any particular mold and require ad hoc creation of an organizing scheme. For example, a fifth-grade student with substantial organizational impairment after TBI was asked to write an autobiographical description. His product was a short and rather disorganized list of things and people he liked or did not like (e.g., "I like football; I like my friend Tom; I do not like schoolwork; I like being an altar boy in church."). His special educator expressed disappointment in this piece of writing and told the student that he should have elaborated more and organized things in a clearer way.

In this case, the student might have profited from an advance organizer such as that depicted in Figure 11-6. Indeed, the teaching interaction would have been ideal had the educator spent a few brief moments exploring the kinds of things the student wanted to say about himself and then *collaboratively* creating something similar to the organizer in Figure 11-6. Discussions of the type of organization to use to complete a specific task are an ideal context for the types of master-apprentice interaction that, within a vygotskyan developmental perspective, lead to internalized cognitive schemes. Assuming the student followed the guide and produced an adequately long, interesting, and well-organized description of his likes and dislikes, the teacher could have then praised him for excellent work and highlighted the value of the organizing scheme.

With a little creativity, organizing schemes of this sort can be developed for nearly any discourse task (read or written), not only improving the individual's performance on that task but also gradually improving organizational functioning in general. For individuals at a higher level of functioning, ideas can be written on index cards that can then be arranged and rearranged to suggest a variety of organizational possibilities with the same material. In the absence of attention to graphic advance organizers of this sort, disorganized children and adolescents predictably fail when required to accomplish organizationally demanding tasks. Therefore, hospital staff should begin this process of teaching organizing schemes but should also ensure that school staff members are aware of the disorganized child's ongoing needs for organizational support and the teaching process we have just described.

Graphic Organizers: Special Considerations. We have included several illustrations of graphic organizers and have emphasized their importance in helping children and adolescents with TBI acquire or reacquire organizing schemes and become better organized in their thinking, talking, remembering, and acting. Graphic advance organizers also help to facilitate consistency in instruction among staff. In creating graphic organizers, one must seriously consider the organization of the organizer. The ultimate goal is that the child will internalize the graphic organizer as an automatic cognitive organizer. Therefore, the tool must be as effective as possible in depicting the true organization of the material.

The story grammar graphic organizer (see Figure 11-4) appears to meet this standard: That is, it starts at the top with a box for the title (i.e., the main idea or unifying theme of the story) and then proceeds to boxes for the characters, place, and time, all on the same level. This is followed by a downward progression of boxes representative of the serial progression of narrative structure that generally exists in the narratives of mainstream American children. (See Gutierrez-Clellen et al., 1995; Westby, 1994; and Westby and Roman, 1995, for a discussion of narrative organization in other cultures.)

We have also seen narrative structure diagrams that fail to meet this standard. For example, one that appeared in a whole-language workbook was circular rather than linear and placed the box for characters (generally the first component of a narrative) in the lower left corner of the circular diagram. To present serially ordered discourse components in a circular guide or to place the starting point on the lower left corner of the page is counterproductive.

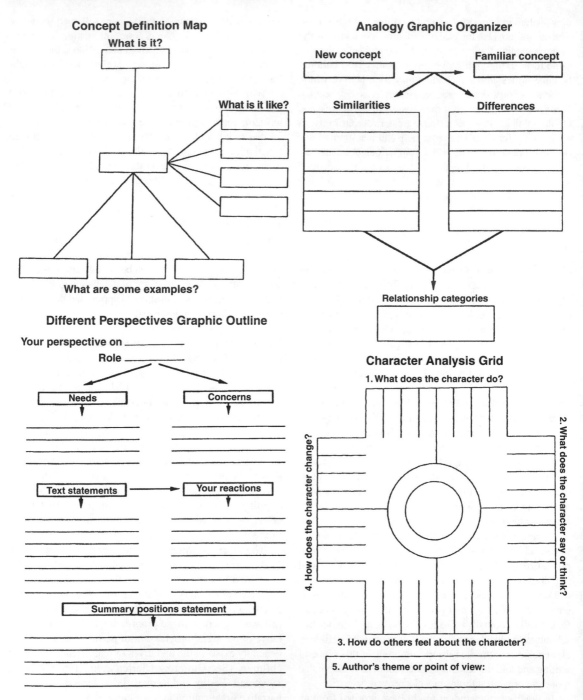

Figure 11-5. Variety of graphic advance organizers for complex cognitive and language tasks. (Reproduced with permission from D Buehl [1995]. Classroom strategies for interactive learning. Madison, WI: Wisconsin State Reading Association.)

The first edition of this book included a graphic organizer (the sun diagram) that similarly used a circular structure (exploiting the rays-of-the-sun metaphor) to organize information that might be linear in organization. Our experience with this diagram has suggested that it can be confusing when used with narrative material. Although this is certainly not a fatal error, it is problematic if children are exposed to a thinking structure that does not accurately mirror the structure of what they are thinking about.

Figure 11-6. Ad hoc graphic advance organizer for a brief auto-biographical sketch. The student wrote a short and disorganized sketch without the organizer. Using the organizer, he wrote an adequately elaborated and organized sketch.

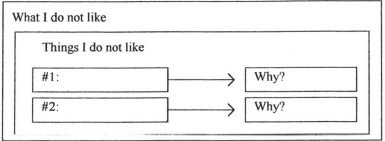

The general point is that graphic organizers should be developed with great care, ensuring that the organization on paper captures the organization in reality. In the next section, we present a graphic organizer for semantic feature analysis (Figure 11-7). In this case, Szekeres chose a circular pattern because the representation of meaning in semantic memory probably is not linear. Nevertheless, having a consistent structure is important for keeping track of the thought process in exploring concepts and for developing a sense for orderliness that can be used in systematic circumlocution when words are difficult to find. We suggest that the diagram be used like a clock, beginning at 12:00 with what often is most strongly associated with an object (its category) and then proceeding clockwise in a way that captures important dimensions of meaning of common nouns.

In addition to attending to the organization of the organizer, one must restrict the number of graphic organizers to which an individual with organizational impairment is exposed at any given time. Disorganized children and adolescents easily confuse the purpose of one organizer with that of another, resulting in heightened disorganization and fragmentation, the opposite of the intended effect.

Organization and Word Retrieval

Word-retrieval problems are associated with a wide variety of causes and locations of acquired brain injury as well as with congenital language disability. The frequency of word-retrieval problems may be related to the fact that the networks and systems of networks of neural connections that underlie word meaning are widespread in the brain: That is, words can be triggered by other words with which they are definitionally associated (e.g., *chair* might be triggered by *furniture, sit, couch, table*), by visual images and stimuli, by phonemes, by sounds and smells, and by other associations. Neurologically, these associations probably correspond to a large number of neural connections—both close and distant—that comprise a word's meaning (from a neuropsychological perspective) and facilitate word retrieval. Damage to varied parts of the brain could, therefore, interfere with the efficiency of word retrieval by eliminating some of these connections. Alternatively, word-retrieval problems could result from generally impaired retrieval processes (e.g., disorganized searches of memory), poorly controlled attention, lack of initiation, weak monitoring, and failure to proceed strategically when faced with word-retrieval difficulties.

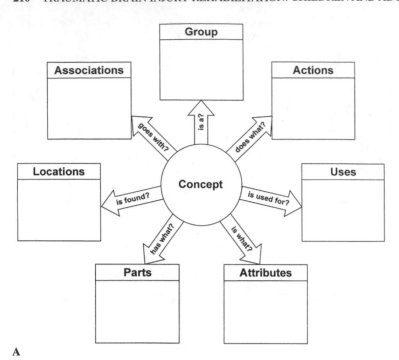

Figure 11-7. A. A guide for semantic feature analysis. B. A completed analysis of an animate object (horse).

A

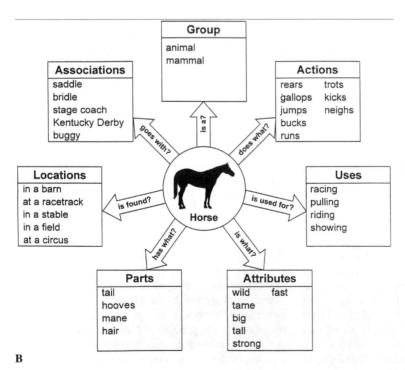

B

Difficulty retrieving words, if severe, can seriously interfere with all types of communication. If less severe, word-retrieval problems can still seriously affect classroom performance and social success. Because stress generally exacerbates word-finding problems, people usually perform worst when they need to perform best, thereby creating considerable frustration. For children with word-finding problems, classroom recitation and timed classroom tests may be the contexts that present the greatest difficulty, a difficulty that may be unexpected, considering only the child's performance on language tests in a nonstressful environment.

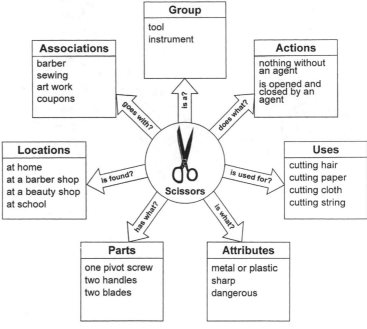

C

Figure 11-8. A portion of the semantic network. A. The concept Robin has been activated and is shown in boldface.

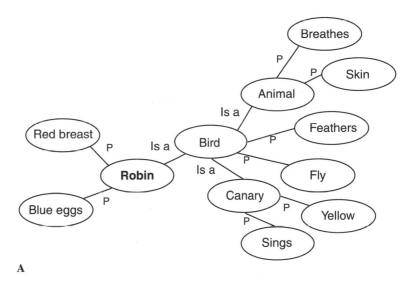

A

The approach to intervention for word-retrieval problems presented in this section is based on the popular network theory of meaning, which was suggested earlier. According to this view, word meanings are networks—and systems of networks—of associations with other words, concepts, images, or stored contents of some other sort. A highly simplified and schematized representation of one such network (including only word associations) is presented in Figure 11-8. In the semantic knowledge base of mature adults, thousands of connections among points in these meaning trees probably exist, and the points are not restricted to other words. The strength and organization of these networks and systems of networks are believed to be related to the efficiency of word-retrieval: That is, if there are very few connections with the stored representation of a given word, that word is less likely to be triggered quickly and efficiently when needed, whereas if there are many connections but they are wholly disorganized or the individual lacks inhibition, the triggering of another word is equally likely. Therefore, appropriate goals of intervention are (1) to ensure that the individual

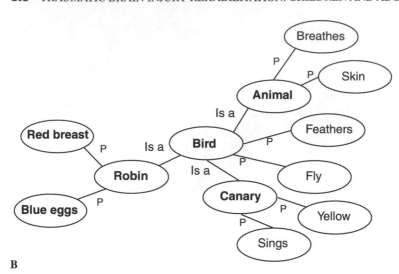

Figure 11-8. *Continued* B. Robin primes (P) its associates and has activated concepts linked to Robin—for example, the boldface Bird, Red breast, and Blue eggs. C. The continued spread of activation that originated from Robin is depicted. (Reprinted with permission from M Ashcraft [1994]. Human Memory and Cognition. Reading, MA: Addison-Wesley, Longman.)

B

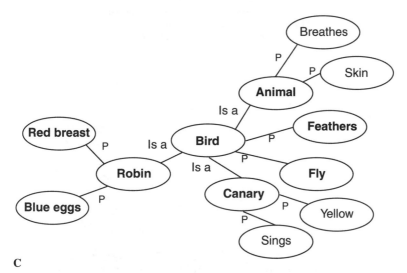

C

has an adequately rich and connected semantic knowledge base; (2) to ensure that networks of concepts are as organized as possible; and (3) to help the individual make deliberate use of this organization if word retrieval must be effortful or if he or she must circumlocute to communicate a desired point.

Kail and colleagues (1984) suggested two hypotheses for word-retrieval difficulties: that the child's lexical storage is impoverished or poorly organized (the storage hypothesis) and that the child cannot efficiently access stored words (the retrieval hypothesis). Kail's group found that children with congenital language disability often have relatively few word entries and weaker links between those words in their semantic memories, partially explaining their inefficiency in word retrieval on the basis of the storage hypothesis. Recent work by McGregor and Windsor (1996), based on the popular semantic priming research paradigm, supports the view that nam-

ing difficulties in preschoolers with word-finding deficits are related to weak organization and elaboration within their lexical systems. The authors concluded that intervention that addresses semantic elaboration, such as the intervention discussed later, is probably most effective for this group of children. In contrast, Lahey and Edwards (1996) failed to find support for the hypothesis that slow naming in somewhat older children with specific language impairment is a consequence of poor lexical organization or elaboration.

Probably a combination of factors affect word finding in children with TBI, and different children may have very different sources of difficulty. Children with TBI often score within normal limits on the Peabody Picture Vocabulary Test, suggesting an adequate stockpile of words. However, the unusual associations and strange twists and turns in conversation frequently observed in these children suggest a change in the networks and systems of networks of associations in the semantic knowledge base (possibly combined with failure to inhibit inaccurate responses based on activation of words that are part of an organized network of meanings but that are not relevant to the issue at hand). This would be consistent with an impaired storage system explanation of word-retrieval problems. However, individuals with TBI also often exhibit general retrieval problems and general slowness in responding, suggesting that at least part of the problem might be at the level of retrieval or be attributable to slowed information processing.

Fortunately, semantic feature analysis intervention can attack the problem at the levels of disorganized storage *and* ineffective retrieval. At different stages of recovery, this type of intervention can be used to achieve different combinations of the following goals: (1) deliberate control of attention; (2) self-monitoring of knowledge of a topic; (3) organized retrieval of information and of words; (4) organized descriptions of objects and of words (possibly as a compensation for ongoing word-retrieval problems); (5) practical use of retrieved information in problem-solving and other functional activities; and (6) functional use of resources, such as dictionaries (Szekeres, 1992). On the assumption that word-retrieval problems of the child with TBI may result in part from disruption of neural connections (associations) that make up a word's network, feature analysis activities may help to reactivate or recreate the connections in an organized manner. On the alternative assumption that the individual is not using an organized retrieval procedure, the activities may re-establish organized searches on an automatic level. Finally, if word-retrieval problems persist and the individual needs to compensate deliberately for the problem, feature analysis activities may teach a system for self-cueing or for circumlocuting and therefore communicating effectively without the target word.

Feature analysis exercises begin with the clinician or teacher guiding the children through an exploration of a familiar object (e.g., cat, car). We use the feature analysis guide (see Figure 11-7) for this exploration—always proceeding in a clockwise fashion, beginning at 12:00—because the point of the exercise is to ensure that networks of concepts and searches for words are as organized as possible. Those objectives would be difficult to achieve if the form and the organization of the activity changed from exercise to exercise. Children are asked to produce as much relevant information as possible in each of the feature categories. For confused children with fleeting attention, the main goal may simply be to attend to the object under discussion for increasing periods. Information is written in the boxes and then evaluated for relevance and completeness. The clinician encourages the children to ask questions and to use references if they are unable to give reasonably complete information about an object. For children functioning at a higher level, information in the boxes can be elaborated (e.g., discussion of when, where, why, by whom, how).

Feature analysis activities are ideal for group sessions, because groups generate more ideas and associations than do individuals, and group members can evaluate one another's contributions for relevance and accuracy. Initially, children are expected simply to focus on the object under discussion, search their memories for relevant information, and inhibit irrelevant information. Subsequently, they are expected to learn to use the guide itself as a procedure for organizing information, for finding words, or for circumlocuting in the event of serious word-retrieval problems. Once the children have learned the procedure, a facilitator can elicit word-retrieval problems with stressful naming tasks (e.g., very rapid naming of pictures), always encouraging the child to use the feature analysis as a mental guide when specific words cannot be found.

As with all cognitive and language intervention activities, clinicians must connect the exercise with practical activities to which it might be relevant. For example, having completed a feature analysis, children may write a descriptive paragraph about the object, using the information and its organization. Subsequently, they might complete a second analysis of a related concept and then perform a similarities and differences exercise, using the information from the two feature analyses. Finally, the group might complete a problem-solving activity, again using the information retrieved and organized during the feature analysis exercise.

For adolescents who evidence similar semantic organizational difficulty, similar feature analysis procedures can be used, incorporating age-appropriate and possibly higher-level concepts for analysis. For example, the procedure might be used for preteaching the vocabulary involved in history or social studies lessons. Elaborating meaning in this organized manner has a decided advantage over multi-trial vocabulary drill in that it promotes storage of semantic information in organized systems, thereby making it more readily accessible. Social skills groups can use the procedure to analyze aspects of social interaction (e.g., conversation). Prevocational groups can use the procedure to gain clarity about important work-related concepts such as boss, interview, and performance appraisal.

Concept exploration, including graphic representation of the word connections, is a common activity in the early grades. However, as used by many regular education teachers, the goal is divergent or creative thinking—that is, identifying as many related concepts as possible. The product may be a "word web" that illustrates many connections but not their organization. The advantage of semantic feature analysis for students with organizational impairment is that the exploration is structured in a consistent manner to achieve the goal of re-establishing organized networks of concepts and words. For children who are capable of divergent thinking but continue to struggle with organization and, in general, with convergent thinking, the facilitator might wish to restrict contributions to one or two words per feature analysis category, insisting that the entries be *the* most important features.

Finally, feature analysis may be a facilitating context for promoting recovery of reading skills. On reviewing a completed analysis that includes words that children have just retrieved and dictated to the clinician, the children will likely retrieve the same words again when asked to read what they have dictated, making "reading" relatively easy (i.e., the words have been primed). Furthermore, if the students are asked to dictate a descriptive paragraph using the information, their "reading" of that paragraph should be facilitated by the fact that they just dictated it.

Feature analysis activities and the feature analysis guide, as we have described them, are among the many highly organized and useful approaches to language intervention for people with significant organizational impairment. German (1994) discussed word-finding difficulties in children with congenital language-learning disability and presented a useful framework for assessment and intervention. Her tests are among the best available tools for exploring word-finding ability in children and adolescents (German, 1986, 1990, 1991). She has also developed a comprehensive intervention program (German, 1993) that includes a number of useful procedures and activities.

Use of Technology in Compensating for Impaired Organization and Memory

The rapidly developing field of rehabilitation technology offers an increasing number of practical answers to questions posed by ongoing cognitive disability (Parenté and Anderson-Parenté, 1991). In Chapter 8, Henry and colleagues discuss issues related to the application of technology for children and adolescents with TBI, including the need for comprehensive and integrated planning that considers needs in all domains, among them mobility, self-care, communication, and cognition. In this section, our goal is to highlight software and devices designed to help individuals compensate for impaired organization and memory. Well-selected devices can complement cognitive intervention programs and increase independent functioning, reducing reminders from adults.

Decisions about using technological compensations are based on several important considerations. In the absence of careful planning, apparently useful devices might be recommended and dispensed but shortly consigned to the closet shelf because they were too difficult to learn, too difficult to use, awkward and stigmatizing, or ineffective in relation to the individual's specific needs. Therefore, careful "head fitting" is required to ensure that the learning needs, aesthetic sensitivities, and functional outcomes of individual students are met. The following questions guide decision making in relation to technological supports:

- *Needs*: What tasks will the student be expected to accomplish that will require compensation due to impaired organization and memory? In what environment will the student be expected to perform these tasks?
- *Cognitive profile:* What is the student's general learning style? How efficient is procedural learning? Is it necessary to simplify the teaching and provide ongoing visual cues? Does the student have adequate judgment to use expensive equipment safely? Is he or she aware of ongoing disability?
- *Physical (sensorimotor) profile:* What is the student's current and projected ability to access the equipment? Will adaptations be needed to operate standardized equipment? Will cognitive prostheses have to be integrated into a larger package of prosthetic equipment?
- *Familiarity:* Did the student have preinjury competence with computers or other technological devices?
- *Motivation and willingness to use technological compensations:* Does the student want to use equipment to compensate for ongoing disability? Is he or she willing to devote time and effort to practicing its use? Is the student concerned about aesthetics and the possible stigmatizing effects of equipment?
- *Environmental support:* Do parents and teachers understand the need for equipment and are they willing to work with the student to establish efficient use and effective maintenance of the equipment?

In Chapter 12, Ylvisaker and colleagues outline procedures that are useful in teaching any compensatory strategy or behavior, including the functional use of cognitive prostheses. Because using equipment can be difficult and time-consuming, a critical element in the teaching process is engaging the student in establishing the need for technological compensations and in monitoring the effectiveness of such compensations. In other words, students must understand that the equipment meets an important need and that it helps them achieve functional goals. Because some students are quick to make final judgments about the usefulness of a compensatory procedure and are also frustrated easily, a student might require considerable time to play with a new piece of equipment and to gain facility with its operation before it is introduced into real-world tasks. Although this advice appears to be contrary to our repeated recommendation that meaningful, real-world contexts be a primary training ground for people who have difficulty transferring, in this case it would be unwise to jeopardize the long-term use of helpful compensations by having the student associate failure and embarrassment with the equipment.

Computer Software

A laptop computer can be developed into a multifunction system to help students with time management, routine reminders, word processing, organized writing, and other possible areas of need. Software currently available for time management includes Ascend 5.0 (Franklin Quest Co., Salt Lake City, UT), Track Day Organizer (Wix Technology, Inc., Arlington, VA), and Stay Organized Quick and Easy Individual Software (Pleasanton, CA). Because these programs were designed for business application, they require some modification for use by students with a disability. These programs include "to do" lists and methods for planning. The computer can be programmed so that the to-do list appears first on the screen, helping the student remain focused on what needs to be done without relying on adult reminders.

Increasingly, commercially available word processors incorporate icons and other cueing systems for students with impaired memory. Question cues prior to leaving documents or deleting files help careless students avoid disastrous loss of files. On-line information searches via the Internet create access to worlds of information that students with physical or organizational disability might otherwise have difficulty accessing. FL90 Windows/Timex Data Link Compatible Organizer (Timex Corp.) is a portable memory system that can be interfaced into a personal computer (with a Windows 95 operating system and a CD-ROM).

External Memory Devices and Cueing Systems

The products described in this section are designed to help individuals remember to do what they need to do. Because problems with organization and memory (including prospective memory) are common after TBI and because many people with TBI, particularly adolescents, react negatively to repeated reminders and cues from adults (i.e., nagging), cognitive prostheses should be explored with the goal of enhancing independence and reducing the risk of escalating behavioral problems. We list a sampling of available products with caution. By the time this book is printed, new products will undoubtedly be available and possibly superior to those described here. The critical message is that there are prosthetic devices that meet a variety of cognitive needs and there will be more. Clinicians must remain informed about these developments to serve their clients effectively.

NeuroPage

NeuroPage (Hersh and Treadgold, Inc., San Jose, CA) is an integration of computer and paging technologies that enables people with memory, planning, organization, attention, or initiation problems to receive predictated reminders through an alphanumeric pager (Hersh and Treadgold, 1994). The system can receive and send to the pager single or multiple reminders that are either ongoing (e.g., "Check daily planner.") or are offered only one time (e.g., "Call mom, 555-7243, about tickets."). At the predetermined time, a computer sends information by modem to a transmitter; then the message is converted into a radio signal and is sent to the client's pager. The client can both view the current message and review previous messages (up to 120 numbers and letters per message). The system is particularly useful for adolescents and young adults who are committed to independence but who need ongoing reminders to remain focused and to remember to do what needs to be done and at the appropriate time. The reminders can be generated by the student, by adults (e.g., therapists or parents) or, more likely, by both students and adults working together. Pagers have the advantage of being inconspicuous, if that is desirable, or they can be prominently displayed if the individual's culture attaches prestige to pagers. Recent developments of this system include a voice-based receiver. In addition, it is possible to create a closed-loop system that requires the user to acknowledge that the message was received (Lynch, 1995).

At the Centre for Traumatic Brain Injury Rehabilitation in Toronto, NeuroPage has been used by children as young as 8. The system was particularly useful for a 13 year old who was dependent on others to follow a schedule and attend therapies during the confused stages of his recovery. A written schedule was insufficient because he typically forgot to consult it at the appropriate times. Within a week of initiating the use of NeuroPage, he began arriving at scheduled therapy sessions independently and on time. In addition to the subjective value for the young man associated with this accomplishment, staff spent less time searching for him and more time engaged in productive therapeutic activities (S Hayman, personal communication, 1996).

Voice It Personal Note Recorder

The Voice It Personal Note Recorder (Voice It Technologies, Inc., Fort Collins, CO) is a simple and relatively inexpensive credit card–sized device that allows for recording and playback of messages up to 120 seconds in length. Its features include icon-labeled access buttons (play, record, erase) and a flashing red light to indicate that a message is waiting.

Yak Back

The Yak Back (YES Technologies, Bozeman, MT) is an inexpensive device that is available in discount stores and can record single messages up to 60 seconds long. The messages can be "locked" into the recorder. The Yak Back can be carried inconspicuously in a pocket but typically requires an additional cue to remind the user to push the button.

Voice Organizer

The Voice Organizer (Voice Powered Technology International, Inc., Canoga Park, CA), a small and moderately priced device with a 4-Mb memory, can record up to 100 names, 400 telephone numbers, 99 individual notes, and 99 reminders. Information is recorded in the user's own voice and access is direct. Notes are entered by stating the title before entering the text. Retrieval is accomplished by reciting the title or description. The device must be "trained" to recognize the user's voice.

MotivAider Personal Achievement System

The MotivAider Personal Achievement System (Behavioral Dynamics, Inc., Thief River Falls, MN), a pager-based system, has been augmented with reminder software designed for children (The MotivAider Method of Cue-Directed Behavior Change for Children). The user wears a pager set on vibrator mode. At predesignated times or time intervals, messages are delivered to the child (e.g., "Check your assignment book"). A teacher's manual accompanies the device.

Case Study

At age 17, and 8 years after her injury, Sarah continued to experience, as a result of her injury, severe motor and cognitive slowness; moderate fatigue; moderate hemiplegia, ataxia, and apraxia; moderate impairment of memory, cognitive organization, and perceptual organization; impaired new learning and generally reduced academic functioning; difficulty writing (motor speed as well as compositional organization); weak self-monitoring; poor safety judgment; and frequent off-task behaviors.

Sarah had a power wheelchair but required continuous adult supervision due to her impaired judgment. She was always accompanied by an adult as she moved from one room to another in her high school. Because of problems with organization and memory, her teaching assistant kept track of and ensured that she completed her assignments, took notes for Sarah, and did all of Sarah's writing for her, including tests. Her teachers were concerned about her inability to express herself in writing, frequent deletions of information when she tried to use a word-processing program, poor time management and inability to remember assignments, failure to complete homework, and poor judgment. The overarching concern was Sarah's near-total dependence on adults as she approached adulthood and the end of her school years.

After consultation from a specialist in brain injury rehabilitation, the staff at Sarah's school developed a comprehensive program designed to increase her independence. Compensations for impairment of organization and memory included the following:

1. *Organization and daily routines:* Ascend 4.0 software was added to Sarah's laptop computer to assist her with time management and task completion. It was programmed so that a to-do list appeared first on the screen when she turned on the computer. Several individual training sessions were devoted to making her use of this system automatic. Her daily routine then came to include sessions in the morning and evening during which daily activities were planned and information was added or deleted. Sarah's family helped her type in plans for non-school activities. One hour each evening was set aside for homework, with all other activities scheduled around homework.

2. *Word processing:* Sarah was provided with a newer word-processing system that incorporated a Windows platform, which provided sufficient cues to prevent unwanted deletion of information and files.

3. *Home-school consistency:* Sarah passed a proficiency test in the care of the equipment and her parents agreed to sign a responsibility waiver so that she could take her laptop home, thereby ensuring that she could use the same organization and reminder systems at home and at school.

4. *Independence in academic work:* To reduce dependence on the teaching assistant, test formats were programmed into the computer, as were math and vocabulary software, so that Sarah could take tests and practice academic skills independently.

5. *Participation in class discussion:* A voice output program was installed in Sarah's laptop so that she could preprogram answers to questions that would be asked during class discussion.

6. *Reminders:* Two Yak Backs were purchased. At school, the message was, "Check your schedule!" The home message was, "What do you have to do for homework?"

Once these supports and compensations became part of Sarah's routine, her independence increased sharply, thereby improving her sense of her own competence as well as adults' perception of her abilities as a student and of her potential for competitive employment and independent living after high-school graduation.

Collaborative Approach to Cognitive Rehabilitation

In this chapter, we have emphasized a collaborative approach to intervention, making use of any activities and all everyday people in the child's life as the deliverers of the service. Specialists in cognitive rehabilitation play an indispensable role in understanding the child's needs, through various assessments and diag-

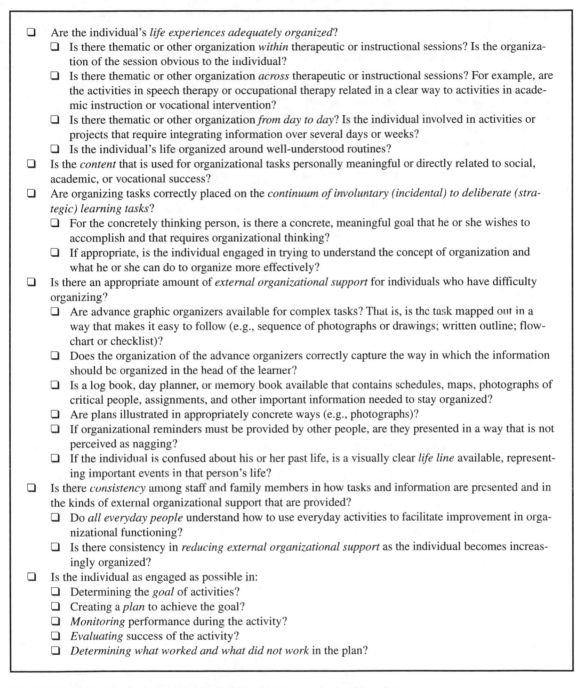

- ❑ Are the individual's *life experiences adequately organized*?
  - ❑ Is there thematic or other organization *within* therapeutic or instructional sessions? Is the organization of the session obvious to the individual?
  - ❑ Is there thematic or other organization *across* therapeutic or instructional sessions? For example, are the activities in speech therapy or occupational therapy related in a clear way to activities in academic instruction or vocational intervention?
  - ❑ Is there thematic or other organization *from day to day*? Is the individual involved in activities or projects that require integrating information over several days or weeks?
  - ❑ Is the individual's life organized around well-understood routines?
- ❑ Is the *content* that is used for organizational tasks personally meaningful or directly related to social, academic, or vocational success?
- ❑ Are organizing tasks correctly placed on the *continuum of involuntary (incidental) to deliberate (strategic) learning tasks*?
  - ❑ For the concretely thinking person, is there a concrete, meaningful goal that he or she wishes to accomplish and that requires organizational thinking?
  - ❑ If appropriate, is the individual engaged in trying to understand the concept of organization and what he or she can do to organize more effectively?
- ❑ Is there an appropriate amount of *external organizational support* for individuals who have difficulty organizing?
  - ❑ Are advance graphic organizers available for complex tasks? That is, is the task mapped out in a way that makes it easy to follow (e.g., sequence of photographs or drawings; written outline; flowchart or checklist)?
  - ❑ Does the organization of the advance organizers correctly capture the way in which the information should be organized in the head of the learner?
  - ❑ Is a log book, day planner, or memory book available that contains schedules, maps, photographs of critical people, assignments, and other important information needed to stay organized?
  - ❑ Are plans illustrated in appropriately concrete ways (e.g., photographs)?
  - ❑ If organizational reminders must be provided by other people, are they presented in a way that is not perceived as nagging?
  - ❑ If the individual is confused about his or her past life, is a visually clear *life line* available, representing important events in that person's life?
- ❑ Is there *consistency* among staff and family members in how tasks and information are presented and in the kinds of external organizational support that are provided?
  - ❑ Do *all everyday people* understand how to use everyday activities to facilitate improvement in organizational functioning?
  - ❑ Is there consistency in *reducing external organizational support* as the individual becomes increasingly organized?
- ❑ Is the individual as engaged as possible in:
  - ❑ Determining the *goal* of activities?
  - ❑ Creating a *plan* to achieve the goal?
  - ❑ *Monitoring* performance during the activity?
  - ❑ *Evaluating* success of the activity?
  - ❑ *Determining what worked and what did not work* in the plan?

Figure 11-9. A checklist for intervention for individuals with organizational impairment.

nostic therapy, and in working with other professionals, paraprofessionals, and family members to ensure that cognitive goals and objectives are pursued meaningfully throughout the day. Furthermore, cognitive specialists identify the types of support the child needs to be successful and help staff and family members provide those supports and systematically remove them as the child improves.

This collaboration is not limited only to a variety of individuals in one facility at one stage of recovery. Rather, hospital and school staff must think of collaboration as occurring over time, with people from the two systems working together to achieve optimal outcomes. This intense collaboration faces many obstacles—historical, institutional, emotional, and logistic. In Chapter 20, Ylvisaker and Feeney address these issues.

Summary

We have addressed the issue of cognitive organization from a variety of perspectives, including ADLs, other everyday routines, play, perception, general organizational schemas, and language. In each case, we recommend providing necessary organizational support, contextualizing intervention so that it is meaningful in terms of content and activities that the child needs to organize, collaborating with others to provide consistent and well-organized intervention, and recruiting everyday people to use everyday activities to encourage improved organizational functioning in children and adolescents with TBI. Figure 11-9 presents a checklist that staff or family members can employ to evaluate their use of a child's life experiences and daily activities from an organizational standpoint.

References

Baddeley AD (1995). The Psychology of Memory. In AD Baddeley, BA Wilson, FN Watts (eds), Handbook of Memory Disorders. New York: Wiley, 3.

Bartlett FC (1958). Thinking. London: Allen & Unwin.

Baumeister A, Smith S (1979). Thematic elaboration and proximity in children's recall, organization, and long term retention of sectorial materials. J Child Psychol 28;231.

Bjorklund D (1985). The Role of Conceptual Knowledge in the Development of Organization in Children's Memory. In M Pressley, C Brainerd (eds), Basic Processes in Memory Development. New York: Springer, 103.

Bower G (1972). A Selective Review of Organizational Factors in Memory. In E Tulving, W Donaldson (eds), Organization of Memory. New York: Academic, 93.

Brown AL (1975). The Development of Memory: Knowing, Knowing About Knowing, and Knowing How to Know. In HW Reese (ed), Advances in Child Development and Behavior, vol 10. New York: Academic, 103.

Brown AL (1978). Metacognitive Development and Reading. In RJ Spiro, BC Bruce, GW Brewer (eds), Theoretical Issues in Reading Comprehension. Hillsdale, NJ: Lawrence Erlbaum, 77.

Brown AL (1979). Theories of Memory and Problems of Development, Activity, Growth, and Knowledge. In FIM Craik, L Cermak (eds), Levels of Processing and Memory. Hillsdale, NJ: Lawrence Erlbaum, 225.

Bruner J (1975). The ontogenesis of speech acts. J Child Lang 2;1.

Case R (1978). Intellectual Development from Birth to Adulthood. In R Siegler (ed), Children's Thinking: What Develops? Hillsdale, NJ: Lawrence Erlbaum.

Case R (1985). Intellectual Development: Birth to Adulthood. Orlando, FL: Academic.

Ceci SJ (1980). A developmental study of multiple encoding and it's relationship to age related changes in free recall. Child Dev 51;892.

Ceci SJ, Howe MJ (1978). Age-related differences in free recall as a function of retrieval flexibility. J Exp Child Psychol 26;432.

Chi MTH (1978). Knowledge Structures and Memory Development. In R Siegler (ed), Children's Thinking: What Develops? Hillsdale, NJ: Lawrence Erlbaum, 73.

Damasio AR, Tranel D, Damasio H (1991). Somatic Markers and the Guidance of Behavior: Theory and Preliminary Testing. In HS Levin, HM Eisenberg, AL Benton (eds), Frontal Lobe Function and Dysfunction. New York: Oxford, 217.

DeLoache J (1985). Memory-Based Searching by Very Young Children. In HM Wellman (ed), Children's Searching: The Development of Search Skill and Spatial Representation. Hillsdale, NJ: Lawrence Erlbaum, 151.

Deutsch D, Deutsch JA (1975). Short-Term Memory. New York: Academic.

Fivush R, Reese E (1992). The Social Construction of Autobiographical Memory. In MA Conway, DC Rubin, H Spinnler, WA Wagenaar (eds), Theoretical Perspectives on Autobiographical Memory. Amsterdam: Kluwer Academic, 115.

Flavell J (1979). Metacognition and cognitive monitoring: a new era of cognitive developmental inquiry. Am Psychologist 34;907.

Flavell J, Miller P, Miller S (1993). Cognitive Development. Englewood Cliffs, NJ: Prentice Hall.

German DJ (1986). National College of Education Test of Word Finding (TWF). Chicago: Riverside.

German DJ (1990). National College of Education Test of Adolescent/Adult Word Finding Skills (TAWF). Chicago: Riverside.

German DJ (1991). National College of Education Test of Word Finding in Discourse (TWFD). Chicago: Riverside.

German DJ (1993). Word Finding Intervention Program (WFIP). Tucson, AZ: Communication Skill Builders.

German DJ (1994). Word Finding Difficulties in Children and Adolescents. In G Wallach, K Butler (eds), Language Learning Disabilities in School-Age Children and Adolescents. Columbus, OH: Merrill, 323.

Grafman J, Sirigu A, Spector L, Hendler J (1993). Damage to the prefrontal cortex leads to decomposition of structured event complexes. J Head Trauma Rehabil 8;73.

Groden J, LeVasseur P (1995). Cognitive Picture Rehearsal: A System to Teach Self-Control. In KA Quill (ed), Teaching Children with Autism: Strategies to Enhance Communication and Socialization. Albany, NY: Delmar Publishers, 287.

Gutierrez-Clellen VF, Pena E, Quinn R (1995). Accommodating cultural differences in narrative style: a multicultural perspective. Top Lang Disord 15(4);54.

Hagen J, Jongeward R Jr, Kail R (1975). Cognitive Perspectives in the Development of Memory. In HW Reese (ed), Advances on Child Development, vol 10. New York: Academic.

Hallowell EM, Ratey JJ (1994). Driven to Distraction. New York: Pantheon Books.

Hersh N, Treadgold L (1994). NeuroPage: the rehabilitation of memory dysfunction by prosthetic memory and cueing. Neurorehabilitation 4;187.

Horowitz L, Lampel A, Takanishi R (1969). The child's memory of unitized scenes. J Psychol 8;365.

Johnston J (1982). Narratives: a new look at communication problems in older language disordered children. Lang Speech Hear Serv Schools 13;144.

Kail R (1990). The Development of Memory in Children (3rd ed). New York: Freeman.

Kail R, Hale CA, Leonard LB, Nippold MA (1984). Lexical storage and retrieval in language-impaired children. Appl Psycholinguistics 5;37.

Kavale K, Mattson P (1983). "One jumped off the balance beam": meta-analysis of perceptual-motor training. J Learn Disabil 16;165.

Lahey M, Edwards J (1996). Why do children with specific language impairment name pictures more slowly than their peers? J Speech Hear Res 39;1081.

Levin HS, Goldstein FC, Williams DH, Eisenberg HM (1991). The Contribution of Frontal Lobe Lesions to the Neurobehavioral Outcome of Closed Head Injury. In HS Levin, HM Eisenberg, AI Benton (eds), Frontal Lobe Function and Dysfunction. New York: Oxford University, 318.

Lhermitte F (1986). Human autonomy and the frontal lobes: II. Patient behavior in complex and social situations: the environmental dependency syndrome. Ann Neurol 106;237.

Light P, Butterworth G (eds) (1993). Context and Cognition. Hillsdale, NJ: Lawrence Erlbaum.

Lynch WJ (1995). You must remember this: assistive devices for memory impairment. J Head Trauma Rehabil 10;94.

MacDonald J (1989). Becoming Partners with Children: From Play to Conversation. Chicago: Riverside.

Mandler G (1967). Organization in Memory. In KW Spence, JT Spence (eds), The Psychology of Learning and Motivation, vol 1. New York: Academic, 327.

Markowitsch HJ (1995). Anatomical Basis of Memory Disorders. In MS Gazzaniga (ed), The Cognitive Neurosciences. Cambridge, MA: MIT Press, 765.

McCabe A, Peterson C (1989). Strategies for Developing Narrative Structure in a Preschool Setting. Paper presented at the annual meeting of the American Educational Research Association, November 8, San Francisco, CA.

McCabe A, Peterson C (1991). Getting the Story: A Longitudinal Study of Parental Styles in Eliciting Narratives and Developing Narrative Skills. In A McCabe, C Peterson (eds), New Directions in Developing Narrative Structure. Hillsdale, NJ: Lawrence Erlbaum, 217.

McCabe A, Rollins PR (1994). Assessment of preschool narrative skills. Am J Speech Lang Pathol 3;45.

McGregor KK, Windsor J (1996). Effects of priming on the naming accuracy of preschoolers with word-finding deficits. J Speech Hear Res 39;1048.

Meichenbaum D (1993). The "potential" contributions of cognitive behavior modification to the rehabilitation of individuals with traumatic brain injury. Semin Speech Lang 14;18.

Moely B (1977). Organization of Memory. In R Kail, J Hagen (eds), Perspectives on the Development of Memory and Cognition. Hillsdale, NJ: Lawrence Erlbaum, 203.

Nelson K (1992). Emergence of autobiographical memory at age 4. Hum Dev 35(3);172.

Norman DA, Shallice T (1986). Attention to Action: Willed and Automatic Control of Behavior. In RJ Davidson, GE Schwartz, D Shapiro (eds), Consciousness and Self-Regulation, vol 4. New York: Plenum.

Ochipa C, Rothi LJG, Heilman KM (1989). Ideational apraxia: a deficit in tool selection and use. Ann Neurol 25;190.

Ornstein P, Baker-Ward L (1983). The Development of Mnemonic Skill. Paper presented at the meeting of the Society for Research in Child Development, Detroit, MI.

Parenté R, Anderson-Parenté J (1991). Prosthetic Memory and Cognitive Orthotics. In R Parenté, J Anderson-Parenté (eds), Retraining Memory: Techniques and Applications. Houston, TX: CSY Publishing.

Patterson K, Hodges JR (1995). Disorders of Semantic Memory. In AD Baddeley, BA Wilson, FN Watts (eds), Handbook of Memory Disorders. New York: Wiley, 167.

Paul R, Smith RL (1993). Narrative skills in 4-year-olds with normal, impaired, and late-developing language. J Speech Hear Res 36;592.

Pellegrino J, Ingram A (1978). Processes, Products and Measures of Memory Organization [Learning Research Development Center report]. Pittsburgh: University of Pittsburgh.

Reese E, Fivush G (1993). Parental styles of talking about the past. Dev Psychol 29;596.

Reese E, Haden CA, Fivush R (1993). Mother-child conversations about the past: relationships of style and memory over time. Cogn Dev 8;403.

Schneider W, Pressley M (1989). Memory Development Between 2 and 20. New York: Springer.

Schwartz MF, Mayer NH, Fitzpatrick-DeSalme EJ, Montgomery MW (1993). Cognitive theory and the study of everyday action disorders after brain damage. J Head Trauma Rehabil 8;59.

Shimamura AP (1995). Memory and Frontal Lobe Function. In MS Gazzaniga (ed), The Cognitive Neurosciences. Cambridge, MA: MIT Press, 803.

Singley MK, Anderson JR (1989). Transfer of Cognitive Skill. Cambridge, MA: Harvard University.

Slifer KJ, Tucker CL, Gerson AC, et al. (1996). Operant conditioning for behavior management during posttraumatic amnesia in children and adolescents with brain injury. J Head Trauma Rehabil 11;39.

Smirnov A (1973). Problems in the Psychology of Memory. New York: Plenum.

Sohlberg M, Mateer C (1989). Introduction to Cognitive Rehabilitation: Theory and Practice. New York: Guilford.

Stuss DT, Benson DF (1986). The Frontal Lobes. New York: Raven.

Szekeres S (1988). Organization and Recall in the Young Language Impaired Child. Doctoral dissertation, University of Pittsburgh, Pittsburgh, PA.

Szekeres S (1992). Organization as an intervention target after traumatic brain injury. Semin Speech Lang 13;293.

Tranel D, Damasio AR (1995). Neurobiological Foundations of Human Memory. In AD Baddeley, BA Wilson, FN Watts (eds), Handbook of Memory Disorders. New York: Wiley, 27.

Tulving E (1995). Organization of Memory: Quo Vadis? In MS Gazzaniga (ed), The Cognitive Neurosciences. Cambridge, MA: MIT Press, 839.

Vygotsky LS (1978). Mind in Society: The Development of Higher Psychological Processes. Edited and translated by M Cole, V John-Steiner, S Scribner, E Souberman. Cambridge, MA: Harvard University.

Wellman H, Fabricius W, Sophian C (1985). The Early Development of Planning. In HM Wellman (ed), The Development of Search Skill and Spatial Representation. Hillsdale, NJ: Lawrence Erlbaum, 123.

Wellman HM, Ritter R, Flavell JH (1975). Deliberate memory behavior in the delayed reactions of very young children. Dev Psychol 11;780.

Westby CE (1994). The Effects of Culture on Genre, Structure, and Style of Oral and Written Texts. In G Wallach, K Butler (eds), Language Learning Disabilities in School-Age Children and Adolescents. Columbus, OH: Merrill, 180.

Westby CE, Roman R (1995). Finding the balance: learning to live in two worlds. Top Lang Disord 15(4);68.

Ylvisaker M, Feeney T (1996). Executive functions after traumatic brain injury: supported cognition and self-advocacy. Semin Speech Lang 17;217.

Ylvisaker M, Szekeres S, Hartwick P (1992). Cognitive Rehabilitation Following Traumatic Brain Injury. In M Tramontana, S Hooper (eds), Advances in Child Neuropsychology, vol 1. New York: Springer, 168.

Ylvisaker M, Szekeres SF, Hartwick P, Tworek P (1994). Cognitive Intervention. In R Savage, G Wolcott (eds), Educational Dimensions of Acquired Brain Injury. Austin, TX: PRO-ED, 121.

Chapter 12

Cognitive Rehabilitation: Executive Functions

Mark Ylvisaker, Shirley F. Szekeres, and Timothy J. Feeney

In this chapter, we discuss themes that are traditionally presented separately for cognitive rehabilitation specialists, educators or special educators, speech-language pathologists, neuropsychologists, school psychologists, occupational therapists, social workers, recreational therapists, vocational specialists, and others. These professionals are the primary intended audience for this chapter. As in Chapter 11, we have elected to address the themes in an integrated rather than a discipline-specific manner for two important reasons. First, the difficulty that many children and adolescents with traumatic brain injury (TBI) experience in controlling and efficiently using their cognitive abilities in learning contexts; controlling their behavior (including communication behavior) in social contexts; doing what it takes to translate cognitive, academic, and physical skills into vocational success; and in other ways directing themselves to do what they are capable of doing and what needs to be done to achieve their goals typically results from the same underlying executive system weakness. Second, to present these themes in separate chapters for different groups of professionals runs the risk of suggesting that a fragmented intervention program can meet the needs of children and adolescents whose internal fragmentation requires intensely integrative and collaborative rehabilitation and special education programs. Although members of the physical restoration team, nursing staff, and family members are not the primary audience for this chapter, they are certainly primary deliverers of cognitive rehabilitation services and as such a strong commitment to collaboration with those with special expertise in the cognitive dimensions of behavior is required.

We recommend that this chapter be read in conjunction with Chapters 9–14. At several points in this chapter, we make the assumption that the reader either is familiar with material in those chapters or will read them to pursue specific themes in greater depth. We especially hope that the reader will study Chapter 9. Many of the practical recommendations made in the current chapter are based on theoretical and empirical supports discussed in that chapter. Themes detailed in Chapter 11, too, intersect with those discussed in this chapter. Indeed, organizing as a cognitive activity is often included in the general category of executive functions.

Because of dramatically decreasing lengths of stay in pediatric rehabilitation centers, many of the issues discussed in this chapter may not be relevant for children and adolescents during their period of inpatient rehabilitation. Rehabilitation activities that took place in inpatient settings when lengths of stay after severe TBI were counted in months now take place, if at all, in homes or schools, because rehabilitation lengths of stay for children with comparable injuries are now typically counted in days or weeks. Nevertheless, it is critical that inpatient staff have solid expertise in the areas of executive system intervention, because it is the staff members' job to ensure that family members and staff at the next level of rehabilitation or education are as well oriented and trained as possible to carry on the rehabilitation efforts begun in a medical setting. Indeed, from a cognitive perspective, orienting and training those people who will be involved with the child in the future, and collaborating with them in developing effective reintegration programs, are often the most important contributions of cognitive specialists who work in inpatient rehabilitation facilities (see Chapter 20). In today's health care climate, inpatient staff typically play a more critical role as consultants to and educators of family members and subsequent professionals than as direct providers of cognitive rehabilitative services. This theme cannot be overemphasized and guides much of our thinking about cognitive rehabilitation.

In the early sections of this chapter, we plot out the territory and clarify our general orientation to executive system rehabilitation. We believe that this background information merits careful study because it provides the theoretical support for the practical intervention suggestions that follow. In the absence of solid theoretical and empirical grounding, intervention suggestions are justifiably seen as laundry lists of procedures that may be useful but that also may be more passing fancy than scientifically defensible rehabilitative measures. In the sections devoted to assessment and intervention, we present procedures and recommendations that we hope will guide clinicians and teachers in their search for practical and effective interventions and supports for children and adolescents with TBI. These sections should be used as a clinical resource rather than read as continuous text. Also in this chapter is a checklist that clinicians and teachers can use to develop and evaluate their interventions as they relate to executive functions.

Foundations of Executive System Rehabilitation

Intervention Premises

The selection of themes to be discussed in this chapter and the intervention activities and procedures that we recommend are based on a small set of premises. Several of these premises are discussed at greater length in Chapter 9.

Executive Control Functions

Premise I states that the executive system includes a variety of control functions that are responsible for directing and regulating cognitive as well as social behavior. The executive system comprises those mental functions involved in formulating goals, planning how to achieve them, carrying out the plans, and revising those plans in the event of failure (Lezak, 1982). The same set of control functions operates in relation to cognitive behavior (e.g., paying attention in the presence of distractions), communication behavior (e.g., planning an organized way to express a complex thought), social behavior (e.g., directing oneself to be polite around irritating people), academic behavior (e.g., efficiently studying for a difficult examination), and vocational behavior (e.g., planning a day at work to complete all of the assigned tasks). An operational definition of executive functions is given in the next section.

Problems with Executive Function After TBI

Premise II holds that problems with executive functions are common after TBI in children and adolescents and have far-reaching effects. Executive functions are associated with frontal (or prefrontal) regions of the brain, which are the most vulnerable brain structures in closed head injury in children and adults, whether the injuries are mild, moderate, or severe (Levin et al., 1991a, 1993; Stuss and Benson, 1986). Therefore, issues associated with executive system impairment are frequently encountered during rehabilitation and special education after

TBI. Executive system impairment can be devastating for a child or adult. First, specific cognitive, academic, vocational, and linguistic skills are of little benefit if the individual cannot efficiently use them in real life. Second, executive system weakness is often associated with behavioral and psychosocial problems, which are the most difficult problems for loved ones, peers, and professionals. Third, if executive functions are seriously impaired, then the individual is unlikely to be actively engaged in rehabilitation and his or her ability to compensate strategically for any disability, including executive function disability, is compromised. The frequency and impact of executive system problems after TBI place them at center stage in the planning of rehabilitative and special education services.

Delayed Executive System Problems

According to premise III, executive system consequences of TBI in children and adolescents are often delayed and may worsen over time. This is one of the dominant themes in the growing literature on frontal lobe injury in young children. Delayed developmental consequences are presumably related to some combination of slow maturation of prefrontal parts of the brain (i.e., the child "grows into" the disability because part of the neurologic makeup needed for future development is injured), behavioral and emotional responses to disability, and ineffective education and behavior management after the injury. In adolescents also, this theme appears to apply, although in this group it is less well documented. The possibility of delayed consequences requires that a long-term monitoring system be put in place for children with TBI and that rehabilitation and education professionals think in terms of preventive intervention before problems escalate. This theme of delayed consequences is elaborated later in this chapter.

Linking Intervention to Normal Executive Function Development

Premise IV states that normal development of executive functions yields insights for intervention. Increasingly, developmental cognitive psychologists have recognized the early onset (in infancy) of development of executive functions and the simultaneous and reciprocal development throughout childhood and adolescence of all components within the entire domain of cognitive processes and systems. Both of these findings support an early and ongoing focus on executive functions throughout the postcoma stages of recovery after brain injury and throughout the childhood years. Furthermore, observation of normally developing children reveals that executive functions develop in ways that are tied concretely to specific contexts and domains of content. This finding supports a highly contextualized approach to rehabilitation for people with executive system impairment. Finally, executive functions develop in part as a result of routine interactions between children and their parents, teachers, and others who possess more mature executive functions. This vygotskyan theme (Vygotsky, 1978) is critical for planning rehabilitation for children and is elaborated in Chapter 20.

Variable Impairment Depending on Type of Brain Injury

Premise V holds that different types of brain injury can result in differential impairment of executive functions. Whereas neurologists and neuropsychologists once spoke of a frontal lobe syndrome, they now recognize a large number of distinguishable executive system problems associated with differential damage to the frontal lobes. The most common division is between problems related to impaired inhibition and problems related to impaired initiation. However, a wide variety of cognitive, communicative, and behavioral problems and combinations of problems is possible (Levin et al., 1993). An effort is currently under way to identify distinguishable components of executive system impairment by means of factor analysis of test results from children with TBI and other neurologic disabilities (e.g., Levin et al., 1996; Taylor et al., 1996). Clearly, there is sufficient variety in impairment to render a general executive system "curriculum" for children and adolescents with TBI an ill-conceived contribution to rehabilitation.

Beyond Formal Testing

According to premise VI, assessment of executive functions requires contextualized exploration beyond the use of formal tests. Formal assessment of executive functions is a potentially paradoxical enterprise. The paradox is illustrated by juxtaposing the following two statements:

1. Executive system assessment includes the attempt to understand how effectively an individual can size up a possibly confusing situation, decide what to do to achieve meaningful goals, plan how to do it, do it and stick to it until it is done, pay attention to how effectively it was done, and identify a clever way to do it better if necessary.
2. In a testing situation, in contrast, tasks are presented clearly in a sterile environment; the goal and ground rules are set by the evaluator; the evaluator provides the motivation, initiation, and encouragement and takes responsibility for evaluating performance; and rarely is there an opportunity for the tested individual to try the task again, having learned from the experience of the first try.

Not surprisingly, many people with frontal lobe injury perform misleadingly well on tests, including purported tests of frontal lobe functioning. On the other hand, some people with executive system impairment—and very likely people with executive system immaturity (e.g., infants, toddlers)—perform better in their real worlds than would be predicted by test performance, because the routines and familiar stimulus cues of the real world guide their behavior. In light of these findings, it is necessary to systematically explore the executive dimensions of behavior in real-world contexts and with real-world tasks and stressors. The theme of contextualized assessment is elaborated later in this chapter and in Chapter 10.

An Integrated Executive System Orientation

Premise VII states that in related areas of disability intervention that have a longer history than does TBI rehabilitation, there has been a steady move away from an exclusive focus on specific skills toward an integrated executive system orientation. The early history of program development after disability categories such as mental retardation, specific learning disability, and attention deficit disorder were identified focused on exercises designed to remediate deficits at the lowest possible level of cognitive functioning (e.g., attention, perception, basic organization) (Mann, 1979). Since the 1970s, steadily increasing attention has been given to helping students to compensate strategically for disability that in many cases cannot be fully eliminated through remedial exercises. The more recent and more compressed history (i.e., same stages, less time) of cognitive rehabilitation for people with TBI has followed a similar course, moving from an enthusiastic focus on hierarchically organized remedial exercises designed to restore cognitive skills and eliminate deficits to an acknowledgment that chronic disability requires intensive efforts to maximize individuals' executive functions in natural contexts, thereby enabling them to strategically achieve goals that may appear unachievable because of disability.

Intervention in the Context of Everyday Routines

Premise VIII holds that intervention for impaired executive functions is ideally provided in the context of everyday routines and is designed to influence those routines. For several reasons, it is critical to provide intervention in everyday contexts and to attempt to influence everyday routines, emphasizing the executive components of those routines. First, studies in cognitive science and developmental cognitive psychology yield the important conclusion that executive functions and other cognitive skills, although inherently generalizable, nevertheless do not transfer readily to tasks and settings that are very different from the tasks and settings in which the skill was acquired (Singley and Anderson, 1989). This domain specificity of executive functions is especially true of young children and individuals who are concrete thinkers as a result of frontal lobe injury or immaturity. Second, the number of learning trials a child receives is increased if people who interact daily with the child (so-called everyday people) use everyday routines as the context for facilitating improvement in executive functions. Third, intervention becomes better integrated if it focuses on everyday people consistently encouraging improvement of executive functions. Finally, close work with everyday people helps to ensure that improvements in executive functions will not be lost because some adults behave in ways that are incompatible with executive system improvement (e.g., doing everything for the child, solving all of the child's problems).

Intervention as a Collaborative Enterprise

Premise IX states that executive system intervention is a collaborative enterprise, in which everyday people are the ideal providers of services and supports. This premise is actually a corollary of premise VIII but is worth highlighting because its implications are not always embraced by practicing clinicians. Because of time constraints, logistic difficulties, documentation problems, or other less concrete forces that drive professionals into insularity, it is all too common for rehabilitation and special education professionals to attempt to address their discipline-specific domain of goals in relative isolation. For reasons mentioned in connection with premise VIII, this isolationist approach results in inefficient intervention at best, particularly in an age of shrinking lengths of stay and reduced funding for medical rehabilitation. One of the goals of this chapter is to promote a collaborative approach to executive system rehabilitation, in which all professionals and everyday people are identified as the critical providers of services and supports and everyday routines are the critical context of intervention. For example, for a child interested in sports, the most important facilitators of executive system improvement may be the physical therapist, coach, and parents.

Clinicians' Self-Perceptions as a Potential Roadblock

Finally, premise X holds that clinicians' perceptions of themselves may be an obstacle to sound intervention. Many rehabilitation professionals are trained to think of themselves (metaphorically) as a cross between a surgeon (i.e., diagnosing and treating medical disorders in medical settings) and a trainer (i.e., formulating behavioral objectives and subjecting clients to large numbers of carefully planned learning trials to equip them with needed behaviors). These powerful metaphors, although applicable to some aspects of rehabilitation, can block development of real-world coaching, consulting, and apprenticeship relationships necessary for effective facilitation of the recovery and maturation of executive functions. This theme is elaborated in Chapter 20.

The Executive Control System

From a practical, everyday perspective, executive functions, based on the metaphor of a business executive's role in relation to the functioning of a company, include (1) knowing enough about oneself to know what is easy and what is difficult to do, (2) setting reasonable goals based on this knowledge, (3) planning and organizing behavior to achieve the goals, (4) initiating behavior toward achievement of the goals, (5) inhibiting behavior that would interfere with achieving the goals, (6) monitoring and evaluating performance in relation to the goals, and (7) thinking strategically and solving problems flexibly if obstacles arise. These processes can operate deliberately (e.g., when a mature adult forgoes a short-term pleasure in pursuit of a long-term goal). More commonly, though, they operate automatically (e.g., when one maintains a topic in conversation despite the many diverse thoughts that move through one's consciousness).

Later in this chapter, we offer some suggestions for addressing separately the components of executive functioning, because it is possible for brain injury to affect specific components differentially, leaving some components relatively intact. However, the components of the executive system are linked in important ways and together determine whether one will be a mature, responsible, strategically thinking, self-controlled human being across a variety of domains of functioning—that is, maintaining an appropriate problem-solving set for attainment of future goals and profiting efficiently from feedback in the pursuit of those goals (Luria, 1966; Welsh and Pennington, 1988). Therefore, a dominant theme of this chapter is that there is a profound advantage in addressing executive functions in an integrated functional manner, targeting all components simultaneously and crossing all relevant contexts.

Executive Functions and Cognition

Presumably the same control functions are responsible for directing and regulating both cognitive and social-interactive behavior. However, much of the research and theoretical literature in this area has focused on regulation of *cognitive* functions. For example, the tests that are often used to assess executive functions include those that measure control of attention (e.g., Gordon Diagnostic System [1988]), flexibility in shifting from one cognitive or perceptual set to another (e.g., Wisconsin Card Sorting Test [Chelune and Baer, 1986]; Trail Making B of the Halstead-Reitan Battery [Reitan, 1987]; and strategic problem solving (e.g., Tower of London [Levin et al., 1991b]). Furthermore, at the same time that professionals in the fields of neuropsychology and adult rehabilitation were developing a conceptual framework around the concept of executive functions, educational psychologists (e.g., Borkowski et al., 1986, 1990; Brown, 1975; Deshler and Schumaker, 1988; Pressley and El-Dinary, 1992; Pressley et al., 1989) and developmental cognitive psychologists (e.g., Flavell et al., 1993) were exploring the related concept of metacognition from theoretical and practical perspectives. These historical observations help to explain the disproportionate emphasis on cognition in discussions of executive functions. The current chapter similarly focuses on executive control of cognitive functions. However, in Chapter 13, we continue the executive system theme as it applies to behavior and social-interactive competence.

It is likely that educators are more familiar with executive function themes in discussion of metacognition, which includes components of the knowledge base as well as the executive system. There is a *static*, knowledge-based aspect of metacognition (e.g., knowing about one's cognitive functioning; understanding what factors affect performance from a cognitive perspective; knowing that there are procedures [strategies] that can be used to make cognitive processes more efficient) as well as a *dynamic executive control* aspect. For educators, the executive component includes knowing when one needs help, checking one's work, and deliberately controlling attempts to solve problems, study, and learn (Brown, 1975). People who know that certain cognitive functions are weak (e.g., organization) and that there are procedures that can be used to compensate for the weakness (e.g., outlining strategies) but who fail to put this knowledge to use in relevant tasks have what Flavell and coworkers (1993) called a "production deficiency"—that is, weak executive control over cognitive functions. Research in this area has formed the foundation for investigations of strategy intervention, which is popular in current educational practices (Pressley, 1993; Pressley et al., 1990; Pressley and Levin, 1983a, b).

Executive Functions and Social Behavior

Less attention has been paid to the concept of executive functions in relation to social-interactive behavior than in relation to cognition. Although self-regulation of behavior has received increasing attention in recent years among behavioral psychologists, rarely is this important topic discussed within the broader confines of executive functions. However, observation of normally developing preschoolers as well as older children with frontal lobe injury reveals the very real possibility that people may know the rules, roles, and routines that apply to a social situation yet behave inappropriately—without being oppositional or defiant: That is, people with immature or impaired executive systems may know what to do but fail to do it because they are distracted, fail to suppress intervening impulses, fail to correctly interpret the situation in which they find themselves, or fail to select the correct routine or action schema for a given task. This executive system failure is an important phenomenon in understanding and managing behavior after TBI (Feeney and Ylvisaker, 1995, 1997; Ylvisaker and Feeney, 1994, 1996, in press).

Furthermore, specific prefrontal lesions are capable of reducing an individual's ability to profit from feedback (i.e., to respond to reinforcements and punishments) in traditional behavior management programs focused primarily on managing consequences of behavior. People with this type of brain injury may fail to "mark" memories in a way that makes them helpful in guiding future decisions and behavior. They may behave as though they have no regard for potential rewards or punishments (Tranel and Damasio, 1995). Perhaps for this reason, classic descriptions of children (e.g., Ackerly, 1964; Eslinger et al., 1992) and adults (e.g., Stuss and Benson, 1986) with frontal lobe injury emphasize social-behavioral impairment and the affected individuals' reduced ability to learn from the social consequences of their behavior. Therefore, behavioral psychologists are well advised to attend to the neuropsychological aspects of frontal lobe injury, the consequences of executive system impairment, and intervention procedures that facilitate development of executive functions.

Similarly, during the last 20 years in the field of communication disorders, emphasis on pragmatics of communication, metalinguistic development, and language as a tool in problem solving and self-regulation has brought this profession squarely into the domain of executive functions, despite infrequent explicit use of the concept (see Ylvisaker, 1992, 1993; Ylvisaker and Feeney, 1996; Ylvisaker and Szekeres, 1989). Within pediatric discussions, perhaps the most substantial recognition of executive functions as a unifying theme has occurred in discussions of attention deficit hyperactivity disorder (ADHD) (e.g., Barkley, 1997; Hallowell and Ratey, 1994; Pennington, 1991; Shue and Douglas, 1992). An increasing number of researchers and clinicians have brought together under the executive-function heading the diverse list of challenges common to many children with ADHD (e.g., poorly controlled attention, lack of sustained effort, impulsiveness, disorganization in thinking and acting, socially immature behavior, reduced self-insight).

In our judgment, grouping these separate aspects of development and intervention under the same theoretical umbrella is profoundly advantageous, especially in working with individuals with frontal lobe injury and associated executive system impairment. First, the intervention efforts of diverse professionals can be integrated. Most of the proposals we offer in this chapter are intended for all professionals and everyday people who interact regularly with children with TBI. This integration increases the child's learning opportunities and facilitates generalization and maintenance. Second, it is important to recognize (potentially) common executive system roots of problems that are as diverse as lacking initiative, performing badly on a test despite understanding the material, behaving impulsively or inappropriately in social context, failing to understand assigned readings for class despite scoring normally on tests of reading comprehension, being inattentive in class, conversing in ways that are tangential and difficult to follow, pursuing unrealistic goals, and persisting with behavior that has failed repeatedly in the past. All these problems could be symptoms of a general executive system impairment.

Executive System Impairment After TBI

Executive functions are associated with frontal (or prefrontal) regions of the brain, which are the most vulnerable brain structures in closed head injury (whether mild, moderate, or severe) in children and adults (Levin et al., 1991a, 1993; Stuss and Benson, 1986). To make our point here, we simplify the complex pathophysiology of closed head injury: When a rapidly moving skull strikes a stationary object (e.g., windshield, road, floor), the brain continues to move due to inertial forces. Linear inertia causes the brain to hit the skull and compress and decompress both at the site of impact and (because of a rebound effect) on the opposite side of the skull. These coup and contrecoup injuries depend on the impact's location and may be associated with a variety of neuropsychological impairments, though the frequency with which prefrontal structures are damaged cannot be explained completely by these impacts alone. However, because most people reflexively turn away from the impact, rotational inertial forces are also present at the moment of impact, causing the brain to twist and turn within the skull.

These combined forces explain surface contusions and lacerations as well as deeper axonal shearing in places where the brain is adjacent to bony prominences within the skull, including prefrontal areas. Furthermore, the sharp bones that separate frontal from anterior, inferior, and medial temporal lobe structures can cause damage to the nerve fibers that connect these two parts of the brain. This type of injury can contribute to poorly regulated emotional reactions and to breakdowns in memory and strategic learning. Therefore, issues associated with executive system impairment figure prominently in rehabilitation after closed head injury.

If severe, executive system impairment can be devastating for a child or adult. For example, the individual may have adequate cognitive skills, as revealed by structured tests, but may fail to make effective use of those skills in everyday academic and social contexts. He or she might fail to regulate attention (short attention span, distractibility, inflexibility in shifting and dividing attention), to control and organize perceptual processes, to use appropriate encoding and retrieval strategies in learning contexts, to apply organizing schemes to complex tasks, and to think strategically and solve problems effectively. Together, these executive system problems can reduce the individual's effectiveness dramatically in academic and vocational contexts, despite the retention of adequate specific motor and cognitive skills necessary to succeed in school and on the job.

Communicative competence might be lost despite preservation of specific skills and knowledge. Types of communication impairment that are potentially associated with prefrontal injury include (1) reduced initiation or activation, resulting in a paucity of communication despite adequate specific speech and language skills; (2) reduced inhibition, possibly resulting in socially inappropriate language, volatility, and perseveration; (3) reduced social perception, resulting in socially awkward interaction; (4) difficulty with abstract and indirect language, including comprehension of verbal abstractions, figures of speech, metaphor, irony, sarcasm, and humor; (5) difficulty in organizing thoughts and language for effective comprehension and expression of extended units of language; and (6) difficulty in retrieving needed linguistic units, including words (Alexander et al., 1989). Speech and language skills are of marginal benefit if the individual does not use them efficiently in everyday interaction. Closely related to communication impairment are the behavioral and psychosocial problems associated with executive system weakness. These are typically the most troubling issues for loved ones, peers, and professionals alike.

If executive functions are seriously impaired, then the motivation to participate in rehabilitation and the ability to compensate strategically for ongoing disability, including executive function disability, are compromised. For this reason, attention to executive functions must be a high priority for rehabilitation and special education professionals.

Not all symptoms of executive system weakness are a result of TBI. It is common for adults (both professionals and parents) to assume responsibility for the executive or control aspects of behavior after a life-threatening injury in a child, thereby contributing to passivity or learned helplessness in the child. Helping adults divest themselves of this "prosthetic frontal lobe" role is a primary goal of staff and family training (Meichenbaum, 1993). For all these reasons, executive control functions are at the heart of rehabilitation and special education for most children and adolescents with severe TBI.

Delayed and Increasing Executive System Disability

A central theme that has emerged from research in the area of frontal lobe injury in children since the mid-1980s is the frequency with which consequences emerge late or grow in severity months or years after the injury (Benton, 1991; Eslinger et al., 1992; Grattan and Eslinger, 1991, 1992; Lehr, 1990; Marlowe, 1992; Mateer and Williams, 1991; Thomsen, 1989). This same phenomenon has been observed in experimental animals (primates) with early frontal lobe lesions (Goldman, 1971; Goldman and Alexander, 1977). Because anatomic and physiologic development of the frontal lobes is slow and protracted, extending into adolescence, an injury might have minimal developmental consequences until the function subserved by the injured part of the brain is expected to mature: Thus, the child may "grow into" the disability.

These delayed or worsening consequences are likely a result of the injury itself, of emotional and behavioral reactions of the individual to life's circumstances after the injury, and possibly of ineffective teaching and behavior management. Whereas the neuropsychological literature tends to emphasize the organic contributors to impairment (e.g., Grattan and Eslinger, 1992), some evidence supports the clinically more productive view that manipulable environmental factors contribute substantially to these delayed consequences (Feeney and Ylvisaker, 1995). This view holds that serious behavioral and psychosocial problems are not biological inevitabilities after severe frontal lobe injury in children and adolescents.

Delayed consequences of prefrontal injury are most readily observable in young children. For example, a 3 year old who is impulsive, a concrete thinker, egocentric, short-tempered, silly, and frequently socially inappropriate is simply a card-carrying 3 year old. However, if the child does not mature substantially in those domains by first grade (which may be the case in a child with serious prefrontal injury), he or she will stand out as having a cognitive and psychosocial disability at that time. Similarly, a first grader who is focused largely on the present, relies on adults for most planning, adds and subtracts by counting fingers, has difficulty following stories that are longer than a few pages, and has difficulty organizing discourse (spoken or written) beyond a few sentences is simply a typical first grader. However, these characteristics would signal a significant disability in a sixth grader.

Although less obvious, delayed consequences of frontal lobe injury in adolescents can similarly interfere with subsequent development and long-term academic and vocational success (Feeney and Ylvisaker, 1995; Williams and Mateer, 1992; Ylvisaker and Feeney, 1995). Table 12-1 lists critical developmental issues at each of three grossly distinguishable stages of adolescence; common cognitive, psychosocial, and communicative concerns with TBI at each stage; and common symptoms with delayed onset at that stage. From a neuropsychological perspective, ongoing development during adolescence is largely in the areas of executive functions and content knowledge. Therefore, it is not surprising that most of the concerns listed in Table 12-1 fall loosely into the category of executive functions.

Normal Development of Executive Functions

An Early Beginning, a Long Course, and Interdependence on Other Aspects of Cognitive Development

Particularly in discussions of rehabilitation, the term *higher-order* is commonly included in references to executive functions. Identifying executive functions as higher-order is often associated with a hierarchical view of cognition, according to which there are basic or lower-order processes (typically including attention and perception) and higher-order processes (typically including reasoning, problem solving, and executive functions).

Occasionally, this view of cognition is tied to a correspondingly hierarchical or serial-order-progression view of cognitive development in infancy and childhood.

Careful observation of young children and examination of recent literature in developmental cognitive psychology yield the inescapable conclusion that cognitive development is not a serial progression from acquisition of one component of cognition to another (Bjorklund, 1990; Flavell et al., 1993). For instance, young children do not master attentional skills before acquiring perceptual skills, followed by organizational skills, followed by memory skills, followed by problem-solving and reasoning skills, followed by executive control over cognitive functions (Bjorklund and Harnishfeger, 1990). In contrast, at every age and developmental level, evidence exists of at least simple and developmentally early forms of all cognitive processes and systems, each developing in ways that are linked intimately with the development of other processes and systems (Bjorklund and Harnishfeger, 1990; Flavell et al., 1993; Siegler, 1991). For example, 2 year olds possess attentional, perceptual, learning, organizational, problem-solving, and executive skills superior to those of 1 year olds but inferior to those of 3 year olds, and so on for the entire period of development. Furthermore, development in each area facilitates development in the others throughout childhood. For example, as the knowledge base grows and as organizational skills improve, so does a child's ability to maintain attention, filter out distractions, divide attention, and assimilate and encode new information efficiently. In a reciprocal fashion, as attentional skills mature, the ability to acquire and organize knowledge likewise matures.

For cognitive rehabilitation, this theme of interrelated development of components of normal cognition implies that it is unwise to organize intervention—for children or adults—around a curriculum that focuses first on socalled lower-order processes (for an extended period or at a designated stage of recovery) and subsequently on so-called higher-order processes. Rather, in rehabilitation as in normal development, the creative engagement of all cognitive processes and systems in ways that exploit their interaction and that are consistent with the individual's current level of functioning is most valuable. Furthermore, executive functions should be a primary target of intervention throughout recovery after TBI because they are so commonly impaired and because individuals with disability rely more heavily on executive functions than do other people in their efforts to succeed at everyday tasks by compensating for their disability.

Domain-Specific Development

Recent studies of transfer of cognitive skill have shown that cognitive skills in general are acquired in a way that ties them to a (broader or narrower) context or domain of content (Singley and Anderson, 1989). For example, a 4 year old who learns to guide his or her behavior appropri-

Table 12-1. Immediate and Delayed Consequences of TBI in Adolescence

Stage of Development	Key Developmental Issues	Common Concerns with TBI	Common Delayed Symptoms Related to Earlier Injury
Early adolescence			
Social, emotional, and behavioral issues	Emerging personal identity associated with short-term future goals, often involving physical accomplishments Emphasis on following a rigid code of behavior and on punishment in moral thinking Development of a cognitive map of social networks, with primary emphasis on same-gender peers • Emergence of fixed friendships, along with crowds and cliques • External locus of control, with deference to the approval or disapproval of peers	Social vulnerability • Related to separation from the clique • Related to socially awkward behavior (associated with frontal lobe injury) Role confusion and psychogenic problems ("I am not who I was"), possibly associated with physical changes caused by the injury Likelihood of behavior problems associated with vulnerability to environmental stressors (especially with frontal lobe injury)	Behavior problems associated with decreasing external control and an inability to meet the expectation for increasing behavioral self-regulation Inability to meet increasing social demands associated with puberty
Cognitive and academic issues	Increase in abstract thinking and hypotheticodeductive reasoning Increase in ability to use organizing schemes deliberately to process large amounts of information (e.g., for reading texts and writing essays)	Increasing concerns with the academic curriculum • Associated with cumulative effects of new learning problems • Associated with difficulty organizing large amounts of information • Associated with difficulty with increasingly abstract information	Increasing academic problems • Associated with cumulative effects of new learning problems • Associated with difficulty organizing large amounts • Associated with difficulty with increasingly abstract information
Middle adolescence			
Social, emotional, and behavioral issues	Increasing awareness of changes associated with puberty Increasingly heterosexual social networks Increasing need to experiment and take risks Increasing ability to manage environmental stressors, profit from feedback, and make flexible and autonomous decisions Increasing ability to read social cues	Discontinuity of personal identification due to physical and cognitive changes Breakdown in social grouping associated with communication and other changes Difficulty managing increasing environmental stressors; ongoing rigidity in responding; inability to profit from feedback Experimentation and risk taking at dangerous levels Possible "hyperegocentrism," with focus on the injury Difficulty reading social cues	Continued rigidity and dependence on external control while peers become increasingly flexible and autonomous Hypersexuality Social withdrawal
Cognitive, academic, and vocational issues	Decreasing egocentrism, resulting in increasing ability to communicate varied thoughts and feelings competently in varied social settings	Difficulty with increasingly demanding curriculum Possibly increasing incongruity between vocational goals and vocational	Increasing academic failure due to cumulative effect of new learning problems Difficulty achieving communicative effectiveness in

Stage of Development	Key Developmental Issues	Common Concerns with TBI	Common Delayed Symptoms Related to Earlier Injury
	Emerging vocational goals and long-range goal planning	potential after the injury	varied social settings requiring varied social registers General difficulty with divergent thinking and flexible problem solving
Late adolescence			
Social, emotional, and behavioral issues	Loosening and shifting of social networks, based on vocational and social needs Reduction in risk taking Increasing ability to identify sources of stress and adjust behavior accordingly (self-management) Continued reduction in egocentrism and growth in attention to the needs of others (a lifelong process) Increasing romantic relationships focused on companionship and love Solidification of communication styles	Regression to rigid behavior, egocentric perspective, and dependence on external control; difficulty considering alternative perspectives Inability to anticipate and recognize stressors and alter behavior accordingly Loss of social networks; possible dependence on old social networks In sexual relations, persistent focus on physical aspects	Retention of concrete thinking and rigid responding Immature social skills; continued dependence on cliques while peers move on Continued dependence on same-gender peers for support; relations with opposite gender possibly characterized by hypersexuality Possible perception of differences between self and others as representing a psychiatric problem
Cognitive, academic, and vocational issues	Solidification of vocational and academic goals; organization of behavior in pursuit of these goals Increasingly mature understanding of academic and vocational potential	Regression to rigid and concrete communication; loss of subtlety, abstractness, and flexibility in communication Incongruity of previous academic or vocational goals and current abilities	Possible failure in college or on the job due to the elimination of the supports provided in high school

Note: By *delayed consequences* we mean symptoms associated with an earlier injury (probably incurred at the previous developmental stage), often observed in adolescents whose recovery had earlier appeared to be generally good.
Source: Modified with permission from M Ylvisaker, T Feeney (1995). Traumatic brain injury in adolescence: assessment and reintegration. Semin Speech Lang 16;32.

ately through the routines of preschool and even to make good flexible decisions in the event of deviations from routines in that context may remain wholly incapable of guiding his or her behavior and making good decisions in another setting. Failure of broad transfer of cognitive skill is one reason for the growing skepticism about Piaget's structuralist theory of cognitive development.

At a higher developmental level, a college student who learns to reason effectively and to avoid common fallacies in logic class might continue to commit the very same fallacies in political science or physics classes. Broad transfer of cognitive skill appears to be strikingly difficult for most human beings. Of course, some abstract thinkers are able to induce highly general cognitive principles, rules, or representations and apply them flexibly

to multiple domains of content (for example, applying a subtle piece of baseball strategy to economic policy). However, most people, particularly those with immature or damaged prefrontal regions of the brain, operate with cognitive representations, including rules of self-regulation, that are more concretely associated with specific domains of content and context.

This domain specificity of executive functions in children is illustrated by a 6 year old who, while being videotaped, was given a miniature candy bar to share with her 3-year-old sister. "I can share," she said as she broke the candy. "Oh, no; these aren't even pieces. Well, I know what I can do. I will give the bigger piece to my sister because she is littler than me, she likes candy more than I do, and I don't want to hurt her feelings." Then the camera was turned off and the girls' father, who was in the room at the time, said, "What you need to know is that there has never been anything remotely like this event in the history of our family." Under normal circumstances in the house, he said, the two sisters would have fought tooth and nail for the larger piece. In the thick of battle, the 6 year old was unable to govern her behavior with the rules of socially appropriate behavior she had learned. However, with the camera on, she slipped easily into a script she had learned thoroughly as a result of patient coaching and innumerable reminders from her parents.

Professionals in the field of TBI rehabilitation can easily produce many analogues to this developmental phenomenon. For example, a 29-year-old woman with frontal lobe injury was told, during an assessment, that she could have a dollar if she selected it on the first try after it had been hidden in one of 12 identical containers and spun on a lazy Susan. The remaining rule was that she could use whatever was on the table (there were stickers on the table) to assist her. She replied, "You mean I can use one of these stickers? Easy!" The dollar then was hidden and the evaluator paused, waiting for the woman to place the sticker on the container in which the dollar had been placed. However, she did nothing. When reminded that she was going to do something, she said, "I am; I'm using my memory" (which certainly would not help), and later, "I'm counting them" (which would be equally unhelpful). Like the 6 year old, this woman had preserved knowledge of how to solve a problem but failed to act on this knowledge when it was most important to do so. When pressed to act, she opted for solutions that were ineffective or absurd. As expected, this woman was very successful in her "talk therapy" sessions but, on the nursing unit, she had developed a reputation as a short-tempered, combative, and often confused person (like the 6 year old who would fight with her little sister).

An analogous context dependency is illustrated by a 10 year old with a history of brain injury (having suffered anoxia at age 5). Staff members at his school were very concerned about his safety judgment at school and on the playground and were worried about the freedom given to the boy at home. When playing or moving through the halls, he often seemed unable to attend to more than one stimulus at a time and consequently placed himself in harm's way if he were not carefully monitored. Furthermore, although he had been at the same school for 3 years, he still had difficulty remembering the basic routines of his classroom. A visit to his farm home, however, revealed that he was very secure in his daily routines, including chores with the animals, and was not at risk in a familiar environment that held more apparent dangers than did his school environment.

This domain specificity of executive functions has implications for assessment that are explored in Chapter 10 and that are reviewed briefly later in this chapter. Equally important are the implications for intervention. For example, von Cramon and Matthes–von Cramon (1994) described the cognitive rehabilitation of a physician (pathologist) with discrete bilateral frontal lobe injury and consequent executive system dysfunction. Before his rehabilitation, which began 9 years after injury, he was unable to hold a job, largely because he could not deal effectively with nonroutine problems in novel or unpredictable situations and seemed not to benefit from external feedback or prompts. His cognitive rehabilitation occurred entirely in a pathology laboratory (i.e., an extended work trial) and focused on helping this physician develop a routine (or "metaroutine") for dealing with problems, including novel problems, that arise in the laboratory. Despite no change in his basic cognitive competence after the 12 months of training (a result that was expected), the subject acquired a routine of using problem-attack and problem-solving strategies sufficient to succeed *in that setting* and was therefore able to maintain his (supported) employment for another 2 years.

The case study of this physician illustrates the important theme of domain specificity of executive functions, particularly in people who are concrete thinkers as a result of frontal lobe injury. There is every reason to believe that this theme is even more applicable to children whose executive functions are immature before injury. The implications for rehabilitation of this domain specificity of cognitive processes was highlighted in Schacter's now classic critique of traditional decontextualized cognitive retraining (Schacter and Glisky, 1986). Case illustrations of contextualized executive function rehabilitation were presented by Ylvisaker and Feeney (1996).

Assessment: Contextualized Exploration of Executive Functions

During the last 10 years, neuropsychologists have been active in developing and validating tests for use in evaluating executive system functioning in children. Some of these tests are downward extensions of tests previously developed for adults (e.g., Levin et al., 1991b, 1996), whereas others are existing developmental tests that have been given a neuropsychological interpretation (e.g., Dennis, 1991; Welsh and Pennington, 1988; Welsh et al., 1991) or are tests newly developed specifically to evaluate components of executive functioning in children (e.g., Dennis and Barnes, 1990). This work holds considerable potential for deepening our knowledge of executive system development in children and of consequences of frontal lobe injury.

In Chapter 10, Ylvisaker and Gioia emphasize the use of collaborative, contextualized hypothesis-testing assessment as the most critical procedure if the goal is to learn how to help a child improve and succeed in school, social life, and other challenging tasks. They offer several reasons for this emphasis, including the well-documented fact that many children and adults with prefrontal injury maintain relatively good performance on standardized tests, including those tests specifically designed to detect the effects of prefrontal injury, though they have difficulty performing effectively on real-world tasks in stressful contexts, such as school (Benton, 1991; Bigler, 1988; Dennis, 1991; Eslinger and Damasio, 1985; Grattan and Eslinger, 1991; Mateer and Williams, 1991; Stelling et al., 1986; Stuss and Benson, 1986; Welsh et al., 1991). Ylvisaker and Gioia cite Lezak's (1982) "paradox of executive system assessment," the paradox inherent in presenting brief and highly structured tasks in a highly controlled environment to determine how effectively the individual can set goals, plan and organize behavior in pursuit of those goals, pay attention to performance, remain focused over time, and flexibly solve problems that arise in the context of unstructured and challenging tasks in complex real-world contexts. The evaluator and evaluation context easily become the prosthetic frontal lobes for the individual with frontal lobe injury (Stuss and Benson, 1986). Alternatively, children may perform better in real-world contexts than is predicted by their performance on formal tests because their performance in context is supported by well-rehearsed routines and well-established stimulus cues. In either case, test performance must be validated by systematic observation of performance in important real-world contexts.

Furthermore, prefrontal injury (and executive system impairment) may have as its primary symptom social disability, including disinhibited, overly familiar, and otherwise socially inappropriate behavior; lack of social initiation; difficulty in reading social cues and interpreting social situations; difficulty in organizing complex social responses; rigid social behavior; awkward behavior in novel situations; and failure to respond to feedback from communication partners in social situations (Brown et al., 1981; Fletcher et al., 1990; Marlowe, 1992; Mateer and Williams, 1991; Perrott et al., 1991; Petterson, 1991; Price et al., 1990; Thomsen, 1989). Because it may not be possible to detect these symptoms outside natural social contexts, assessment of social-interactive competence requires, at a minimum, observation of the individual in a variety of social contexts and in the presence of a variety of social stressors.

We recommend that you read Chapter 10 for considerable detail regarding executive system assessment, particularly the use of collaborative, contextualized hypothesis-testing assessment. In the current chapter, we wish to augment the discussion in that chapter by highlighting four aspects of assessment that have particular relevance to executive system intervention: executive function interviews, negotiated assessment, self-assessment, and executive function rating scales.

Executive Function Interviews

Engaging individuals in dialogue about their abilities as a part of everyday routine is useful. Before an activity, children can be asked whether the task will be easy or difficult and why. If relevant, children can be asked for a prediction of how well they will do and what they plan to do to succeed. During the task, specific opportunities for initiation and inhibition can be created. Furthermore, children can be asked to report on how well they are doing as they proceed. After completing the task, children can be asked to describe how well they did and how that performance compares to the prediction. In addition, they can be asked what special procedures they used to succeed. It might be necessary to give children some options and to ask whether they used any of them. In addition to yielding important assessment information, these conversations, which can be used by all staff and family members and which should be natural and nonthreatening, encourage engagement of the child's executive functions throughout the day.

Negotiated Assessment

A useful strategy, particularly for the adolescent who refuses to accept professionals' judgments about his or her limitations, is to engage the individual (and possibly also family members) in identifying a way to settle the conflict. The gist of the communication to the adolescent is, "You and I seem to disagree about your strengths and needs at this point. What can you do to prove to me that I'm wrong and you're right, that you can succeed in areas where I am afraid you can't succeed now?" For example, if the student is returning to school, it might be possible to teach some academic content currently being taught in school and then to administer the school's test. Finding such a litmus test is not always possible but, when it is possible, the results of the experiment generally are more meaningful to the individual and family than are specialized test results.

Often patients in a rehabilitation facility are simply told in an authoritative fashion that they are unable to succeed in a regular classroom or to take care of themselves with no adult supervision or to safely resume favored recreational activities, an appeal to authority that predictably alienates and angers many people. In contrast, the process of negotiating assessment tasks, even if unsuccessful, carries the potential to promote collaborative and collegial relationships and to educate the individual and family about the practical consequences of the injury. In addition, the possibility always exists that staff members have assumed an overly pessimistic view and will be proved wrong.

Self-Assessment

Figure 12-1 presents a protocol for formulating an individualized education plan (IEP) that relies on a self-assessment instrument, presented in Figure 12-2. Both were developed for use with adolescents with

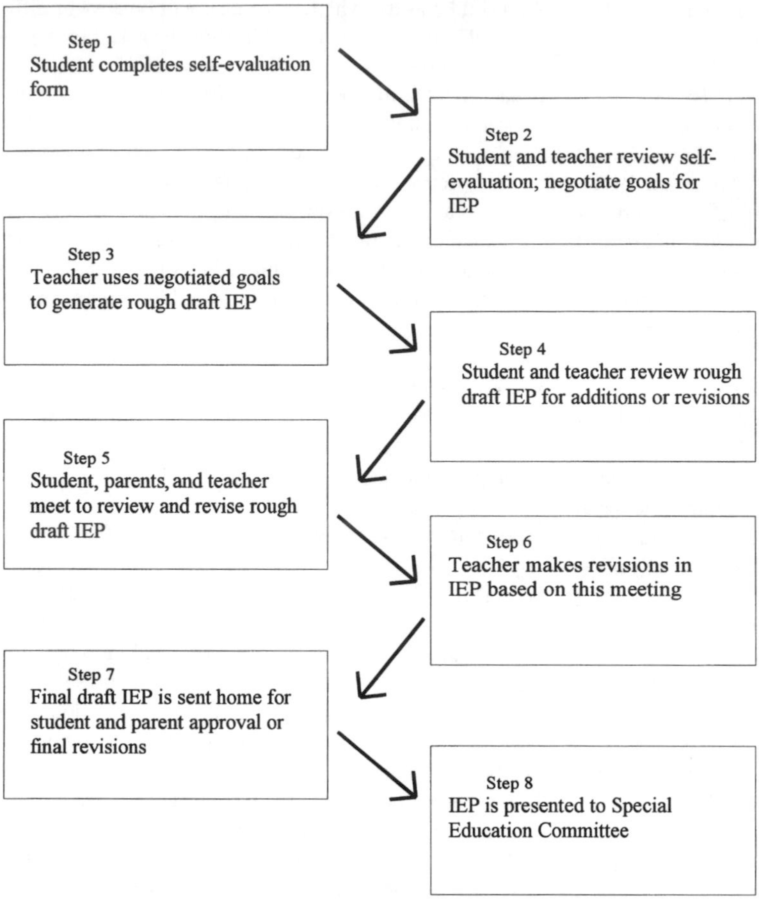

Figure 12-1. Flowchart representing sequential stages in the development of student-generated individualized education plans (IEPs). (Copyright 1994, K Ylvisaker.)

learning disabilities served in a high-school resource room. The point of the self-assessment process is to help adolescents with cognitive and social disability gain greater insight into their strengths and needs, become more engaged in their education, and take greater responsibility for their academic program. Areas identified by the student as areas of need (perhaps with some guidance) can then be stressed in the IEP and intervention program, whereas areas identified as strengths can be exploited in the development of compensations. If students are encouraged to participate in their assessment, the likelihood is increased that they can be engaged in collaboratively identifying solutions to their academic problems. Because many students with TBI have a similar or more pronounced unawareness of their strengths and needs, this self-assessment process can also serve an important educational and counseling purpose for them.

Executive Function Rating Scales

Figure 12-3 presents a rating scale that can be used to alert diverse staff and family members to important components of executive functions. Under each heading in the table, raters have the opportunity to give a child or adolescent a grade-level rating and to rate the degree to which that component of executive functioning actually interferes with classroom success. In the few clinical trials to which this rating system has been subjected, we have found that staff members who work with grade-school–age students have little difficulty with the grade levels; however, grade-level placement is more difficult for middle-school and high-school teachers, who seem to prefer rating the degree of problem represented by the component of executive functioning. In either case, a primary advantage of scales of this sort is that they communicate a vocabulary and conceptual framework to staff who might otherwise be inattentive to executive functions.

The scales are intended to teach staff about important areas of executive functioning and to track general improvement rather than to acquire psychometrically sound assessment data for diagnostic purposes. As long as the scales are used only for this clinical or educational purpose and staff in a particular setting achieve general consistency in the application of these scales, the absence of solid reliability information is not troubling.

Student's name: _____

Form completed by: _____ Date: _____

Study skills

I'm pretty good or very good at	I'm okay but not great at	I have a hard time	
❏	❏	❏	understanding what I'm good at and what I'm not good at.
❏	❏	❏	setting reasonable goals for myself.
❏	❏	❏	listening to directions in class.
❏	❏	❏	remembering to bring materials to class.
❏	❏	❏	keeping my class materials organized.
❏	❏	❏	keeping track of assignments.
❏	❏	❏	knowing how much time tasks will take.
❏	❏	❏	getting started on assignments soon enough.
❏	❏	❏	remembering to bring homework home.
❏	❏	❏	taking time to do my assignments and homework well.
❏	❏	❏	knowing what to do when I get stuck on assignments when I'm at home.
❏	❏	❏	completing homework.
❏	❏	❏	completing assignments on time.
❏	❏	❏	remembering to turn in my assignments.
❏	❏	❏	understanding what I'm reading.
❏	❏	❏	answering questions about what I have read.
❏	❏	❏	summarizing what I have read.
❏	❏	❏	working with the teacher on something that's difficult for me.
❏	❏	❏	telling my resource room teacher what I need to work on.
❏	❏	❏	making good use of resource room support, assistants, or other support.
❏	❏	❏	using the library for assignments or research.

Tests and test taking

I'm pretty good or very good at	I'm okay but not great at	I have a hard time	
❏	❏	❏	knowing what to study for tests.
❏	❏	❏	knowing how to study for tests.
❏	❏	❏	spending enough time studying for tests.
❏	❏	❏	reading all of the words on examinations.
❏	❏	❏	understanding the questions on examinations.
❏	❏	❏	finishing examinations within the class period at school.
❏	❏	❏	remaining relaxed and focused during examinations.

Others:

❏	❏	❏	_____
❏	❏	❏	_____

Written expression

I'm pretty good or very good at	I'm okay but not great at	I have a hard time	
❏	❏	❏	taking notes in class or from reading assignments.

Figure 12-2. Student self-evaluation for developing an individualized education plan. (Copyright 1994, K Ylvisaker.)

❑	❑	❑	thinking of topics for open assignments or assigned essays.
❑	❑	❑	knowing exactly what the teacher is asking for in writing assignments.
❑	❑	❑	getting started on a composition.
❑	❑	❑	expressing my ideas clearly in writing.
❑	❑	❑	elaborating on my thoughts and making my papers long enough.
❑	❑	❑	organizing my ideas and topics in a paper.
❑	❑	❑	dividing my writing into paragraphs.
❑	❑	❑	forming good sentences.
❑	❑	❑	using correct punctuation, grammar, and spelling.
❑	❑	❑	proofreading and checking my written work before handing it in.
❑	❑	❑	completing writing assignments on time.

Others:

❑	❑	❑	_____
❑	❑	❑	_____

General school issues and behavior

I'm pretty good or very good at	I'm okay but not great at	I have a hard time	
❑	❑	❑	attending school regularly and consistently.
❑	❑	❑	getting to classes on time.
❑	❑	❑	expressing my concerns and needs clearly to my teachers.
❑	❑	❑	paying attention in class.
❑	❑	❑	understanding what the teacher is talking about.
❑	❑	❑	working with other students.
❑	❑	❑	finding other students with whom to work on group projects.
❑	❑	❑	doing presentations in front of the class.
❑	❑	❑	asking questions in class.
❑	❑	❑	asking for help when I need it.
❑	❑	❑	getting along with my teachers.
❑	❑	❑	organizing my time to get everything done.
❑	❑	❑	motivating myself to do what I know I need to do.
❑	❑	❑	following the rules in class and in school.
❑	❑	❑	thinking about what I do before I act.

Social and interpersonal skills

I'm pretty good or very good at	I'm okay but not great at	I have a hard time	
❑	❑	❑	finding people I enjoy as friends.
❑	❑	❑	relating easily to new acquaintances.
			listening to others.
❑	❑	❑	talking to others about my ideas, thoughts, and feelings.
❑	❑	❑	feeling that other people understand me or care about me.
❑	❑	❑	helping other people.
❑	❑	❑	congratulating others when something good happens to them.
❑	❑	❑	losing graciously, without complaining or pouting.

Figure 12-2. *Continued*

❑   ❑   ❑   taking directions or criticism.
❑   ❑   ❑   making decisions.
❑   ❑   ❑   treating others, even people I don't like, with
                      respect.
❑   ❑   ❑   being happy more often than being sad.
❑   ❑   ❑   feeling good about or comfortable with who I am.
❑   ❑   ❑   participating in organizations or clubs.
❑   ❑   ❑   feeling like I belong here in this school.
❑   ❑   ❑   having a positive attitude about school.
❑   ❑   ❑   controlling my temper.

Others:

❑   ❑   ❑   _____
❑   ❑   ❑   _____

Specific school-related issues

List the subjects you currently are taking and, for each, answer the questions.

Class	How are you doing in this class?	What about this class is easy?	What about this class is difficult?
_____	_____	_____	_____
_____	_____	_____	_____
_____	_____	_____	_____
_____	_____	_____	_____
_____	_____	_____	_____
_____	_____	_____	_____

Which have been your favorite subjects in school?
1. _____   Why? _____
2. _____   Why? _____

Which have been your least favorite subjects in school?
1. _____   Why? _____
2. _____   Why? _____

How many nights per week do you do homework?
_____

About how many hours per week do you spend on homework?
_____

Do you have a quiet place at home to do homework?
_____

Does anyone at home check to see that you've done your homework?
_____

Is there a time set aside every day to do your homework? _____

Do you feel pressure at home about school? _____

Do your parents have reasonable expectations for you? _____

Describe your strengths. What do you do best in school, sports, social life, and other aspects of your life?
_____
_____
_____
_____

Describe your weaknesses. With what do you have the greatest difficulty, both in and out of school?
_____
_____
_____
_____

Student's name: _____ Student's age: _____

Student's school, grade : _____ Special-ed classification:_____

Person completing this rating: _____

Relationship to the student: _____

How long have you worked with the student?_____

Instructions

In each of the following categories, circle the developmental level that, in your judgment, best fits the student's typical behavior. If a student uses special supports (e.g., a planning book, a monitoring log, an advance organizer for writing projects), rate that student's behavior with the supports in place.

Exact placement of the student at a grade level will be very difficult. Please make the best estimate you can make, based on your experience with this student and your understanding of typical maturation. *Positive behaviors* and *negative behaviors* are listed under each category simply to focus your attention on the types of behaviors that are relevant to your consideration about that category.

Planning and organizing

PS   K   1   2   3   4   5   6   7   8   9   10   11   12   PHS

Negative impact of behavior in this area on success in school:

    1   2   3   4   5   6   7

No negative impact   Major negative impact

Illustrations of problem behaviors in this area:_____

_____

_____

Positive behaviors: stores school materials and personal articles in an organized manner; formulates a plan before beginning a complex task; produces well-organized artwork, craft projects, and the like; speaks in an organized manner; produces well-organized stories or essays

Negative behaviors: stores materials in a disorganized way; if given no reminders, begins tasks without a plan or without the needed materials; produces disorganized arts and crafts projects; can express only single thoughts; extended discourse (speaking and writing) is disjointed or incoherent

Initiation

PS   K   1   2   3   4   5   6   7   8   9   10   11   12   PHS

Negative impact of behavior in this area on success in school:

    1   2   3   4   5   6   7

No negative impact   Major negative impact

Illustrations of problem behaviors in this area:_____

_____

_____

Positive behaviors: starts tasks with no reminders or cues; when stuck or finished with a task, asks for help or, in some other way, proceeds; starts interaction with peers

Negative behaviors: needs cues or reminders to start tasks; when stuck or finished with a task, stops and needs new reminders to continue; waits for peers to initiate interaction

Inhibition

PS   K   1   2   3   4   5   6   7   8   9   10   11   12   PHS

Negative impact of behavior in this area on success in school:

    1   2   3   4   5   6   7

No negative impact   Major negative impact

Illustrations of problem behaviors in this area:_____

_____

_____

Figure 12-3. Executive function rating scale. This scale is *not* to be used for formal diagnostic purposes but rather to identify important areas of functioning that may need attention in rehabilitation or special education programs. (PS = preschool; K = kindergarten; 1, 2, 3, 4, 5, etc. = grade level; PHS = post–high school [typically mature young adult after high school]).

Positive behaviors: stops and thinks before acting; controls emotions; continues schoolwork in the presence of distractions

Negative behaviors: acts impulsively; says or does things without thinking (e.g., talking in class without permission); has tantrums; insults others without intending to; is easily distracted by things going on in the environment; does the same thing over and over, even when it is clearly inappropriate

Independence (include perseverance, task completion)

| PS | K | 1 | 2 | 3 | 4 | 5 | 6 | 7 | 8 | 9 | 10 | 11 | 12 | PHS |

Negative impact of behavior in this area on success in school:

| 1 | 2 | 3 | 4 | 5 | 6 | 7 |

No negative impact   Major negative impact

Illustrations of problem behaviors in this area:_____

_____

Positive behaviors: completes work without help or cues; sticks to a task even when difficult; uses needed resources without help or reminders; can work alone

Negative behaviors: needs reminders to begin and continue work; needs reminders and help to use resources; has difficulty working alone

Orientation to task and flexibility

| PS | K | 1 | 2 | 3 | 4 | 5 | 6 | 7 | 8 | 9 | 10 | 11 | 12 | PHS |

Negative impact of behavior in this area on success in school:

| 1 | 2 | 3 | 4 | 5 | 6 | 7 |

No negative impact   Major negative impact

Illustrations of problem behaviors in this area:_____

_____

Positive behaviors: easily learns and adapts to new classroom and other routines; understands how to complete a task with minimal direction; stays oriented to tasks over time; shifts easily from activity to activity and class to class

Negative behaviors: has difficulty adjusting to new situations; often does not know what to do; needs frequent reminders to stay on task; has difficulty shifting from class to class and from activity to activity

Understanding of task difficulty

| PS | K | 1 | 2 | 3 | 4 | 5 | 6 | 7 | 8 | 9 | 10 | 11 | 12 | PHS |

Negative impact of behavior in this area on success in school:

| 1 | 2 | 3 | 4 | 5 | 6 | 7 |

No negative impact   Major negative impact

Illustrations of problem behaviors in this area:_____

_____

Positive behaviors: correctly identifies (verbally or in some other way) some tasks as being easy and others as being difficult for him or her; can state what makes a task difficult; sets reasonable goals; can list or describe own strengths and weaknesses

Negative behaviors: misidentifies difficult tasks as easy or easy tasks as difficult; begins difficult tasks, expecting to succeed; cannot list or describe own strengths and weaknesses; sets unrealistic goals

Self-monitoring and self-evaluating

| PS | K | 1 | 2 | 3 | 4 | 5 | 6 | 7 | 8 | 9 | 10 | 11 | 12 | PHS |

Negative impact of behavior in this area on success in school:

| 1 | 2 | 3 | 4 | 5 | 6 | 7 |

No negative impact   Major negative impact

Illustrations of problem behaviors in this area: _____

_____

_____

   Positive behaviors: checks work for mistakes; notices mistakes; accurately evaluates the quality of a product or activity in relation to a goal; can identify what worked and what did not work after completing a task; notices the effects of behavior on others
   Negative behaviors: does not check work or notice mistakes; inaccurately evaluates the quality of work (overly optimistic or overly pessimistic); cannot identify what worked and what did not work after completing a task; fails to notice the effects of behavior on others

Strategic behavior
PS   K   1   2   3   4   5   6   7   8   9   10   11   12   PHS
Negative impact of behavior in this area on success in school:
        1   2   3   4   5   6   7
No negative impact   Major negative impact
Illustrations of problem behaviors in this area: _____

_____

_____

   Positive behaviors: when a task (physical, academic, communicative, cognitive, social) is difficult, tries a variety of approaches; suggests interesting solutions to practical problems and acts on those suggestions
   Negative behaviors: when a task is difficult, either gives up or persists with ineffective plan; rarely tries varied solutions to problems; rarely suggests meaningful solutions to practical problems; talks about strategic solutions, but does not act on that talk.

Figure 12-3. *Continued*

Intervention: An Everyday Approach to Executive Functions

Insights from Related Disability Groups

Cognitive rehabilitation after TBI has a relatively brief history as a specialized area of intervention. The first decade of intensive program development, from approximately 1975 to approximately 1985, focused on programs of remedial exercises, often targeting cognitive processes or skills as though they existed as independent and hierarchically organized faculties of the mind that could be strengthened much as one rebuilds weakened muscles. This approach bore striking resemblance to nineteenth-century efforts to remediate cognitive deficits in students with congenital learning problems or mental retardation (Mann, 1979) and to the early decades of modern special education (1950s and 1960s), with its focus on decontextualized remedial exercises, largely targeting attentional, perceptual-motor, rote memory, and basic organizational faculties (reviewed by Mann, 1979). Indeed, some of the exercises recommended for cognitive rehabilitation in the 1980s were identical to those that were popular in the nineteenth century but were unable to withstand empirical scrutiny.

   For many reasons that exceed what can reasonably be reported here, this remedial cognitive exercise approach in special education has largely given way to a combination of intensive contextualized efforts to teach relevant academic and vocational content and important life skills and attempts to help students with disability to capitalize on strengths in compensating for weaknesses that are likely to persist, in one form or another, indefinitely. The latter, often referred to as a *metacognitive approach to special education*, is closely related to what we refer to as *executive system intervention* and is increasingly delivered in the context of content instruction rather than as a separate intervention. The shift in special education was due in no small measure to the accumulation of evidence that exercises at the level of basic cognitive processes, even if successful at that level, had little impact on generalized cognitive functioning in real-world contexts or on academic success (Kavale and Mattson, 1983). In a parallel fashion, careful scrutiny of the effectiveness of cognitive rehabilitation exercises has led many practitioners to conclusions that had already been embraced in special education (e.g., Ponsford, 1990; Schacter and Glisky, 1986; Ylvisaker and Urbanczyk, 1990). The intervention framework and suggestions presented in this chapter are based in part on a large and impressive body of research in adult cognitive psychology (e.g., Singley and Anderson, 1989), developmental cognitive psychology (e.g., Flavell et al., 1993; Light and Butterworth, 1993), educational psychology (e.g., Pressley et al., 1990), and special education (e.g., Deshler and Schumaker, 1988), all supporting a contextualized, everyday approach to cognitive intervention.

General Executive System Intervention

During an interview that focused on executive functions, a 10-year old fifth grader was asked, "What do you have trouble with in school?" He replied, "Social studies is kind of hard." The interviewer then asked, "What makes it hard?" The student said, "To get a good grade on the tests, you have to know specific facts. You might have the general idea, but if you don't know the facts, you won't do well. That's kind of hard." "So what do you do to help yourself?" the interviewer asked. The student responded, "Well, I really try to concentrate on the words in italics, because the teacher always asks questions about those words. So when I read a new chapter, I find the words in italics and then read around them to find out what is important about that thing or person. Then I think of a question that she might ask and see if I can answer it. Then I go on." Other questions and tasks revealed similarly exceptional development of strategic thinking and behavior.

Clearly, this young man had very well-developed executive functions, at least in relation to cognitive and academic tasks. He knew a good deal about himself (what was easy and difficult for him, and what to do when tasks were difficult), he took responsibility for doing what needed to be done to succeed, he paid attention to what worked and what did not work for him, and he used this knowledge to do a bit better the next time.

What could explain this remarkable level of development in a 10 year old? Although it is impossible to answer this question with certainty, two features of this young man's life stand out as especially relevant: First, his parents were very good at modeling, coaching, and expecting this kind of behavior. Second, the boy had a medical condition that required him to pay close attention to his physical state and to engage in strategic behavior in the event of trouble signs, or he would suffer severe medical consequences. This child's case illustrates two critical characteristics of environments that foster development of executive functions: First, people in the culture (especially parents) *value* executive functions (i.e., they provide many occasions for practicing these functions, expect that children will take responsibility for their behavior (within appropriate developmental expectations), model executive functions in their interactions with the child, and richly reward successful performance in these areas). Second, there are genuine and important *consequences* associated with successful or unsuccessful performance in these areas.

One of our goals in this chapter is to outline procedures that everyday people can use to create an environment or culture that facilitates development of executive functions. From a theoretical perspective, this approach to intervention is based on the rich developmental theories of Vygotsky, summarized in Chapter 9. Within this tradition, covert cognitive processes and a variety of other rules that guide behavior have their origin in interpersonal interaction and routines involving young children and their caregivers. What appear in older children and adults to be highly abstract internal cognitive representations and rules are transformed and internalized versions of highly structured everyday social-interactive routines. In this sense, young children serve an apprenticeship in their interaction with people, including parents, who possess greater expertise than do the children.

This developmental principal is perhaps most intuitively obvious in tracing the origin of complex conversational rules and skills to simple repetitive social communication games that prelinguistic infants play with their parents (Bruner, 1975). In recent years, a number of investigators have found support for the hypothesis that episodic memory and the ability to organize thoughts and express them in organized discourse develop during the preschool years as a function of the type of conversational interaction children have with their parents as they collaboratively construct narratives about the past (McCabe and Peterson, 1991; Reese et al., 1993; Reese and Fivush, 1993). The adults' role in fostering development is to provide the necessary scaffolding (Bruner, 1978) for children to be successful and then either to withdraw aspects of the scaffold systematically as the child matures or to add complexity to the interaction. For example, in talking with 2 year olds about experiences they have shared, parents provide most of the content as well as the connections and interpretations. In discussing shared experiences with 5 year olds, parents may choose either to let the child provide most of the narration or to engage the child in higher levels of discussion about explanations, interpretations, reactions, and the like. In either case, parents are using enjoyable, everyday social interactions to help children improve their ability to search memory actively, to organize the items found in memory (in a variety of ways; see Chapter 14), and to express these thoughts in an organized manner.

A theme of the current chapter is that executive or self-regulatory functions are similarly grounded in structured interaction between children and others with more mature executive functioning (adults or older children). This vygotskyan theme, depicted in Figure 12-4, is one of the theoretical pillars of the approach to intervention that we propose.

Focus on Executive Functions Throughout the Continuum of Recovery

In the following sections, we discuss procedures for implementing an environmental approach to executive system intervention during each of three broad phases of cognitive recovery. These phases should be understood as artificial divisions in what is better represented as a continuum of recovery (see Chapter 9). Similarly, executive system intervention procedures and expectations for independent performance should develop gradually as the child recovers cognitive function.

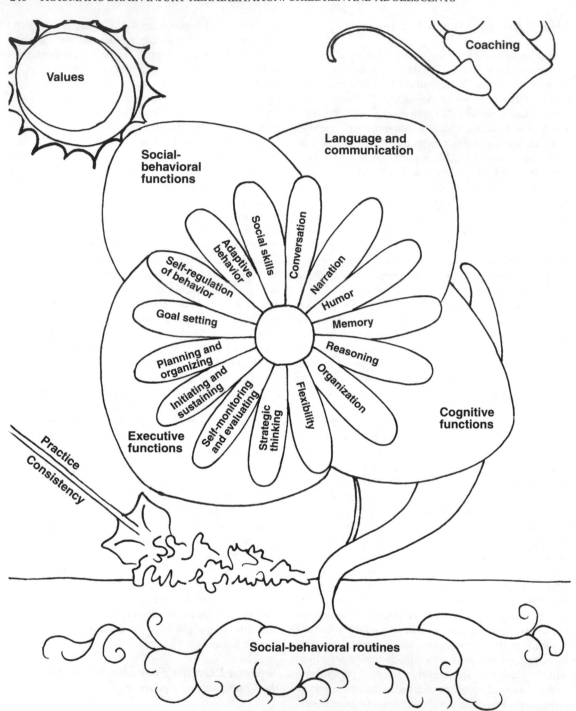

Figure 12-4. Development of cognitive and related executive and communication functions from everyday interactive routines. In environments in which the functions are valued, coaching and supported practice are liberally provided. This is a graphic representation of Vygotsky's interactionist view of cognitive and communication development. (Copyright, M Ylvisaker, Ph.D.)

Early Phases of Cognitive Recovery

Emergence from coma in children and adolescents with very severe TBI can be a protracted process, lasting many weeks in some cases. On the surface, it would appear that there is no meaning to executive system intervention for children who respond minimally to environmental events and who exhibit no goal-directed activity. However, just as it is a mistake to suppose that, in normal development, executive functions emerge only after maturation of other cognitive functions, so also it is a mistake to understand cognitive rehabilitation in a rigid hierarchical fashion. Rather, there is a developmentally appropriate application of the concept of executive functions at all phases of recovery after resumption of some level of alertness and at least minimal attention to external events.

During the early phase of recovery, promotion of *agency* in the child by family and staff is valuable. Often, children emerging from coma are treated as though they are little more than passive recipients of medical, nursing, and rehabilitative care and stimulation: They are not considered agents who act; rather, they are simply acted on, the passive objects of others' actions. Within a culture that respects executive functions, children would be encouraged and prompted to act. Such assistance may take the form of physical prompts (hand over hand, if necessary) to participate in activities of daily living (e.g., brushing one's hair, washing one's face) and other familiar behavior. In this way, the child emerges into a world of familiar routines and agency, particularly if all everyday people (especially parents and nursing staff) take advantage of all everyday routine events to prompt active, functional behavior.

Furthermore, from a neurologic stimulation perspective, sensorimotor neural loops are activated as opposed to sensory receptors alone. Activating sensorimotor loops by causing the child to engage in familiar activity may add importantly to the positive effect of sensory stimulation (Dru et al., 1975; Ferchmin et al., 1975; Will, 1977). In addition, if at this early stage family members and staff adopt a framework within which the child is an *agent*, it is more likely that they will be respectful of choice making and other aspects of executive functions later in recovery.

A second and logistically more complicated procedure during the early phases of recovery (if protracted) is to attempt to engage the child in remote switch control of environmental events. Staff and family identify an electronically controllable event that the child would presumably like to control (e.g., favorite music, videos, an electronic toy) and a movement with which the child could control a switch (negotiated with the physical and occupational therapists). The switch arrangement can be set up in the child's room so that nursing staff and family members can prompt the movement (hand over hand, if necessary) many times daily. If the child does emerge from coma, then he or she emerges into a world of action and favored activities. Furthermore, it is a world in which everyday people respect the child's need to be an agent and to be as independent as possible.

If the child does *not* emerge from coma, possibly the most effective way for family members to understand the realities of persistent unresponsiveness is to have them attempt (unsuccessfully) to prompt the child's control over desirable events. Parents of children in a state of persistent unresponsiveness often believe that the child's mind remains active in a body that is not working. When staff simply argue with parents about this belief, the effect is often alienation and hostility. When the parents are invited to be collaborators and are allowed to experience first-hand the child's lack of responsiveness, they may find it easier, intellectually and emotionally, to grasp the realities of their child's condition.

Middle (Confused) Phases of Recovery

A traditional rehabilitation prescription for children who are alert but very confused and easily agitated is to create a highly structured and consistent environment in which the children are not required to make even simple choices. The typical rationale for withholding choices is that an open-ended, unstructured world of free choices can induce confusion, anxiety, and agitation.

Although elimination of the sources of confusion and agitation is sound practice, the potentially negative impact of choice making is easily overestimated. In our experience, most confused children are capable of making at least some simple choices without becoming additionally confused or agitated. These choices might be presented during activities of daily living: For example, do you want to wear this shirt or this shirt? Do you prefer to drink milk or soda? Similarly, children can be engaged in selecting therapy activities from a limited set of choices: For example, do you want to try walking first, or do you want to do mat work?

If therapists have photographs of the child engaged in routine therapeutic activities, the photographs representing the day's choices can be placed on a planning board and referred to as the *day's plan*. As each activity is completed, the child can remove the representative photograph from the planning board and can place it in a "completed" stack. At the end of the session, the therapist should review the completed plan with the child. In this simple and highly supported (i.e., scaffolded) manner, children with severe cognitive impairment can be engaged in choosing, planning the near-term future, and reviewing the recent past—without exposure to the confusion and anxiety associated with completely open choices and lack of structure. Simple choosing and highly facilitated planning not only begin the long process of improving the child's ability to make intelligent choices and to plan; they have the added benefit of reducing resistance to therapeutic activities. Choice making has been found to increase participation in and enjoyment of activities in other populations of children with serious cognitive limitations, for example, children with developmental disabilities (Harchik et al., 1993).

Late Phases of Recovery

As children and adolescents gradually increase both their orientation to the world around them and the appropriateness of goal-directed behavior, the entire domain of executive functions is opened to rehabilitation efforts consistent with the child's age and developmental level.

Environmental Executive System Intervention

In this section, we first describe environmental practices that address executive functions generally. We then discuss intervention options for specific components of the executive system. Finally, we offer recommendations for teaching compensatory strategies.

Goals, Activities, Procedures, and Coaches

The *goals* of environmental executive system intervention are to help children (1) know what they are good at and what is difficult for them, (2) know that there are special things that can be done when tasks are difficult, (3) make plans for getting the work done, (4) pay attention to how well they are doing, and (5) try a new approach if they are not successful. *Procedures* include modeling and coaching within the context of everyday routines and everyday conversational interaction. Appropriate *activities* include anything that interests the child and requires some effort. *Coaches* include all adults, and possibly older children, who regularly interact with the child.

The overriding goal for the rehabilitation program is to create a culture within which there is a developmentally appropriate focus on executive functions throughout the day. The following dialogue between a 5-year-old child recovering from TBI and her mother illustrates this culture:

Child: *(Attempts unsuccessfully to take a lid off a vitamin container; becomes frustrated.)*
Mom: How're ya doing?
Child: Can't do it; hate this thing!
Mom: It's hard to do, huh?
Child: Dumb thing!
Mom: What have you tried?
Child: Turning; it doesn't work.
Mom: I see. So you need to think of something else. I wonder what else you could do?
Child: You do it.
Mom: Okay, that's one possibility. You could get me to do it for you. That would work. But

let's see if we can find out what the problem is. Oh, look. There is writing here. It says, "Push down and turn." Now we know what the problem is. You have to be able to read to do this, and you haven't learned how to read yet. Here, let's try it together.
Child: *(Opens the container with mom.)* Thanks, Mom.
Mom: Great job. That was hard, but we thought about it and figured it out.

This simple everyday conversation—involving facilitated perception of task difficulty, identification of the nature of the problem, consideration of alternative possible solutions, selection of a successful strategy, and reflection on the positive outcome—is a good illustration of the vygotskyan theme that cognitive processes are based in social interaction between children and caregivers. In this case, the child contributed very little, but children's contributions can incrementally increase with age or recovery after TBI. The support or scaffolding provided by the adult can be systematically withdrawn as the child improves. Alternatively, adults can maintain a relatively high level of support but increase the difficulty level of the task and associated problems that need to be solved. In normal development, interaction of this sort is common, beginning with the child's acquisition of language comprehension around the first birthday and proceeding throughout the developmental years with steady increases in complexity of tasks and expectations for independent functioning.

More generally, a culture that recognizes the importance of executive functions is one in which adults routinely seek out natural opportunities for the following types of exchange throughout the day:

1. "You want to try . . . ? Fine. Do you think it will be difficult or easy? . . . Why do you think it will be easy? . . . How'd you do? . . . Was it difficult or easy? Did you need to do anything special?"
2. "Oops, we've got a problem here. What do you suppose we can do to fix this? . . . Good idea, try it. . . . How'd it work? Can you think of anything else?"
3. "So you want to . . . . Okay, what's your plan? Why do you think that will work?"
4. "You think you can walk all the way down the hall? Great! How long do you think it will take? . . . How long did it take? Oops, why do you suppose it took twice as long as you thought it would? I wonder how you could do it faster."
5. "Do you think you can remember where to go without writing it in your memory book? Fine, try it, but I am going to write down here that you don't think you need the book. . . . So you forgot where to go? This time let's write it in your book; see if that helps. . . . Great! This time you remembered. Writing it in the book helped, didn't it?"

If staff and family members manage to find only one meaningful occasion per half hour for such scaffolded executive function facilitation, that still totals 30 learning trials during a 15-hour waking day. At this rate, the child receives 210 learning trials per week, 840 per month, 9,080 per year, and 90,800 (almost 100,000!) during the course of 10 years. From the perspective of executive system maturation, this approach is incomparably preferable to the all-too-common institutional environment in which professionals serve as prosthetic frontal lobes, identifying the child's needs, setting the goals, making the plans, initiating activity, monitoring and evaluating performance, and solving all the problems that arise. The latter culture is classically associated with the evolution of shallow self-insight in the individuals served, along with some combination of learned helplessness and oppositional behavior.

Executive Function Routines

The point of environmental executive system intervention is to improve the executive dimensions of behavior in everyday routine actions. Everyday routines are used as the context to improve the way children engage in those routines. As is true of other important general educational and rehabilitation goals (e.g., communication goals), targeting executive function goals throughout the day in the context of everyday activities and routines is better than targeting these goals in highly specialized therapy or instructional periods. An executive system focus is desirable in all activities, including nursing unit, classroom, therapeutic, and recreational activities, and activities of daily living at home. This approach may take little additional time or effort once staff and family members have developed appropriate habits in this area. For example, any activity can include the following aspects:

1. An initial decision about or choice of a *goal*. ("What are you trying to accomplish?")
2. A decision about how *easy or difficult* it will be to accomplish the goal. ("Is this going to be hard or easy?")
3. Development of a *plan*. ("What materials do we need? Who will do what? In what order do we need to do these things? How long will it take?")
4. Some planned (e.g., in which staff members ensure that problems arise) or unplanned *coaching* of the students in *problem solving and strategic thinking* as issues arise (see Executive Function Routines).
5. A quick *review* of the goal, plan, and accomplishments at the end. ("What were you trying to accomplish? How did you do? How did you do it?")
6. A summary of *what worked and what didn't work*; a summary of *what was easy and what was difficult*—and why.

Clearly, young or more seriously impaired children require more support or scaffolding than older and less impaired children. Initially, children's participation in these executive system routines may be minimal, and adults may need to model, conversationally, most or all components of the routine. As children recover cognitive function and mature developmentally, support can be systematically reduced so that the children are as independent as possible in implementing these executive system routines.

Because young children and children with executive system weakness are often concrete thinkers, use of a task organization map of some sort can help to make these executive system processes concrete and visually apparent. Figure 12-5 presents a form that can be used by staff and family members to organize their focus on the executive dimensions of behavior. Such a form can serve as an executive system map for children and staff alike. Making modifications to fit individual needs, we have used this general form with a large number of individuals with TBI, ranging in age from preschoolers to young adults.

While using the executive function map presented in Figure 12-5, staff can help children associate concrete meaning with important words such as *goal, plan, materials, equipment, sequence* or *steps, problem, solution, idea, think, organize, good at* or *easy, not good at* or *difficult, do something special, review, predict, works, does not work*, and many other terms related to the ability to think about and regulate one's behavior.

When children fail to achieve their predicted level of success, review interaction can help to teach them that a limited set of options is available to people who fail to achieve their goals:

- Change the prediction or goal
- Practice
- Modify the task
- Modify the manner of performing the task
- Modify the environment
- Ask for help
- Increase the reward for achieving the goal (i.e., motivation)

With children or any concrete thinker, this set of options is easiest to teach in the context of physical activities. For example, if a boy says he will walk 10 steps in physical therapy but walks only three, he could do any combination of the following to achieve his goal: (1) reduce the current goal; (2) practice walking and try again; (3) change the task from walking to getting from here to there in another way; (4) use some kind of support (e.g., a cane); (5) try walking on a smoother surface or in a quieter environment; (6) ask for help from the therapist; or (7) increase the reward so motivation is heightened.

These general categories of options, which apply to all types of behavior, can be printed on a piece of paper so the child can habitually look at the same list of options when he or she must find some way to change failure into success in any therapeutic or daily activity.

Goal

What do I want to accomplish?

Plan

How am I going to accomplish my goal?

Materials and equipment	Steps or assignments
1.	1.
2.	2.
3.	3.
4.	4.
5.	5.

Prediction

How well will I do? How much will I get done?

Do

Problems	Solutions
1.	1.
2.	2.
3.	3.

Review

How did I do?
Self-rating:

1 2 3 4 5 6 7 8 9 10

Other rating:

1 2 3 4 5 6 7 8 9 10

What worked?	What didn't work?
1.	1.
2.	2.
3.	3.

What will I try next time?

Figure 12-5. A guide for targeting the executive components of any task.

We sometimes use fun activities (e.g., shooting baskets) to teach these executive components of activity (i.e., predict performance, make a plan, monitor and evaluate performance, act strategically if actual performance falls short of predicted performance) and then work to generalize the system to more meaningful activities (Ylvisaker et al., 1992).

Case Illustration

DJ sustained a severe closed head injury as a 17-year-old senior in high school. After prolonged acute care and rehabilitation hospitalization, he was discharged to home and enrolled in an outpatient program. At that point (almost 1 year after his injury), he had moderate physical disability (e.g., dysarthric but intelligible speech, slow and labored gait) and cognitive and academic disability (e.g., grade-school level scores in most academic areas). He had a reasonable understanding of his physical deficits but minimal insight into his cognitive and psychosocial challenges. DJ's personal goal, which was to complete his graduate equivalency diploma (GED) and enter college, was considered by staff to be unrealistic. When the gap between his goal and current functioning levels was concretely illustrated for him, DJ generally became upset and blamed therapists for not using effective procedures that would restore him to preinjury levels of ability. He also blamed his former friends for his current social isolation.

Staff agreed that the executive system contributors to DJ's disability were most critical to his long-term success or failure in academic, social, and vocational life and had to be addressed in a comprehensive manner. Because DJ had been an athlete in high school, staff changed the operative metaphor from "executive" to "self-coaching" functions and tried to turn most therapy sessions into self-coaching training sessions. At the beginning of each session, DJ identified his goal (e.g., "I want to speak clearly and without tightness") and the problem or obstacle to achieving the goal (e.g., "I tighten up, especially when I'm nervous and don't use breath support efficiently"). He then gave himself a plan, instructions for how he would address the problem he had identified. He audiotaped or videotaped his practice sessions and reviewed the tape (like a coach reviewing game films). Each review included an overall evaluation of his performance, a judgment about what was working and what was not working, and a revision of the plan. DJ used a form similar to that illustrated in Figure 12-5 to ensure that he routinely addressed all relevant dimensions of self-coaching functions. Throughout this process, he explicitly referred to himself as his own coach. Staff remained available to keep him on the right track with respect to specific exercises and also to provide guidance and encouragement as he worked at being a coach for himself.

Initially, staff members had hoped that DJ would use his growing self-coaching ability to realize that his college dream was unrealistic and, as a consequence, that he would accept a more modest vocational track. However, because of his extraordinary perseverance and commitment to his goal, and because his family was willing and able to support him indefinitely, DJ continued to work toward his initial goal of attending college. Nonetheless, an important change occurred. As he became better at self-coaching, DJ blamed others less and increasingly accepted responsibility for the hard work that would be needed to achieve his goal. In addition, he creatively sought out a variety of avenues to achieve his goals. He added home tutoring to his rehabilitation program, purchased GED preparation software for independent practice, and worked in a more collaborative manner with the outpatient therapists. Two years later, DJ had passed his GED examinations and was slowly accumulating credits at a community college. Meanwhile, he worked as a volunteer assistant instructor at a YMCA swimming program for children. Despite substantial residual disability after his life-altering injury, DJ's life became more satisfying and his efforts more productive as he increasingly made self-coaching thought patterns and behaviors part of his daily routines.

Measurable Objectives

One of the objections frequently raised against this environmental approach to executive function intervention is that insurance companies, special education administrators, and others demand evidence that the child or adolescent is achieving specific, measurable treatment objectives. The objectives listed here are illustrations of how the general concept of executive functions can yield measurable objectives. We have chosen arbitrarily to use the name John to represent any child or adolescent in this context. Creative clinicians will undoubtedly conjure up many more illustrations and customize them to fit the needs of specific individuals. These should be considered transdisciplinary, collaborative objectives. However, it generally is wise to designate one staff person to take responsibility for documentation, basing such reports on conversations with other staff and family members.

1. Self-awareness
   a. John will accurately identify tasks that are easy or difficult for him.
   b. Given a difficult task, John will (verbally or nonverbally) indicate that it is difficult.

c. John will accurately explain why some tasks are easy or difficult for him.

d. John will request help when tasks are difficult.

e. John will offer help to another when he is more capable than the other child.

2. Goal setting

a. John will accurately predict how effectively he will accomplish a task. For example, he will accurately predict whether he will be able to complete a task; how many (of something) he can finish; his grade on a test; how many problems he will be able to complete in a specific time period; and the like.

b. John will participate with teachers and therapists in setting instructional and therapeutic goals (e.g., to be able to read this book; hit a baseball across the gym; write my name so mom can read it; talk to grandma on the phone).

3. Planning

a. Given an everyday routine (e.g., snack), John will indicate what items are needed (e.g., plates, cups, crackers, juice, napkins) and the order of the events.

b. Given a selection of six activities for a therapeutic or instructional session, John will select three, indicate their order, create a plan on paper (e.g., with photographs), and stick to the plan.

c. Given a task that he correctly identifies as difficult for him, John will create a plan for accomplishing the task.

d. Having failed to achieve a predicted grade on a test, John will create a plan for improving performance for the next test.

4. Organizing

a. John will create a system for organizing personal items in his room or locker.

b. To tell an organized story, John will place photographs in order and then narrate the sequence of events.

c. John will select and use a system to organize his assignments and other schoolwork.

d. Given a complex task, John will organize the task on paper, including the materials needed, the steps to accomplish the task, and a time frame.

e. John will prepare an organized outline or semantic map before proceeding with writing projects.

5. Self-initiating

a. When John does not know what to do, he will ask an adult for help.

b. With no prompting from adults, John will begin his assigned tasks, initiate work on his plan, and the like.

6. Self-monitoring and self-evaluating

a. John will keep a journal in which he records his plans and predictions for success and also records his actual level of performance and its relation to his predictions.

b. John will identify errors in his work without a teacher's assistance.

c. John's rating of his performance on a 10-point scale will be within 1 point of the teacher's rating.

7. Problem solving

a. When faced with obstacles to accomplishing educational or other objectives, John will offer a number of suggestions for actions he could take to overcome the obstacle, give reasons for and against each, choose the best, do it, and evaluate its effectiveness.

b. John will offer a number of possible solutions to everyday problems as they arise over the course of the school day.

Intervention for Specific Components of the Executive System

In the sections that follow, we offer suggestions for focusing intervention on one or more specific components of the executive system. This runs the risk of fragmenting what should be an integrated system of functions and a correspondingly integrated intervention plan. However, because they are often differentially impaired, individual components may require relatively greater or lesser emphasis in rehabilitation.

Self-Awareness

Weak self-awareness of strengths and weaknesses is a common phenomenon after TBI and may result from some combination of organically based unawareness, denial, and simple developmental immaturity. Individuals with frontal lobe injury (and other possible locations of brain injury) often fail to perceive their neurologically based deficits or to recognize the implications of those deficits (i.e., *anosognosia*). It is important to distinguish this phenomenon from *denial*, which results from a psychological or emotional inability to confront and deal with troubling realities. Professionals all too commonly assert, mistakenly, that a person is in a state of denial—an assertion often associated with a recommendation for stronger confrontation; organically based unawareness is frequently a more accurate diagnosis and less likely to be resolved with confrontation. In the case of children with TBI, these two phenomena, one neurologic and the other psychological, combine with the developmental fact that children only gradually come to have some degree of this awareness over the entire span of the developmental years. In some cases, an additional (and avoidable) contributor to unawareness is the natural tendency of some parents and some professionals to guarantee (by offering unreasonably high levels of support) that a child with disability is always successful, thereby creating the illusion that the child has no special needs.

Table 12-2. Intervention Options for a Child with Significantly Impaired Self-Awareness of Strengths and Needs

Relatively low-confrontation options

1. Negotiated assessment tasks (e.g., "What can you do to prove to your therapists, teachers, parents, or others that you can do more than they think you can do?") and self-assessment (see text).
2. Daily conversational interaction and coaching designed to help the child to understand that some tasks are difficult and others easy; to identify which tasks are difficult and which are easy; and to appreciate that when tasks are difficult, there are special things one can do to succeed. For example, "Wow, you are really good at that; that's easy for you, isn't it? But this is hard, isn't it? Why do you think this is so hard? I bet there's something you can do to make it easier! Oh look; this worked! You did it! But it was hard to do, wasn't it?"
3. Identification of "special experts" within a rehabilitation group or class, with every child being an expert in something but also needing help from others in something else.
4. Facilitated "product-monitoring" tasks to encourage self-discovery. For example, "Try to accomplish this task without any help; now try it a different way, using helpful procedures. Which worked better? Why?"
5. Self-monitoring system. For example, "Keep a log of all of your classes, assignments, and other important tasks that you wish to accomplish. In each case, before you start indicate how well you think you will do and, later, how well you actually did. Compare your prediction with your actual performance."
6. Natural consequences of failure or impaired performance (including clinicians, teachers, and others evaluating the student, using their standard criteria and giving honest feedback).
7. Peer teaching (to gain proficiency in identifying strengths and needs in others, thereby improving the ability to identify strengths and needs in oneself).
8. Student engagement in orienting and training the student's staff (e.g., self-advocacy video).
9. Student engagement in planning intervention (e.g., positive futures planning).
10. Passage of time.

Relatively high-confrontation options

1. Verbal recitation of deficits.
2. Direct presentation of low test results.
3. Peer confrontation (in or out of therapy).
4. Self-observation on video (taped while attempting challenging tasks).

Note: Options should be selected in light of the child's age, length of time since the injury, emotional fragility, and other factors discussed in the text.

Whatever its cause, unawareness creates frustrations for staff and family members alike. In the case of rehabilitation and special education, unawareness of deficits blocks individuals' active engagement in rehabilitation and remedial education and reduces the likelihood that they will work to compensate for residual deficits: If there is no deficit, why work to compensate for it? Impaired self-awareness reduces people's motivation to engage in effortful strategic behavior, despite their need to be more strategic than others because of their newly acquired disability.

Table 12-2 presents a number of procedural options for use with people who need to be more acutely and accurately aware of their strengths and needs. These options are grossly divided into those that are relatively confrontational and those that are relatively nonconfrontational (although it may be better to think of intervention options as falling on a continuum of confrontation). The risks of premature confrontation include an increase in the individual's sense of perplexity, an increase in a sense of loss and depression, loss of a sense of self-worth, and destruction of the therapeutic relationship between the child or adolescent and the staff member. Therefore, a decision to be confrontational may require the approval of a professional trained to make such judgments (e.g., psychiatrist, clinical psychologist, or psychiatric social worker). For example, some rehabilitation facilities require authorization before subjecting a person with a newly acquired brain injury to potentially threatening self-observation on videotape.

Deciding on Appropriate Interventions: Confrontational Versus Nonconfrontational Approaches. Where staff and family members should be on the continuum of confrontational options at any given time depends on many factors. Because unawareness often gives way gradually to denial, making decisions about appropriate intervention is extremely difficult.

AGE.   Other things being equal, the older the individual, the greater the rationale for confrontational options. Young children simply cannot be expected to have a clear and accurate perception of their strengths and needs, particularly their cognitive needs. However, by the use of supportive, nonconfrontational options, self-awareness may be accelerated beyond normal developmental expectations if the child has a disability that must be brought to a level of conscious awareness.

LENGTH OF TIME SINCE THE INJURY.   Other things being equal, the longer the time elapsed since the injury, the greater the rationale for confrontational options. Many adolescents (and their family members) have reported that they needed 2 full years to begin to adjust to a new self with altered capabilities. Serious confrontation before this time may simply generate anger and alienation. Furthermore, in the early months after TBI, making confident predictions about long-term outcome is difficult, adding to the inappropriateness of early confrontation.

SEVERITY OF UNAWARENESS.   If the child or adolescent has the type and severity of brain damage that makes acquisition of a clear perception of deficits virtually impossible, the risks of confrontation may outweigh its potential benefits.

EMOTIONAL FRAGILITY.   Other things being equal, the greater the child's emotional fragility, the greater is the need to avoid potentially destructive confrontation. For example, there is potential danger in forcing emotionally unstable people to view themselves (on videotape) struggling with tasks that should be easy (based on their pre-trauma standards).

CONSEQUENCES OF UNAWARENESS.   Generally, the greater the consequences of unawareness, the greater the rationale for confrontation. Often, young children comply with assigned tasks without recognizing their necessity. Therefore, confrontation may serve no useful purpose. On the other hand, unawareness or denial in older adolescents may result in fierce resistance to parents and staff, failure in school, and unacceptable risk taking. In these cases, confrontational options may be required.

AVAILABLE RESOURCES.   There is less reason to be confrontational if a family has the resources to pursue options (e.g., specialized treatments or educational programs) that staff members judge to be wasteful or overly expensive, as compared to the family that lacks these resources and that might squander what little they have on programs that offer little realistic potential for improvement in the child.

Nonconfrontational Procedures.   In general, during the early months after a brain injury, it is wise to focus on the here and now, to help the individual experience as much success as possible, and to supportively introduce compensations using nonconfrontational procedures. However, if persistent unawareness or denial combines with ongoing disability, confrontational procedures might be valuable, as might reduction of supports for the individual (while maintaining a safety net) so that he or she experiences the natural consequences of failure. In the following sections, we highlight four relatively nonconfrontational procedures that might be useful for some children and adolescents in gaining an increasingly accurate understanding of their strengths and needs: self-assessment, peer teaching, self-advocacy videotapes, and positive futures planning.

SELF-ASSESSMENT.   Earlier we discussed the advantages of engaging children and adolescents in their own assessment, and we presented a self-assessment form that could facilitate this process for adolescents. Including students, particularly adolescents, in planning their own assessment and generating their own goals is not only respectful; it also contributes over time to these individuals' growing awareness of those things they do well and those things with which they need help.

PEER TEACHING.   In rehabilitation settings, we have tried to engage children and adolescents in helping other patients. Possibilities range from simple physical assistance (e.g., pushing another child's wheelchair; helping another child with snack or other daily living activities) to tutoring a younger child who is getting ready to return to school. A good option for adolescents with relatively good cognitive recovery is to support them in reviewing younger children's log books at the end of a day. Typically, this review includes not only the events of the day but also the rationale for the various therapeutic activities. In discussing with the tutoring child how to conduct these reviews, the reasons for them, and the functional disability in the child being helped, staff can meaningfully emphasize corresponding strengths and needs in the case of the tutoring child. In this way, children are given a framework for thinking about their own needs after the injury and are also invited to focus on another person's needs, which may help to move them beyond the egocentrism often present during the early months after brain injury. Helping other children to understand themselves and to regulate their behavior as a step toward understanding oneself and regulating one's own behavior is consistent with Vygotsky's developmental theory, in which regulation of others precedes and facilitates the development of self-regulation.

SELF-ADVOCACY VIDEO.   As part of a general focus on executive functions in rehabilitation and special education, children and adolescents with TBI, working collaboratively with staff and parents, can create a videotape that has as its primary purpose to orient and train staff in how to teach, help, treat, and otherwise work with the student. This can be a project for the last 2 or 3 weeks of the child's rehabilitation program or can be completed in the spring of the school year as a tool to train and orient the staff in next year's classroom. In either case, the children are engaged in a meaningful and important project that has a concrete and very legitimate goal—to help others understand their strengths and weaknesses and become oriented to the teaching or therapeutic procedures that are most helpful. Secondary purposes for this project include helping the children gain insight into those areas in which they do well, those areas in which they need help, and those strategies that they are going to have to use to help themselves. In other words, they must process this information about themselves in order to teach someone else.

GENERAL PROTOCOL.   A general protocol for producing self-advocacy videos (that can and should be modified to meet the needs of specific individuals and situations) and its rationale are presented in Table 12-3. On several occasions, we have engaged children, their families, and their staff in developing a product of this sort. In our experience, the product is a useful training tool (its ostensible purpose) but, more importantly, the children and their families learn a great deal about their needs over the course of its production. Having children and their parents view the child on videotape and decide what to tell the school staff about the child's needs is sometimes very powerful. Furthermore, the participants generally enjoy the process, are grateful for the respect implicit in the invitation to participate in the project, and experience an important sense of empowerment upon its completion. We have used the process with individuals ranging in age and level of functioning from early grade school to young adult.

In selected cases, the self-advocacy videotape might have as one of its goals—or as the only goal—advocating for oneself to oneself. For example, some adolescents and young adults choose not to present themselves to others on videotape but agree to be videotaped while making a strong statement about themselves, their goals, their plans, their strengths, and their needs, with the qualification that only they will watch the tape. Some of these individuals have reported that they watched the videotape repeatedly, learned about themselves from their own statements, and drew strength from the insights that they had revealed on the tape.

Case Illustration

TK, described in Chapter 11 as an illustration of a child whose severe executive system and organizational impairment masqueraded as a primary attentional deficit, was helped to produce a training videotape as he was finishing fifth grade and moving up to middle school, which entailed a change of schools and staff. The process began with a meeting between a brain injury consultant and TK, his mother, and his resource room teacher. The purpose of the meeting was to develop a shared understanding of the videotape, its purposes and its contents. Both TK and his mother were pleased that they could play a leading role in orienting and training staff at the next level of his education.

Although he had been using his customized planning, organizing, and monitoring book for several weeks (with great success; see Chapter 11), TK needed considerable help from his mother and his teacher to identify important content and strategies to pass on to sixth-grade staff. The discussion was collaborative, however, and none of the participants dominated.

After general decisions had been made about important content, TK used school time to prepare for the videotaping. He made some graphics in art class, wrote script in language arts class, used math class to organize some data regarding his improvement, and spent some social time discussing a role in the videotape for a friend. The video came to include the following segments: (1) an introduction, in which TK and his friend showed an opening graphic and invited the viewer to "sit back, relax, and enjoy the show"; (2) a segment in which TK demonstrated how he used his task assignment checklists followed by self-ratings and peer ratings of performance; (3) a segment in which TK demonstrated weak writing performance when simply instructed to write a summary, followed by demonstration of success when given a helpful graphic advance organizer to use in writing the summary; (4) a discussion between his mother and resource room teacher about important components of his program; and (5) a discussion between his regular education teacher and a paraprofessional aide about important components of his program. TK introduced each of these segments with a few comments designed to orient the viewer to the point of the next segment.

Figure 12-6, modified from Meichenbaum (1993; personal communication, 1994), illustrates an important feature of these self-advocacy videotapes and, more generally, of support for people with disability. The figure highlights four important dimensions of skill development: level of task difficulty and complexity (from easy to difficult or complex), context (from acquisition to application or transfer), mastery (from acquisition through consolidation to consultation), and support needed (from maximal support to independent performance). The ultimate goal of skill development is that individuals will be able to independently perform difficult tasks in a variety of settings and to master the skill to such a degree that they could serve as consultants to other people. Without special supports, few people master many skills to this extent and, if they do, generally years of effort have been expended. With appropriate support, however, people can quickly be brought to the upper levels of each of the other three dimensions.

In TK's case, he was asked to do something extremely difficult (i.e., teach strangers about cognitive disability and how to teach a very complex child—himself); he was asked to do it in an unfamiliar context (i.e., his new school with new staff); and he was expected to play the role of consultant, a role that very few professionals can play effectively. Finally, he was asked to do this as a fifth grader with significant disability and given only 1 month of preparation time. In fact, TK did a very effective job because he was given appropriate support—namely, help in developing his training material and a video procedure to compensate for the context challenges.

Table 12-3. Transitional or Self-Advocacy Videotape: Rationale and Procedures

Goals

Primary goal: To produce a videotape that can be used to orient and train people (e.g., school staff, employers, baby-sitters, others) who may need to be trained in how to teach, interact with, or manage the student.

Associated goals

1. Students will gain a sense of empowerment, of control over their lives.
2. Students will gain progressively more insight into their strengths and needs.
3. Students will become progressively more strategic in their thinking about themselves and their rehabilitation and school careers.
4. Parents will gain a sense of empowerment.
5. Parents will gain progressively more insight into the child's strengths and needs and will share their insights with staff.
6. Parents will gain an appreciation of the importance of executive functions and the student's participation in goal setting, planning, and strategic thinking.
7. Staff will strengthen their collaborative relationships with other team members (including parents) as they work together to produce the videotape.
8. Staff will gain greater appreciation for the perspective of students and parents.

Procedures (subject to considerable variation in individual cases)

1. Several weeks before the end of the rehabilitation admission, school year, or other transitional time, staff, student, and parents hold a *planning meeting*. The purposes of this meeting are:
   a. To decide what *content* would be most important to demonstrate on videotape. It is critical that *strengths* be highlighted and that the *students' and parents' goals* be highlighted. This meeting could be part of an individualized educational plan (IEP) meeting or standard parent conference. Alternatively, it could be a separate meeting. This might include:
      - *Physical* strengths, weaknesses, and management issues (e.g., seating, positioning, mobility, dressing, eating).
      - *Cognitive* strengths, weaknesses, and management issues (e.g., types of advance organizers needed; types of environmental or materials modifications needed owing to attentional, perceptual, or other processing problems; types of cues and prompts needed).
      - *Communication* strengths, weaknesses, and management issues (e.g., use of an augmentative communication system; demonstration of partner communication styles that facilitate comprehension).
      - *Behavioral or social* strengths, weaknesses, and management issues (e.g., procedures for preventing behavior problems; ways to diffuse behavioral outbursts; ways to facilitate peer interaction).
   b. To decide what *format and scripts* would be most effective in demonstrating critical points.
      - It often is effective to show the student (a) succeeding at a task at which he or she is good; (b) failing at an important but difficult task when appropriate procedures, modifications, or equipment are *not* in place; and then (c) succeeding when they are in place.
      - It often is effective to communicate content by means of a *conversation* between student and staff or between staff and parents—as opposed to simply videotaping a "talking head."
      - It is ideal to videotape the student's own orientation to and commentary about the videotape segments and then to edit these into the tape as orientation for the viewer. This videotaping can be done after the student has watched the other segments.
   c. To decide *who should play what role* in the videotape. If possible, the student should play a leading role (possibly with considerable support). We often have parents of young children make introductory comments about the child.
   d. To work out *logistics* of videotaping and editing. The student and parents may be more or less involved in this planning, depending on many factors.
2. During the following weeks, students can be engaged in planning this videotape project in many of their therapeutic and instructional sessions. For example, development of scripts can be part of language arts or speech-language therapy sessions; development of presentation of strengths and needs can be part of counseling sessions; development of physical demonstrations can be part of physical, occupational, speech-language, and other therapies; development of instructional demonstrations can be part of instructional sessions; and summaries of performance data can be part of math class. Alternatively, if staff believe that these therapy and instructional times would not be wisely spent in such preparatory activities, the videotape could be less carefully planned and still serve a useful purpose.
3. The actual videotaping can be a simple matter of setting up a camera in a therapeutic or instructional session and proceeding with the demonstration. If other students are present, they must present signed releases. Ideally, the videotape will be edited (if staff members have time and two videotape cassette recorders). However, this is not necessary.

Advantages of this end-of-the-year or transitional routine

1. *Incidental learning—student:* Students acquire important information about themselves and about their rehabilitation or education program by being engaged in an enjoyable, product-oriented activity.
2. *Incidental learning—staff:* Staff members acquire important information about the student, family, and their own program by being engaged in an enjoyable, product-oriented activity.
3. *Incidental learning—parents:* Parents acquire important information about the student and the program by being engaged in an enjoyable, product-oriented activity.
4. *Efficient, nonthreatening, nonpunishing training and orientation for current staff:* Staff currently working with the child may acquire important insights from other staff or from family members.
5. *Meaningful training and orientation for future staff:* Staff at the next level of care or education receive orientation to the child that goes beyond what can be communicated in written reports.
6. *Development of a shared conceptual framework:* The team refines its own shared conceptual framework by being engaged in an enjoyable, product-oriented activity.
7. *Fun:* Producing this videotape can actually be enjoyable.
8. *Permanent record:* If this practice becomes an annual routine, the student and family will have an invaluable permanent record of the student's educational history.
9. *Student and parent satisfaction:* In general, students and parents are very pleased when staff accord them the respect that is implicit in this activity. Indeed, this can be a vehicle for overcoming an adversarial relationship, if one exists.

Figure 12-6. The four main contributors to successful performance of a task: (1) the difficulty level of a task (from easy to difficult), (2) the context in which the task is performed (from controlled training context to unlimited contexts), (3) the amount of support that is provided (from intense support to no support), and (4) the level of mastery (from beginner's level through mastery to consultant level). In this case, the task is difficult; it is performed in a training context; a moderate amount of support is provided; and performance is at a mastery level, but the learner is not yet able to teach another. (Based on D. Meichenbaum, personal communication, 1994.)

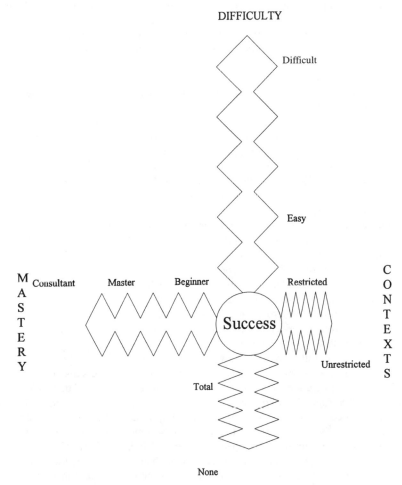

In Figure 12-6, the lines are drawn in accordion fashion to illustrate how clever supports can enable a person to move with surprising ease toward the upper end of the dimensions. This concept of support is analogous to Vygotsky's concept (discussed earlier) of social-interactive support used to help young children engage in otherwise difficult cognitive and executive function behaviors.

POSITIVE FUTURES PLANNING.　Understood as an intervention procedure, positive futures planning could legitimately be classified as goal setting, planning, and problem solving. We have chosen to discuss it along with other options designed to increase self-insight because it is an ideal framework for addressing commonly occurring conflicts among students (especially adolescents), their parents, and rehabilitation or education staff. Positive futures planning (Mount and Zwernik, 1986; O'Brien and Lyle, 1987) and related approaches (e.g., the Magill Action Planning System; Vandercook et al., 1989) evolved from attempts to help people with developmental disabilities articulate their dreams for the future and identify means to achieve those dreams. Academic, vocational, social, and residential goals are addressed comprehensively by each individual with disability, professionals who work with those individuals, the individual's family members, and others who may have an important stake in the person's life, possibly including peers and friends.

The process, the completion of which may take several hours over more than one session, typically involves an honest examination of the past (i.e., How did we get to where we are today?), the present (i.e., What is your life like today? What is good about it and what bad?), and the future (Where do you want to be 5 or 10 years from now and how do you plan to get there? What are the obstacles and how do you plan to overcome them?). Conflicts in perception of the past and present and in vision of the future inevitably arise, requiring a skilled facilitator to maintain control while also encouraging frank airing of differences. If the adolescent, possibly supported by the family, envisions a future that staff members believe is out of the question, the group can at least identify small steps required to achieve the long-term goal and to create a plan with many steps that can be monitored along the way. It is possible that the individual will succeed beyond everybody's wildest dreams. Alternatively, if the vision of the future has to be altered, the alterations can result in part from self-discovery.

This process is unlikely to be productive during the first 2 years (or so) after severe TBI, if only because long-term outcome remains relatively open. On the other hand, the process should be commenced at least 2 years before the individual leaves school, thereby allowing time to make adjustments in the academic or vocational training program depending on the outcome of the futures planning process. Because the futures planning process is threatening, natural resistance to getting started is the norm. This resistance should be anticipated and meetings calmly rescheduled if necessary.

Goal Setting

Helping individuals improve their ability to set goals for themselves can involve routine use of the everyday planning and monitoring system described earlier. Positive futures planning may also be part of this process. In rehabilitation hospitals, patients may passionately embrace what staff consider fiercely unrealistic goals. In these cases, staff are well advised (1) to creatively structure meaningful intervention around the individual's goals or components of those goals; (2) to request provisional acceptance of temporary rehabilitation goals while supporting the individual's pursuit of ultimate goals; and (3) to illustrate connections between long-term goals and current rehabilitation activities. In the early months after a severe injury, asking the individual to be a realistic goal setter is inappropriate. However, low-keyed adjustment counseling may help the child or adolescent deal with fears about the future.

Meanwhile, staff should engage the individual in frequent goal-setting practice. For example, for every activity in any therapy session, the individual can set a goal: For example, "Today, I will walk three steps with no help. By the end of the week, I will walk the entire staircase." In addition to setting dates for accomplishment, the individual should create a plan for achieving the goal and keep records of his or her progress. Goals and progress should be recorded so the individual is routinely oriented to his or her goals and progress toward achieving those goals. Revisions in the goals should be encouraged as required by reviews of performance data.

Peer teaching is another meaningful context in which to target goal setting. In rehabilitation and special education programs, we have paired higher- and lower-functioning individuals. One of the jobs of the peer teacher is to help set reasonable goals for the other person based on an understanding of that person's limitations. Having achieved some skill in connecting ability levels with goals in connection with another person, the individual may find it easier to apply the same thought processes to himself or herself.

Planning

In discussing environmental intervention, we recommended that children and adolescents be engaged in planning throughout the day and that a system that highlights the activity of planning be used. When every activity begins with a plan, it becomes part of the routine, which is ideal. However, for those who have special difficulty grasping the idea and components of planning, more specialized instruction may be relevant. In this case, it may be useful to employ activities that are engaging and relatively easy (so resistance is minimized and the child is not focused on the difficulty of the activity) and that have distinct steps that can be numbered. The activity begins with the creation of a plan, with some concrete object or photograph placed on a number card to signify the place in the plan for that object. The number cards are placed in sequence, representing the plan.

As the activity progresses, the clinician makes frequent reference to the plan and conversationally highlights its importance: For example, "We need to stick to the plan. When we stay organized, we get things done. That's why it's good to have a plan." If the children become distracted or deviate from the plan, they must be redirected to the agreed-on plan: For example, "Remember, this is your plan. Let's stick to your plan." On the other hand, if there is good reason to deviate, then taking a moment to formulate a new plan is probably worthwhile.

Initiating

People with severe initiation impairment lack activation across all domains. They are not candidates for strategy intervention because they would simply fail to initiate the strategy just as they fail to initiate other behavior. Furthermore, if frontal lobe injury is sufficiently severe, practice may fail to affect performance. Perhaps for this reason, frontal lobe patients were once considered inappropriate candidates for rehabilitation. However, individuals with severe initiation impairment may profit from well-conceived environmental support and prosthetic initiators. For example, an adolescent who is alert but who does not initiate interaction may have an attractive sign on his lap tray that invites others to engage him or her in conversation on a favored topic, play a game, listen to music, or engage in another favored activity. The sign on the tray serves as a sort of prosthetic initiator. The objective of such a system is to improve the quality of life of a person who may never recover this component of executive functioning.

Other options are available for individuals with mild to moderate initiation impairment. Most important is that everyday people, including teachers and parents, understand the critical difference between initiation impairment and laziness or lack of motivation. When people with initiation impairment are labeled as lazy, relationships are poisoned and everybody experiences unnecessary frustration. In addition, rehabilitation staff should help family members and others understand the degree of initiation impairment involved in everyday activities. For example, unstructured conversations are very demanding and therefore tend to make people with initiation impairment feel anxious. In contrast, board and card games that are highly structured with rules that govern each turn require little ongoing initiation. With an understanding of initiation demands of activities, family members are in a better position to help the child enjoy a rich set of activities without experiencing undue frustration. Also valuable is orienting peers to the child's needs and inviting them to assume the initiator role more than would naturally be their inclination.

For some adolescents, prosthetic initiators (e.g., an alarm watch) may be of some use. For adolescents and young adults with initiation and memory impairment, the NeuroPage system (Hersh and Treadgold, Inc., San Jose, CA) can be extremely helpful (see Chapter 11). With this system, reminders and other messages are telephoned into a central office, where they are logged into a computer. At predesignated times, the individual is paged, and the reminder or message appears on the pager.

Self-Monitoring and Self-Evaluating

The general executive system routine depicted in Figure 12-5 includes evaluation ("How did I do?") and review ("What worked? What didn't work?") segments. Depending on the amount of support provided by others, this routine can profitably be used by individuals from toddlers to sophisticated adults. When they do not pay attention to how effectively they perform a job, people are much less likely to profit from the natural feedback inherent in the actual outcome of their efforts. Many people with frontal lobe injury do not automatically attend to their level of success and therefore need to be encouraged to engage in this activity deliberately.

Older children and adolescents should keep their own records of performance, starting with nonthreatening tasks (e.g., win-lose performance in social games) and moving to academic and other tasks. Graphs of improvement can be very motivating for children who are frustrated by slow progress. Alternatively, graphs showing minimal improvement may be necessary objective feedback for those who need help in understanding their limitations. In either case, self-monitoring and self-evaluating are best approached by building these routines into everyday activities.

Teaching Compensatory Strategies

Background

For people with chronic disability, whether congenital or acquired, it may be possible to achieve goals by using equipment and procedures not needed by people whose automatic or unaided behavior serves them well. In the case of physical disability, this includes the entire domain of prosthetic equipment, including wheelchairs for people who cannot walk, augmentative communication devices for people who cannot talk, and the like. For people with cognitive disability, there is an analogous domain of compensatory equipment and procedures, some of which are described in Chapters 8 and 11. Discussions of compensatory procedures fall into the domain of executive functions because the ultimate goal is not simply to equip cognitively impaired people with a few compensatory behaviors that might be helpful but more importantly to help them to think and behave as strategically as possible in pursuit of their goals. In other words, being effectively strategic and having mature executive functions are more or less equivalent in one's everyday functioning.

Early work with cognitive strategy intervention in educational psychology can be thought of as the *quick-fix phase*. Experimenters trained students with and without disability to use specific procedures to improve performance on specific tasks in laboratory settings. On the basis of pretesting and post-testing on tasks similar or identical to those being trained, many of the early research reports were optimistic about the effectiveness of such intervention (e.g., Flavell, 1976). For example, students were trained successfully to use mental rehearsal in word list–learning tasks, with improved performance in the laboratory. However, it soon became clear that maintenance of strategic behavior over time and transfer of strategic procedures to more meaningful academic or other tasks were much more difficult to achieve (e.g., Brown and Barclay, 1976; Butterfield and Belmont, 1977; Keeney et al., 1967; Pressley and Levin, 1983a, b). These outcomes parallel results of so-called memory improvement training of normal adults: Improvements are noted after training programs but are rarely maintained or transferred to practical life, even when the trained subjects are specialists in cognitive psychology (Hermann and Searleman, 1992).

Partly as a consequence of these findings, discussions of strategy instruction in educational psychology and special education since the early 1980s have emphasized the following critical features of successful intervention (Flavell et al., 1993; Hermann et al., 1992; Pressley et al., 1990):

1. Strategy intervention must be embedded in meaningful academic or social context and must not be considered a laboratory or purely clinical enterprise.
2. To have a long-term effect on student performance, contextualized cognitive strategy intervention must be intensive and ongoing (at least 2 years [Pressley, 1993]).
3. Strategy intervention is more than equipping a person with a strategic procedure. The intervention must also address the individual's motivation, self-knowledge, attribution (reasons why one succeeds or fails), knowledge base, environment, and other factors that critically affect outcome.
4. Many procedures must be built into the intervention to support generalization and maintenance.

Strategy intervention for people with TBI has followed a similar course in the recent past: a period of enthusiastic teaching of specific compensatory procedures, followed by a realization that generalization and maintenance are unlikely without a comprehensive focus on executive functions and environmental factors (Ylvisaker et al., 1994).

In this discussion, we emphasize the importance of meaningful context and the long-term aspect of strategy intervention. We do this at the risk of discouraging rehabilitation staff from beginning the process of strategy intervention. After all, a rehabilitation hospital is a most unusual setting, and the limited time (generally, a few weeks) that a child or adolescent might receive services in this setting is relatively minimal as compared to the many months of instruction necessary to have a meaningful effect on the child's strategic behavior in the real world. The answer to this challenge is that rehabilitation staff should initiate a process of strategy exploration and intervention that ideally continues without interruption as the child reenters school. This demands a commitment to collaboration across systems of service delivery, as discussed earlier in this chapter.

Defining a Cognitive Strategy

As we use the term, a *cognitive strategy* is a procedure or operation (i.e., something that is done) that goes beyond the processes that are a natural consequence of carrying out the task, that is used to achieve a cognitive goal, and that is at least potentially conscious or controllable. For example, a student who wants to follow the teacher's instructions but who has serious auditory processing difficulties may ask the teacher to write the instructions. If the student does this routinely, it may become a habit and therefore not a conscious decision on every occasion. However, according to our definition, *potentially* conscious use (*not* conscious use) of a special procedure is required.

Some argue that this last clause of the definition should simply be eliminated, thereby permitting the organized, effortful, goal-directed behavior of infants to be characterized as strategic. In our opinion, there is value in viewing the problem-solving behavior of infants as the first stage in a long process of thinking and behaving increasingly and more self-consciously strategically over the many years of childhood and adolescence. In normal development, a child does not *abruptly* enter the domain of strategic thinkers and doers. However, in discussions of teaching specific strategies, there is reason to consider only those strategic procedures that are potentially conscious and controllable.

Strategies may involve the use of *external aids* (e.g., calculator, printed schedule, memory book, graphic task organizer), *overt behavior* (e.g., asking for information to be repeated or clarified, repeating information aloud), or *covert behavior* (e.g., mentally rehearsing, organizing and elaborating information, guiding oneself through a task with covert self-instructions). In normal development and also in recovery from brain injury, strategic behavior progresses from prompted use of simple external aids to internally directed use of elaborate mental procedures. Whichever procedure is chosen, the strategy is what the student does, *not* what the therapist or teacher does (i.e., instructional strategies).

Strategic Versus Antistrategic Strategy Intervention

Compensatory strategy intervention that is not part of a broader focus on executive functions typically has the

Table 12-4. Characteristics of Good Strategy Users

Goals	Good strategy users have goals to which strategies are relevant.
Metacognition: self-knowledge	Good strategy users know that their performance needs to be enhanced (in certain areas), that strategies enhance performance, and that they are capable of using strategies.
Metacognition: awareness of task difficulty	Good strategy users are capable of perceiving the difficulty level of tasks and the consequent need for special effort.
Metacognition: strategy-specific knowledge	Good strategy users know when, where, how, and why to use specific strategies.
Initiation and responsibility	Good strategy users take responsibility for their successes and failures and initiate strategic behavior when it is necessary.
Self-monitoring	Good strategy users can monitor the effectiveness of their performance with strategies so that improved performance can be its own reward and ineffective performance can be changed.
Flexibility	Good strategy users know several strategic procedures and can select the procedure that is useful for a specific problem.
Automaticity	Good strategy users use strategies as a matter of routine so that many strategic procedures become automatic and require little effort or planning.
Working memory	Good strategy users have adequate working memory so that they can think about the task at hand and about strategic procedures at the same time.
Impulsiveness	Good strategy users are not so impulsive that they act before taking critical information into account and considering strategies.
Anxiety	Good strategy users are not so anxious about performance that they neglect strategies because of an overriding fear of failure.
Support	Good strategy users receive support from teachers, parents, and others for the use of strategies.
Content knowledge	Good strategy users know enough about the subject that they can meaningfully apply strategies within that content domain.

Source: Adapted from M Pressley, F Goodchild, J Fleet, et al. (1989). The challenges of classroom strategy instruction. Elem School J 89;301.

following structure: The clinician or teacher diagnoses the child's problem, identifies a strategic procedure that can be used to compensate for the problem, trains the student to use the procedure under specific circumstances, evaluates the student's performance with the procedure in place, and makes modifications as needed. The student's job is to comply and practice. For example, many grade-school arithmetic teachers teach regrouping (i.e., borrowing and carrying) in this manner. The procedures that the students learn may be useful for the task at hand and may be maintained if practiced to habituation. However, there is no reason to believe that this type of instruction will cause the student to be increasingly strategic in attacking difficult problems that do not resemble the training problems. On the contrary, if teachers and clinicians assume responsibility for all strategic thinking, *they* might become increasingly strategic thinkers over time, but their clients or students are likely to become increasingly dependent on others and nonstrategic in their cognitive functioning. *Strategic strategy intervention*, in contrast, engages the child in as much of the strategic thinking and decision making as possible.

Levels and Scope of Strategy Intervention

In normal development, strategic behavior follows a continuum from the wholly nonstrategic behavior of newborns to the extremely strategic behavior of clever, busy college students. Similarly, in rehabilitation, there are many levels on which compensatory behavior can be addressed and many domains of behavior that might need to be targeted in a comprehensive program of strategy intervention. Table 12-4 presents a list of characteristics of people who are proficient users of strategies (Pressley et al., 1989).

An operational definition of the sort suggested in Table 12-4 gives clinicians and teachers a vision of the ultimate goal of strategy intervention and helps them to identify what areas might require attention and how far a person is from being an independently strategic person. Because the 13 variables listed in Table 12-4 are relatively independent of one another and occur in degrees, many different profiles of people exist with respect to strategy needs, receptiveness to strategy intervention, and the focus of that intervention. At one extreme is the simple preparatory work appropriate for preschoolers

Table 12-5. Important Considerations in Selecting Specific Strategies for Specific Students

Negotiation with the student	The probability of generalized use of strategies is increased if the student is involved in selecting the procedure.
Spontaneous use	Other things being equal, procedures that a student uses spontaneously are preferable to essentially new procedures.
Complexity and abstractness	Simple, concrete, externally focused, and possibly externally cued procedures are preferable for young or significantly impaired students.
Difficulty of use	Difficult and time-consuming procedures are appropriate only if the payoff is substantial. Strategies should be as simple as possible.
Domain of applicability	Depending on the purpose of the strategy, either task-specific strategies (e.g., an outlining procedure for processing narrative text; mnemonics to remember people's names) or highly generalizable strategies (e.g., asking for clarification, checking one's work) may be selected.
Neuropsychological strengths	Strategies should capitalize on the student's strengths.
Metacognitive requirements	Strategies that require a high degree of self-insight or subtle situational discrimination and perception of task demands are not appropriate for young or significantly impaired students.
Personality fit	For example, strategies that involve social-interactive behavior that is potentially stigmatizing (e.g., asking for help) are appropriate only for students who find this behavior emotionally acceptable.

(described in Chapter 14). At another extreme is the dispensing of study and writing strategies observed daily in college and university study skills offices. After TBI in adolescents, strategy intervention may cover this entire developmental continuum.

The characteristics of good strategy users listed in Table 12-4 can be considered a list of potential goals for individuals with TBI. Diagnostic teaching of strategies is often the most effective way to identify areas that require specific attention. For example, individuals who are unaware of their cognitive limitations will predictably not see the point of compensatory procedures; therefore, the emphasis of their intervention may be self-awareness procedures (described earlier). Because TBI is often associated with poor self-awareness of strengths and weaknesses, intervention frequently focuses on self-awareness for these students.

A similar case can be made for transforming each of the variables in Table 12-4 into an intervention goal for selected individuals. People who lack goals are rarely willing to exert the effort implicit in strategic behavior. People who erroneously perceive tasks as easy or impossible are unlikely to shift into a strategic mode to accomplish the task successfully. Those individuals who do not have strategies that work for specific tasks will probably discontinue strategic behavior. People who have an initiation impairment or who believe that their success or failure is a consequence of factors outside of themselves will not use strategies. People who rigidly apply the same procedure to every task or who get bogged down in special effort because none of their strategic procedures become habitual are unlikely long-term users of strategies. Those individuals who are extremely impulsive will probably act long before they remember that there is a strategic

way to accomplish the task. People who are very anxious are likely to be focused on something other than strategic possibilities when they face challenging tasks.

Environmental support for strategy use warrants special attention. Just as parents may understandably be unreceptive to compensations for physical impairment (e.g., communication aid) on grounds that the prosthetic alternative may interfere with the recovery of normal physical function, some parents may react negatively to cognitive prostheses or strategies on grounds that they might interfere with cognitive recovery. Similarly, teachers may not be supportive of compensatory classroom procedures because their student with TBI may score within normal limits on tests when returning to school and so appear to be fine. Parents and teachers may need to be educated about the consequences of TBI combined with sensitive counseling about the role of compensatory procedures in recovery and long-term success.

Selecting Strategic Procedures

We have already highlighted the importance of engaging the child as much as possible in identifying the need for strategic behavior and in selecting useful strategies to get the job done. Table 12-5 lists considerations important in making the selection.

Facilitating Functional Use of Strategic Procedures

In many respects, teaching strategies is similar to teaching other skills. Therefore, general principles of good teaching apply to this process. For example, complex tasks must be analyzed into manageable components, teaching must progress from simple to complex, cues and prompts are liberally provided to ensure success and then are systematically faded, goals are limited so that the student can experience success, target behaviors are clearly described and modeled so that the student knows exactly what to do, and the child is encouraged to practice until the strategy becomes relatively effortless.

In Table 12-6, we highlight several special goals and procedures designed to address areas of weakness frequently observed in students with TBI and to avoid the trap of antistrategic strategy intervention. Helping people to be functionally strategic in their daily lives is more than teaching specific behaviors, however helpful those behaviors may be. Therefore, Table 12-6 includes procedures designed to heighten metacognitive awareness, to underscore the value of functioning strategically, to engage students in selecting compensatory behaviors, and to maintain and generalize these behaviors. These are the critical areas in strategy intervention for people with TBI. In Appendix 12-1, we list a wide range of cognitive strategies that may be helpful for some people in overcoming obstacles imposed by their cognitive impairment after TBI.

Generalization, Maintenance, and Supported Cognition

Table 12-6 includes several procedures that are important if generalization and maintenance of strategic behavior are to be realistic expectations. As is the case with most types of intervention, acquiring a behavior in a training context is considerably easier than maintaining the behavior over time and generalizing its use to a variety of relevant contexts and tasks. With considerable attention to generalization procedures, some individuals with TBI can become independently strategic and can succeed in academic and vocational life by compensating for ongoing cognitive disability.

However, professionals who have followed a large number of people with TBI over several years after their injuries often report that ongoing support, reminders, cues, and the like continue to be necessary indefinitely for many students. In Chapter 11, we describe MS, a teenager who appeared initially to be very successful in her use of strategies to comprehend and remember extended text but who continued to need special support 9 years later to use her strategies to succeed in her academic work. Because of injury to her frontal lobes, MS remained a relatively concrete thinker and had shallow insight into her cognitive strengths and weaknesses. However, she was highly motivated and retained reasonable academic skill and therefore was able to complete her college education. Throughout her 5 years of college, she was enrolled in a learning disabilities program that mandated 8 hours per week of coached study hall. By her own admission, MS would not have succeeded without this support. At each stage of her rehabilitation and education, a primary contribution of staff who knew her well was to pass along to the staff at the next stage an understanding of the procedures that MS needed to succeed and the support she needed to use her procedures effectively.

MS illustrates the important concept of *supported cognition,* an approach to cognitive rehabilitation that, in our judgment, has received insufficient attention in the literature. In the educational psychology and rehabilitation literature, *independence* is often the unambiguous goal of intervention. Therefore, persistent dependence is viewed as failure. However, for many people such as MS, complete cognitive independence, particularly in nonroutine contexts, is not a realistic goal. In these cases, professionals must go to great lengths to ensure that relevant supports, analogous to MS's coached study hall, are available as the individual progresses through the educational system and into vocational life. Success of the intervention then would not be determined by independence but by achievement of goals with the help of the most natural and unobtrusive supports possible.

Executive System Intervention and Collaboration: Everyday People as the Ideal Providers of Services and Supports

Throughout this chapter, we have emphasized the importance of contextualizing executive system intervention, using real-world activities throughout the day and considering everyday people as the primary deliverers of the service. This is not a specialized therapeutic approach that is the territory of one or two rehabilitation professions. Because there is an executive dimension to all human behavior, all activities can be made the context for coaching and the service must be seen as an intensively collaborative service.

The obstacles to this approach are numerous and include the self-perception and self-definition of many rehabilitation professionals (discussed in the next section). Furthermore, helping everyday people to play this role effectively requires time and professional competence. In Chapter 20, we outline procedures that are useful in orienting and training everyday people.

In Figure 12-7, we present a checklist that can be used by all staff and family members to evaluate and adjust intervention from the perspective of executive functions. If the people who are most involved with the life of the child or adolescent with TBI would try to fashion their interaction with the child so that as many boxes as possible could be checked, then they will have created an "executive system culture." Within such a culture, children and adolescents are encouraged to achieve their highest possible level of executive or self-regulatory functioning.

Table 12-6. Procedures Useful in Teaching Compensatory Strategies

I. Phase 1: General strategic thinking
    A. Metacognitive awareness. Note that these metacognitive discoveries are facilitated if the activities are personally meaningful and intimately connected to the student's goals.
        1. Goals: Students will discriminate effective from ineffective performance; become aware of their strengths and weaknesses; and recognize implications of their deficits.
        2. Rationale: Given the frequency of frontal lobe injury in traumatic brain injury (TBI), self-awareness often is compromised. Individuals are unlikely to acquire and use procedures designed to compensate for problems that they do not recognize as problems.
        3. Procedures
            a. Objective: Improve the student's perception of successful versus unsuccessful task performance.
            Procedure: Illustrate successful and unsuccessful performance of a functional task through role playing or on videotape. With the student, analyze the performances in sufficient detail that the student can identify the features that account for successful versus unsuccessful performance.
            b. Objective: Improve the student's ability to perceive functional cognitive disabilities.
            Procedures: Individually, request that the student make note of specific deficits of other students in the program or of individuals observed on tape. Discuss these observations. Planned peer teaching is useful. Discuss the effects of TBI on cognitive and social functioning. If appropriate, read and discuss literature on the effects of TBI.
            c. Objective: Improve the student's awareness of his or her strengths and weaknesses.
            Procedures: (See other sections of this chapter for other procedures.) Videotape the student in activities designed to reveal strong and weak areas of functioning. (Alternatively, use role playing.) Review the tapes (beginning with strong performance), first without commentary and subsequently inviting comments about what was done well and what needs improvement. Gradually turn over to the student the responsibility for stopping the tape when problems are noted. Note that considerable desensitizing may be needed before videotape self-viewing is possible.
            d. Objective: Improve the student's understanding of the relation between deficits and long-term goals.
            Procedures: Discuss in detail the individual's long-term goals and expectations. Jointly create a list of specific skills and resources needed to achieve these goals. Jointly identify the skills that are present and those that are weak relative to this goal.
    B. Value of functioning strategically
        1. Goal: Students will recognize the importance of thinking and acting strategically and will identify the characteristics of strategic people.
        2. Rationale: Because the ultimate goal of this intervention is to promote strategic thinking and strategic behavior in general—not simply to teach specific strategic behaviors as routines—it is important that the student understand what it is to function strategically and that these are valuable attributes.
        3. Procedures
            a. Objective: Improve the student's understanding of strategy.
            Procedures: Using games, sports, or other relevant models, clarify the concept of strategy as something that people do to achieve goals when there are obstacles.
            b. Objective: Heighten the student's appreciation of strategic behavior.
            Procedures: Together with the student, identify several individuals who are known to think and behave very strategically (e.g., legendary sports figures, military heroes). Discuss why these people are considered heroic. Clinicians should also clearly model their own strategic behavior and discuss the value of their own strategies.
            c. Objective: Improve the student's understanding of the behaviors that are part of functioning strategically.
            Procedures: Using models relevant to the student (e.g., military, sports, or business analogies), brainstorm about the characteristics of people who are known to be very strategic, among them a high level of motivation and initiative, the ability to identify and clarify obstacles to goals, the ability to plan procedures to overcome obstacles, the ability to monitor and evaluate performance, and a willingness to engage in ongoing problem solving.
II. Phase 2: Selecting specific strategic procedures
    A. Goal: Students will identify specific procedures useful in overcoming important personal obstacles.
    B. Rationale: It is important that students participate in the selection of strategic procedures that they will use and that the procedures be truly useful in achieving the students' goals.
    C. Procedures
        1. Use group brainstorming procedures to identify possible strategies.

2. Use product-monitoring tasks to test the value of strategies: Have the student perform a task with and without the strategy or with a variety of different strategies. Objectively compare the results. (Videotape analysis may be useful here.)

3. Have advanced students demonstrate the value of certain procedures or offer testimonials.

4. Discuss the widespread use of compensatory procedures (lists, memos, tape recorders, and so forth) by people who do not have brain injury.

III. Phase 3: Teaching specific strategies—procedures. Note that if the discovery procedures in phase 2 (e.g., brainstorming and product monitoring) are effective, there may be little need for specific teaching procedures.

    A.   Task analysis, modeling, and rehearsal: The steps in the strategy can be modeled by the therapist or by a peer, or by means of videotape or other media. Modeling is accompanied initially by overt verbalization of the strategy by the model. The student then rehearses the strategy with gradually decreasing cues and self-talk.

    B.   Direct instruction: The carefully programmed behavioral teaching procedures of direct instruction can be used to teach strategies. However, if this is the only approach used, it is likely that the best result will be the acquisition of a learned sequence of behaviors (which may be a desirable outcome), without positive movement in the direction of becoming a strategically thinking person.

    C.   Functional practice: However the strategy is acquired, it must be frequently rehearsed in natural settings using functional activities.

IV. Phase 4: Generalization and maintenance. Generalization of strategic behavior beyond the context of training is a combined consequence of the perceived utility of the strategy for the individual, the inherent generalizability and utility of the strategy, widespread environmental support for strategic behavior and thinking, and specific teaching procedures designed to enhance generalization.

    A.   Notes

        1. Generalization includes generalized use of specific strategies as well as strategic behavior in general.

        2. Generalization may not be a separate phase if the acquisition stage takes place in the context of functional activities and natural settings. This is particularly important for very concretely thinking people (including young people and people with serious cognitive impairment).

        3. Generalization may be a relatively unimportant phase of intervention if the individual has acquired a strategic attitude and actively seeks occasions for transfer.

        4. Some individuals may need to be reminded indefinitely (with environmental reminders) to use their strategic procedures.

    B.   Objective: Improve the student's discrimination of situations that require or do not require a given strategy. Procedures

        1. Use videotaped scenes or role playing to illustrate the correct use of a strategy in an appropriate situation, inappropriate use of the strategy, and failure to use the strategy when appropriate. Discuss the conditions that require the strategy.

        2. Use short, videotaped scenes to train the student in efficient and accurate judgments as to whether a strategy is appropriate in a context.

    C.   Objective: Increase the student's spontaneous use of strategies in varied situations. Procedures

        1. Include family members, work supervisors, and teachers in strategy intervention to (a) provide varied opportunities for the use of specific strategies and of strategic behavior in general, (b) reinforce the student's use of strategies, and (c) model strategic behavior.

        2. Ask students to keep a log in which they record their successes and failures in strategy use. Make generalization an explicit goal.

    D.   Objective: Increase the student's acceptance of strategic behavior. Procedures

        1. Ensure that the student is successful using strategies.

        2. Promote emotional acceptance of strategic behavior by using whatever motivating procedures work (e.g., personal images or metaphors, testimonials).

Note: The phases of intervention listed in this table are not necessarily hierarchical or mutually exclusive.

Source: Modified with permission from J Haarbauer-Krupa, K Henry, S Szekeres, M Ylvisaker (1985). Cognitive Rehabilitation Therapy: Late Stages of Recovery. In M Ylvisaker (ed), Head Injury Rehabilitation: Children and Adolescents. Boston: Butterworth–Heinemann, 318–319.

General considerations

❏   Is intervention in the areas that fall into the category of executive functions structured around the individual's *meaningful goals*?

❏   Is intervention infused into *everyday activities*? Are all *everyday people* oriented to how they can facilitate improved executive functions? Are all everyday people aware of the dangers of *learned helplessness*?

❏   Are everyday people aware of the strategies that the individual is being taught or is expected to use?

❏   Is successful performance in the areas classified as executive functions richly and naturally *rewarded*? Is the individual held *responsible* for effective strategic performance?

❏   Is the individual given *ample opportunity* to identify and solve his or her own problems (with guidance, if necessary)?

❏   For individuals who are young or very concrete thinkers, are executive function tasks structured around *concrete physical activities* (vs. *abstract or purely cognitive activities*)?

❏   Do everyday people in the environment routinely *model* expert use of executive functions?

❏   Is the individual given sufficient *practice* so that strategic behavior becomes *automatic*?

❏   Are everyday people in the environment *supportive* of strategic or compensatory ways to accomplish tasks?

❏   Does the individual *respect* a strategic or compensatory approach to everyday problems? If not, is appropriate help or counseling provided?

❏   Are everyday people in the individual's environment fully *aware of possible limitations* in the individual's executive functions (especially initiation and inhibition) so that they do not misinterpret behavior?

Appropriateness: level of development and level of recovery

Level of development

❏   *Preschoolers:* Are preschoolers introduced to relevant vocabulary, including *difficult or easy to do; plan; do something special; review; what works and what doesn't work*? Are they actively engaged in identifying what is difficult and easy for them (especially physical activities)? Are they actively engaged in identifying clever ways to accomplish difficult tasks? Are they richly and naturally rewarded for clever solutions to difficult everyday problems?

❏   *Grade-school-age children:* Are grade-school-age children actively engaged in identifying what is difficult and easy for them (including cognitive and academic activities)? Are they actively engaged in identifying clever ways to accomplish difficult tasks? Are they actively encouraged to seek help on their own when tasks are difficult? Are they richly and naturally rewarded for clever solutions to difficult everyday problems? Are they encouraged to help one another solve problems?

❏   *Older students and adults:* See entire checklist.

Level of recovery

❏   *People who are minimally responsive:* Is the individual prompted (physically, if necessary) to engage in familiar activities (e.g., activities of daily living), so that he or she is *acting*, not just being acted on? Has every attempt been made (e.g., remote switch control) to enable the individual to control meaningful events? Do everyday people in the environment *respond* to the individual as an agent?

❏   *People who are alert but confused:* Is the individual given *choices* whenever possible (short of increasing confusion)? Is the individual thoroughly *oriented to the purposes* of intervention activities? Do staff *negotiate* activities with the individual? Does the individual have opportunities to experience *natural consequences* of choices?

❏   *People who are no longer seriously confused:* See entire checklist.

Self-awareness of strengths and needs

❏   Is the individual maximally engaged in *identifying what is easy and difficult to do* and in determining what makes activities easy or difficult?

❏   Is the individual given opportunities to *compare performance* when an activity is completed in a usual way versus when it is completed with special strategic procedures?

❏   Does the individual keep a *journal* in which strengths and needs are recorded?

Figure 12-7. A checklist for intervention for individuals with executive system impairment.

❑   Is the individual given opportunities to *identify strengths and needs in others and strategic procedures* that others may use (e.g., peer teaching)?

❑   Is the individual given appropriate informative *feedback* (e.g., peer feedback, video feedback, confrontational feedback if appropriate)?

Goal setting

❑   Is the individual routinely asked to *predict* how well he or she will do on activities?

❑   Are predictions recorded in journals and *compared with actual performance*?

❑   Does the individual maximally participate in rehabilitation and special-education *goal setting*? Is adequate support provided if this is difficult?

❑   Are intervention activities structured around the *individual's personal goals*?

Planning

❑   Does the individual participate maximally in *planning his or her intervention activities*?

❑   Is a *planning guide* available, if needed?

❑   Does the individual begin the day by *preparing a plan* on a planning board or in a journal? Does the individual begin each activity by preparing a plan?

❑   Do therapeutic activities include attempts to plan meaningful complex events (e.g., parties, outings)?

❑   Does the individual participate maximally in *long-term future planning,* rehabilitation planning, and development of the individualized education plan?

Organizing: See the organization checklist in Chapter 11.

Self-initiating

❑   Do everyday people give the individual *opportunities to initiate* and then wait an appropriate length of time? Are *signals* available to remind the individual to initiate activities?

❑   Do the activities in which the individual engages make *appropriate demands* on the individual's ability to initiate? (For example, board games may require little initiation, whereas conversations may require much initiation.)

❑   Are all forms of institutional *learned helplessness* avoided?

❑   Are *prosthetic initiators* available if needed (e.g., alarm watch, NeuroPage)?

❑   If initiation cues are necessary, are they provided as much as possible by peers as opposed to staff? Is nagging avoided?

Self-inhibiting

❑   Do everyday people give the individual *opportunities to inhibit* impulsive or inappropriate behavior that are realistic in their demands?

❑   Do the activities in which the individual engages make *appropriate demands* on the individual's ability to inhibit? (For example, unstructured and unfamiliar activities in a distracting environment require considerable inhibition.)

❑   If inhibition cues are necessary, are they as subtle as possible and provided as much as possible by peers as opposed to staff? Is nagging avoided?

Self-monitoring and evaluating

❑   Do everyday people give the individual *opportunities to self-monitor and evaluate* performance? If cues are necessary, are they subtle? Is nagging avoided?

❑   Is the individual maximally involved in *charting* his or her own performance; in keeping a *journal* in which performance is recorded; and in graphing performance?

❑   Is the individual routinely asked to fill in a form regarding his or her own performance: *What works and what doesn't work*?

Problem solving and strategic thinking

❑   Is the individual maximally involved in *solving everyday problems* as they arise? Are *everyday people* thoroughly oriented to the importance of problem solving?

❑   Is the individual maximally engaged in *selecting strategies* to overcome obstacles and achieve important goals?

❑   Is there an appropriate amount of *external support for strategic thinking*?
   ❑ Does the individual have a *form* that cues the appropriate kind of strategic thinking?
   ❑ Do everyday people in the environment *expect and cue strategic performance*?
   ❑ Do everyday people in the environment avoid *learned helplessness*: That is, do they resist solving all of the individual's problems?
❑   Is there *consistency* among staff and family members in how problem-solving tasks are presented and in the kinds of external problem-solving supports that are provided? Is there consistency in *reducing external support* as the individual becomes increasingly independent in problem solving?

Figure 12-7. *Continued*

A Final Word About Clinicians' Self-Perception

Assuming value of the everyday approach to executive system intervention described in this chapter, many obstacles to implementing the approach still remain. Among these obstacles are inadequate training of many professionals and a rehabilitation and special education system that often focuses on *specific* motor, cognitive, communicative, academic, and vocational skills and behaviors to the exclusion of general executive functions, which span all disciplines and therefore have no natural professional home.

Perhaps more important than any of these obstacles, however, is the natural resistance to everyday approaches to intervention created by the self-perception of many rehabilitation professionals. Many of us are taught (perhaps incidentally) in our training programs to think of ourselves as a cross between a surgeon and an animal trainer (see Chapter 20). The surgeon metaphor is associated with the medical model of rehabilitation, which specifies a goal (cure, restoration, remediation of deficits), an authority structure (the professional as the expert who retains all rights to making decisions and setting goals), values (value of the technical expertise of the professional), a process (diagnosis of the disorder and prescription of a treatment program with which the patient is expected to comply), a setting (clinical setting wherein treatment is provided), and a vocabulary (e.g., *patient, diagnosis, prognosis, treatment, treatment plan, treatment room, cure*).

The animal trainer metaphor carries with it a narrowly defined behavioral model, which is also associated with a goal (elimination of dysfunctional behaviors, establishment of a repertoire of positive behaviors), an authority structure (the trainer as expert and decision maker), values (value of the technical expertise of the trainer), a process (identification of present and absent behaviors and prescription of a regimen of training exercises with which the trainee is expected to comply), a setting (a specialized training setting), and a vocabulary (e.g., *trainer, training, skill hierarchy, shaping, cueing, fading, learning trials, percent correct, reinforcement*

contingencies, acquisition, stabilization, and generalization phases).

These two metaphors or models are useful for some of the interventions provided by rehabilitation professionals. However, for people with chronic cognitive disability, particularly if that disability is related to executive system dysfunction, these metaphors quickly become counterproductive for two important reasons. First, if professionals accept full responsibility for (1) identifying the individual's strengths and weaknesses, (2) setting goals for the individual, (3) planning and organizing the individual's rehabilitation activities, (4) initiating activity and inhibiting inappropriate activity, (5) monitoring and evaluating the individual's performance, and (6) identifying compensatory strategies for the individual, then the professionals have become their client's prosthetic executive system, and a reasonable expectation is increasing learned helplessness or oppositional behavior over time. Second, if professionals restrict their interaction with clients to professional encounters in specialized treatment settings, then transfer to functional settings and tasks is seriously jeopardized, and everyday routines will likely not be exploited or ultimately changed for the better.

Therefore, rehabilitation professionals are well advised to adopt a new set of metaphors to guide and enliven their professional activity. In the professionals' interaction with individuals with chronic executive system weakness, a combination of mentor, coach, consultant, and master craftsperson metaphors yields much more productive intervention than does the traditional combination of surgeon and animal trainer metaphors. These alternative metaphors are explored in Chapter 20. More importantly, individuals with chronic disability would be well served by professionals who acted as consultants to design such individuals' entire lives so as to promote incremental improvements in their daily performance of executive functions. This role requires a willingness to relinquish authority, to work collaboratively (including family members, paraprofessionals, and peers), to leave clinical settings and enter everyday settings, and to recognize that individuals' everyday routines in their real worlds are the beginning and end of good rehabilitation.

Summary

In this chapter, we have attempted to explain and illustrate an approach to cognitive rehabilitation that is particularly important for people with TBI because of the frequency of executive system impairment in this population. The premises with which we began the chapter highlight the theoretical themes underlying the framework that we have strengthened during the course of many years of serving children and adolescents with TBI. The intervention suggestions and protocols that compose the bulk of the chapter illustrate concrete approaches that we have used successfully with many children and that have received increasingly positive support in the research literature devoted to a variety of disability groups.

References

Ackerly SS (1964). A Case of Paranatal Frontal Lobe Defect Observed for Thirty Years. In JM Warren, K Ackert (eds), The Frontal Granular Cortex and Behavior. New York: McGraw-Hill, 192.

Alexander MP, Benson DF, Stuss DT (1989). Frontal lobes and language. Brain Lang 37;656.

Barkley RA (1997). Behavioral inhibition, sustained attention, and executive functions: constructing a unifying theory of ADHD. Psychol Bull 121;65.

Benton A (1991). Prefrontal injury and behavior in children. Dev Neuropsychol 7;275.

Bigler ED (1988). Frontal lobe damage and neuropsychological assessment. Arch Clin Neuropsychol 3;279.

Bjorklund DJ (1990). Children's Strategies: Contemporary Views of Cognitive Development. Hillsdale, NJ: Lawrence Erlbaum.

Bjorklund DF, Harnishfeger KK (1990). Children's Strategies: Their Definition and Origins. In DF Bjorklund (ed), Children's Strategies: Contemporary Views of Cognitive Development. Hillsdale, NJ: Lawrence Erlbaum, 309.

Borkowski JG, Carr M, Rellinger E, Pressley M (1990). Self-Regulated Cognition: Interdependence of Metacognition, Attributions, and Self-Esteem. In BF Jones, L Idol (eds), Dimensions of Thinking and Cognitive Development. Hillsdale, NJ: Lawrence Erlbaum, 53.

Borkowski JG, Johnston MB, Reid MK (1986). Metacognition, Motivation, and the Transfer of Control Process. In SJ Ceci (ed), Handbook of Cognitive, Social, and Neuropsychological Aspects of Learning Disabilities. Hillsdale, NJ: Lawrence Erlbaum.

Brown AL (1975). The Development of Memory: Knowing, Knowing About Knowing, and Knowing How to Know. In HW Reese (ed), Advances in Child Development and Behavior, vol 10. New York: Academic, 103.

Brown AL, Barclay CR (1976). The effects of training specific mnemonics on the metamnemonic efficiency of retarded children. Child Devel 47;71.

Brown G, Chadwick O, Shaffer D, et al. (1981). A prospective study of children with head injuries: III. Psychiatric sequelae. Psychol Med 11;63.

Bruner J (1975). The ontogenesis of speech acts. J Child Lang 2;1.

Bruner J (1978). How to Do Things with Words. In J Bruner, A Garton (eds), Human Growth and Development. Oxford: Oxford University.

Butterfield E, Belmont J (1977). Assessing and Improving the Executive Cognitive Functions of Mentally Retarded People. In I Bialer, M Sternlicht (eds), The Psychology of Mental Retardation: Issues and Approaches. New York: Psychological Dimensions, 277.

Chelune GJ, Baer RA (1986). Developmental norms for the Wisconsin Card Sorting Test. J Clin Exp Neuropsychol 8;219.

Dennis M (1991). Frontal lobe function in childhood and adolescence: a heuristic for assessing attention regulation, executive control, and the intentional states important for social discourse. Dev Neuropsychol 7;327.

Dennis M, Barnes M (1990). Knowing the meaning, getting the point, bridging the gap, and carrying the message: aspects of discourse following closed head injury in childhood and adolescence. Brain Lang 39;428.

Deshler DD, Schumaker JB (1988). An Instructional Model for Teaching Students How to Learn. In JL Graden, JE Zins, MJ Curtis (eds), Alternative Educational Delivery Systems: Enhancing Instructional Options for All Students. Washington, DC: National Association of School Psychologists, 391.

Dru D, Walker JP, Walker JB (1975). Self-produced locomotion restores visual capacity after striate lesions. Science 187;265.

Eslinger PJ, Damasio AR (1985). Severe disturbance of higher cognition following bilateral frontal lobe oblation: patient EVR. Neurology 35;1731.

Eslinger PJ, Grattan LM, Damasio H, Damasio AR (1992). Developmental consequences of childhood frontal lobe damage. Arch Neurol 49;764.

Feeney TJ, Ylvisaker M (1995). Choice and routine: antecedent behavioral interventions for adolescents with severe traumatic brain injury. J Head Trauma Rehabil 10(3);67.

Feeney TJ, Ylvisaker M (1997). A Positive, Communication-Based Approach to Challenging Behavior After TBI. In A Glang, G Singer (eds), Children with Acquired Brain Injury: The School's Response. Baltimore: Paul Brookes.

Ferchmin PA, Bennett EL, Rosenzweig MR (1975). Direct contact with enriched environment is required to alter cerebral weights in rats. J Comp Physiol Psychol 88;360.

Flavell J (1976). Metacognitive Aspects of Problem Solving. In LB Resnick (ed), The Nature of Intelligence. Hillsdale, NJ: Lawrence Erlbaum, 231.

Flavell J, Miller P, Miller S (1993). Cognitive Development (3rd ed). Englewood Cliffs, NJ: Prentice Hall.

Fletcher JM, Ewing-Cobbs L, Miner M, Levin HS (1990). Behavioral changes after closed head injury in children. J Consult Clin Psychol 58;93.

Goldman PS (1971). Functional development of the prefrontal cortex in early life and the problem of neuronal plasticity. Exp Neurol 32;366.

Goldman PS, Alexander GE (1977). Maturation of prefrontal cortex in the monkey revealed by local reversible cryogenic depression. Nature 267;613.

Gordon Diagnostic System (1988). Model III Instruction Manual. DeWitt, NY: Author.

Grattan LM, Eslinger PJ (1991). Frontal lobe damage in children and adults: a comparative review. Dev Neuropsychol 7;283.

Grattan LM, Eslinger PJ (1992). Long-term psychological consequences of childhood frontal lobe lesion in patient DT. Brain Cogn 20;185.

Hallowell EM, Ratey JJ (1994). Driven to Distraction. New York: Pantheon Books.

Harchik AE, Sherman JA, Sheldon JB, Bannerman DJ (1993). Choice and control: new opportunities for people with developmental disabilities. Ann Clin Psychiatry 5;151.

Hermann DJ, Searleman A (1992). Memory Improvement and Memory Theory in Perspective. In DJ Hermann, H Weingartner, A Searleman, C McVoy (eds), Memory Improvement: Implications for Memory Theory. New York: Springer, 8.

Hermann DJ, Weingartner H, Searleman A, McVoy C (eds) (1992). Memory Improvement: Implications for Memory Theory. New York: Springer.

Kavale K, Mattson P (1983). "One jumped off the balance beam": meta-analysis of perceptual-motor training. J Learn Disabil 16;165.

Keeney T, Cannizo S, Flavell J (1967). Spontaneous and induced verbal rehearsal in a recall task. Child Dev 38;953.

Lehr E (1990). Psychological Management of Traumatic Brain Injuries in Children and Adolescents. Gaithersburg, MD: Aspen Publishers.

Levin HS, Culhane KA, Hartman J, et al. (1991b). Developmental changes in performance on tests of purported frontal lobe functioning. Dev Neuropsychol 7;377.

Levin HS, Culhane KA, Mendelsohn D, et al. (1993). Cognition in relation to magnetic resonance imaging in head-injured children and adolescents. Arch Neurol 50;897.

Levin HS, Fletcher JM, Kufera JA, et al. (1996). Dimensions of cognition measured by the Tower of London and other cognitive tasks in head-injured children and adolescents. Dev Neuropsychol 12;17.

Levin HS, Goldstein FC, Williams DH, Eisenberg HM (1991a). The Contribution of Frontal Lobe Lesions to the Neurobehavioral Outcome of Closed Head Injury. In HS Levin, HM Eisenberg, AI Benton (eds), Frontal Lobe Function and Dysfunction. New York: Oxford University, 318.

Lezak MD (1982). The problem of assessing executive functions. Int J Psychol 17;281.

Light P, Butterworth G (eds) (1993). Context and Cognition. Hillsdale, NJ: Lawrence Erlbaum.

Luria AR (1966). Higher Cortical Functions in Man (2nd ed). Translated by B. Haigh. New York: Basic Books. (Original work published 1962.)

Mann L (1979). On the Trail of Process: A Historical Perspective on Cognitive Processes and Their Training. New York: Grune & Stratton.

Marlowe WB (1992). The impact of a right prefrontal lesion on the developing brain. Brain Cogn 20;205.

Mateer CA, Williams D (1991). Effects of frontal lobe injury in childhood. Dev Neuropsychol 7;359.

McCabe A, Peterson C (eds) (1991). New Directions in Developing Narrative Structure. Hillsdale, NJ: Lawrence Erlbaum.

Meichenbaum D (1993). The "potential" contributions of cognitive behavior modification to the rehabilitation of individuals with traumatic brain injury. Semin Speech Lang 14;18.

Mount B, Zwernik K (1986). It's Never Too Early, It's Never Too Late. St. Paul, MN: Metropolitan Council (pub. no. 421-88-109).

O'Brien J, Lyle C (1987). Design for Accomplishment. Decatur, GA: Responsive Systems Associates.

Pennington B (1991). Diagnosing Learning Disorders: A Neuropsychological Framework . New York: Guilford.

Perrott SB, Taylor HG, Montes JL (1991). Neuropsychological sequelae, familial stress, and environmental adaptation following pediatric head injury. Dev Neuropsychol 7;69.

Petterson L (1991). Sensitivity to emotional cues and social behavior in children and adolescents after head injury. Percept Mot Skills 73(3 pt 2);1139.

Ponsford J (1990). The Use of Computers in the Rehabilitation of Attention Disorders. In RL Wood, I Fussey (eds), Cognitive Rehabilitation in Perspective. London: Taylor and Francis, 48.

Pressley M (1993). Teaching cognitive strategies to brain-injured clients: the good information processing perspective. Semin Speech Lang 14;1.

Pressley M, et al. (1990). Cognitive Strategy Instruction That Really Improves Children's Academic Performance. Cambridge, MA: Brookline Books.

Pressley M, Borkowski JG, Schneider W (1989). Good information processing: what it is and what education can do to promote it. Int J Educ Res 13;857.

Pressley M, El-Dinary PB (1992). Memory Strategy Instruction That Promotes Good Information Processing. In DJ Herrmann, H Weingartner, A Searleman, C McEvoy (eds), Memory Improvement: Implications for Memory Theory. New York: Springer, 79.

Pressley M, Levin JR (eds) (1983a). Cognitive Strategy Training: Educational Applications. New York: Springer.

Pressley M, Levin JR (eds) (1983b). Cognitive Strategy Training: Psychological Foundations. New York: Springer.

Price B, Doffnre K, Stowe R, Mesulam M (1990). The comportmental learning disabilities of early frontal lobe damage. Brain 113;1383.

Reese E, Fivush G (1993). Parental styles of talking about the past. Dev Psychol 29;596.

Reese E, Haden CA, Fivush R (1993). Mother-child conversations about the past: relationships of style and memory over time. Cogn Dev 8;403.

Reitan RM (1987). Neuropsychological Evaluation of Children. Tucson, AZ: Neuropsychology Press.

Schacter DL, Glisky EL (1986). Memory Remediation: Restoration, Alleviation, and the Acquisition of Domain-Specific Knowledge. In B Uzell, Y Gross (eds), Clinical Neuropsychology of Intervention. Boston: Martinus Nijhoff, 257.

Shue KL, Douglas VI (1992). Attention deficit hyperactivity disorder and the frontal lobe syndrome. Brain Cogn 20;104.

Siegler R (1991). Children's Thinking (2nd ed). Englewood Cliffs, NJ: Prentice Hall.

Singley MK, Anderson JR (1989). Transfer of Cognitive Skill. Cambridge, MA: Harvard University.

Stelling MW, McKay SE, Carr WA, et al. (1986). Frontal lobe lesions and cognitive function in craniopharyngioma survivors. Am J Dis Child 140;710.

Stuss DT, Benson DF (1986). The Frontal Lobes. New York: Raven.

Taylor HG, Schatschneider C, Petrill S, et al. (1996). Executive dysfunction in children with early brain disease: outcomes post *Haemophilus influenzae* meningitis. Dev Neuropsychol 12;35.

Thomsen IV (1989). Do young patients have worse outcomes after severe blunt head trauma? Brain Inj 3;157.

Tranel D, Damasio AR (1995). Neurobiological Foundations of Human Memory. In AD Baddeley, BA Wilson, FN Watts (eds), Handbook of Memory Disorders. New York: Wiley, 27.

Vandercook T, York J, Forest M (1989). The McGill Action Planning System (MAPS): a strategy for building the vision. J Assoc Pers Severe Handicaps 14;205.

von Cramon DY, Matthes-von Cramon G (1994). Back to work with a chronic dysexecutive syndrome? [A case report.] Neuropsychol Rehabil 4;399.

Vygotsky LS (1978). Mind in Society: The Development of Higher Psychological Processes. Edited and translated by M Cole, V John-Steiner, S Scribner, E Souberman. Cambridge, MA: Harvard University.

Welsh MC, Pennington BF (1988). Assessing frontal lobe functioning in children: views from developmental psychology. Dev Neuropsychol 4;199.

Welsh MC, Pennington BF, Groisser DB (1991). A normative-developmental study of executive function: a window on prefrontal function in children. Dev Neuropsychol 7(2);131.

Will BE (1977). Methods for Promoting Functional Recovery Following Brain Damage. In SR Berenberg (ed), Brain: Fetal and Infant. The Hague: Martinus Nijhoff, 330.

Williams D, Mateer CA (1992). Developmental impact of frontal lobe injury in middle childhood. Brain Cogn 20;196.

Ylvisaker M (1992). Communication outcome following traumatic brain injury. Semin Speech Lang 13;239.

Ylvisaker M (1993). Communication outcome in children and adolescents with traumatic brain injury. Neuropsychol Rehabil 3;367.

Ylvisaker M, Feeney T (1994). Communication and behavior: collaboration between speech-language pathologists and behavioral psychologists. Top Lang Disord 15(1);37.

Ylvisaker M, Feeney T (1995). Traumatic brain injury in adolescence: assessment and reintegration. Semin Speech Lang 16;32.

Ylvisaker M, Feeney T (1996). Executive functions after traumatic brain injury: supported cognition and self-advocacy. Semin Speech Lang 17;217.

Ylvisaker M, Feeney T (in press). An Integrated Approach to Brain Injury Rehabilitation: Positive Everyday Routines. San Diego: Singular Press.

Ylvisaker M, Szekeres S (1989). Metacognitive and executive impairments in head-injured children and adults. Top Lang Disord 9(2);34.

Ylvisaker M, Szekeres S, Hartwick P (1992). Cognitive Rehabilitation Following Traumatic Brain Injury. In M Tramontana, S Hooper (eds), Advances in Child Neuropsychology, vol 1. New York: Springer, 168.

Ylvisaker M, Szekeres S, Hartwick P, Tworek P (1994). Cognitive Intervention. In R Savage, G Wolcott (eds), Educational Dimensions of Acquired Brain Injury. Austin, TX: PRO-ED, 121.

Ylvisaker M, Urbanczyk B (1990). The efficacy of speech-language pathology intervention: traumatic brain injury. Semin Speech Lang 11;215.

Appendix 12-1

Examples of Compensatory Strategies for Students with Cognitive Impairments

I. Attention and concentration
  A. External aids
    1. Use a timer or alarm watch to focus attention for a specified period.
    2. Organize the work environment and eliminate distractions.
    3. Use a written or pictorial task plan with built-in rest periods and reinforcement; move a marker along to show progress.
    4. Place a symbol or picture card in an obvious place in the work area as a reminder to maintain attention.
    5. Alternate low-interest tasks with high-interest tasks.
  B. Internal procedures
    1. Set increasingly demanding goals for self, including sustained work time.
    2. Self-instruct. (For example, "Am I wandering? What am I supposed to do? What should I be doing now?") Written cue cards may be needed during training period.
II. Orientation (to time, place, person, and event)
  A. External aids
    1. Use a log book or journal or tape recorder to record significant information and events of the day.
    2. Refer to pictures of persons who are not readily identified (carry pictures attached to log book).
    3. Use appointment book or daily schedule sheet.
    4. Use alarm watch set for regular intervals.
    5. Refer to maps or pictures for spatial orientation; make maps that depict landmarks.
  B. Internal procedures
    1. Select anchor points or events during the week and then attempt to reconstruct either previous or subsequent points in time. (For example, "My birthday was on Wednesday and that was yesterday, so this must be Thursday.")
    2. Request time, date, and similar information from others, when necessary.
    3. Scan environment for landmarks.
III. Input control (amount, duration, complexity, rate, and interference)
  A. Auditory control
    1. Give feedback to speaker (e.g., "slow down," "speed up," "break information into smaller chunks").
    2. Request repetition in another form. (For example, "Would you please write that down for me?")
  B. Visual control
    1. Request longer viewing time or repeated viewings; request extra time for reading.
    2. Cover parts of a page and look at exposed areas systematically, as in a clockwise direction or from left to right.
    3. Use finger or index card to assist scanning and to maintain place.

Source: Reprinted with permission from J Haarbauer-Krupa, K Henry, S Szekeres, M Ylvisaker (1985). Cognitive Rehabilitation Therapy: Late Stages of Recovery. In M Ylvisaker (ed), Head Injury Rehabilitation: Children and Adolescents. Austin, TX: PRO-ED, 317–319. Copyright 1997, Butterworth–Heinemann.

    4. Use symbol to mark right and left margins of written material or use top and bottom segments as anchors in space.

    5. Use large-print books or talking books.

    6. Request a verbal description.

    7. Remove an object from its setting to examine it; then return it to the original setting and view it again.

    8. Place items in best visual field and eliminate visual distracters.

    9. Turn head to compensate for field cut.

IV. Comprehension and memory processes

    A. Use self-questioning. (For example, "Do I understand? Do I need to ask a question? How is this meaningful to me? How does this fit with what I know?") Periodically look for gaps, misconceptions, or confusion by summarizing or explaining and checking back with a speaker, a written source, or reference material.

    B. Build "frames" or background for new information that is of particular significance or interest. Read summaries and general textbooks and ask knowledgeable persons about topics of special interest (a procedure in building frames).

    C. Use a study guide for extended discourse material (e.g., survey, question, read, recite, review—the SQ3R procedure).

    D. Make charts and graphs of important relationships in textual material.

    E. Use external memory aids (e.g., tape recorder, log book, notes, memos, written or pictured timelines).

    F. Use rehearsal: covert or overt; auditory-vocal or motor (pantomime).

    G. Use organization cues: Scan for or impose some order on incoming information.

    H. Use mnemonics: method of loci, rhymes, imagery (meaningful and novel associations).

    I. Use diagrams or forms that facilitate deeper encoding of information and its subsequent retrieval.

    J. Relate the information to personal life experiences and current knowledge. Use semantic knowledge of basic scripts (e.g., going to a restaurant, buying groceries) to help reconstruct previous events.

    K. Project and describe situation in which target information will be needed or used.

    L. At retrieval, reconstruct environment in which information was received.

    M. Verbalize visuospatial information. (For example, "X is to the left of Y.") Visualize verbal information in graphs, pictures, cartoons, or action-based imagery.

    N. Keep items in designated places.

V. Word retrieval

    A. Search lexical memory according to various categories and subcategories (e.g., person, family).

    B. Describe the concept; circumlocute (talk about or around subject) using a feature analysis.

    C. Use the feature analysis guide (see Chapter 11).

    D. Use gestures or signs.

    E. Attempt to generate a sentence or use a carrier phrase.

    F. Search letters or sounds of the alphabet (more effective in retrieving items in a limited category, such as names).

    G. Describe perceptual attributes and semantic features of the concept.

    H. Draw the item.

    I. Attempt to write the word.

    J. Create an image of the object in a scene; then attempt to describe the scene.

    K. Attempt to retrieve the overlearned opposite.

    L. Engage in free association, having an image in mind.

    M. Associate persons' names with physical characteristics or a known person of the same name.

VI. Thought organization and verbal expression

    A. Use a structured thinking procedure (e.g., the graphic advance organizers in Chapter 11).

    B. Use knowledge of scripts to generate real or imagined descriptions of experiences (narratives).

    C. Construct a timeline to maintain appropriate sequence of events.

    D. Note topic in any conversation; self-question about the main point of expression; alert others before shifting a topic abruptly.

    E. Watch others for feedback as to whether your words are confusing: Watch facial expression and so forth or directly ask listeners, "Am I being clear?"

    F. Rehearse important comments or questions and listen to self.

    G. Set limits of time or allowable number of sentences in any one turn.

VII. Reasoning, problem solving, and judgment

    A. Use a problem-solving guide.

    B.   Use self-questioning for alternatives or consequences (e.g., "What could I do?" "What would happen if I did that?").

    C.   Look at possible solutions from at least two different perspectives.

    D.   Scan environment for cues as to appropriateness or inappropriateness of a behavior (e.g., facial expression of others; signs such as "No Smoking"; formality versus informality of setting).

    E.   Set specific times or places for behaviors that are appropriate only in specified situations.

    F.   Actively envision situations to which successful procedures can be generalized.

    G.   Work with others in deriving useful solutions to problems.

VIII. Self-monitoring

    A.   Use symbols or signs placed in obvious places or use alarms that mean "pause" or "stop" or ask oneself, "Am I doing what I should be doing?"

    B.   Use book or notebook into which cards with self-monitoring cues (e.g., "Summarize what you read") are inserted at selected places.

    C.   Pair specific self-instruction with the associated emotion (e.g., "calm down" when angry).

  IX. Task organization

    A.   Use task organization checklist: materials, sequenced steps, timeline, evaluation of results. Check each task when completed.

    B.   Prepare work space and assign space as task demands.

Chapter 13

Social-Environmental Approach to Communication and Behavior

Mark Ylvisaker, Timothy J. Feeney, and Shirley F. Szekeres

Socially skilled people—people who are liked and have a high degree of social-interactive competence in their chosen social contexts—are people who are able to affect other people positively and with the effect that they intend and who are capable of being affected positively by others the way the others would like to affect them. This broad definition of the territory covered in this chapter has many important implications.

First, it suggests that social skills include a variety of general competencies as well as specific goal-directed, situationally appropriate, verbal and nonverbal behaviors. Second, it highlights the important fact that the characteristics comprising social-interactive competence must be defined in relation to specific social contexts and communication partners and that the competencies of the partners are critical contributors to an individual's social success.

Third, this definition brings together many professional disciplines within the domain of one integrated clinical enterprise: teaching social skills to children with disability. Traditionally, this work has been the professional domain of classroom and special education teachers, social workers, and in some clinical settings, occupational therapists. Focusing on the language (i.e., the pragmatic) dimensions of social skills brings speech-language pathologists squarely into this shared territory. Focusing on the behavioral dimensions introduces behavioral psychologists and the useful framework of applied behavior analysis. Recognizing the impact of emotional adjustment on social-interactive competence introduces counseling psychologists and social workers. The powerful impact of cognitive functioning (general as well as social cognition, social perception, social attribution, and social perspective taking) on social success brings cognitive rehabilitation specialists into the domain. The importance of partner competencies gives a critical role to family counselors and peer trainers. The need for meaningful and enjoyable social activities brings in the skills of recreation therapists. The well-documented impact of social-interactive competence on vocational success means that vocational specialists must also be considered critical members of the team of professionals whose goal is helping people with disability to achieve satisfying social, educational, and vocational lives by becoming effective communication partners with those who matter.

We hope that this chapter will be helpful for the professionals and others who interact regularly with children and adolescents with traumatic brain injury (TBI) (i.e., everyday people) and who share a legitimate stake in their social success. The need for a consistent and integrated perspective on behavioral and psychosocial issues in TBI rehabilitation is underscored by the complexity of the issues for this population. For example, an adolescent with serious frontal lobe injury can experience satisfactory recovery in physical, intellectual, and academic domains but have the ability of a young child in regulating behavior (including both cognitive and social behavior). It is very difficult for adults and peers to understand the behavior of such individuals in appropriate developmental terms and to avoid unhelpful personal responses to their objectionable behavior. Complicating this even more is the possibility of damage to other parts of the frontal lobes that can result in surprisingly weak learning from feedback. In this case, traditional behavior modification (i.e., rewarding appropriate behavior and ignoring or punishing inappropriate behavior) will be inefficient at best, staff and family members will have great trouble understanding the behavior as other than willful, and the individual's behavioral course is likely to deteriorate rather than improve.

This chapter has the following structure: After outlining possible contributors to behavioral and social-communication problems after TBI, we describe 12 premises that serve as the foundation for the approaches to intervention discussed later in the chapter. These premises are derived from research in a variety of professional domains (e.g., behavioral psychology, communication disorders, developmental cognitive psychology), involving a variety of disability groups. This section includes references to important literature supporting our approach to intervention. We intend the remainder of the chapter to serve as a resource for clinicians, teachers, and others seeking guidance in their attempts to help children and adolescents with TBI to overcome obstacles to achieving satisfying lives as effective communicators in their chosen social contexts. It includes an extended case illustration along with intervention protocols, forms, checklists, and other materials. It would not be wise to read the resource section of the chapter as connected prose but rather to use it as a source of potentially useful intervention ideas. The clinical perspectives presented in this chapter are complemented by those in Chapters 9–12, which focus more specifically on the cognitive dimensions of behavior, and in Chapter 5 (psychopharmacology), 15 (counseling), 17 (school reentry), 18 (classroom intervention), and 14 (preschool intervention).

Behavioral and Psychosocial Consequences of TBI

After severe TBI in children and adolescents, virtually any outcome is possible, depending on a large number of factors, most notably the characteristics of the children and their families before the injury and its nature and severity. Some children enjoy a remarkably favorable outcome, succeeding in school and social life with few special services or supports. Others experience severe and persistent disability across a wide range of functional domains. Despite this enormous variation within the population, investigators and clinicians agree that changes in behavior and difficulties in psychosocial adaptation are common and often the most troubling long-term consequences of severe brain injury for family members, friends, teachers, employers, and the injured children themselves (Brown et al., 1981; Fletcher et al., 1990; Papero et al., 1993; Perrot et al., 1991; Petterson, 1991; Ylvisaker, 1993; Ylvisaker and Feeney, 1995). In Chapter 2, Ewing-Cobbs and colleagues summarize recent research into the nature and frequency of cognitive, behavioral, and psychosocial disturbances after TBI in children and adolescents. In this section, our goal is simply to highlight the variety of possible contributors to behavioral and psychosocial challenges after TBI, summarized in Figure 13-1.

Preinjury Social, Behavioral, and Learning Problems

In many cases, challenging behavior after injury is continuous with or perhaps an exaggeration of preexisting behavior or communication problems. Disproportionate numbers of children and adolescents who experience TBI

were at risk for the injury because of challenging environmental circumstances (e.g., inadequate supervision at home, dangerous neighborhoods, abusive parents) or of personal characteristics that placed them at risk (e.g., a history of maladaptive or risk-taking behavior, abuse of alcohol and drugs, impaired judgment and self-regulation) (Asarnow et al., 1991; Brown et al., 1981; Fletcher et al., 1990; Greenspan and MacKenzie, 1994). In addition, many children with TBI had preexisting communication or learning disabilities that placed them at risk for problems in the development of effective and satisfying social interaction before their brain injury. Although it is certainly a mistake to assume that something is suspicious about the preinjury life of a child or adolescent who incurs a brain injury, the frequency with which predisposing circumstances are discovered should motivate a thorough exploration of all aspects of the child's life in developing a comprehensive plan to support the child after the injury.

Pathophysiology and Social-Behavioral Outcome

In many cases, particularly in the early weeks and months after severe TBI, challenging behaviors are a *direct* result of the injury. For example, damage to prefrontal areas, the most common site of lesion in closed head injury (Levin et al., 1991; Mendelsohn et al., 1992), can have a variety of effects on behavior and social interaction. For example, fronto-orbital injuries can result in transient or persistent disinhibition, impulsiveness, lability, reduced anger control, aggressiveness, sexual acting out, perseveration, and poor social judgment despite normal physical appearance and psychological test profiles (Stuss and Benson, 1986; Varney and Menefee, 1993). Additionally, ventromedial prefrontal injury is believed to reduce an individual's ability to associate normal feeling states ("somatic markers") with memories for events, thereby reducing the efficiency of learning from consequences (Damasio, 1994; Damasio et al., 1990). That is, to profit from a negative experience, one must store an intellectual representation of the circumstances or action to be avoided in the future *along with a persistent marker that this is something to avoid*. It is precisely such markers that seem not to be stored and activated effectively in people with ventromedial prefrontal injury. Further, damage to dorsolateral or medial parts of the prefrontal lobes can result in failure to initiate activity, including social interaction (Daigneault et al., 1997); rigid adherence to behavioral routines; and impaired perception and interpretation of social cues (particularly right-hemisphere damage). Anterior temporal lobe injury, also common in closed head injury, can contribute to weak regulation of behavior. Damage to limbic regions, specifically the hippocampus and amygdala, appears to reduce one's ability to "unlearn" emotional responses to frequently encountered situations that provoke fear or anxiety. People with these

Figure 13-1. A highly simplified model of possible contributors to behavior problems after traumatic brain injury.

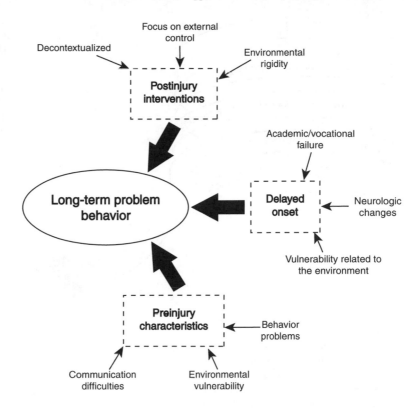

injuries tend to revert to established patterns of response even when they possess ample evidence that the fear response is unwarranted (Adolphs et al., 1995; Allman and Brothers, 1994; Bechara et al., 1995; LeDoux, 1993).

Each of these types of injuries (which, of course, occur in degrees of severity) has a direct effect on social competence. Taken together, they not only render a child vulnerable in relation to behavioral outcome but call into question the usefulness of consequence-oriented behavior management programs. Children or adolescents who are impulsive and disinhibited (much like a young preschooler), inefficient in profiting from feedback, and unlikely to initiate behavior—even knowing that it is important at the time—do not respond well to intervention that focuses mainly on providing rewards for desirable behavior and providing punishment, "time out," or neutral responses for undesirable behavior. If the individual's physical, language, and academic outcome yields no obvious evidence of brain injury, these characteristics, combined with predictably ineffective traditional behavior management, produce a potentially volatile mix. Parents, teachers, and others typically set high standards for behavior and for quick responses to rewards and punishments. If their expectations are not met, they understandably heighten their attempts to control the child and intensify negative consequences for undesirable behavior. Although these adult responses are natural, they may be the opposite of what is needed for children with the com-

bination of injuries common in closed head injury, with the long-term consequences being steadily deteriorating behavior over the years following the injury (Feeney and Ylvisaker, 1995; Ylvisaker and Feeney, 1995).

Behavior and Communication Problems Secondary to Other Disability

Behavior and social interaction problems can also be an *indirect* result of an injury. For example, general cognitive weakness (e.g., difficulty in planning and organizing behavior, in paying attention and staying on task, in remembering what to do, in shifting flexibly from activity to activity, in predicting the consequences of an action, and in recognizing one's limitations) may be associated with behavior problems, particularly if teachers, parents, and others have inappropriate expectations for the child (e.g., expecting a child with difficult-to-detect cognitive weakness to meet preinjury levels of performance in school). Impaired social cognition, including loss of knowledge of social concepts, rules, roles, and routines; difficulty in drawing appropriate inferences about causes of behavior; and impaired perception of social cues, have an obvious impact on social-interactive competence. Specific speech and language problems may also interfere with social interaction, but these problems are relatively uncommon in TBI and tend to affect social relationships less than personality and behavior changes (Ylvisaker, 1993).

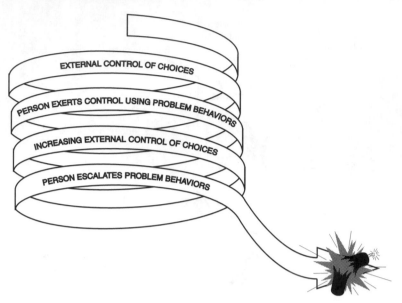

Figure 13-2. The classic negative cycle of control. (Reproduced with permission from TJ Feeney, M Ylvisaker [1997]. A Positive, Communication-Based Approach to Challenging Behavior After TBI. In A Glang, G Singer, B Todis [eds], Children with Acquired Brain Injury: The School's Response. Baltimore: Paul H. Brookes, 229.)

Many children act out or withdraw as a reaction to the changes in their life circumstances associated with disability. For example, it is natural for adolescents who cannot perform adequately in school, sports, or social life to lose friends. This loss, in turn, easily results in anger or depression, which are associated with behaviors that only exacerbate the problem.

Behavior Problems Secondary to Inappropriate Management

Ill-conceived responses to the child's behavior—infantilizing older children and adolescents; punishing children for behavior over which they have minimal control; responding to outbursts in the confused stages of recovery in a way that transforms them into learned escape communication or learned access communication; excusing children and failing to hold them responsible for behavior that they can control—are capable of creating otherwise preventable behavior problems over time. Similarly, socially challenging behaviors may represent the individual's protest against adult-imposed restrictions on behavior or other negative life circumstances (e.g., protracted hospitalization, placement in a special class, special restrictions) that are considered unacceptable (Feeney and Ylvisaker, 1995).

The classic negative cycle of control effectively illustrates this theme, particularly in the case of adolescents with TBI (Figure 13-2). Accustomed to considerable autonomy before an injury, the adolescent attempts to exercise this autonomy by doing something inconsistent with adult wishes. Possibly with the best intentions, the adult exercises control and imposes restrictions. Naturally, the adolescent reacts negatively to the restrictions,

causing the adult to become irritated and to tighten control, which triggers an intensified negative reaction, which confirms the adult's suspicion that the adolescent is incapable of making good judgments—and a full-blown negative cycle of control is unleashed. To be sure, many adults are skilled at avoiding this cycle. Our current point is simply that professionals and caregivers must be alert to the frequency with which they contribute to preventable behavior problems after TBI.

When adults respond inappropriately to behaviors that are uncomfortable but expected after TBI, the child may learn to communicate important messages with undesirable behavior. For example, if screaming or hitting routinely results in escape from painful therapy procedures, or if acting aggressively routinely results in desirable adult attention, it is likely that children will add these behaviors to their repertoire of communication acts designed to get what they want and to avoid what they do not want (Burke, 1990; Carr et al., 1993, 1994; Durand, 1990). If such behaviors are easiest and most effective, the child has little reason not to use them. Our point here is not that adults should simply refuse to react to challenging behavior; the solution is considerably more complicated: Rather, all adults must be alert to their role in promoting positive communication and in teaching positive communication alternatives to challenging behavior.

Delayed Psychosocial and Behavioral Consequences

In many cases, behavioral and psychosocial problems increase over the years after a disabling injury (1) because earlier neurologic injury prevents an injured child from maturing in social and behavioral domains; (2) because the cumulative emotional effect of considerable social and academic failure is anger, hostility, depression, withdrawal, or some other negative psychological reaction; (3) because the individual has no goals, activities, or friends to give meaning to life; or (4) because caregivers, teachers, and others inadvertently contribute to the problems through poorly planned interaction and intervention. Delayed behavioral consequences are easiest to understand in preschoolers with frontal lobe injury. For example, a 3-year-old child with prefrontal injury may experience excellent recovery in physical, intellectual, and communication functioning. The child's impulsiveness, rigidity, poorly regulated behavior, egocentricity, aggressiveness, and poor response to situational social cues can easily be interpreted as developmentally appropriate in a 3-year-old child. However, if substantial maturation has not taken place in these areas by first grade, the child surely will be judged to have a serious behavior problem (Benton, 1991; Eslinger et al., 1989; Eslinger et al., 1992; Grattan and Eslinger, 1992; Marlowe, 1989, 1992).

Although somewhat more difficult to detect and interpret, delayed behavioral and psychosocial consequences are also common in adolescents injured during their late childhood or early adolescent years (Feeney and Ylvisaker, 1995; Williams and Mateer, 1992; Ylvisaker and Feeney, 1995). Although some investigators have suggested that behavioral deterioration over time may be largely a neurobiological phenomenon minimally influenced by intervention or life circumstances (Grattan and Eslinger, 1992), it is our conviction, based on our work with children and adolescents with behavioral challenges after TBI, that long-term behavioral consequences of TBI can, in most cases, be prevented or reduced through intelligent use of the behavioral, cognitive, and social supports described in this chapter.

It is very likely that a complex and evolving combination of these preinjury, injury, and postinjury factors—some environmental and some internal to the individual—is operative in most cases, necessitating a flexible and multifaceted approach to helping children and adolescents with TBI to achieve a satisfactory degree of social-interactive competence and behavioral adjustment. This fact is one reason for our addressing the broad territory of social-communicative and behavioral intervention in one integrated chapter.

Foundations: Premises Supporting Integrated, Contextualized, Antecedent-Focused Intervention

The following 12 premises form the basis for the approach to behavior and social-interactive competence described in this chapter. The premises are based on recent research involving other disability groups (e.g., children and adolescents with emotional disturbance, language-learning disabilities, attention deficit hyperactivity disorder) and on

the authors' combined 50-plus years of clinical experience with children and adolescents with TBI. Together, these sources of clinical wisdom have led us increasingly to an integrated, contextualized, and functional approach to intervention. Later in the chapter, all the intervention premises are illustrated by descriptions of a young man severely injured at age 10 and followed to age 19.

Careful Delineation of the Nature of the Problem

Premise I states that effective intervention requires careful differential diagnosis of the nature of the problem. After the phase of profound confusion and disinhibition has passed, children with TBI may behave in awkward or troubling ways for a variety of reasons. Some children fall into the "can't do" category: They lack the knowledge or cognitive abilities necessary to do what others would like them to do (items 1 and 2 in the following list). Other children fall into the "won't do" category: They are oppositional and defiant or have learned to communicate in ways that are undesirable but that work for them (items 3 and 4). Still others fall into the "doesn't do" category. Such children, including many with TBI, know the rules and are not oppositional but fail to do what we would like them to do because of significant impairment of inhibition or initiation related to their brain injury (items 5 and 6). Of course, most children with behavior problems do not fall neatly into only one of these general categories. However, intervention will be ineffective if the child's mix of issues is not understood well.

1. *Cognition: knowledge base.* Some children fail to do what we want them to do because they have lost—or had never acquired—knowledge of the rules, roles, routines, and scripts that define socially acceptable behavior in specific contexts. Such children may be candidates for traditional role-play social skills training, assuming adequate motivation to achieve social success as defined by their social group and assuming contextualized coaching is available as a second phase of the intervention.
2. *Cognition: social perception.* Some children have difficulty perceiving social cues accurately in context, including interpretation of others' responses to them, and may need ongoing situational coaching.
3. *Learning history: oppositional behavior.* Some children are oppositional and defiant. Social skills training and coaching are unlikely to be helpful in this case. Rather, reasons for the opposition must be identified and addressed.
4. *Learning history: challenging behavior as communication.* Some children have learned to use challenging behavior as the most efficient means of communicating their intentions. They require a systematic approach to teaching positive communication alternatives to their challenging behavior.

5. *Frontal lobe injury or immaturity: disinhibition.* Some children behave badly because they lack the neurologic wherewithal to inhibit impulsive behavior. Rather than needing decontextualized skills training, these children require environmental and other antecedent supports, including patient understanding on the part of people in their communication environment.
6. *Frontal lobe injury: lack of initiation.* Some children fail to do what we want them to do because of a neurologically based impairment of activation or initiation, again necessitating environmental and other antecedent supports.

Ongoing, Collaborative, Contextualized Functional Assessment of Behavior

Premise II holds that functional assessment of behavior is ongoing, collaborative, and contextualized. Many approaches to behavior and social competence are available in the professional fields that intersect to form the domain covered in this chapter: applied behavior analysis, social skills intervention, speech-language pathology, counseling psychology, and others. Each approach is capable of contributing to a full assessment in individual cases. Most critical, however, is that assessment be ongoing, collaborative, appropriately contextualized, and driven by customized tests of hypotheses that are directly relevant to planning intervention for the individual (Dumas, 1989; Dunlap et al., 1991; Haring and Kennedy, 1990; Kern et al., 1994). This approach to assessment is described in greater detail in Chapter 10.

Assessment must be *ongoing* because neurologic recovery, situational changes, and possibly delayed consequences of an injury may combine to change intervention and support needs during the months and years after the injury. *Collaboration* in assessment among professionals and between professionals and everyday communication partners not only increases the pool of data available for decision making; it helps to ensure cooperation in implementing intervention plans. Using *real-world contexts* (settings, people, activities, stressors) for assessment is necessitated by the well-documented contextual variability in behavior associated particularly with early childhood and with frontal lobe injury in older children and adolescents. *Actively testing hypotheses* regarding changes that might affect behavior renders assessment directly relevant to planning intervention in a way that passive accumulation of observational data, standardized testing, and use of standardized questionnaires are not. Finally, because effective social interaction is a consequence of the behavior of both parties to an interaction, assessment of the behaviors and competencies of everyday communication partners is also necessary.

Focus on Antecedents

Premise III states that effective intervention for children and adolescents with TBI focuses more on antecedents than on consequences. Traditional behavior modification highlights contingency or consequent management (i.e., attaching a positive consequence to desirable behavior and ignoring or attaching a negative consequence to undesirable behavior). Although attention to consequences of behavior is critical for all people, no matter how young or how cognitively impaired, the lower the potential for self-control of behavior, the greater the reliance on antecedents to behavior and proactive intervention procedures. This principle is illustrated best by typically developing toddlers and young preschoolers who are clearly capable of learning from consequences but whose behavior is managed best by (1) childproofing the environment to eliminate triggers for challenging behavior, (2) establishing well-understood routines and scripts that help to maintain the appropriateness of behavior, (3) preparing the child in advance for any deviation from routines, (4) making demands only when the child is in a psychological state to deal appropriately with the demands, and (5) redirecting the child at the first sign of disruptive behavior.

All these antecedent control procedures (in a very broad sense of "antecedent") are critical when children with TBI are in the confused and disinhibited stages of recovery. Beyond these stages, if children or adolescents have the type of injury that reduces self-control, these procedures continue to be critical and can be complemented by attempts to teach individuals to manage their antecedents (e.g., making plans in advance for methods to deal with a stressful situation, leaving a stressful situation before it gets out of control). A growing body of literature supports this approach for individuals with TBI (Feeney and Ylvisaker, 1995, 1997; Ylvisaker and Feeney, 1996; Slifer et al., 1996).

Principle of Setting Events

People in a generally positive state when presented with a stressful task are typically able to respond positively and effectively; on the other hand, people in a generally negative state are more likely to respond negatively and ineffectively (Colvin and Sugai, 1989; Michael, 1982, 1989; Vollmer and Iwata, 1991; Wahler and Fox, 1981). Background setting events that can influence the behavior of a child or adolescent with TBI include (1) a variety of internal states of the individual, including neurologic states (e.g., overactivation of the limbic system), other physiologic states (e.g., pain, illness, over- or under-stimulation), cognitive states (e.g., confusion, disorientation), and emotional states (e.g., anger, anxiety, depression, sense of loss); (2) task difficulty as perceived by the child; (3) the presence or absence of specific people; and (4) other environmental stressors (e.g., activity levels,

Figure 13-3. Negative setting events and their effect on behavior. (Reproduced with permission from TJ Feeney, M Ylvisaker [1997]. A Positive, Communication-Based Approach to Challenging Behavior After TBI. In A Glang, G Singer, B Todis [eds], Children with Acquired Brain Injury: The School's Response. Baltimore: Paul H. Brookes, 229.)

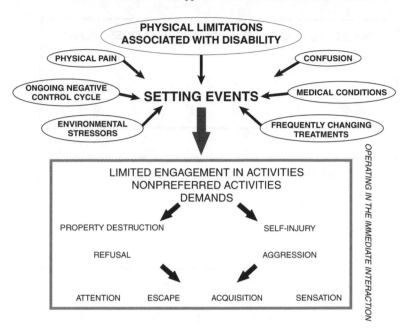

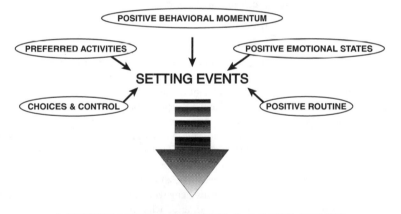

Figure 13-4. Positive setting events and their effect on behavior. (Reproduced with permission from TJ Feeney, M Ylvisaker [1997]. A Positive, Communication-Based Approach to Challenging Behavior After TBI. In A Glang, G Singer, B Todis [eds], Children with Acquired Brain Injury: The School's Response. Baltimore: Paul H. Brookes, 229.)

background noise). Although under-represented in the traditional behavioral literature on grounds that they may be unobservable and difficult to control, setting events have received increasing attention and are critical in managing the behavior of children and adolescents with TBI.

Some internal setting events can be manipulated pharmacologically (see Chapter 5). Others may be manipulated indirectly (Conroy and Fox, 1994; Fox and Conroy, 1995; Kennedy and Itkonen, 1993). For example, confusion and disorientation may be reduced by creating familiar routines and providing a rich set of external orientation supports (see Chapters 11 and 12). Anxiety and frustration may be reduced by ensuring that the child is capable of succeeding and has support available in the event of difficulty. Anger, resentment, and control battles may be minimized by providing the child with greater opportunity for choice and control.

When children with TBI are given difficult tasks coupled with a background of physical pain, confusion, frustration, depression, failure on preceding tasks, and the like, the predictable consequence is more failure, refusal, and increasingly negative behavior. In contrast, when the same tasks are presented with a background of clear orientation, understanding of routines, success on preceding tasks, and a sense of competence and control, the likelihood of engagement in and successful completion of the task is increased. This principle of setting events (illustrated in Figures 13-3 and 13-4) has been validated experimentally in the developmental disabilities literature (e.g., Kennedy and Itkonen, 1993; Vollmer and Iwata, 1991). Because of

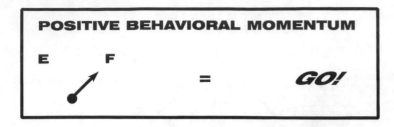

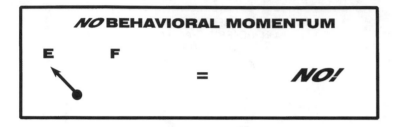

Figure 13-5. Behavioral momentum seen as the fuel needed to complete difficult tasks. (Reproduced with permission from TJ Feeney, M Ylvisaker [1997]. A Positive, Communication-Based Approach to Challenging Behavior After TBI. In A Glang, G Singer, B Todis [eds], Children with Acquired Brain Injury: The School's Response. Baltimore: Paul H. Brookes, 229.)

the strong likelihood of negative internal setting events after TBI, this principle must play a leading role in managing behavior and facilitating social-interactive competence.

Principle of Behavioral Momentum

Positive and successful behavior generates more positive and successful behavior; negative and unsuccessful behavior likewise generates more negative and unsuccessful behavior. Technically a component of the more general principle of positive setting events, the principle of positive behavioral momentum has been singled out for special discussion and investigation by behavioral psychologists (e.g., Fowler, 1996; Mace et al., 1990; Mace et al., 1986; Nevin, 1988). The basic principle is easy to appreciate: If an individual faces a stressful task with a backlog of success, rewards, positive engagement in choice making, and a clear understanding of what is required, the demands and stress of the new task will be easier to deal with (Horner et al., 1990; Horner et al., 1993; Kennedy, 1994). Conversely, if the individual comes to the stressful task with a backlog of failure, frustration, punishment, and absence of choice in the matter, dealing with the demands and stress of the new task will be more difficult.

This principle holds many important implications for intervention. As much as possible, staff must create a series of successes before presenting difficult tasks, must structure rehabilitation and education as much as possible around the individual's strengths, and must provide the cognitive supports necessary to ensure that the individual is oriented and is clear about what is expected. Furthermore, counselors must work closely with other professionals to ensure that genuine successes can be brought to the table in helping individuals with TBI to restore a positive sense of self. Children and adolescents with generally good cognitive recovery can be taught to

contribute to their self-management by understanding that "the gas tank has to be full" (i.e., they need to have positive momentum on their side) before attacking a difficult task. This useful metaphor is illustrated in Figure 13-5.

Principle of Choice and Control

Like the principle of positive behavioral momentum, the principle of choice and control is part of a broader focus on setting events but deserves individual attention because of its importance after TBI. A large number of studies of individuals with developmental disabilities (reviewed by Harchik et al., 1993) support the following principle: When people are given opportunities for choice and control, their level of willing participation increases, the frequency of challenging behavior decreases, and they rate the activity as more satisfying.

Because of the dramatic restrictions on autonomy associated with acquired brain injury, the principle of choice and control emerges as both critically important and extremely difficult to honor (Condeluci, 1991, 1992; Condeluci and Getz-Laski, 1987). Many restrictions on activity are dictated by physical limitations, others are ordered by physicians and various professionals, and still others are imposed by parents and staff who understandably feel a strong need to protect the child and may also believe that people with TBI are incapable of making responsible decisions for themselves. Under these circumstances, children are pulled easily into the downward control cycle (described earlier), inadvertently giving parents and staff confirmation of their belief that the child requires intensive external control. Too often the long-term result is some combination of bitter control battles and learned helplessness.

The antidote to this negative outcome is a general culture in which parents and staff provide the child with as many opportunities for choice and control as possible, consistent with important goals that all parties agree are a high priority for the child. For example, it may not be possible for children to refuse physical therapy, but they may easily be given control over activities within the therapy session and possibly even over the location of the session. Children who have difficulty in making choices may need special supports (e.g., a choice board and photographs representing the activities from which the child can choose). In addition, children may need to learn that, in some situations, they have no choice; that such situations are not arbitrarily designated; and that resistance to them will not benefit them. Teaching "no choice" to a child is much easier if the teaching occurs within a context of rich opportunities for choice.

Positive Roles, Routines, and Scripts

In everyday life, positive behavior is maintained largely by routines and scripts attached to the person's various social roles (e.g., student, employee, son, sister, boy scout, athlete). Recent work on the development of social skills and interactive competence in preschoolers has highlighted the important contribution of script knowledge to social-interactive competence (Hudson, 1993). Scripts include roles, places, sequences of events, and conversational turns and specific language that accompanies those turns. Young children learn a number of positive scripts, including those that govern behavior at the dinner table, in classrooms, in restaurants, at birthday parties, on the playground, during doctor visits, and in many more contexts.

A critical setting event associated with *negative* behavior after TBI is the loss of meaningful roles and associated scripts that dictate positive behavior. In rehabilitation hospitals, for example, a patient might feel that the only two roles available are (1) be good and do whatever people tell me to do even if I have no idea why I am doing it, and (2) resist and oppose with all my might. Given these options, many young people with TBI—especially adolescents who may have been somewhat oppositional before the injury—predictably choose the latter.

After returning home, the old roles (e.g., class officer, paper deliverer, concert master, prize mathematics student, captain of the football team, party animal) may not be available. New roles will inevitably be created to fill the vacuum. Staff and family members are well advised to facilitate the development of positive and important roles at every stage of improvement after a child emerges from coma. For example, in a rehabilitation hospital, children can be given simple but important jobs, such as lunch assistant or group leader. Similarly, better-recovered children can be asked to help less-well-recovered children with mobility, orientation, or other needs. Because children with TBI find themselves so consistently at the receiving end of help, it is easy for them to begin to think of themselves as helpless or as victims and to retain a thoroughly egocentric perspective on life. Therefore, such children must be encouraged to adopt roles that include a helping component and a script that focuses on the needs of others.

When a child is back in school, other roles become possibilities. It is helpful for the student to have some sort of job that is doable and important. If the student is willing, special roles can capitalize on experiences gained because of the injury, such as helping the health teacher with the brain injury or injury-prevention component of the curriculum. Many possibilities exist. The important point is that adults must be creative in helping children to develop roles and associated scripts that are positive and personally satisfying.

Communication Alternatives to Challenging Behaviors

According to premise IV, changing negative behavior often requires teaching communication alternatives to those behaviors. One of the most important principles yielded by years of research in applied behavior analysis is that very few behaviors are truly maladaptive. That is, no matter how unusual or objectionable a behavior may be, it is likely that it serves an important purpose for the individual. Stated as a principle of communication, this principle asserts that virtually all behavior (whether fully intentional or not) communicates something to someone, and challenging behavior is typically an important part of a person's communication ecology. Early in recovery, behavior (e.g., screaming, hitting) may be driven neurologically but, like the unintentional behaviors of a young infant, without appropriate treatment can easily become an intractable part of the child's communication system if responded to inappropriately (Ylvisaker and Feeney, 1994).

A communication interpretation of challenging behavior dictates that the goal of intervention is not simply to eliminate or extinguish the behavior but rather to substitute a communication alternative that is at least as effective as the undesirable behavior and is easier for others to accept (e.g., requesting a break as an alternative to throwing the math book across the room) (Carr et al., 1994, Durand, 1990; Reichle and Johnston, 1993; Reichle and Wacker, 1993; Ylvisaker and Feeney, 1994). Later in this chapter, we provide elaboration of this important approach to challenging behavior. Appendix 13-1 is an integrated communication and behavior plan written for a grade-school-age boy with rapidly deteriorating behavior that was clearly central to his communication system.

Integration of Behavioral and Cognitive Perspectives

Premise V states that effective intervention integrates behavioral and cognitive perspectives. After TBI, challenging behaviors are often associated with cognitive weakness. For children with cognitive impairment that has not been diagnosed adequately, acting out may be an expression of frustration related to the difficulty of tasks, a means to escape tasks that are difficult, or a response to the cumulative effects of failure. Difficulty in planning and organizing behavior, in remembering what to do, in remaining focused, and in shifting focus appropriately may result in undesirable behavior, which in turn leads to adults assuming increasing control over the child or adolescent's behavior, which may in turn initiate a negative cycle of control. Unrelenting academic failure (from the child's perspective) based on cognitive weakness may also set in motion a downward emotional spiral, resulting in withdrawal and depression.

Problems with social-interactive competence may also be more directly related to cognitive weakness. For example, perseveration and memory problems often conspire to produce irritating, repetitive conversation. Organizational impairment is associated with wandering, tangential discourse that creates social vulnerability.

Furthermore, some problems may be related more specifically to social cognition and social perception. Children who have lost knowledge of social rules, roles, scripts, and routines may benefit from direct instruction in social skills and social scripts, an approach commonly used with children who have developmental disabilities and whose social problems are related clearly in part to inadequate social knowledge (Goldstein et al., 1980; Walker et al., 1988a, b). Other children whose knowledge base may be adequate to the social tasks they face in everyday life may nevertheless have difficulty in perceiving and interpreting social cues, including indirect messages in the communication of others (Chapman et al., 1997; Dennis and Barnes, 1990), which predictably results in behavior that is socially awkward and increases the likelihood of social alienation and associated problem behaviors. This impairment in social perception tends to be more difficult to deal with than loss of knowledge and lends itself to situational coaching and counseling of communication partners in the child's environment so that they understand all the hidden contributors to the child's behavior.

Many people with TBI—children and adults alike—are considered egocentric and unwilling or unable to consider the perspectives of others in making decisions about how to behave (Price et al., 1990). Egocentrism in typically developing preschoolers is a cognitive, not a moral phenomenon. That is, preschoolers are in the process of creating for themselves a "theory of mind," an understanding of people as having distinct minds and therefore possessing distinct perspectives on the social and nonsocial world (Flavell et al., 1993). In the absence of such an understanding of other people, it is natural for young children to act as though their interests were the only interests to consider in deciding how to behave. People with TBI, especially those with frontal lobe injury, may have similar difficulty with cognitive egocentrism, either because they have lost the abstract thinking ability to place themselves in another person's shoes or because limitations on working memory make it difficult to simultaneously consider a variety of perspectives on an issue. Egocentrism associated with cognitive impairment may be exacerbated by the natural human tendency to focus on ourselves and our needs during periods of illness, injury, or stress.

In general, promoting improved social-interactive competence in children injured during the developmental years may require attention to all aspects of the development of social cognition (Flavell et al., 1993).

- Social thinking moves from surface considerations to inferences about the underlying beliefs, intentions, and needs of others.
- Children experience a gradual release from "centration" or fixation on the most salient feature of things and people.
- With development comes growth in understanding that people have stable characteristics despite day-to-day changes in behavior.
- A key to social cognitive development is the gradual development of a theory of mind combined with a growing "sense of the game," which posits that other people have ideas, beliefs, intentions, and emotions that they may express directly or try to hide and that value is in looking for clues with which to "read" the mental state of others.
- Closely connected to the growing sense of other "selves" is a maturing sense of oneself. One of the child's most difficult challenges after TBI is the creation of a new, accurate, and positive sense of self, a challenge made particularly difficult because of the incomplete development of a sense of self and others before the injury.
- Children gradually learn about causes of behavior and become increasingly accurate in explaining both their and others' behavior (attribution). After TBI, attribution is often complicated by the natural tendency to feel victimized (i.e., it is always "somebody else's fault") or to think of oneself as completely incompetent (i.e., "I can't do anything right").

In light of these and other possible interactions between cognitive and behavioral difficulties, it is critical for professionals to integrate the two perspectives in serving individuals with TBI. In some cases, what appears to be a chronic behavior problem that would ordinarily be expected to require intensive, long-term, remedial behavior management, can be eliminated quickly with the provision of appropriate cognitive supports (e.g., organizational support, support designed to enable the individual to remain oriented or to participate in decision making). In many cases, a good justification for involving a cognitive rehabilitation specialist in planning a child's educational program is that intelligent educational planning from a cognitive perspective is required to prevent the evolution of behavior problems over time (Feeney and Ylvisaker, 1997; Ylvisaker and Feeney, 1996).

From External Control to Internal Self-Control of Behavior

Premise VI holds that improvement after TBI progresses from external control to internal self-control of behavior, a component of the development of executive functions. In normal child development, control of behavior (including both covert cognitive behavior and overt social behavior) proceeds from largely external control to increasingly internal control (Flavell et al., 1993). For example, the cognitive focus of a 12-month-old child is in the here and now, largely determined by the most salient or novel event in the environment at that time. Similarly, social behavior is largely a function of biological needs or salient characteristics of the objects, events, and people in the immediate environment. Progression from this heavy dependence on biological and external stimuli in early childhood to the controlled self-direction (under ideal conditions) of mature adults involves many intervening steps, supported in part by the slow physical maturation of the frontal lobes and best represented as a continuum.

Similarly, when children and adolescents emerge from coma after TBI, they tend to act without inhibition in response to internal biological states or salient features of the immediate stimulus environment and only gradually re-establish (or, if young children, establish) self-control. This important progression drives intervention goals and procedures, which move in small steps from external control procedures (e.g., childproofing the environment to prevent undesired behaviors, creating a carefully modulated stimulus environment, redirecting the child at the first sign of challenging behavior, ensuring that everyday people understand the child's limited self-control) to facilitation of planned, deliberate, self-controlled behavior in real-world settings with real-world stressors. Driven by a strongly felt need to protect the injured child or by a perception of the child as incapable of making good decisions, adults often fail to facilitate this progression after severe brain injury.

It is useful to place this aspect of behavioral and social intervention in the broader context of executive system intervention. Because Chapter 12 is devoted to this topic, it is given short shrift in this discussion of behavior and social skills. However, a wise and integrated approach to behavioral intervention is one in which the executive system routines described in Chapter 12 are integrated into the attempt to help children and adolescents to develop increasing self-regulation of social behavior (Ylvisaker and Feeney, 1996, in press).

Routines in a Social-Communicative Context

Premise VII states that effective intervention occurs in social-communicative contexts and is designed to influence routines in those contexts. For several reasons, intervention is ideally delivered in real social-communicative contexts with everyday people as communication partners, at least in large part (Ylvisaker et al., 1993a, 1993b; Ylvisaker and Feeney, in press). The most important lesson learned from decades of research on the effectiveness of behavioral and social skills intervention with a variety of clinical populations is that behaviors trained outside of natural social contexts are unlikely to be transferred to meaningful social contexts in the absence of heroic efforts to effect that transfer (McIntosh et al., 1991; Reichle and Wacker, 1993; Zaragoza et al., 1991). In a review of social skills intervention, Hill Walker, historically associated with decontextualized direct instruction of positive social behaviors, strongly emphasized the importance of situational coaching to effect transfer of skills acquired in an instructional setting (Walker et al., 1994). Walker and colleagues (1994, p. 79) added pessimistically that this critical second phase of social skills instruction "is rarely implemented by school personnel, yet it is probably more important than Part One in determining the magnitude and persistence of social skills training effects."

Failure of transfer or generalization is particularly common in the case of people who are relatively concrete thinkers and are stimulus bound (Horner et al., 1988), including those with frontal lobe immaturity (e.g., young children) or impairment (e.g., many people with TBI). For example, it would obviously be unwise to teach a toddler a social behavior in a decontextualized training setting as opposed to the social setting in which the behavior is required. Similarly, many people who are concrete thinkers after TBI profit most from intervention that is delivered primarily or exclusively in real social settings (Ylvisaker et al., 1993a; Ylvisaker and Feeney, in press).

Furthermore, a quick calculation of the waking hours of people with TBI in rehabilitation hospitals or any other setting reveals that most of the time and potential learning trials of these people occur in nonprofessional settings with nonprofessional people. Therefore, efficiency of intervention requires that these everyday settings and interactions be made as therapeutic as possible, which mandates that professionals get into real-world contexts and work closely with everyday people so that everyday interactions are the keystone of the intervention program (Ylvisaker and Feeney, in press).

The point here is not simply physical settings. Ineffective interventions can be delivered in places that appear to be natural for the child; similarly, important dimensions of effective intervention (e.g., exploring alternative scripts and developing self-knowledge via carefully designed feedback) can be delivered in settings that may not seem natural for the child (e.g., "pull-out" therapy). Quiet, nonthreatening settings may also be the best place to develop an intimate and trusting relationship with the child. Ultimately, however, the focus of intervention must be on effective interaction in natural contexts that include activities, partners, topics, and places.

Integration and Collaboration

According to premise VIII, TBI rehabilitation requires an integrative, collaborative approach to social-interactive competence. The variety of types and sources of behavioral and social-communicative challenge after TBI requires that intervention be integrated among many professionals and everyday people. Ineffective social interaction may have its source in poor emotional adjustment (the domain of counseling psychology, social work); in weak processing of information, including social information (the domain of cognitive rehabilitation, special education); in learned undesirable behavior (the domain of behavioral psychology); in impaired pragmatics of language (the domain of speech-language pathology); in poor grooming and hygiene (the domain of nursing, occupational therapy); or in ineffective communication partners (the domain of family professionals and others). Furthermore, because the most powerful learning occurs in meaningful social context, everyday communication partners (e.g., family members, paraprofessionals, peers) must be considered the primary agents of change. With potentially so many people having a legitimate interest in promoting improved social interaction, it is critical for all to follow the same recipe and to recognize themselves as collaborators contributing to the same project.

Crisis Management

Premise IX holds that crisis management is not behavior management. Although specific concerns about behavior are often identified as a result of behavioral crises, which give rise to a legitimate need to know how to manage those crises, it is critical to draw a sharp distinction between managing crises and teaching positive behaviors. To be sure, learning can occur during and after a crisis; however, such learning is typically negative (e.g., by hitting you, I can get out of physical therapy) and difficult to ameliorate. Fear-associated learning, without explicit consciousness of its origin, is particularly resilient (LeDoux, 1993). Furthermore, behavior plans that exclusively target negative behaviors for extinction run the profound risk of escalating that behavior or substituting a behavior that is even less desirable because the original behavior served a communication purpose that had to be served.

We have described a variety of teaching and antecedent control procedures that, in our experience, together constitute effective behavior management for children and adolescents with TBI. However, the question remains: What should be done about behavioral crises? Rule 1 in crisis management is to prevent crises. This is often possible with efficient antecedent control procedures and creative redirection during the very early stages of a behavioral episode. Redirection (i.e., breaking a psychological set and positively re-engaging an individual) is a particularly useful skill in working with people with TBI, because the explosive combination of impulsiveness, perseveration, and memory problems predictably dictates failure for the alternative procedure, planned ignoring. Therefore, staff must be well-trained in the technique of *redirection without reinforcement*. Although it may be tempting to use a powerfully reinforcing event to quickly redirect a person who is beginning to engage in challenging behavior, it runs too great a risk of increasing the likelihood of the original challenging behavior. The key is to redirect to a neutral event and redirect quickly, ending the episode without running any risks.

Of course, both prevention and redirection fail at times. Rule 2 in crisis management is to survive and defuse the crisis, keeping everybody safe and using a minimum of force or restraint. Important competencies and skills are associated with crisis management (see Figure 13-6), discussed in a variety of useful texts (e.g., Colvin and Sugai, 1989). However, our point here is simply that this is not behavior management. The emphasis of behavior programs should be on facilitating positive behavioral routines, not reacting to negative behavioral routines.

Long-Term Supports

Premise X states that long-term, flexible, and frequently adjusted supports may be needed to prevent behavior problems and facilitate social development. Long-term outcome after severe TBI cannot be predicted in detail. Children with TBI—like Ben, described later in this chapter—often surprise even seasoned professionals both with their accomplishments and with their changing needs for supports during the years after the injury. Changes in levels and types of needed support may be dictated by changes in life circumstances (e.g., moving from grade school to middle school), in people (e.g., moving from a teacher who is flexible to one who is inflexible), in stressors (e.g., divorce in the family), in expectations, and in many more changes. The general point is that severe TBI often renders the child vulnerable to problems evolving in the area of behavior and psychosocial functioning, necessitating alert monitoring over time and requiring flexible adjustments of supports.

The phenomenon of changing needs over time is not unusual. Parents of normally developing children know that needs intensify at certain predictable times, such as in the transition from grade school to middle school. Parents and staff routinely anticipate and attend to these needs with increased levels of psychosocial support without suggesting that anybody, including the child, has failed. The same orientation should apply to children with TBI, the difference being that the needs may be more intense and the occasions for changing needs more frequent. If possible, plans for heightened support should be formulated before problems arise; waiting and reacting are ill-advised (see Ben's history later in this chapter).

Beyond Medical and Training Models of Intervention

According to premise XI, professionals must move beyond narrow medical and training models of intervention. An appropriately functional and contextualized approach to social-interactive competence requires professionals to regard themselves as working within more than a combination of the traditional medical and behavioral-training models (see Chapter 20). That is, in the former model, the professional diagnoses a disorder and provides treatment designed to remediate the disorder. In the latter, the professional targets a behavior to be acquired or eliminated and subjects the individual to a series of learning trials designed to achieve the target behavior, with carefully designed schedules of reinforcement for successful performance. Moving beyond these narrow professional self-definitions includes creating an alliance with everyday people (including the child or adolescent, when that becomes possible) to identify desirable goals and changes in behavior and then serving as a problem solver to help those everyday people to achieve their goals and to effect the desirable changes. Professionals may need to regard themselves as some combination of consultant, coach, mentor, and master craftsperson rather than as a combination of surgeon and animal trainer. Particularly in an era of managed care and decreasing funding for rehabilitation, specialists must think of themselves as support people for an individual with disability and for everyday people in that individual's environment.

Meaningful Engagement in Chosen Life Activities

Premise XII states that in the absence of meaningful engagement in chosen life activities, all interventions will fail. Despite excellent rehabilitation, some adolescents with TBI are depressed, withdrawn, angry, or hostile because they simply do not have a life they consider meaningful. Old friends may have gone separate ways; preinjury activities, such as sports, that were rewarding may now be impossible; and academic success (in the eyes of the individual) may be unattainable. Social skills training, state of the art behavioral intervention, and disability counseling cannot be expected to generate social-interactive competence and a satisfying social life under these tragic circumstances. People cannot be expected to interact positively with others when they have no reason to get out of bed in the morning, have no satisfying social relationships, experience uninterrupted failure, have generally low self-esteem, and have little control over their lives.

Professionals have a limited but important role in helping individuals create meaning in their lives. First, professionals must realize that *functional* is a relative term and that they must, therefore, provide rehabilitative services that are functional *in relation to goals that an individual genuinely embraces.* Second, a significant part of rehabilitation is the systematic search for meaningful activities and satisfying peer relationships that fit the individual's new level of functioning. Professionals might help by identifying a potential support group of youngsters who have a similar history of life-altering brain injury and who—more so than professionals or family members—may be in a position to help the newly injured person to begin creating a new, meaningful life. Chapter 15 addresses related issues in counseling children and adolescents with TBI.

Summary of Intervention Premises

These premises support a communication, behavior, and social-competence approach that is somewhat novel in its emphasis on temporally contiguous and remote antecedents, on the integration of cognitive and behavioral perspectives, and on the importance of everyday people. It is a perspective that has evolved over the course of many years working intensively with children and adolescents with TBI. This perspective is gaining steadily greater acceptance in working with other groups of children with disability. In the remainder of the chapter, we offer case illustrations of the premises and materials that may assist professionals in implementing the approach.

Illustration of Intervention Premises

Case Study: Ben

Before his brain injury at age 10, Ben, a popular fifth grader, was a good student (getting Bs with little effort) and a good athlete who participated in several sports and enjoyed a wide network of friends. He divided his home time between his mother (who was remarried) and his father, who had frequent disagreements with his former wife about how to raise Ben and his two siblings (an older sister and a younger brother). Ben had no identified disability before his injury. He was characterized as stubborn, but not unusually so, by his mother.

Toward the end of fifth grade, while delivering newspapers, Ben was struck by a car and received severe bilateral frontal lobe injury and posterior right and left hemisphere injury. Right frontal and parietal regions were obliterated almost completely. Ben was in an acute-care hospital for 6 months: 6 weeks in intensive care and a total of 4 months in a state of minimal responsiveness (coma).

Six months after the injury, Ben was transferred to inpatient rehabilitation, during which phase he improved very slowly. As part of his neurologically based agitation associated with emergence from coma, Ben began to rub the right side of his head (which had been crushed in the accident and undoubtedly was the source of discomfort). Videotapes made at the rehabilitation hospital reveal that staff focused on this behavior and tried to extinguish it with verbal prompts and by physically removing Ben's hand from his head. In retrospect, it is likely that this seemingly innocent and well-intentioned intervention was the beginning of Ben's use of head hitting as a form of communication. That is, an initially reflexive behavior that was not deliberately communicative appears to have evolved into an effective, albeit negative, component of Ben's communication system, in part because of the response it generated from communication partners.

After 3½ months of inpatient rehabilitation (approximately 9 months after onset), Ben's parents withdrew him from the program (against professional advice) because they were impatient with his slow progress. At that time, he was quadriplegic (unable to walk) and unable to talk or use his arms and hands effectively as a result of severe oral and limb apraxia. He was fed through a gastrostomy tube because of a gradually resolving pharyngeal swallowing disorder. He was alert and comprehended simple language directed at him but had no expressive communication modality other than gross, undifferentiated vocalization and gestures.

For 3 months, Ben received tutoring and therapeutic regimens (physical, occupational, and speech therapy) at his home, usually totaling 3 hours per day of structured stimulation and intervention. During this phase of his recovery, Ben began to resist tasks—particularly physical and occupational therapy exercises—that were difficult or painful for him. He communicated this resistance by screaming or rubbing his head more forcefully than previously. Staff initiated a consequence-oriented behavior modification program (rewards for participation in therapy activities and termination of interaction in response to his screaming or rubbing his head). Although well-intentioned, this program had the effect of increasing the challenging behavior, in effect teaching Ben that the most effective way to terminate an undesirable activity was to scream or hit his head. The behaviors became so extreme that tutoring and therapies were terminated temporarily.

Approximately 1 year after onset, Ben began to attend school in a classroom for children with severe, multiple developmental disabilities. None of the children in his class spoke or communicated effectively. Ben expressed considerable displeasure at being placed with students with mental retardation, a sentiment shared by his mother but not by his father. During the several months in this classroom, Ben's self-injurious behavior escalated to frequent and intense head hitting. The behavior management system in the classroom focused exclusively on consequences: token economy, including response cost (i.e., Ben lost points for bad behavior). When Ben refused to participate in assigned activities, staff attempted to force compliance physically. His challenging behavior escalated. At the same time, school staff attempted to have Ben resume oral eating, using contingency procedures (e.g., loss of privileges for refusing food). This program was unsuccessful and contributed to Ben's increasing use of challenging behavior to communicate his desire to escape.

Because of the severity of his challenging behavior, Ben was transferred to a classroom that served students with behavior problems. The class consisted of eight students, one teacher, one aide, and one behavior aide assigned exclusively to Ben. Staff in this program believed that Ben's noncompliance was not related directly to his brain injury but rather was a result of learning and manipulativeness associated with insufficiently rigorous behavioral programming since the injury. In response to behavioral crises and in an attempt to force compliance, physical intervention was used repeatedly in the class. Ben's self-injurious behavior continued to escalate, and positive communication was rare.

Ben was transferred to a third classroom where the staff were accustomed to working with students with autism by engaging them in highly repetitious drills, hand-over-hand if necessary. Ben's challenging behavior continued to escalate, resulting in his mother's increasing discouragement with Ben and with her own ability to serve him effectively. Consequently, he moved in with his father, who was convinced that external control, including physical control whenever necessary, was the appropriate management system for his son. Now more than 2 years after injury, Ben's challenging behaviors continued to escalate.

Ben was transferred next to a private school for students with behavior problems (his fourth school placement since the injury). As with his previous programs, this school chose to manage behavior almost exclusively with consequences (rewards and punishments). After several weeks of observing lack of improvement in Ben's behavior or communication, his mother decided that a more dramatic intervention was needed and had Ben admitted to a specialized inpatient pediatric TBI rehabilitation facility for intensive behavioral intervention. His father reluctantly acquiesced in this decision.

It was in this program that the authors of this chapter came to know Ben and his family and to shape his intervention program. Ben was 13 years old (at 2½ years after onset). On admission, his behavior was characterized by frequent and severe self-injury (hitting his head), aggression toward objects (e.g., overturning chairs and tables), and infrequent aggression toward people. The positive, antecedent-focused, communication-based interventions described later were initiated during this admission, with the effect of increasing positive, socially acceptable communication and—as a consequence—extinguishing self-injurious and aggressive behavior. With the help of the behavioral psychologist in this rehabilitation program, this approach to intervention was reinitiated at important points during the years after Ben's discharge.

Following discharge from this second inpatient rehabilitation program, Ben returned to middle school in a 12:1:1 self-contained special education class (i.e., 12 students, one teacher, one aide). The behavioral psychologist from the rehabilitation hospital spent 2 weeks at Ben's school, orienting and training staff and helping Ben to establish positive routines in the school. After several uneventful weeks, free of major behavioral incidents, Ben began to use former behaviors. The school staff chose to use the consequence-oriented management system with which they were most familiar. The year ended with escalation of Ben's behaviors, including aggressive behavior (e.g., attempts to hit others).

The next September, Ben was promoted to the local high school, where he was taught in a resource room with some mainstreaming for nonacademic classes. At this time, he was able to walk with a walker; to eat independently (a process resumed during his second inpatient rehabilitation admission); to follow everyday conversation (including relatively abstract content); to read words that were functional and frequently repeated in natural communication contexts; to perform basic arithmetic calculations; and to communicate with basic signs and gestures, a picture-symbol board, and drawing. He had demonstrated the ability to use an electronic communication aid (Dynavox, Sentient Systems, Pittsburgh, PA) but found it cumbersome and undesirable in natural communication contexts. Relative to general cognitive abilities revealed by his receptive language and sense of humor, Ben's organizational abilities were very weak. He routinely got lost or

disoriented in the middle of even moderately complex tasks. For example, it was difficult for him to walk from one room to another at school, in the presence of the distractions presented by other students, without becoming lost or forgetting what he was supposed to be doing. Because most staff believed that he should be able to perform such simple tasks, they easily became irritated by his failures and communicated their irritation, triggering strong behavioral reactions from Ben.

At the beginning of this first high school year, his program was fragmented and disorganized, including few consistent routines. Ben's negative behavior immediately escalated; aggression now was directed at other students, who were frightened. Ben's father was hired to show school staff how to manage his behavior—largely with firm demands and punishment for noncompliance. Ben's negative behavior escalated even further.

Recognizing the seriousness of this behavior, school staff contacted the rehabilitation behavioral psychologist for consultation. The psychologist engaged staff in collaborative hypothesis testing about Ben's behavior (see Chapter 10), which resulted in a return to the types of routine, choice, and positive-escape communication that had been successful earlier. Within 2 weeks, incidents of challenging behavior again had returned to zero. At the same time, staff decided (with Ben's parents' consent) to shift the program to a greater vocational focus. Ben was given a meaningful job (stacking racks and other back-room tasks in a bagel shop) with a job coach. The school year ended on a very positive note.

In summer school, the cycle was repeated. It began with (1) a frequently disrupted, confusing, nonroutine schedule, which elicited (2) behavioral escalation, followed by (3) unsuccessful management with consequences (including punishment), followed by (4) consultation with the rehabilitation center psychologist, who reinstituted (5) collaborative hypothesis testing regarding Ben's behavior, which again yielded (6) positive antecedent-focused, communication-based intervention, which resulted in (7) reduction in noncompliance and challenging behavior, resumption of effective vocational and academic performance, and satisfying social interaction.

The next school year, this vicious cycle began to repeat itself again but was caught by Ben's mother within the first 2 weeks of school. With a positive behavior program in place, Ben's behavior was minimally problematic during the first half of the year. After the December break, the vocational component of Ben's program was increased. He completed the year with few incidents of challenging behavior. At age 18, Ben is completing his formal high school education, spending the bulk of his time in two supported work settings. He continues to have severe multiple disability caused by his brain injury. However, because of intensive efforts focused on the cognitive, behavioral, communication, and psychosocial aspects of his disability, he looks forward to a future that contains meaningful, paid work; community living with reasonable supports; and generally satisfying interaction with others in his environment.

In the following sections, we illustrate the intervention premises articulated earlier in this chapter, using successful components of Ben's rehabilitation and special education program as they evolved during 9 years after his severe brain injury. Ben's injury was at the extreme end of the severity continuum; therefore, his disability and the issues with which he struggled are more obvious and extreme than those of most children and adolescents with TBI. However, the successes and failures of intervention applied in Ben's case clearly illustrate all our intervention premises. We invite readers to be creative in modifying their application of these premises for individuals with less severe disability.

Premise I: Careful Delineation of the Nature of the Problem

Ben's severe social and behavioral difficulties were a result of a complex and evolving interaction of cognitive and communication impairment, executive system weakness, negative communication behavior learned as a result of years of mismanagement, frustration with restrictions and lack of control, and anger. To be effective, programs of intervention had to address each of these issues in an integrated manner and had to evolve as Ben's situation, needs, and abilities evolved. Interventions that failed did so for reasons that are relatively easy (in retrospect) to identify:

1. Behavior modification programs based exclusively on consequences were insensitive to Ben's severely restricted self-regulatory abilities (e.g., disinhibition and impulsiveness related to fronto-orbital injury), his need for cognitive support (related to severe organizational impairment), and his relative inability to profit from feedback (possibly related to presumed ventromedial prefrontal injury).
2. Extinction programs designed exclusively to eliminate challenging behaviors were insensitive to the communication value of those behaviors for Ben and to the associated need for him to communicate those intentions in some effective way.
3. The practice of social skills outside the context of everyday social-interactive routines was insensitive to the extreme difficulty Ben had both in seeing the point of out-of-context role playing and in transferring skills from training to application context.
4. Behavior management programs based exclusively on external control versus choice were insensitive to Ben's sense of self, developed before his injury as a very independent, willful young man.
5. Programs that lacked routine and consequently were confusing for Ben were insensitive to his need for meaningful routines and scripts within those routines to remain oriented and positively goal directed.

In settings in which Ben's behavior was managed poorly and in which his social interaction deteriorated, assessments tended to be unrelated to his everyday behavior in social context. Considerable testing took place and involved delineation of neuropsychological strengths and weaknesses, but this information was not connected to the real world of his interaction with others. Furthermore, despite considerable observation of his behavior and documentation of the frequency and intensity of his challenging behaviors, subsequent analysis was not driven by an attempt to understand the behavior's communication function and the role of communication partners in maintaining the behaviors.

Premise II: Ongoing, Collaborative, Contextualized Functional Assessment

When Ben was admitted to his second inpatient rehabilitation program (2½ years after onset), assessment of behavior and social-communication competence began with collaborative brainstorming about the potential functions (including communication functions) of his behaviors. All rehabilitation team members, including Ben's mother, his case manager, and all the clinicians, participated in this brainstorming and subsequent testing of hypotheses. Several hypotheses emerged, most of which were found to have some merit in developing his rehabilitation program. The hypothesis that his challenging behavior was in part escape communication was confirmed by dramatic decreases in self-injurious and aggressive behavior when staff prompted and honored a positive signal for "stop" (see premise IV). The hypothesis that his challenging behavior was in part an expression of a need for control was confirmed by decreases in challenging behavior associated with experiments designed to give Ben control over activities in his life (see premise III). The hypothesis that his challenging behavior was related in part to an accumulation of negative setting events was confirmed by experiments in which challenging behavior decreased when staff systematically introduced difficult or less preferred activities only when Ben had a backlog of successes and was in a generally positive state (see premise III).

Procedures and benefits of collaborative, contextualized hypothesis-testing assessment are discussed at length in Chapter 10. The point here is that this type of assessment is the basis for developing effective intervention programs for complex individuals such as Ben. Furthermore, because the evolution of needs and abilities after severe TBI is largely unpredictable—particularly in relation to changing settings and demands over time—this type of contextualized experimental assessment must be ongoing.

Premise III: Focus on Antecedents

Here, we use the term *antecedent* broadly to include immediate antecedents (events continuous with the behavior in question) and temporally more remote events that may be related in important ways to the behavior and internal states of the individual.

Setting Events

For Ben, perhaps the most critical setting event proved to be a meaningful daily routine that he had helped to formulate. In the absence of a well-understood, concrete routine that was apparent to Ben, he became easily confused and disoriented, which gave rise to associated increases in anxiety and behavioral outbursts. In the absence of his participation in formulating the routine, he felt coerced and often responded with oppositional behavior. Ben now begins each day in his vocational placement by working with his aide to formulate his plan (i.e., routine) for the day, given the constraints of the work that must be done.

In addition, staff and family use a 1–10 rating scale for evaluating Ben's general readiness for difficult or non-preferred tasks. On certain days, possibly related to internal neurologic events or physical pain, Ben's tolerance for stress or failure is limited severely. The agreed-on plan for such days is that he remain at home. In the event of less extreme negative internal states, both staff and family work hard to create positive setting events (including building positive behavioral momentum) before introducing stressful tasks.

Behavioral Momentum

During the intensive behavioral programming of Ben's second inpatient rehabilitation admission, staff made sure that the daily routine progressed systematically from preferred and relatively easy tasks to nonpreferred and more difficult tasks. For example, Ben hated to shower and routinely resisted the demand to do so when it came early in the morning. Therefore, because it was an important goal of rehabilitation to decrease resistance to showering, this activity was moved from the morning to a time in Ben's daily routine when it was important to take a shower (e.g., immediately after intense physical exercise) and after a series of successful interactions. It simply made no sense to begin the day with a nonpreferred, stressful task, risking resistance and conflict and an associated negative effect on subsequent tasks throughout the day. Similarly, therapies that included potentially painful or difficult activities were scheduled late in the day, and every attempt was made to build a series of successes and positive experiences before introducing the potentially threatening activities.

Choice and Control

Like most people (including most people with disability), Ben reacted and continues to react negatively to a steady diet of demands, directions, and restrictions. In the settings in which external control was most extreme and overt, Ben's behavior deteriorated most quickly, and his self-injurious and aggressive behavior was most intense. After reviewing more than 100 studies of the effects of choice on individuals with developmental disabilities, Harchik and colleagues (1993) concluded that opportunities for choice and control have the general effect of increasing compliance, increasing engagement in tasks, and increasing enjoyment of the activities. Very little reflection is required to appreciate the value of this principle for people with no identified disability. However, for people such as Ben, accustomed to a life of relative autonomy and ability to make countless genuine choices daily, acquired brain injury—and the restrictions it imposes on choice and activity—easily creates a crisis of autonomy.

In the control-oriented school programs that Ben attended, staff frequently fell into the trap known as the *negative cycle of control* (see Figure 13-2):

1. The adult imposes demands and restrictions, believing that Ben is incapable of making good choices for himself.
2. Ben reacts negatively to the demand and refuses to comply.
3. The adult becomes more assertive, believing that it is important to exercise firm authority.
4. Ben digs in his heals and escalates his resistance.
5. The adult increases the level of demand and external control, interpreting noncompliance as confirmation for his view that Ben is incapable of making good choices.
6. Ben's behavior spirals out of control. Unfortunately, this downward spiral can be observed daily in schools and institutions serving people with behavior problems.

In his second inpatient rehabilitation admission, choice was a key component of Ben's daily routines. His day began by formulating his plan (i.e., his routine for the day) with staff, allowing some flexibility for including his choices. In addition (as described under the next premise), the process of teaching communication alternatives to challenging behavior included routines in which Ben was allowed (for a time) to terminate any activity by signaling "stop." Staff made a point of returning to important activities that Ben terminated in this manner, but at least he experienced considerable control over his activities. In his current vocational training setting, Ben begins each day at work by formulating a plan for the day. To be sure, expectations detail what he will accomplish and set limits on what he is allowed to do in that setting. However, it is critical for him to have a legitimate sense that he is directing himself and choosing what to do to meet his goals for himself.

Positive Scripts and Positive Roles

In high school, Ben has two special and desirable roles: He takes attendance and distributes the attendance sheets, and he distributes other mail in the building. Because these jobs are meaningful for him, he does them willingly and has never engaged in challenging behavior while discharging these responsibilities. Furthermore, he efficiently performs the communication acts associated with these and other meaningful activities. Similarly, Ben's behavior and communication are exemplary at his two places of work. He has had no episodes of challenging behavior at work, and he continues to be enthusiastic about the work and the associated social interaction. Ben serves as a clear illustration of the power of roles and scripts in facilitating positive behavior and communication.

Childproofing

We use the term *childproofing* cautiously, with no intention to communicate that older children, adolescents, or adults be treated disrespectfully. However, because the concept of childproofing an environment is clear to everybody who has cared for children, the term is useful in capturing a wide variety of environmental control procedures designed to keep impulsive people out of trouble. Examples that were important in working with Ben included efforts of his middle-school staff to help peers to understand Ben's needs and to interact with him in a way that was positive and nonprovoking. In high school, staff initially placed Ben next to a youngster whom Ben did not like and who was in a wheelchair. This placement gave Ben a target for his anger during a tough transitional time. Staff quickly learned that in the classroom, wise physical placement based on social relationships was a critical childproofing procedure for Ben.

Premise IV: Communication Alternatives to Challenging Behavior

In our account of Ben's history since his injury, we deliberately emphasized the evolution of self-injurious behavior (head hitting) as escape communication. Clearly, it was not so easy to understand this evolution in its initial stages. However, by 2½ years after onset, when Ben was admitted to our rehabilitation program, it was clear that his head hitting indeed served an important communication purpose: escape from undesirable tasks or situations.

The test that confirmed this hypothesis was the following. In half of Ben's therapy and instructional sessions, staff were instructed to look for the first sign of escape-motivated behavior. At its appearance, they took his hand (before he had a chance to hit his head) and quickly shaped it into a gross gesture for "stop." Staff then thanked Ben for telling them that he wanted a break, and they respected his wishes (i.e., discontinued the activity). In those experimental sessions, the frequency of head hitting was reduced quickly to zero. In those therapy and instructional sessions in which staff did *not* prompt and respect the "stop" communication, Ben's frequency of head hitting remained high. Therefore, in the first 2 weeks of his admission, a facility-wide program was implemented to teach Ben to use his gesture for "stop" rather than head hitting as an effective way to communicate his desire to escape. Subsequently, the teaching program was expanded to include other communication situations and acts. The general assumption was that Ben's negative behaviors were communication acts and that, with few exceptions, they communicated either *escape* (i.e., a desire to escape an activity, a demand, a person, or a place) or *access* (i.e., a desire for access to an activity, a person's attention, a place, or simply increased stimulation).

Some staff members voiced the concern invariably expressed at this stage of teaching positive communication alternatives: This teaching would turn Ben into "an escape monster." That is, if staff and family members invariably respect his wishes when he gestures "stop," would he not learn that he can escape any task he wanted to escape? The question is natural and legitimate. Fortunately, the answer—as in Ben's case—is relatively simple. Teaching communication alternatives to challenging behavior does not produce escape monsters or access monsters (i.e., people who get whatever they want when they use positive escape or request communication), if the teaching is accompanied by other positive intervention procedures and by a clear distinction between choice and no-choice situations. In Ben's case, it was critical to add intensive use of antecedent control procedures (including positive setting events, positive behavioral momentum, and choice).

With all these management procedures in place, staff were able to reintroduce less desirable and more difficult tasks. For example, Ben did not like potentially painful physical therapy procedures. During the period of intensive teaching of his gesture for "stop," staff invariably respected this gesture and Ben escaped the difficult physical therapy tasks. Once the positive escape communication had been learned, staff reintroduced physical therapy exercises by preceding them with high-success tasks (maintaining behavioral momentum), by ensuring that Ben was in a generally good state (using positive setting events), and by giving him a choice of physical therapy exercises (offering choice). Ben still had a sense of control and knew that if he persisted in gesturing "stop," his wishes would be respected. Within a relatively short period, all Ben's therapeutic regimens and instructional sessions had been resumed. Furthermore, all staff members were pleased with Ben's heightened engagement and the increased effectiveness of their interventions.

This teaching process was repeated when Ben's behavior deteriorated after several months back in school. Later, staff and family members added a variety of other communication gestures for escape (no, quit, leave me alone) and other communication acts for requesting access to things, activities, and people (e.g., raising a hand for access to people's attention).

For Ben and for many children with behavior problems, comprehensive intervention also requires careful teaching of the important distinction between *choice* and *no-choice* situations. For example, going to school or—in Ben's current situation—going to work may be a *no-choice* situation, whereas the school or workday may include many opportunities for choice and many occasions in which staff know that they should honor positive escape or access communication. During his inpatient rehabilitation, with a primary focus on teaching communication alternatives to challenging behavior, Ben was always given choices regarding activities and places in which to engage in those activities. When he returned to school, staff routines included presenting embedded choices along with no-choice demands. For example, Ben had no choice about getting on the school bus, but he was reminded routinely of his choices once on the bus (e.g., where to sit, what music to listen to, and the like). Ben is working now to recognize his physiological and emotional states (e.g., headache, anger) and to use specific signs and gestures to communicate these feelings rather than using simple lashing out to communicate negative feelings and smiling to communicate positive feelings.

Because of the importance of this communication perspective on challenging behavior, we have included a communication and behavior report written for another child whose behavior was deteriorating badly in a grade-school setting (see Appendix 13-1). This report, which was written collaboratively by a speech-language pathologist and a behavioral psychologist, may serve as a useful model in developing comparable intervention programs for students with severe challenging behavior after TBI.

Premise V: Integration of Behavioral and Cognitive Perspectives

Behavioral Reactions to Cognitive Failure

Much of Ben's challenging behavior during the years since his injury has been in response to tasks that, from a cognitive perspective, were too difficult for him. Although the severity of Ben's global impairment is obvious, his comprehension of language and his rather sophisticated sense of humor have led staff to consistently overestimate his organizational abilities. For example, in the early years after his injury, he frequently got lost in the middle of tasks (e.g., brushing his teeth), though others were convinced he had mastered them. Then staff or parents would nag, and Ben would become upset, which likely would result in a consequent behavioral outburst.

This pattern continues to this day, although with reduced frequency because of the many cognitive supports that have been put in place for Ben. For example, in his high school recently, he was in an elevator with his paraprofessional aide and a visitor. The aide waited for Ben to select the appropriate floor and activate the elevator, which is his routine responsibility. Ben simply stood with his walker, attending to the visitor. The aide waited. Nothing happened. Finally, the aide turned to the visitor and said, "I don't know why he's just standing there. He knows full well what to do." Ben became upset, and some effort was expended to get him back on track.

Of course, Ben "knew what to do." When routines are uninterrupted, he performs well and independently. However, one of the common cognitive consequences of prefrontal injury is what Shallice (1988) has termed *supervisory attentional system distractibility syndrome* (i.e., surprisingly severe difficulty in remaining focused and organized when well-rehearsed routines are disrupted). This type of organizational impairment is often more severe than are other aspects of cognitive disability after TBI, leading to breakdowns in performance, punitive responses from staff and others, and systematically deteriorating behavior. In Ben's case, and in the case of many children with TBI, cognitive intervention and support are a major component of behavior management.

This connection between severe behavior disorders and organizational impairment was highlighted by Feeney and Ylvisaker (1995) in their experimental validation of a combined behavioral and cognitive intervention for three adolescents with severe aggressive behavior after TBI (with prefrontal focus). Like Ben, these adolescents were surprisingly disorganized (relative to their other cognitive abilities) and, therefore, had difficulty in completing tasks, a behavior that staff interpreted as willful. With photographic advance organizers (and subsequently written advance organizers), combined with greater staff appreciation of the importance of setting events, behavioral momentum, and choice, aggressive behavior was reduced to near zero, and all three subjects successfully completed their academic-vocational programs and acquired paying jobs.

Intervention for individuals with organizational impairment is discussed at length in Chapter 11. Our point is that this type of intervention is often a critical component of intervention for individuals whose primary presenting disability is behavioral or psychosocial. Predictable routines and organizational supports, including drawn or written plans, have become staples in Ben's menu of critical supports. With these external advance organizers in place, his behavior is generally orderly and appropriate.

Social Cognition and Social Perception

Ben's injury included significant loss of neural tissue in right frontal and right temporal areas of the brain, those associated with perception and interpretation of a variety of social cues. Because he is able to interpret only extreme manifestations of emotion (e.g., laughter representing positive emotion and crying representing negative emotion), he frequently misinterprets others' behavior and emotions. For example, if somebody says to him something that is intended to be ironic or sarcastic or metaphoric, Ben is likely to interpret the words literally and to become confused or possibly upset. Ben's mother is more aware than are others that it is critical to tell him directly how she is feeling and not to expect that he will correctly interpret even fairly obvious cues. She also counsels staff to do the same. In Ben's case, the most critical intervention in this area is providing scripts to communication partners so that they know how to interact with him, explaining their emotional states and clarifying indirect meanings.

Related to his difficulty in perceiving social cues is his difficulty in receiving feedback from others regarding his behavior. For example, Ben enjoys being tickled and tickling others. His memory impairment, combined with a tendency to perseverate and a difficulty in reading feedback cues from others, results in his persisting with tickling to the point of seriously alienating potential friends. Currently under way is intervention that combines clarifying information for communication partners (so that they understand Ben's behavior) with a script for Ben that begins with his request, "Is it okay if I touch you?"

Ben is also receiving contextualized instruction in identifying somewhat-higher-level emotional states (e.g., *frustrated, stressed out, excited*) and important related concepts (e.g., *obnoxious* and *interesting*). These feelings and concepts are brought up for discussion only when Ben or someone in the environment is actively experiencing that state. Predictably, attempts to teach the concepts via workbook exercises (e.g., identifying the emotion represented by drawn faces) and role playing have failed.

Other Options

Many children and adolescents with TBI have residual social cognition and social perception deficits that are much less severe than are Ben's; in such cases, other intervention options are available. For example, many packaged social skills training programs are available, most of which rely on role playing as a means of learning prosocial behaviors (Goldstein et al., 1980; Walker et al., 1988a, 1988b). Social skills training may be useful for those individuals who do not know the rules, roles, and scripts that underlie socially acceptable behavior and who

have some ability to transfer learned behaviors from training context to application context. Many children with acquired brain injury know the rules (from before the injury) but fail to govern their behavior by those rules in stressful real-world action contexts. Traditional social skills training is *not* useful for such children. However, even in the case of those for whom decontextualized social skills training is relevant as the first stage of intervention, it is important to heed the wise counsel of Walker and colleagues (1994) and to reinforce out-of-context training with contextualized coaching in the social context.

Some children and adolescents with social perception deficits less severe than Ben's may profit from the types of video and role-playing exercises described by Ylvisaker and colleagues (1987). For example, video illustrations of various speech acts (language used to tease, encourage, compliment, insult, scare, threaten, warn, entertain, punish, and the like) can be played, followed by discussion of the clues that enable one to interpret the speaker's intent. This activity can be followed by role-playing practice with the conventions that are used to send and receive these distinct intentions. Students with relatively mild impairment sometimes profit from these exercises. Those with somewhat more severe impairment may not improve their ability to interpret speakers' intent with these exercises but may at least learn that this aspect of communication is difficult for them and that they may need to ask speakers to explain their intent.

Videotape Feedback

Adolescents with mild-to-moderate impairment in social interaction may benefit from videotape analysis of their interaction with others, followed by practice to improve performance and further videotape analysis. Interpersonal Process Recall (IPR) (Kagan et al., 1969) is one of the few intervention approaches that has been validated experimentally for use with young adults with TBI (Helffenstein and Wechsler, 1982). IPR is designed to improve social and interactive skills by means of coached self-observation of conversational interaction on videotape. We have used videotape self-observation for a variety of training purposes both with staff and with individuals with TBI. However, important cautions must accompany this recommendation. Emotionally fragile individuals should not be subjected to self-observation, at least not without psychiatric approval and without appropriate desensitization. Confronting oneself on videotape can be threatening, especially for a person who looks and sounds different as a result of the injury.

A reasonable sequence of desensitizing experiences could include (1) self-observation in a mirror, (2) self-observation on audio tape, (3) observation and discussion of others on videotape, (4) videotape observation of oneself engaged in a nonthreatening task, (5) videotape observation of oneself engaged in a more difficult task but with no discussion and, finally, (6) videotape observation of oneself engaged in a difficult task, followed by analysis of the performance. It is also wise to have videotape equipment routinely available in the environment for desensitizing purposes and for the clinician to engage in self-scrutiny with the clients before expecting the same of clients. A variety of applications of videotape technology in psychology are presented in Dowrick and Biggs (1983), including a review of videotape applications in social skills training (Hosford and Mills, 1983).

Premise VI: From External Control to Internal Self-Control of Behavior

Just as typical child development proceeds from external to internal (deliberate) control of behavior, so also recovery after severe brain injury follows the same pattern. Adults, possibly including both parents and professionals, often fail to facilitate this progression actively. Their failure may be motivated by an understandable need to protect a child who already has been injured seriously and by a belief that the child or adolescent is incapable of making good decisions and, therefore, requires external control. In these cases, it is useful to point out that in normal development, thousands of intervening steps occur between the total external control of a newborn to the internal control of a mature adult. Similarly after TBI, it is always possible to identify reasonable and safe small steps in the direction of internal control.

In Ben's case, staff faced a serious dilemma. He responded negatively to overt external control but seemed incapable of planning and organizing his behavior internally to achieve important rehabilitation and educational goals. His life after the injury was punctuated by frequent and mutually damaging control battles with adults. We do not suggest that this control dilemma is solved easily. However, some intervention approaches are useful in at least partially resolving the dilemma. The process of teaching positive communication alternatives to challenging behavior (described earlier) is one of these approaches.

In addition, a major component of Ben's intervention for several years has been directed at teaching him to make good plans and to follow them with minimal adult intervention. The process of teaching children to make, follow, and review plans is described in Chapters 12 and 14 in the sections dealing with executive system intervention. Several of the intervention procedures described in those chapters were used with Ben. Currently, he is responsible for making his plans for the day both at school and at work. His aide initiates the routine by asking Ben for his plan to accomplish the work that must be done. Alternatives are available to Ben in the form of printed words that he can read. Then he draws pictures to represent the sequence of his plan for that day. At the end

of his day at school or work, he reviews his plan, checks off the items that were satisfactorily completed and, if necessary, discusses reasons for incompleted components of the plan.

In addition, efforts are under way to teach Ben to recognize the need for help in difficult tasks and then to ask for such help. This step is critical in phasing out the support of his paraprofessional aide, which must occur if Ben is to be a candidate for work that is supported only partially. Ben's earlier special education programs did not help him to understand the characteristics of tasks that are easy and difficult for him. In the early stages of Ben's current program, his aide noticed the increase in difficulty for Ben and asked him whether he needed help and what kind of help he needed. The goal was gradually to fade the cue question in response to improvement in Ben's ability to notice the need for help. In his two familiar work settings, Ben has come to recognize certain tasks as difficult and to request help from his work supervisor without cues. This improvement has allowed the aide to reduce his presence at these two sites.

Identification of task difficulty is a presupposition of strategic behavior: If you do not recognize a task as difficult, you will not be motivated to use special strategic procedures to succeed. More generally, recognizing the difficulty level of tasks and knowing what to do when presented with difficult tasks are prerequisites to Ben's ultimately taking control of the supports that he probably will need indefinitely. The alternative is learned helplessness, the opposite of Ben's goal of independence and internal control.

Premise VII: Routines in a Social-Communicative Context

All the interventions that have proved to be effective for Ben have occurred in real social-communicative contexts and have been designed to influence routines and scripts in those contexts. Ben is a very concrete thinker who has difficulty in perceiving meaning in activities or exercises not directly related to goals that he embraces. He also has difficulty in transferring behaviors or skills from the acquisition to the application context. With these dominant characteristics as background, it is understandable that he resisted training on the Dynavox, which was introduced and used exclusively in pull-out speech-language therapy sessions by staff who were not well trained in its use. He failed to see the benefit of this potentially useful augmentative communication device, a failure probably attributable in part to the manner in which it was introduced. In addition, decontextualized training in social skills and social perception has failed consistently to yield generalizable changes in behavior, whereas Ben has learned and continues to use many positive social behaviors taught in the context of social routines and designed to be part of those routines.

Table 13-1. DOs and DON'Ts in Managing
Behavioral Crises

Crisis DOs

Do help an individual to identify personal feelings.
Do remember to look as if you know what you're doing.
Do be certain that your behavior clearly indicates that you
  are trying to help.
Do remember to look stone-faced.
Do remember that this too shall pass.
Do find your "buttons" and hide them.
Do ask yourself, "Is it really worth making an issue of this?"
Do choose your battles wisely.
Do ensure that everybody is safe and defuse the crisis as
  quickly and efficiently as possible.

Crisis DON'Ts

Don't plant the suggestion of a problem behavior.
Don't threaten consequences.
Don't present commands as questions or pleas.
Don't have more than one person speak at the same time.
Don't restart a confrontation by demanding immediately
  that a person begin a difficult activity.
Don't rehash the incident in front of a person.
Don't "climb ladders."
Don't "teach lessons."
Don't confuse crisis management with behavior management.

Premise VIII: Integration and Collaboration

The most critical member of Ben's rehabilitation and special education team has been his mother. In the early years after his injury, she was not invited warmly to participate as a member of the team, an act of neglect that resulted both in her growing despair and alienation from professionals and in fragmented services for Ben.

In Ben's second inpatient rehabilitation program, every attempt was made to overcome barriers that had been created. For example, the rehabilitation team spent hours with Ben's mother, using her as a critical resource in learning about Ben and his needs and about interventions that both had and had not worked. In effect, staff served an apprenticeship with Ben's mother during the first week of his admission, a joint effort that generated trust sufficient to render her, in turn, subsequently willing to serve an apprenticeship with them. In that time, she mastered the positive, antecedent-focused approaches to communication and behavior that were used in this program and that proved to be effective with Ben. In addition, staff called Ben's mother every day after she returned to her home and, in general, demonstrated such a level of commitment to Ben that she was able to feel comfortable as a team member.

Additionally, integration and collaboration were fostered by having a single rehabilitation plan that covered cognition, communication, behavior, and psychosocial functioning. Involved in this program were several staff members, including a special education teacher, a speech-language pathologist, a behavioral specialist, and a social worker. However, they were convinced that these areas of functioning were inextricable in Ben's case, so much so that they worked together to create one integrated rehabilitation plan with one documentation and reporting system. Furthermore, they sought frequent opportunities to serve Ben by working elbow-to-elbow with one another and with everyday people, including nursing staff and family members.

Integration and collaboration continue in Ben's program, with the focal point being his aide. Ben's teachers, therapists, and psychologist agree that the key figure in facilitating growth in cognition, communication, behavioral self-regulation, social interaction, and vocational development is the paraprofessional aide. Therefore, every attempt is made to speak with one voice in guiding the aide's activity and in modifying Ben's program in response to his improvement. Understanding their primary role as consultants to Ben, to his mother, and to his aide has contributed to staff willingness to collaborate among themselves and, consequently, to integrating Ben's intervention program.

Premise IX: Crisis Management

An examination of Ben's 9 years since the injury clearly reveals that whenever the focus of behavior management was extinction of "maladaptive" behaviors, his behavior worsened. In contrast, when the focus was preventing crises and teaching positive behaviors, his behavior improved.

Two simple principles guide the management of behavioral crises. The first is to prevent crises. However, if a crisis is under way, the second principle is to keep people safe and to defuse the crisis as quickly and painlessly as possible, with minimal restraint and without rewarding negative behavior.

With respect to prevention, all the antecedent-focused behavioral interventions discussed earlier, including the teaching of positive communication alternatives to challenging behavior, can be seen in part as crisis-prevention procedures. As part of crisis prevention, Ben's current program includes involving him in rating his internal state (on a scale of 1–10) and in making decisions about the tasks and settings appropriate for that day on the basis of this rating. As Ben becomes increasingly proficient in assigning himself a rating, he will be the keystone in his own crisis-prevention system.

We do not suggest a cavalier attitude toward behavioral crises. Staff who work with individuals with severe behavior disorders certainly must be equipped with specialized skills to deal effectively with crises. (The crisis *dos* and *don'ts* in Table 13-1 are a summary of some of these skills.) Rather, our point is that *crisis management is not behavior management.* Crisis times are not teaching times. Lessons can be learned during crises, but they usually are negative lessons (e.g., "If I hit hard enough, I get out of physical therapy"; "I hate that person"). Ben learned powerful lessons when staff thought that they could "teach him lessons" during crises. For example, he learned that he could escalate self-injurious behavior to a level at which he could escape any task that he did not like. However, he never learned a positive lesson from a person whose state of mind at the time was revealed by a statement such as, "I am very angry with you, and I plan to teach you a lesson you won't soon forget." That state of mind should serve as a signal to adults to leave the battlefield to regain their control before resuming interaction with the individual with disability.

Premise X: Long-Term Supports

Ben's history since his injury illustrates the unpredictability of long-term outcome and also of the need for supports along the way. At one time, knowledgeable professionals predicted that he would never walk (though now he walks with a walker), would never eat (though he eats all textures with ease), and surely would never work (though he has two training jobs, and the quality and quantity of his work please his supervisors). To be sure, Ben has severe, irreversible brain injury and associated severe, multiple disability. However, his accomplishments are a remarkable success story in light of the severity of his injury.

These accomplishments are a result of hard work and perseverance on Ben's part. They are also a result of a set of supports that has evolved as Ben has improved and as the demands placed on him have changed. With appropriate supports in place, Ben has prospered. In the absence of appropriate supports, he has invariably regressed behaviorally and in other ways. In some cases, staff simply "fell asleep at the wheel." For example, on his return to school after his second rehabilitation admission, Ben's behavior generally was not a problem and staff usually followed the plan obtained from the rehabilitation staff. After several weeks, staff grew lax, Ben's former negative behaviors crept back into his repertoire, staff resorted to their traditional management methods, and Ben's inappropriate behavior escalated.

In other cases, staff failed to anticipate the need for intensified supports due to changes in setting and demands. For example, Ben's behavior deteriorated when he started attending high school. This transition is stressful for all students and is associated with a need for increased support. Ben's brain injury magnified the stress associated with this transition, thereby creating a need for significantly intensified supports. Because this need was not anticipated, Ben's behavior predictably deteriorated. In Chapter 9 we present a set of delayed negative consequences of TBI in adolescents. In many cases, these consequences are a result of inadequate anticipation by professionals of needs for cognitive, academic, or social support as developmental demands increase.

Premise XI: Beyond Medical and Training Models of Intervention

In Chapter 20, we describe a variety of ways in which professionals can choose to regard themselves and their services. The type of professional service that has proved to be most helpful for Ben—and for many other children and adolescents with TBI—can be understood best as a combination of the coach, consultant, mentor, and apprenticeship models of service delivery. As would coaches, effective professionals worked with Ben on a real playing field—his everyday life; as would consultants, they oriented their services around Ben's goals and distributed their expertise to people most involved in Ben's life; as would mentors, they created a powerful relationship of mutual respect with Ben; as would master craftspersons working with apprentices, they taught by showing Ben in context how to create the "product" that he was supposed to create (e.g., positive social interaction). In contrast, when professionals behaved in ways exemplified by the medical model, their services generally were ineffective. Further, when they behaved in ways characteristic of the animal-trainer model, Ben's behavior generally deteriorated.

Premise XII: Meaningful Engagement in Chosen Life Activities

Meaning and purpose have been and continue to be critical for Ben, as they are for most people. When engaged in activities that he finds meaningful—in part because he has chosen them—Ben's attention is focused, his behavior is positive, and his learning is effective. The best current example of this fundamental principle is Ben's attitude toward work. Because he values his role as worker—and is valued by supervisors as a worker—he has been surprisingly successful in his two work settings, with no episodes of seriously challenging behavior. In contrast, Ben has a rich history of negative behavior when presented with apparently meaningless drill activities enforced with coercive methods of discipline.

Several factors render the principle of meaning particularly critical for Ben and for many people like him with a history of acquired brain injury. First, he still knows himself as the person who was once an active 10-year-old experiencing great success as a student, athlete, paper deliverer, friend, and regular kid. Now, he has a serious disability but is not about to "play dead" in relation to arbitrary decisions of professionals who come and go in his life and who sometimes find it difficult to focus their thinking around him and his long-term goals in life. Second, he is a very concrete thinker who has difficulty in processing professional wisdom such as, "This cognitive exercise is good for you because it will help you think better." Third, exercises meaningless for him may change behavior in the training setting without influencing behavior in Ben's real world. Finally, with the domain of meaningful and satisfying activities severely restricted by his disability, it seems only fair that decision makers in Ben's life exert every effort to tie rehabilitation and education to meaningful activities and to work with Ben in expanding this domain.

Checklist for Planning Behavioral Intervention

In Figure 13-6, we present the approach advanced in this chapter in the form of a checklist that might help clinicians remain focused and attend to all of the activities needed for a successful, antecedent-focused behavioral intervention.

Summary of Effectiveness of Intervention

In our presentation of intervention premises, we cited literature that provides empirical support for most of the principles of positive, antecedent-focused, communication-based intervention embraced in this chapter. With very few exceptions, available studies focus on children and adolescents with diagnoses other than TBI. The research literature dealing with behavioral and psychosocial intervention in children with TBI is in its infancy. Therefore, our clinical orientation is based primarily on our years of clinical experience with this group and on evidence from other populations, neuropsychological considerations, and several of our suggestive single-subject experiments with children and adolescents with TBI (Feeney and Ylvisaker, 1995, 1997; Ylvisaker and Feeney, in press).

Summaries of investigations of the effectiveness of role-play–based social skills intervention for children with developmental disabilities, learning disabilities, and behavior disorders unrelated to TBI are not optimistic (McIntosh et al., 1991; Walker et al., 1994; Zaragoza et al., 1991). Although intensive training has the potential to change interactive behavior in training settings and, with special efforts at generalization, possibly influence adult ratings of a child's behavior, little evidence substantiates that social skills training programs positively influence peer ratings of the individuals receiving the training. Because a primary goal of social skills intervention is to help children to interact effectively with peers and to have friends, this finding is particularly sobering. These summaries are among the many reasons for our emphasis on contextualized intervention combined with training and support for communication partners. Ylvisaker and colleagues (1992) summarized the small but growing literature on social skills intervention with adults with TBI.

Despite the limited empirical support available in the literature and regardless of the rather gloomy picture of social outcome painted in much of the literature regarding pediatric TBI outcome, we leave the reader with a sense of optimism. Ben's life is much more satisfying and holds much greater promise than it would have in the absence of the ongoing, integrated, contextualized, antecedent-focused, communication-based intervention described in this chapter. The same can be said for a large number of other children and adolescents who experienced TBI and with whom we have worked intensively, many of whom were expected to have no meaningful social life because of the severity of their injuries. Certain interventions and supports make a difference. The work is difficult and has no end, but it is work that must be done and holds the promise of enormous emotional rewards for those who want to positively influence the lives of children with TBI.

Assessment

❏ Acquire relevant background information:
  ❏ Preinjury information: interests, levels of development, behavioral functioning.
  ❏ Nature of the injury and associated behavioral vulnerabilities.
  ❏ General medical information.
  ❏ Evolution of behavioral issues since the injury.
  ❏ Critical communication partners and supports in the natural environment.
❏ Identify the cognitive profile in detail, including cognitive contributors to behavior problems (e.g., difficulties with attention, perception, organization, memory, executive functions).
❏ Operationally define problem behavior in concrete behavioral terms.
❏ Perform a functional and ecologically valid assessment.
  ❏ Observe the child in a variety of natural environments, with a variety of communication partners, and with a variety of stressors.
    ❏ What is the child's current daily routine?
    ❏ What are the general environmental conditions present at the time of challenging behavior?

Figure 13-6. Checklist for planning behavioral intervention for children and adolescents with traumatic brain injury.

❑ What specific antecedents and consequences are associated with challenging behavior (i.e., ABC analysis)?

❑ What patterns are associated with the daily routine; with general environmental conditions; with specific antecedents; with medications?

❑ Generate hypotheses about the communication value of challenging behaviors or other possible purposes served by the behavior.

❑ Test the most likely hypotheses, in context (see Chapter 10).

❑ Identify general strengths and skills.

❑ Identify the most effective positive communication alternative to the problem behaviors.

❑ Identify support system in the natural environment.

Intervention

❑ Collaboratively identify meaningful long- and short-term goals. Determine priorities for behavioral intervention.

❑ Facilitate positive behavioral routines:

❑ Create a concrete, meaningful daily routine (events, sequences, people, places, activities).

❑ Provide organizational and other supports needed to compensate for cognitive weakness.

❑ Create positive setting events (external and internal) before requesting performance of difficult tasks.

❑ Create positive behavioral momentum before requesting performance of difficult tasks.

❑ Create as many opportunities for choice and control as possible; teach choice making if necessary.

❑ Create positive scripts and roles for an individual.

❑ Eliminate chronic behavioral provocations in the environment and in the behavior of others.

❑ Ensure that the individual is able to perform all requested activities.

❑ For children with severe behavioral outbursts, ensure that all staff understand emergency scripts for themselves (for use in the event of behavioral crises) and that they possess fall-back plans to avoid severe behavioral disruption.

❑ Teach communication alternatives to challenging behavior.

❑ Collaboratively identify the communication value of challenging behavior.

❑ Operationally define the communication behavior(s) selected to replace the challenging behaviors.

❑ Collaboratively decide the point at which it is acceptable to respond affirmatively to the new positive communication acts for escape or access.

❑ In appropriate contexts, prompt the positive communication alternative; then reward that alternative with escape or access as appropriate. Ensure that a large number of successful learning trials are available daily.

❑ Fade cues and prompts and increase the variety of contexts and tasks in which a child is willing to use communication alternatives.

❑ If necessary, teach relevant social knowledge (rules, roles, routines, and scripts), including specific pragmatic communication acts.

❑ If necessary, teach social perception and social decision making.

❑ Ensure that all regular communication partners are trained and take part in the program.

❑ Do communication partners understand the positive, antecedent-focused program and their role? Do they understand fully that behavior management is facilitating and teaching positive behaviors, not reacting to negative behaviors?

❑ Are communication partners competent in the following areas: setting events, positive behavioral momentum, offering choices and avoiding control battles, positive roles and scripts, redirection without reinforcement of negative behaviors, and management of behavioral crises with minimal intervention and restriction?

❑ Do communication partners have adequate support so that they can continue to play their roles effectively?

❑ If possible, teach the individual to manage personal antecedents.

❑ Create a "minimalist" intervention plan for managing behavioral crises.

References

Adolphs R, Tranel D, Damasio H, Damasio AR (1995). Fear and the human amygdala. J Neurosci 15;5879.

Allman J, Brothers I (1994). Faces, fear, and the amygdala. Nature 372;613.

Asarnow RF, Satz P, Light R, Neumann E. (1991). Behavior problems and adaptive functioning in children with mild and severe closed head injury. J Pediatr Psychol 16;534.

Bechara A, Tranel D, Damasio H, et al. (1995). Double dissociation of condition and declarative knowledge relative to the amygdala and hippocampus in humans. Science 269;1115.

Benton A (1991). Prefrontal injury and behavior in children. Dev Neuropsychol 7;275.

Brown G, Chadwick O, Shaffer D, et al. (1981). A prospective study of children with head injuries: III. Psychiatric sequelae. Psychol Med 11;63.

Burke GM (1990). Unconventional behavior: a communicative interpretation in individuals with severe disabilities. Top Lang Dis 10;75.

Carr EG, Levin L, McConnachie G, et al. (1994). Communication-Based Intervention for Problem Behavior: A User's Guide for Producing Positive Change. Baltimore: Paul H. Brookes.

Carr EG, McConnachie G, Levin L, Kemp DC (1993). Communication-Based Treatment of Severe Behavior Problems. In R VanHouten, S Axelrod (eds), Behavior Analysis and Treatment. New York: Plenum, 231.

Chapman SB, Watkins R, Gustafson C, et al. (1997). Narrative discourse in children with head injury, children with language impairment, and typically developing children. Am J Speech Lang Pathol 6;66.

Colvin G, Sugai G (1989). Managing Escalating Behavior. Eugene, OR: Behavior Associates.

Condeluci A (1991). Interdependence: The Route to Community. Orlando, FL: Deutsch.

Condeluci A (1992). Brain injury rehabilitation: the need to bridge paradigms. Brain Inj 6;543.

Condeluci A, Getz-Laski S (1987). Social role valorization: a model for community re-entry. J Head Trauma Rehabil 2;49.

Conroy MA, Fox JJ (1994). Setting factors and challenging behaviors in the classroom: incorporating contextual factors into effective intervention plans for children with aggressive behaviors. J Prev School Fail 38;29.

Daigneault S, Braun CMJ, Montes JL (1997). Pseudodepressive personality and mental inertia in a child with a focal left-frontal lesion. Develop Neuropsych 13;1.

Damasio AR (1994). Descartes' Error. New York: Avon Books.

Damasio AR, Tranel D, Damasio H (1990). Individuals with sociopathic behavior caused by frontal lobe damage fail to respond automatically to socially charged stimuli. Behav Brain 4;81.

Dennis M, Barnes M (1990). Knowing the meaning, getting the point, bridging the gap, and carrying the message: aspects of discourse following closed head injury in childhood and adolescence. Brain Lang 39;428.

Dowrick PW, Biggs SJ (1983). Using video: psychological and social applications. New York: Wiley.

Dumas JE (1989). Let's not forget the context in behavioral assessment. Behav Assess 11;231.

Dunlap G, Kern-Dunlap L, Clarke M, Robbins FR (1991). Functional assessment, curricular revisions, and severe behavior problems. J Appl Behav Anal 24;387.

Durand VM (1990). Severe behavior problems: communication based intervention. New York: Guilford.

Eslinger PJ, Damasio AR, Damasio H, Grattan LM (1989). Developmental consequences of early frontal lobe damage. J Clin Exp Neuropsychol 11;50.

Eslinger PJ, Grattan LM, Damasio H, Damasio AR (1992). Developmental consequences of childhood frontal lobe damage. Arch Neurol 49;764.

Feeney TJ, Ylvisaker M (1995). Choice and routine: antecedent behavioral interventions for adolescents with severe traumatic brain injury. J Head Trauma Rehabil 10;67.

Feeney TJ, Ylvisaker M (1997). A Positive, Communication-Based Approach to Challenging Behavior After TBI. In A Glang, G Singer, B Todis (eds), Children with Acquired Brain Injury: The School's Response. Baltimore: Paul H. Brookes, 229.

Flavell J, Miller P, Miller S (1993). Cognitive Development (3rd ed). Englewood Cliffs, NJ: Prentice Hall.

Fletcher JM, Ewing-Cobbs L, Miner M, Levin HS (1990). Behavioral changes after closed head injury in children. J Consult Clin Psychol 58;93.

Fowler R (1996). Supporting students with challenging behaviors in general education settings: a review of behavioral momentum techniques and guidelines for use. Oregon Conf Monogr 8;137.

Fox J, Conroy M (1995). Setting events and behavioral disorders of children and youth: an interbehavioral field analysis for research and practice. J Emot Behav Dis 3;130.

Goldstein AP, Sprafkin RP, Gershaw NJ, Klein P (1980). Skillstreaming the Adolescent: A Structured Learning Approach to Teaching Prosocial Skills. Champaign, IL: Research Press.

Grattan LM, Eslinger PJ (1990). Influence of cerebral lesion site upon the onset and progression of interpersonal deficits following brain injury. J Clin Exp Neuropsychol 12;33.

Grattan LM, Eslinger PJ (1992). Long-term psychological consequences of childhood frontal lobe lesion in patient DT. Brain Cogn 20;185.

Greenspan AI, MacKenzie EJ (1994). Functional outcome after pediatric head injury. Pediatrics 94;425.

Harchik AE, Sherman JA, Bannerman DJ (1993). Choice and control: new opportunities for people with developmental disabilities. Ann Clin Psychiatr 5;151.

Haring TG, Kennedy CH (1990). Contextual control of problem behavior in students with severe disabilities. J Appl Behav Anal 23;235.

Helffenstein D, Wechsler F (1982). The use of interpersonal process recall (IPR) in the remediation of interpersonal and communication skill deficits in the newly brain injured. Clin Neuropsychol 4;139.

Horner R, Dunlap G, Koegel R, et al. (1990). Toward a technology of "nonaversive" behavioral support. J Assoc Persons Severe Handicaps 15;125.

Horner R, O'Neill RE, Flannery KB (1993). Effective Behavior Support Plans. In M Snell (ed), Instruction of Students with Severe Disabilities. New York: Merrill, 184.

Horner RH, Dunlap G, Koegel RL (eds) (1988). Generalization and Maintenance: Lifestyle Changes in Applied Settings. Baltimore: Paul H. Brookes.

Hosford RE, Mills ME (1983). Video in Social Skills Training. In PW Dowrick and SJ Biggs (eds), Using Video: Psychological and Social Applications. New York: Wiley, 123.

Hudson JA (1993). Understanding Events: The Development of Script Knowledge. In M Bennett (ed), The Development of Social Cognition. New York: Guilford, 142.

Kagan N, Schauble P, Resnikoff D (1969). Interpersonal process recall. J Nerv Ment Dis 148;365.

Kennedy CH (1994). Manipulating antecedent conditions to alter the stimulus control of problem behavior. J Appl Behav Anal 27;161.

Kennedy CH, Itkonen T (1993). Effects of setting events on the problem behavior of students with severe disabilities. J Appl Behav Anal 26;321.

Kern L, Childs KE, Dunlap G, et al. (1994). Using assessment-based curricular intervention to improve the classroom behavior of a student with emotional and behavioral challenges. J Appl Behav Anal 27;7.

LeDoux JE (1993). Emotional memory systems in the brain. Behav Brain Res 58;69.

Levin HS, Goldstein FC, Williams DH, Eisenberg HM (1991). The Contribution of Frontal Lobe Lesions to the Neurobehavioral Outcome of Closed Head Injury. In HS Levin, HM Eisenberg, AI Benton (eds), Frontal Lobe Function and Dysfunction. New York: Oxford University, 318.

Mace FC, Lalli JS, Shea MC, et al. (1990). The momentum of human behavior in a natural setting. J Exp Anal Behav 54;163.

Mace FC, Page TJ, Ivanck MT, O'Brien S. (1986) Analysis of environmental determinants of aggression and disruption in mentally retarded children. Appl Res Ment Retard 7;203.

Marlowe WB (1992) The impact of a right prefrontal lesion on the developing brain. Brain Cogn 20;205.

Marlowe WB. (1989) Consequences of frontal lobe injury in the developing child. J Clin Exp Neuropsychol 12;105.

McIntosh S, Vaughn S, Zaragoza N (1991). A review of social interventions for students with learning disabilities. J Learn Disabil 24;451.

Mendelsohn D, Levin HS, Bruce D, et al. (1992). Late MRI after head injury in children: relationship to clinical features and outcome. Childs Nerv Syst 8;445.

Michael J (1982). Distinguishing between discriminative and motivational functions of stimuli. J Exp Anal Behav 37;149.

Michael J (1989). Motivative Relations and Establishing Operations. In J Michael (ed), Verbal and Non-Verbal Behavior: Concepts and Principles. Kalamazoo, MI: Western Michigan University, 40.

Nevin JA (1988). Behavioral momentum and the partial reinforcement effect. Psychol Bull 103;44.

Papero PH, Prigatano GP, Snyder HM, Johnson DL (1993). Children's adaptive behavioral competence after head injury. Neuropsychol Rehabil 3;321.

Perrott SB, Taylor HG, Montes JL (1991). Neuropsychological sequelae, familial stress, and environmental adaptation following pediatric head injury. Dev Neuropsychol 7;69.

Petterson L (1991). Sensitivity to emotional cues and social behavior in children and adolescents after head injury. Percept Motor Skills 73;1139.

Price B, Doffnre K, Stowe R, Mesulam M (1990). The comportmental learning disabilities of early frontal lobe damage. Brain 113;1383.

Reichle J, Johnston SS (1993). Replacing challenging behavior: the role of communication intervention. Top Lang Dis 13;61.

Reichle J, Wacker DP (eds) (1993). Communicative Alternatives to Challenging Behavior. Baltimore: Brookes.

Shallice T (1988). From Neuropsychology to Mental Structure. Cambridge, UK: Cambridge University Press.

Slifer KJ, Tucker CL, Gerson AC, et. al. (1996). Operant conditioning for behavior management during posttraumatic amnesia in children and adolescents with brain injury. J Head Trauma Rehabil 11;39.

Stuss DT, Benson DF (1986). The Frontal Lobes. New York: Raven.

Varney NR, Menefee L (1993). Psychosocial and executive deficits following closed head injury: Implications for orbital frontal cortex. J Head Trauma Rehabil 8;32.

Vollmer TR, Iwata BA (1991). Establishing operations and reinforcement effects. J Appl Behav Anal 23;417.

Wahler RG, Fox RM (1981). Setting events in applied behavior analysis: towards a conceptual and methodological expansion. J Appl Behav Anal 14;327.

Walker HM, McConnell SM, Holmes D, et al. (1988). The Walker Social Skills Curriculum: The ACCEPTS Program. Austin, TX: PRO-ED.

Walker HM, Schwarz IE, Nippold MA, et al. (1994). Social skills in school-age children and youth: issues and best practices in assessment and intervention. Top Lang Dis 14(3);70.

Walker HM, Todis B, Holmes D, Horton G (1988). The Walker Social Skills Program: The ACCESS Program. Adolescent Curriculum for Communication and Effective Social Skills. Austin, TX: PRO-ED.

Williams D, Mateer CA (1992). Developmental impact of frontal lobe injury in middle childhood. Brain Cogn 20;196.

Ylvisaker M (1993). Communication outcome in children and adolescents with traumatic brain injury. Neuropsychol Rehabil 3;367.

Ylvisaker M, Feeney T (1994). Communication and behavior: collaboration between speech-language pathologists and behavioral psychologists. Top Lang Dis 15(1);37.

Ylvisaker M, Feeney T (1995). Traumatic brain injury in adolescence: assessment and reintegration. Semin Speech Lang 16(1);32.

Ylvisaker M, Feeney T (1996). Executive functions: supported cognition and self-advocacy after traumatic brain injury. Semin Speech Lang 17;217.

Ylvisaker M, Feeney T (in press). An Integrated Approach to Brain Injury Rehabilitation: Everyday Positive Routines. San Diego: Singular Press.

Ylvisaker M, Feeney T, Urbanczyk B (1993). A social-environmental approach to communication and behavior after traumatic brain injury. Semin Speech Lang 14(1);74.

Ylvisaker M, Feeney T, Urbanczyk B (1993). Developing a Positive Communication Culture for Rehabilitation. In CJ Durgin, ND Schmidt, J Fryer (eds), Staff Development and Clinical Intervention in Brain Injury Rehabilitation. Gaithersburg, MD: Aspen Publishers, 57.

Ylvisaker M, Szekeres S, Henry K, et al. (1987). Topics in Cognitive Rehabilitation. In M Ylvisaker, E Gobble (eds), Community Re-Entry for Head Injured Adults. Boston: Butterworth–Heinemann, 137.

Ylvisaker M, Urbanczyk B, Feeney T (1992). Social skills following traumatic brain injury. Semin Speech Lang 13;308.

Zaragoza N, Vaughn S, McIntosh R (1991). Social skills interventions and children with behavior problems: a review. Behav Dis 16;260.

Appendix 13-1

Proposed Components of an Integrated Communication and Behavior Plan for an Individual with Seriously Challenging Behavior

Teaching Positive Communication Alternatives to Challenging Behavior

The most important focus of John's* communication and behavior plan is a concentrated effort on the part of all staff and family members to teach him positive communication alternatives to his challenging behaviors. This approach to behavior problems is based on the following premises:

Premises

1. *All behaviors communicate something.* Initially, the behavior may be unintentional. However, if communication partners consistently reinforce the behavior, it will likely become intentional.
2. *Most behaviors— however unconventional—are adaptive* in that they effectively communicate intended messages.
3. If a challenging behavior (e.g., hitting, screaming, hair pulling) is part of an individual's communication system, it is critical to *substitute a more acceptable behavior* rather than trying simply to extinguish the challenging behavior. Extinguishing the challenging behavior without teaching a positive communication alternative likely will result in development of a more challenging behavior to communicate the same intention.
4. Ideal teaching of positive communication alternatives occurs *in natural communication contexts with everyday communication partners as the primary agents of change.*

*The name John was selected arbitrarily to represent any child with TBI.

Consistency is one of the keys. Communication partners must develop good communication routines to help the individual acquire good communication routines.

Selection of Communication Intentions to Target

John uses a variety of negative behaviors (e.g., hair pulling, hitting, falling to the floor) to communicate a variety of important messages. Many of the messages that he (at least occasionally) communicates in negative ways fall into two important categories:

1. *Access:* In such cases, John is trying to get something, such as attention, desired activities, desired objects, or stimulation.
2. *Escape:* In such cases, John is trying to escape or avoid something, such as unwanted attention, unwanted activities, unwanted objects, unwanted demands, or unwanted stimulation.

Selection of Positive Communication Alternatives to Teach

Staff and family must work together to select the best communication alternative to promote at any stage in John's intervention. At the outset, it is important that the positive communication alternative have the following characteristics:

1. It is *easy* for John—at least as easy as the negative behavior it will replace.
2. It is *powerful* for John—at least as effective and (it is hoped) more effective in communicating his message successfully than is the negative behavior it replaces.

299

3. It is possible for staff and family to *prompt* the positive communication alternative. This characteristic renders gesturing, signing, and pointing to pictures or symbols more useful at the outset than talking. It is possible to prompt the former, but not the latter, physically.

The specific communication behaviors that John uses to communicate important messages will change over time and will become more complex. Staff and family should decide collaboratively when to move from a less to a more complex or conventional means of communicating his messages (e.g., moving from gesture or sign to speech or an augmentative communication device).

Current Plan: Positive Communication Alternatives

1. *Escape:* Sign finished or say no.
2. *Access attention:* Vocalize calmly or tap the other person on the shoulder.
3. *Access activity or object:* Point to activity or object, point to picture or symbol, or say the word.

Teaching Within Routines of Interaction.   It is critical for staff and family to ensure that John communicates positively and is rewarded for communicating positively much more frequently than communicating negatively and being rewarded for doing so. Teaching positive communication alternatives must become a *routine* for all staff and family. Ideally, during each day, John will have at least 100 rewarded experiences with positive communication to counterbalance the small number of inevitable, inadvertently rewarded negative communications. The key is to make these teaching interactions *routine*. (See illustrations of communication-teaching routines at the end of this chapter.)

Deciding When Escape and Access Are Acceptable. Staff and family should decide collaboratively when it is acceptable for them to honor John's positive communication of escape or access messages. For example, they may decide that communication is a higher priority now than are physical therapy exercises. Therefore, exercise time would be an acceptable and desirable time at which to prompt and honor John's positive escape communication. At certain times, John is *not* free to escape undesired activities or to access desired activities. Staff should prepare for those times with the procedures listed later (positive behavioral momentum). In the early stages of training, it is important for staff to recognize the importance of communication-behavior intervention and avoid scheduling a large number of no-choice situations that carry the inevitable risk of confrontation and negative behaviors, which may be rewarded unintentionally.

Procedures to Use When Escape or Access Is Not Acceptable.   Early in the training, a very large number of times

during the course of the day staff should ensure that John has the opportunity to use his positive access or escape communication to access desired activities or to escape undesired activities. However, staff must be prepared with procedures when placing demands on John that are non-negotiable.

- *Cognitive preparation:* Ensure that John is alerted to upcoming events in his schedule so that negative surprise-based responses are avoided.
- *Positive behavioral momentum:* Ensure that John has experienced a backlog of success (is "on a roll") before introducing potentially difficult or undesirable tasks.
  1. Identify high-success, high-satisfaction tasks.
  2. Identify low-success, low-satisfaction—but *doable* —tasks.
  3. Engage John in three, four, five, six, or more high-success, high-satisfaction tasks (depending on need) before introducing a low-success, low-satisfaction task: That is, ensure that John is feeling relaxed and successful before introducing difficult tasks.
- *Positive setting events:* Try to ensure that John is in a generally positive state (e.g., not sick, tired, or in pain) before asking him to perform tasks that you know are difficult or stressful for him. In addition, make your interaction with him as pleasant as possible and give him as much control as possible.
- *Choice and no-choice:* Teach John the difference between choice and no-choice. For this teaching to be successful, staff and family should use the words *no choice* only for very important times, when it is critical that John comply and when they are willing to persevere in the face of potentially very negative behavior. Make every effort to avoid saying "no choice" and subsequently giving in to him in the face of his fierce resistance. *Choose your battles wisely.* Try to avoid control battles. If you must begin a control battle for some very important reason, ensure that you win it quickly and efficiently; then move on without dwelling on the negative interaction.

Documentation.

- *Focus on positive communication:* Staff and family should try to chart the number of times per day that John both communicates positively without prompting and with prompting. From the beginning, the total number of positive communications should be very large (perhaps requiring considerable prompting). The percentage of unprompted positive communications should rise over time. This increase is the primary measure of success. With an increase in unprompted positive communications will come an inevitable decrease in negative communications (challenging behaviors). It is important for the documentation system to focus on positive communication alternatives as the primary target behaviors and not just on negative behaviors.

- *Progression over time:* Initially, John should be rewarded quite consistently for his positive communication alternatives to challenging behavior. As such alternatives become a more stable part of his communication repertoire and as the frequency of negative communication behaviors decreases, demands on John's compliance can gradually increase again, and less time can be devoted to teaching communication. As with all aspects of the program, this progression must be coordinated well among staff and between staff and family.

Important Conditions Required for This Intervention to Work.

- Staff and family must agree to the principles and practices of this intervention. All staff and family members are teachers of positive communication alternatives. The most important teachers are those who spend the most time with John (his family members and direct-care staff) and, therefore, interact with him more than others do.
- Staff must avoid the temptation to engage John in tests of will. Conflicts should be kept to a minimum. In situations of conflict, John will likely resort to the negative behaviors that he knows have been successful in the past. At least some of these behaviors will likely be rewarded by staff, however good their intentions.

Dealing with Purely Impulsive Behavior

Reportedly, some of John's challenging behavior is purely impulsive, without communicative intent. For example, when unoccupied, on impulse John may touch nearby women inappropriately, with no intent to communicate. The frequency of impulsive negative behaviors must also decrease, because behaviors that begin as purely impulsive can easily become learned components of John's communication system. The two most important procedures in dealing with impulsive behavior are prevention and redirection.

Prevention

To prevent purely impulsive behavior, try to eliminate provocation. For example, women who are not working with John should avoid walking within arm's length of him. Also, try to ensure that John is engaged in meaningful activities as much as possible.

Redirection

When John is beginning to engage in negative impulsive behavior, staff and family members may direct his attention quickly to a neutral activity that breaks the negative behavior pattern. However, redirection must be effected with great caution. If redirection is from a less desired

activity to a more desired activity, negative behavior inadvertently may be rewarded, thereby increasing rather than decreasing the negative behavior.

Reacting to Seriously Challenging Behavior

See the behavior specialist's recommended procedures for reacting to negative behaviors and crises on those occasions when preparation, prevention, and redirection have not worked. These procedures must be followed to ensure that everyone remains safe and that John's negative behavior is not reinforced systematically. However, staff and family members must clearly understand that times of crisis are *not* occasions for teaching. Do not try to teach lessons when either John or you are upset. Teaching positive communication alternatives should occur under conditions of low stress.

Interaction Routines for Teaching Positive Communication Alternatives

Guidelines for Interaction

Successful interaction requires guidelines that include careful attention to (1) the general teaching routine, (2) escape and access communication training, and (3) agreement on and indications for situations in which escape and access are acceptable (both in *natural* communication contexts or *contrived* situations).

1. Carefully observe John and interpret his behavior. Identify times at which he is likely to use challenging behavior to communicate escape or access. Ideally, such times occur when escape- or access-motivated behavior is expected but *has not yet begun*. A second-best alternative is to identify the *first sign* of escape- or access-motivated behavior.
2. *Do not wait until John is using challenging behavior.*
3. Prompt the positive communication alternative (e.g., model, shape hands, point hand-over-hand to symbol).
4. Reward the positive communication alternative with escape or access as appropriate.
5. Make it clear that the reward is for the communication alternative. For example, "Thanks for telling me you don't want to do exercises now. We can come back to it later. Let's take a break."
   a. Act before the challenging behavior occurs. *Timing is critical.*
   b. Never reward the challenging behavior.
6. Fade prompts and practice.

Illustrations

Escape: Contrived Communication Situations. Context: In physical therapy sessions, assume that the exercises are not currently a high priority for staff and not a desired activity for John.

Adult (A): John, how about some exercises?

John (J): *(Looks unhappy but hasn't acted yet.)*

A: It looks like you don't want to do this now. Here, show me "finished."

J: *(Is prompted to use positive communication alternative [PCA].)*

A: OK! Thanks for telling me! Let's not do it now. We can come back to it later. It's great that you tell me that way that you don't want to do this. Let's do . . . *(or,* Show me what you would like to do for a few minutes . . .*).*

This teaching sequence could be repeated several times during a 20- to 30-minute scheduled exercise session.

Escape: Natural Communication Situations

Context: A staff person wants John to carry his lunchbox as he walks down the hall.

A: Here, John, carry your lunchbox.

J: *(Reacts negatively but does not fall to the floor or engage in any other negative communication [NC].)*

A: I bet you don't want to carry the box, do you? Why don't you tell me "no"?

J: *(Is prompted to use PCA.)*

A: Oh!!! Alright! I see you want me to carry it. Thanks for telling me so nicely. Of course I'll carry it when you ask like that.

Access: Contrived Communication Situation

Context: John is with other clients and clearly wants a peer to interact with him. The peer has been alerted to respond when John uses the PCA.

A: John, I bet you would like to talk with Tim. Why don't you tell him? *(Prompts the PCA.)*

J: *(Uses the PCA.)*

Peer: *(Responds to John's PCA.)* Oh, hi, John. I didn't see you. Thanks for letting me know you want to talk.

Access: Natural Communication Situations

Context: John is at home, and it is time for him to do something he likes to do (e.g., watch television).

A: John, I wonder what you want to do. I bet you would like to watch TV. Can you let me know? *(Prompts the PCA.)*

J: *(Uses the PCA.)*

A: *(Responds to John's PCA.)* Okay, great. Here's the remote. Thanks for telling me that you wanted to watch TV.

Chapter 14

Rehabilitation After Traumatic Brain Injury in Preschoolers

Mark Ylvisaker, Carole Wedel Sellars, and Larry Edelman

In this chapter, we highlight selected issues in outcome and intervention for preschoolers with traumatic brain injury (TBI). We have chosen to emphasize cognitive, psychosocial, and family-related themes because they are common areas of concern in this age group, are easily neglected or misinterpreted, are extremely important, and may be inadequately addressed in traditional rehabilitation programs. Fortunately, reinventing the wheel is unnecessary for young children with this diagnosis. For at least three decades, there has been growing interest in early intervention programs for infants and preschoolers with developmental disabilities and for those at risk for academic and social failure as a result of environmental factors. Increasingly these intervention programs have emphasized a family-centered approach, which is equally important in rehabilitation after TBI. The early-childhood and special education literature is a rich source of programmatic ideas and summaries of research into what does and does not work (Dunst et al., 1988; Hanft, 1989; Shelton et al., 1987). Recognizing TBI as a disability category does not require that rehabilitation and educational programs be designed specifically for this group. Indeed, the enormous diversity within the population of preschoolers with TBI would render such an enterprise an exercise in frustration.

This chapter is intended for all rehabilitation, early-childhood, and special education professionals who work with preschoolers with TBI. The themes that we address cut across professional boundaries and call for a collaborative approach to intervention. A major premise of the chapter is that professionals must create collaborative partnerships with family members and other people who function daily in the child's life (so-called everyday people), so that everyday routines and everyday interactions become the context of rehabilitation and ongoing development. Such collaboration is contrasted with short-term or infrequent therapeutic interactions between the child and professionals who are not integral components of the child's life over the long term.

Outcome After TBI in Infants, Toddlers, and Preschoolers

Outcomes after TBI are difficult to predict in children of any age. Some with apparently severe injuries and many with mild injuries enjoy an excellent outcome, whereas others with severe injuries and some with apparently insignificant injuries have long-term disability with lifelong implications. Much of the literature on outcome was reviewed by Ewing-Cobbs and colleagues in Chapter 2. Among the important themes that have emerged from these studies and from increasing clinical experience with this population are the following:

- Contrary to the traditional plasticity hypothesis (Finger, 1991; Kennard and Fulton, 1942), youth is not necessarily an advantage in outcome after TBI. Indeed, many investigators have found infants and toddlers to be particularly vulnerable to the effects of TBI (Lange-Cosack et al., 1979; Mahoney et al., 1983; Raimondi and Hirschauer, 1984). Others have found that outcome in groups of older preschoolers and young grade schoolers is, at best, no better than in comparably injured older children and adults, and is often worse (Brink et al., 1970; Chadwick et al., 1981; Ewing-Cobbs et al., 1987, 1989; Klonoff et al., 1977; Levin et al., 1993). One possible contributor to severe disability after TBI in infants and toddlers is the high frequency of abuse as a cause of these injuries.
- Prefrontal injury, very common in closed head injury, appears to be a particularly strong indicator of negative outcome in young children (Kolb, 1995; Levin et al., 1993; Marlowe, 1992). Injury to the prefrontal brain is compatible with good physical recovery but ongoing difficulties in social, behavioral, and cognitive development.
- Consequences of TBI in young children often worsen over the years after the injury as they "grow

into" their disability (Eslinger et al., 1992; Feeney and Ylvisaker, 1995; Grattan and Eslinger, 1991, 1992; Marlowe, 1992; Mateer and Williams, 1991; Price et al., 1990; Williams and Mateer, 1992; Ylvisaker and Feeney, in press). This is true particularly of consequences related to executive control functions and associated behavioral issues, because prefrontal parts of the brain that support development of executive self-regulation normally mature slowly (Yaklovev and Lecours, 1967). For this reason, a preschooler with damage to the prefrontal brain might be no more impulsive, egocentric, inflexible, concrete in thinking, dependent on others, or disorganized than neurologically intact peers. However, if prefrontal maturation does not take place, these characteristics create substantial disability later in childhood and adult life. In addition, consequences of injury to parts of the brain associated with new learning (versus recovery of knowledge and skill acquired before the injury) may not become apparent for months or years but are more debilitating for young children than for adolescents and adults because of these children's limited preinjury knowledge and skill.

• Lack of understanding of the child's cognitive and behavioral needs, overprotection on the part of parents and other adults, an absence of supported experiences with peers in settings that are as normal as possible, and help that is so intense and pervasive as to create learned helplessness are all avoidable contributors to negative outcomes.

A profound obstacle to measuring outcome in individual cases is the considerable variability in the development of preschoolers, particularly with respect to executive, self-regulatory functions. This variability has both biological and environmental roots. Professionals who work with preschoolers with TBI must have a thorough grounding in normal development, including the extent of normal variability, so that they are at the same time sensitive to possible consequences of the injury and aware of the temptation to overinterpret mildly discrepant behavior.

Only one study has attempted to trace the long-term outcome (into adulthood) of children injured as preschoolers (Koskiniemi et al., 1995). Of 55 children who met entrance criteria (age 1–7 years at injury *and* unconscious for more than 24 hours *or* shorter-term unconsciousness combined with focal neurologic deficit, penetrating injury, or elevated intracranial pressure), 39 were located as adults and agreed to participate. The worst outcome was in the younger group. Furthermore, the investigators asserted that adult outcome was clearly worse than was expected on the basis of initial recovery and early school achievement. Perhaps the most pessimistic finding was that none of the children injured before age 4 was able to work full-time as an adult, in contrast to 29% of those injured between ages 4 and 7 who were employed full-time. Computed tomographic scanning results and electroencephalographic findings were ineffective predictors of functional outcome, and duration of coma and functional outcome were only roughly correlated. Interestingly, the individual's sense of identity was found to be the best indicator of functional adult outcome (Koskiniemi et al., 1995), a finding that highlights the importance of the cognitive, psychosocial, and familial themes emphasized in this chapter.

Cognitive Aspects of Rehabilitation

Frequently Occurring Cognitive Deficits

As we use the term, *cognition* includes the mental processes (e.g., attention, perception, memory and learning, organization, reasoning) and systems (e.g., working memory, the executive system, the knowledge base, and the response system) necessary for the efficient acquisition and use of knowledge. Using this framework, Ylvisaker and Szekeres (Chapter 9) outlined common cognitive deficits during three broad phases of recovery after TBI in children. Although virtually any combination of cognitive strengths and weaknesses is possible after TBI, some common threads are related to severity and location of injury.

Early in recovery, as children emerge from coma, all cognitive processes and systems generally are severely and pervasively disrupted. This disruption begins as minimal intellectual interaction with the world and evolves into a state of alertness combined with gradually decreasing confusion, disorientation and, possibly, hyperreactivity. The nature and severity of residual cognitive deficits are related to the location and severity of an individual's injury. Common cognitive problems in children with TBI are related to common sites of injury. Prefrontal injury predictably results in weak regulation of cognitive processes, especially under novel or stressful circumstances. For example, attention may be poorly regulated (short attention span, distractibility); perception may be disorganized; learning may be inefficient and nonstrategic; the child may have difficulty planning, organizing (e.g., organizing discourse), solving problems, and initiating cognitive behavior; and behavior might be perseverative (difficulty with inhibition) and rigid (difficulty with flexible shifts of cognitive set).

Anterior and medial temporal lobe damage can result in inefficiencies of memory and new learning and in difficulties with emotional control that can negatively affect both internal cognitive behavior and social behavior. Prefrontal injury and widespread diffuse axonal injury can result in slow information processing in all sensory modalities. In addition to these sites of frequent injury associated with common threads in cognitive outcome, specific sites of a child's brain injury might create specific difficulties with language processing, visual perception, academic skills, or any other aspect of cognition.

Important Themes in Cognitive Assessment

In Chapter 10, Ylvisaker and Gioia discuss issues in cognitive assessment and argue for an approach that highlights ongoing, collaborative, contextualized hypothesis testing. Much of the material in that chapter is relevant to the assessment of preschoolers. In this chapter, we simply outline critical features of cognitive assessment particularly important for this age group.

Serial Assessment and Long-Term Follow-Up

After very severe injuries, children may experience uneven neurologic improvement for many months or years. However, young children with moderate to severe TBI may also experience delayed developmental consequences of their injuries (Eslinger et al., 1992; Grattan and Eslinger, 1991, 1992; Mateer and Williams, 1991; Price et al., 1990; Williams and Mateer, 1992; Ylvisaker and Feeney, in press). In some cases, this is also true of apparently mild injuries (Marlowe, 1992). Disability that increases over time is more commonly observed in cognitive and psychosocial development than in physical development. Both of these developmental trajectories (neurologic improvement and delayed developmental consequences) argue for periodic reassessment of preschoolers with TBI and caution in predicting long-term outcome and possible need for services. Indeed, confident predictions about long-term outcome and ongoing development may be impossible until years after the injury.

Contextualized Assessment

In typically developing young children, performance on tasks associated with cognitive and communicative functions tends to depend heavily on context. It is a common lament of parents, for example, that their children do not do in the doctor's office what they do with minimal effort at home. Similarly, the conversational ability of toddlers and preschoolers varies strikingly with different conversation partners and settings. After TBI, this normal contextual variation might be exacerbated by the variety and strangeness of the new contexts in which the child is expected to perform and by frontal lobe injury, which is associated with increased vulnerability in relation to environmental stressors. This context-dependent variability mandates that evaluators acquire valid information about the child's performance from a variety of contexts. Such information acquisition can be accomplished by some combination of observing the child in several contexts (including the use of videotaping); care-

fully organizing a collaborative cognitive assessment; and engaging parents, nursing staff, and others as partners in this assessment.

Assessment of Executive Functions

In Chapter 10, Ylvisaker and Gioia discuss executive system assessment at considerable length. Exploration of executive functions is especially important for children with closed head injury because of the vulnerability of prefrontal regions of the brain, which are associated with executive control functions. Little normative information regarding the development of executive functions in preschoolers, and few tests designed specifically to assess this area of development, are available. Indeed, development varies widely, depending on neurologic maturation and personality variation, family expectations, and preschool experience. Furthermore, some investigators of child development fail to recognize the emergence of executive functions until the child acquires deliberate, conscious control over cognitive behavior during the grade-school years. Perhaps for these reasons, in addition to the contextual variation described in the last paragraph, executive functions are rarely included as an explicit component of preschool assessment.

Given all these qualifications as background, one must carefully observe preschool children's recovery and ongoing development of executive functions, including the children's ability to detect the level of difficulty of tasks; to initiate activity and interaction; to inhibit competing responses and filter out distracting stimuli; to sustain attention to tasks; to organize materials, play, language, and activities of daily living; to pay attention to how well they perform a task; and to try alternative strategies when they fail to accomplish what they want to accomplish. Observations should be compared to developmental expectations and to each child's preinjury functioning as reported by parents or preschool teachers.

For very young children, piagetian tasks related to object permanence and means-ends relations can be interpreted from an executive system perspective (Willatts, 1990). Object permanence tasks (e.g., searching for an object after it has been hidden multiple times) yield information about a child's ability to inhibit impulsive responses (Goldman, 1971), whereas means-ends tasks (e.g., attempting to acquire objects that are out of reach, attempting to activate mechanical toys) provide clues to a child's ability to solve practical problems (i.e., to think and act strategically) (Willatts, 1990). Traditional cognitive developmental tasks have come to be included by some child neuropsychologists in executive system assessment of young children (Roberts and Pennington, 1996). In addition, observation of a child's social development (e.g., ability and willingness to share and appreciate another's perspective) provides clues to ongoing development of executive functions.

Assessment of New Learning

In addition to jeopardizing prefrontal parts of the brain associated with executive functions, closed head injury is associated with damage to medial temporal lobe structures (e.g., the hippocampus) that are involved in consolidating new memories (see Chapter 2). Many children and adults with severe closed head injury, particularly if such an injury is followed by hypoxic-ischemic damage involving medial temporal lobe structures, recover much of the knowledge and skill that they had acquired before the injury but have great difficulty acquiring new knowledge and academic skill. This finding explains, in part, the commonly observed phenomenon of a child's adequate performance on standardized tests a few weeks or months after such an injury (based on recovery of preinjury learning) but inadequate learning and academic performance in preschool and grade school during succeeding years. Therefore, it is critical to assess new learning in as realistic a manner as possible. For example, clinicians can interview parents to identify a unit of content (e.g., information about animals or other relevant preschool content) to which the child was not exposed before the injury. That unit can then be taught, with careful documentation of learning rate (e.g., number of learning trials to mastery) and retention over time. Learning style should also be assessed and documented: For example, is the child a passive or active learner? Does he or she ask questions? Does the child relate new information to old information? Does he or she prefer action-based learning?

Cognitive Intervention

Purposes of Intervention

Cognitive intervention for preschoolers with TBI has several possible purposes. First, engaging children in tasks that challenge without overwhelming their cognitive processes and systems serves the purpose of facilitating recovery and maximizing restoration of function. Second, because young children have just begun their long journey of acquiring knowledge and cognitive skill, cognitive specialists can contribute to long-term outcome by ensuring that everyday people (family members, teachers, and others) are as knowledgeable and skilled as possible in facilitating the child's ongoing acquisition of new knowledge and cognitive skill. To do this effectively, cognitive specialists must thoroughly understand the child's cognitive strengths and weaknesses as well as the most effective teaching approach. Third, cognitive specialists can begin the long process of helping children recognize their residual disability and use strategic procedures to be as successful as possible despite their ongoing cognitive limitations.

Finally, cognitive rehabilitation for preschoolers can be understood as serving a preventive purpose. If cognitive specialists can help everyday people create the supports the child needs to be successful (in school, at play, and in activities of daily living) in the presence of cognitive weakness, the likelihood of behavior problems (associated with failure and frustration) is thereby reduced. At the same time, if cognitive specialists can help everyday people reduce supports as the child acquires greater cognitive competence, the likelihood of long-term learned helplessness is reduced. These, then, are two critical goals for cognitive rehabilitation specialists: to ensure that the child has sufficient cognitive support to prevent failure, frustration, and associated behavior problems, and to ensure that the child is challenged, thereby preventing learned helplessness. Balancing these two goals requires ongoing collaborative reassessment of the child's needs and active communication among specialists, family members, and others.

Context of Intervention

Typically developing preschoolers have a number of cognitive characteristics that may be exacerbated by TBI. For example, they tend to be concrete learners who profit from learning tasks that have a concrete and personally meaningful goal; information or skills are presented as necessary to process in order to achieve the meaningful goal (e.g., learning color words by requesting paints to complete a finger painting). Preschoolers do not generally profit from instructions to "sit still, pay attention, and learn." Even if they were motivated by this instruction (which is most unlikely), young children would probably not be able to orient to the abstract cognitive goals of paying attention and learning and would not have access to cognitive strategies to achieve those abstract goals. For these reasons, it is critical to engage preschoolers in concrete and personally meaningful activities.

In addition, preschoolers acquire cognitive skills in part by internalizing social processes in their everyday interaction with adults or older children (Vygotsky, 1978). (This point is developed later in the discussion of organization.) This theme applies to acquisition of a wide variety of cognitive and social skills, therefore requiring careful attention to the style and content of interaction that everyday communication partners have with young children.

Finally, the most natural context for preschoolers' learning and cognitive growth is play. Therefore, rehabilitation professionals who are accustomed to serving older children and adults using structured and nonplayful therapeutic activities may need to learn how to support children's play, perhaps taking courses or, better still, serving a brief apprenticeship in a child-care program to put themselves in a position to serve preschoolers with TBI appropriately.

Organization and Memory

We have chosen to highlight organization and memory as cognitive domains frequently in need of clinical attention after TBI. Being able to organize one's thoughts and behavior and to remember experiences and lessons are skills that are obviously important for success in school and later in adult life. Unfortunately, these two cognitive domains are often affected by closed head injury because of the vulnerability of prefrontal areas (involved in organization and certain types of memory) and medial temporal areas (involved in explicit, declarative memory).

Because of the extreme importance of organizational knowledge and skill in the developing life of a young child with TBI, we provide several illustrations of how everyday, functional activities can be used to promote recovery and development in this area. The approach we offer is very different from that suggested in some cognitive rehabilitation and preschool curricular materials, in which various components of organization (e.g., categorizing, sequencing, associating) are targeted separately by using decontextualized drills: For example, "Tell me as many ____ as you can think of." "Which of these go together?" "Put these in order." We do not recommend these academic and, from the child's perspective, abstract activities. However, all the components of cognitive processing intended to be addressed by such activities are also addressed in the organizational activities that we recommend, but in a way that is functional, meaningful, appropriately concrete for a preschooler, and associated with everyday routines. Figure 14-1 includes a checklist that staff and family members can use to ensure that there is an appropriate focus on cognitive organization in the child's rehabilitation.

Connection Between Organization and Memory. In Chapter 9, Ylvisaker and Szekeres discuss the bewildering number of aspects of memory, varieties of memory processes or systems, and variables that influence memory. Cutting across all of these important considerations, however, are some simple yet powerful themes that are critical for rehabilitation after TBI. One such theme is that information is more easily remembered if it is meaningfully organized when presented: The better organized the information at the time of encoding, the easier storage and subsequent retrieval of that information is (assuming the organization in the information matches the organization in the head of the learner). Therefore, there is an intimate connection between organization and memory that can be exploited in rehabilitation.

Conversational Style and the Development of Memory and Organization.   Since the mid-1980s, students of child development have witnessed an exciting burst of interest in experimental research on normal development of thought organization and autobiographical memory in preschool children. From our perspective, the dominant theme that has emerged from these studies is support for Vygotsky's view that intrapersonal or covert cognitive processes (e.g., organizational schemas; memory processes) are transformed and internalized versions of interpersonal processes, largely social-interactive routines

involving children and their parents or other people with expertise that exceeds that of the child (Vygotsky, 1986). The role of parents or other adults in this process is to provide children with daily opportunities to rehearse their skills in the context of everyday routine interaction and to provide the scaffolding or support children need to be successful (Bruner, 1978).

In contrast to typical research paradigms in which unfamiliar investigators ask children to perform (e.g., report a past event, tell a story, indicate understanding of specialized vocabulary), early learning and use of cognitive and linguistic skills occur in the context of social-interactive routines with familiar people, typically parents. The upshot of a decade of research is that there are distinct parental styles in talking with children about past events and that these differences in style make a difference in the child's cognitive and verbal development. A helpful interactive style tends to be collaborative (i.e., "we are doing this together" versus "I am having you perform for me"), elaborative (e.g., more extension of topics, more exploration of how things and events in the world go together), and fun (e.g., "we are having a good time talking" versus "I want you to work for me"). This style is similar to what Reese and colleagues called a *high elaborative style* (Reese et al., 1993) and to what Nelson (1973) called a *positive cognitive style of conversation.* In contrast, an unhelpful interactive style in talking about the past is directive, performance oriented, inquisitorial (involving a large number of questions presented as tests), and fragmented (i.e., less elaboration of topics, less help with organizational structure). This style is similar to what Fivush and colleagues referred to as a *low elaborative* or *repetitive style* (Fivush and Fromhoff, 1988; Reese et al., 1993) and to what Nelson (1973) called a *negative social style.*

Young children's ability to organize their thoughts, organize language into coherent narratives, and remember events from their own experience develops in ways that are at least closely correlated with, and probably causally related to, the conversational style of their parents. Mothers with a helpful collaborative and elaborative style have preschool children (ages 3–6) who remember more in their preschool years than do children of nonelaborative mothers (Reese et al., 1993; Reese and Fivush, 1993). Furthermore, these highly elaborative mothers have children who remember more 1 year after an event (McCabe and Peterson, 1991) and even 2½ years later than do children of nonelaborative mothers (Reese et al., 1993). This finding has led some investigators to the cautious conclusion that an elaborative style facilitates the development of memory and cognitive organization (Reese et al., 1993).

Finally, mothers who provide frequent orienting and evaluative statements in coconstructed narratives have children who, 1 year later, similarly provide relatively frequent orienting and evaluative statements in their independent

❏ Are *everyday people* in the child's life (e.g., family members, nurses, teachers, aides, baby-sitters) *thoroughly oriented* to (1) the child's organizational strengths and weaknesses, (2) the importance of engaging the child in organizational activities at his or her level, and (3) procedures for presenting activities (e.g., activities of daily living, play, art, chores, language) in a way that highlights their organizational components?

❏ Are *everyday activities* in the child's life (e.g., play, activities of daily living, chores, conversations about meaningful topics) used as the basis for gradually increasing his or her ability to organize thought, language, and behavior?

❏ Are the child's *life experiences adequately organized?*

  ❏ Is there thematic or other organization *within* therapy and instructional sessions? Is the organization of each session obvious to the child?

  ❏ Is there thematic or other organization *across* therapy and instructional sessions? For example, are the activities in speech therapy or occupational therapy related in a clear way to activities in preschool class?

  ❏ Is there thematic or other organization *from day to day*? Is the child involved in activities or projects that require integrating information over several days or weeks?

  ❏ Is the child's life organized around *consistent routines*? Does the child understand the routines?

❏ Is the *content* that is used for organizational tasks personally meaningful and engaging? Are *concrete and personally meaningful* routines and tasks used as the basis for organizational intervention before more abstract tasks (e.g., categorizing, associating, or sequencing items that are not personally relevant) are used?

❏ Are organizational tasks presented as *involuntary (incidental) learning tasks*? That is, is there a concrete, meaningful goal or product that the child wishes to accomplish and that requires organizational thinking and acting?

❏ Is an appropriate amount of *external organizational support* available for children who have difficulty organizing?

  ❏ Do adults model the organizational activity?

  ❏ Are advance graphic organizers available for complex tasks? That is, is the task mapped out in a way that makes it easy to follow (e.g., a sequence of photographs or drawings to help a child move through a project or routine)?

  ❏ Is a day planner or memory book available that contains pictured schedules, simple maps, photographs of critical people, and other important information that the child needs to stay organized?

  ❏ Are plans and schedules illustrated in appropriately concrete ways (e.g., with photographs)?

  ❏ If organizational reminders must be provided by other people, are they presented in a way that is not perceived as nagging?

❏ Is there *consistency* among staff and family members in how tasks and information are presented and in the kinds of external organizational support that are provided? Is there consistency in *reducing external organizational support* as the child becomes increasingly organized?

❏ Is the child as engaged as possible in the *executive aspects* of organizational activities?

  ❏ Does the child help to determine the *goal* of the activity? (For example, "Let's make a truck out of Legos.")

  ❏ Does the child help to create a *plan* to achieve the goal? (For example, first let's get a picture of a truck to look at; then let's get the pieces we need; then let's put them together.)

  ❏ Does the child help to *monitor* performance during the activity? (For example, "We're doing a good job; it looks like the picture.")

  ❏ Does the child help to *evaluate* success of the activity? (For example, "We're done. We used all the pieces and it looks like a truck.")

  ❏ Does the child help to *determine what did and did not work* in the plan? (For example, "It helped to have a picture to look at; having so many pieces made it hard.")

Figure 14-1. Intervention for preschoolers with organizational impairment: a checklist.

narratives. Parental influence appears to function similarly in children's development of fictional narratives through conversations with parents (Snow and Goldfield, 1981). APPLICATION OF CONVERSATIONAL STYLE PRINCIPLES TO TBI REHABILITATION.   Although the rehabilitation application of these principles of conversational style has not been validated experimentally, the developmental literature is sufficiently persuasive to yield valuable recommendations that contrast sharply with common practices in pediatric rehabilitation programs and special education classrooms. In interacting with children with disability, rehabilitation professionals display an understandable but unfortunate tendency to depart from natural teaching interactions and to assume a directive and pedagogical posture while engaging children in activities that may have nothing to do with their interests or their lives. This is certainly true of most cognitive rehabilitation exercises found in workbooks or other therapy manuals.

In contrast, we recommend that rehabilitation professionals work collaboratively with parents, nursing staff, teachers, aides, and others so that all conversations with the child about the past, however simple, can be transformed—through effective use of scaffolding procedures—into events that facilitate cognitive and social recovery. Table 14-1 presents conversational procedures that should be taught (if necessary) to everyday communication partners of young children with cognitive impairment after TBI. Because of a youngster's cognitive impairment, the use of these procedures may need to be intensified (relative to normal positive parental styles of communicating) and supplemented with concrete support, including photographs of people, places, and things that are part of any narrative that is being constructed.

Because it is easier for parents and others to be elaborative when they know about the events that a child is trying to recall and describe, programs serving children with cognitive weakness must have in place effective log- or memory-book systems. These books, which can be personalized so that they are attractive to the child, should include pictures of family members, relevant staff, and others; schedules and routines; and logs of all events that would be useful for parents or nurses to talk about with the child. From an organizational perspective, perhaps the most useful therapy materials to have in great abundance are photographs of the child engaged in familiar daily routines and in memorable singular events. These photographs can serve as support for elaborated, socially coconstructed narratives about past events, an activity that is meaningful, fun, and facilitative of improved organization and memory.

Many advantages are associated with this approach to memory and organization. First, it assigns the most critical role in rehabilitation to everyday people (parents, siblings, nurses, teachers, aides, etc.). It also dramatically increases the number of therapeutic learning opportunities available to a child. Furthermore, increasing the effectiveness of the interaction that everyday people have with the child contributes to cognitive rehabilitation while facilitating social and behavioral adjustment.

In contrast, when they are not oriented to the value of a collaborative interactive style, everyday people often resort to a directive, interrogational, and pedagogical style that results in a large degree of failure and frustration for the child. If parents, for example, believe it is their job to quiz their child about his or her day in rehabilitation (on the assumption that they are exercising the child's memory), their questions will likely create anxiety in the child and will be answered correctly only a small percentage

of the time (if answered at all). This translates into marked failure for the child and increases the likelihood of negative behavioral reactions to failure. Shifting from an interrogational to a collaborative style of interaction can easily reduce the rate of failure from very high to almost nonexistent while simultaneously increasing the child's ability to organize information and search his or her memory. Long-term outcomes of this emphasis on narrative organization may include a lessening of the child's language impairment (Evans, 1987) and diminished difficulties in school (Roth, 1986), including difficulty learning to read (Paul and Smith, 1993).

MILESTONES OF NARRATIVE DEVELOPMENT. The developmental literature that presents milestones for narrative development in preschool children is not very helpful in setting appropriate expectations for the type of collaborative narration promoted in the previous section. Developmental milestones are typically based on observation of children's independent performances when asked to describe an event or tell a story (Peterson and McCabe, 1983). For example, McCabe and Rollins (1994) outlined a developmental progression during the preschool years that included: "miscellaneous" narratives at age 2 (i.e., bits of information presented in no obvious order but representing some real event); "leap-frog" narratives (i.e., several meaningful events in some semblance of order but omitting important components and deviating from actual order) and "chronologic" narratives (i.e., several meaningful events in correct order) by age 4; and "end-at-highpoint" narratives (i.e., many components of a story but with no resolution) and, finally, "classic" narratives (i.e., stories with characters, setting, initiating event, character's response, plan, action, and resolution) by age 6. These milestones in independent narration can serve as legitimate goals for children but should not cause adults to depart from the social and collaborative narrating activities that help children achieve cognitive and linguistic milestones.

A developmental literature also exists that addresses children's independent performances in understanding metacognitive vocabulary associated with organizing and remembering (e.g., words such as *organize, remember, memory, think, first-next-last, when, why, because*). However, as with independent narrating, this literature is based largely on children's fully developed and independent understanding of these abstract terms. Such understanding develops gradually, in part through conversations with adults who use these important words often and expect children to make some sense out of them long before full comprehension is established. Adults are well advised to use this vocabulary in their collaborative narratives with preschoolers as part of the process of teaching metacognitive understanding.

Organization and Play. In normal development, infants and young children follow a predictable sequence in their play with objects (Piaget, 1974). Newborns show little

Table 14-1. A Positive Collaborative and Elaborative Style of Interaction for Use in Parent-Child Socially Co-Constructed Narratives About Past Experiences

The goal of these interactions is to facilitate development of autobiographical memory, thought organization, and language organization through conversational, collaborative construction of narratives about shared experiences.

Collaboration procedures
Implicit message: "We are doing this together as a cooperative project."

Collaborative style	Noncollaborative style
Collaborative intent	*Teaching or testing intent*
1. Partner shares information; does not just demand it.	1. Partner mainly demands information.
2. Partner uses collaborative talk. (For example, "Let's try to remember the day we . . ."; "I enjoy thinking about these things with you.")	2. Partner talks as would a teacher or trainer.
	3. Partner fails to confirm partner's contributions.
3. Partner confirms partner's contributions. (For example, "That's right, that was next.")	
Cognitive support	*Lack of cognitive support*
1. Partner gives information when needed (within either statements or questions).	1. Partner does not give information when it is needed; continues quiz.
2. Partner makes available memory and organization supports (e.g., photos, memory book, gestures).	2. No resources are available.
3. Partner gives cues in a conversational manner.	3. Partner fails to give necessary cues.
4. Partner responds to errors by giving correct information in a nonthreatening, nonpunitive manner.	4. Partner corrects errors in a punishing manner.
Emotional support	*Lack of emotional support*
1. Partner respects other's concerns.	1. Partner fails to communicate respect.
2. Partner explicitly acknowledges difficulty of the task. (For example, "It's hard to put all these things in order, isn't it?")	2. Partner does not acknowledge difficulty of a given task.
Questions: positive style	*Questions: negative style*
1. When questions are used, they are used in a nondemanding and supportive manner.	1. A high percentage of questions used are nonsupportive and demanding. Questioning is performance oriented (i.e., testing).
2. Partner uses specific questions that include cues, if necessary. (For example, "Did we go swimming next?" vs. "What did we do next?")	2. Questions are insufficiently specific and do not include needed cues.

Elaboration procedures
Implicit message: "I am going to help you organize and extend your thoughts."

Elaborative style	Nonelaborative style
Topics	*Topics*
1. Partner introduces topics of interest, with potential for elaboration.	1. Partner introduces topics of marginal interest, with little potential for elaboration.
2. Partner maintains topic for many turns (e.g., repeats partner; affirms partner's contribution; adds information; asks open questions; reviews topic; expresses interest; if necessary, corrects partner in a nonthreatening manner).	2. Topic is changed frequently.
	3. Partner adds little information.
3. Partner contributes many pieces of information per topic.	4. Partner offers few open invitations to add information.
4. Partner invites elaboration (e.g., "I wonder what happened . . .").	
Organization	*Organization*
1. Partner tries to organize information as clearly as possible:	1. Partner fails to organize information conversationally.
a. sequential order of events (e.g., "First, we . . . , then we . . .")	2. Partner fails to review organization of information.
b. physical causality (e.g., "It broke because you dropped it.")	3. Partner fails to make connections explicit when topics change.
c. psychological causality (e.g., "You ran because you were scared.")	

    d. similarity and difference (e.g., "Yes, they are similar
       because . . .").
    e. analogy and association (e.g., "That reminds me
       of . . . , because . . .").
2. Partner reviews organization of information.
3. Partner makes connections when topics change.

Explanation
1. Partner adds explanations for events.
2. Partner addresses problems and solutions (e.g., "I
   wonder whether we can think of a better way to handle
   this if it comes up again.").

Explanation
1. Partner offers few explanations.
2. Partner does little problem solving.

General procedures

Enjoyment
1. Partner shows enjoyment (e.g., laughs, expresses enjoyment directly, acts animated).
2. Partner talks about fun (e.g., "I really enjoy chatting
   about this.").
3. Partner is playful (e.g., jokes, teases, plays with words).

Language of thinking, remembering, and organizing
1. Partner uses language of memory (e.g., "Let's see how
   much we can remember." "I remember it one way and
   you remember it another.").
2. Partner uses language of thinking and organizing (e.g.,
   "Let's organize these somehow—how do these go
   together?" "I think this was first and that second."
   "You did a great job of thinking of solutions.").

Work
1. Interaction seems more like a quiz than a socially
   enjoyable activity.
2. Partner talks about work.
3. Partner is not playful.

Language of thinking, remembering, and organizing
1. Partner uses little metacognitive language.

---

interest in objects but, by a few months of age, become active in exploring their sensory features. Sensorimotor exploration, which dominates the first year of life, includes actions such as holding objects, mouthing them, patting, dropping, turning, banging, throwing, and the like. By 1 year of age, most children have begun to use at least some objects playfully according to their conventional purpose (e.g., rolling a ball, scribbling with a crayon, stirring in a cup with a spoon). At between 12 and 24 months, most children come to use most household objects functionally, begin to organize objects in representational play (e.g., feed a baby doll with a bottle; put a baby doll to bed and cover it with a blanket; put logs in a toy truck and a driver in the driver's seat and drive off), and begin to use objects symbolically (e.g., pretend that a pot is a hat or that a pencil is a comb). During the preschool years, children also progress systematically in their social play, from little interest in peers to side-by-side play, to cooperative play with peers (using shared objects to achieve shared goals), to sociodramatic play (e.g., "I'll be the daddy and you be the mommy.") and games with defined rules (e.g., Candyland).

After severe TBI, preschoolers often repeat these developmental progressions, in part because normal development reveals a natural progression from less to more complex cognitive activity. This systematic increase in cognitive demands makes normal developmental progressions in play a useful scale by which to measure cognitive

improvement after TBI. From an intervention perspective, play is an ideal learning context for children. Helping children to become better organized in their play with objects can take the form of systematically prompting (as a play partner) developmentally higher levels of play. For example, staff and parents can help the child to progress from exploring the sensory features of a baby doll to holding it, to feeding it with a toy bottle, to bathing and dressing it, to organizing a tea party with dolls. Similarly, play with trucks can progress from sensorimotor exploration to running the truck on a surface, to putting people and things in the truck before pretending to drive it on the road, to using the truck in the context of a complex of props. Interaction during organized representational play with objects should highlight its organizational elements: For example, "The driver goes in the driver's seat and the logs in the back. We could also put these blocks in the back. What else do you think we could haul in our truck? What kind of truck would we need to haul milk?" For children with physical impairment, intervention may require that staff, family members, or older children help the child with hand-over-hand manipulation of objects while the child is enjoying play at the upper end of his or her ability to organize.

Organization and Activities of Daily Living. Both while they are hospitalized and later at home, children with organizational impairment should have well-organized daily routines, including morning routines around dressing and hygiene and evening routines around bath time, storybooks, and a review of the day, depending on family routines and values. All routine activities can become therapeutic from an organizational perspective as adults encourage and systematically expect increasingly independent organizing from the child. For example, for a very disorganized child, participation in dressing may consist of no more than selecting the socks before the shoes. Gradually, the child may be increasingly able to select more of the necessary clothes and put them on in reasonable sequence, with whatever support is needed. Finally, he or she may be able to make selections based on the day's activity, the weather, and other relevant information.

At each stage, parents or nursing staff can up the ante gradually by encouraging somewhat better-organized planning and dressing. If children become stuck at a relatively low level of organizational functioning, external organizers can be tried (e.g., sequenced photographs of the various items of clothing). Furthermore, the routines themselves can be photographed so that the child has a clear visual model of the sequence of activities that compose his or her routine.

Similarly, household chores (e.g., making the bed, putting toys away) can be components of organizational intervention in the hospital and at home. Both nursing staff and parents tend naturally to do these chores for the child, motivated by either an understandable sympathy for the child or a desire to complete the tasks quickly. However, sensitive consultation combined with situational coaching can teach most parents and staff members to appreciate the therapeutic usefulness of these natural activities and to become effective organizational coaches for the child. The use of daily chores in the child's therapeutic program should begin in the hospital so that parents can be shown their value and can be instructed in how to use such chores to facilitate organized thinking and acting.

Figure 14-2 is one example of a daily schedule that can be posted in a child's room and perhaps included in his or her log book. Photographs can be used instead of drawn pictures. As the child scans through his or her schedule, frequent review of the sequence of daily events is useful, as is having the child check off each event as it occurs. Alternatively, the child could place photographs or pictures on Velcro pegs and remove them when an activity is completed. The rationale behind any of these organizing tools is to provide support for disorganized children by representing in a simple and concrete external manner what the children have difficulty representing in their heads.

Cognitive Intervention: Executive Control Functions

The abilities and behaviors grouped within the general category of the executive system include functions that are critical to success in life, especially for a person with a disability. These include (1) knowing about what one can do well and what one has difficulty doing; (2) being able to set reasonable goals for oneself; (3) planning and organizing behavior around achieving those goals; (4) initiating behavior (including thinking) that relates to those goals; (5) inhibiting behavior (including thoughts) that interfere with achieving those goals; (6) monitoring and evaluating one's behavior (and thoughts) to ensure that one is doing well in relation to the goals; and (7) thinking strategically and doing something clever if achievement of the goal is difficult. It is useful to think of these functions as executive *control* functions because their purpose is to enable people to control their behavior, including cognitive behavior, rather than to allow behavior to be purely a function of environmental stimuli and one's history of learning.

These important functions develop gradually from infancy through adulthood. They are associated with the prefrontal parts of the brain, which develop gradually throughout childhood (Yakovlev and Lecours, 1967) and are the most vulnerable part of the brain in closed head injury (Levin et al., 1991). Development of executive functions is often impeded in children with disability, regardless of whether they have suffered frontal lobe injury, because these children may be given little coaching to develop the functions or, worse, professionals and parents block development in this area by assuming all responsibility for executive functions (Meichenbaum, 1993). Learned helplessness is the predictable result when children are not held responsible, in developmentally appropriate ways, for choosing, planning, self-monitoring, problem solving, and other aspects of executive functions.

Because of the importance of well-developed executive functions in the life of a person with a disability, these themes should be addressed as early as the preschool years. As with organization and memory, intervention should be a natural component of everyday activities, not a special type of therapy or a separate component of the curriculum. It is most important for specialists in cognitive development and intervention to work with the child's everyday communication partners so that they habitually inject this executive system focus into activities in a way that keeps up with the child's recovery and ongoing maturation. Figure 14-3 presents a checklist that can help in developing executive function interventions within everyday activities.

Why Executive Functions Are Often Neglected. Despite their increasing popularity in discussions of educational psychology, executive functions are often omitted as goal areas in preschool rehabilitation and special education programs, perhaps because of a misguided hierarchical orientation to cognitive development, within which executive functions are seen as higher-level functions and late developmental acquisitions. Within this

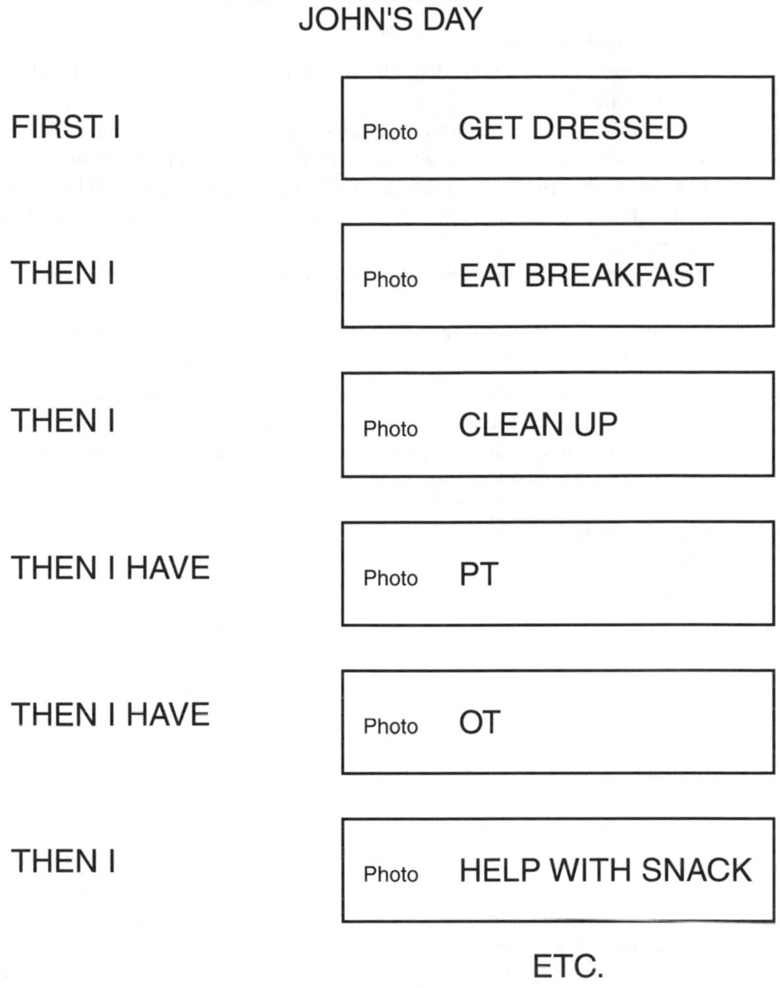

Figure 14-2. Example of a daily schedule that can be posted in the child's room and perhaps included in the log book.

JOHN'S DAY

FIRST I

| Photo | GET DRESSED |

THEN I

| Photo | EAT BREAKFAST |

THEN I

| Photo | CLEAN UP |

THEN I HAVE

| Photo | PT |

THEN I HAVE

| Photo | OT |

THEN I

| Photo | HELP WITH SNACK |

ETC.

framework, preschool cognitive targets are restricted to basic world knowledge (and the language associated with this knowledge) and basic cognitive processes (e.g., attention, perception, memory, and basic organization).

In contrast, recent interpretations of infant and preschool cognitive development suggest very early and gradual development of executive functions (Willatts, 1990), development that can be influenced by experience. For example, a number of neurobiological primate studies by Goldman-Rakic and Diamond (e.g., Diamond and Goldman-Rakic, 1989) suggest that some of the improvements in human cognitive behavior during the first 12 months of life (e.g., intelligent searches for objects) are a result of improved response inhibition, an aspect of executive control. Infants beyond 12 months of age have been shown not only to explore creative solutions to problems but also to store those solutions (Jarrett, 1988). Infants as young as 12 months have been shown to plan three-step solutions to object acquisition problems (Willatts, 1990). In summary, children as young as 1 year have been shown to think strategically in

solving problems, to be able to plan solutions, to remember previously successful solutions, and to inhibit responses that have been found to be unsuccessful.

By age 4–5, children may not yet have the language of executive functions, but they are quite competent at judging which physical tasks are easy or difficult for them and are active in seeking strategies to succeed in difficult physical tasks (e.g., walking on a balance beam). They even create strategies to succeed at some cognitive tasks (e.g., doing something special to remember the location of a prized object). To be sure, fully self-conscious and deliberate strategic behavior, particularly strategic behavior in relation to cognitive versus physical goals, is a much later developmental acquisition. However, there can be no doubt that development in this area begins early and is a legitimate target for preschool intervention programs.

Indeed, a focus on executive functions is a centerpiece of one of the most popular preschool curricula for children at risk for academic failure, the High/Scope Curriculum (Hoffmann and Weikart, 1995). In a High/Scope preschool

General considerations
❑ Is intervention in the areas that fall into the category of executive functions structured around the child's own *meaningful goals*?
❑ Is intervention infused into *everyday activities*? Are all *everyday people* oriented to ways that they can facilitate improved executive functions? Are all everyday people aware of the dangers of *learned helplessness*?
❑ Is successful performance in the areas of executive functions richly and naturally *rewarded*?
❑ Is the child given *ample opportunity* to identify and solve his or her own problems (with guidance if necessary)?
❑ Are executive function tasks structured around *concrete physical activities* (vs. *abstract or purely academic activities*)?
❑ Do everyday people in the environment routinely *model* expert use of executive functions?
❑ Is the child given sufficient *practice* so that strategic behavior becomes *automatic*?
❑ Are everyday people in the environment *supportive* of strategic or compensatory ways to accomplish tasks?
❑ Are everyday people in the child's environment fully *aware of possible limitations* in executive functions (especially initiation and inhibition) so that they do not misinterpret behavior (e.g., misinterpret lack of initiation as resistance or laziness)?

Appropriateness
Level of development
❑ Are preschoolers introduced to relevant vocabulary, including *difficult/easy to do*; *plan*; *do something special*; *review*; *what does/does not work*. Are they actively engaged in identifying what is difficult and easy for them (especially physical activities)? Are they actively engaged in identifying clever ways to accomplish difficult tasks? Are they richly and naturally rewarded for clever solutions to difficult everyday problems?
Level of recovery
❑ *Children who are minimally responsive:* Is the child prompted (physically, if necessary) to engage in familiar activities (e.g., activities of daily living) so that he or she is *acting*, not just being acted on? Has every attempt been made (e.g., remote switch control) to enable the child to *control* meaningful events? Do everyday people in the environment *respond* to the child as an agent?
❑ *Children who are alert but confused:* Is the child given *choices* whenever possible (short of increasing confusion)? Does the child have opportunities to experience *natural consequences* of choices?
❑ *People who are no longer seriously confused:* See entire checklist.
Self-awareness of strengths and needs
❑ Is the child maximally engaged in *identifying what is easy and difficult to do* and what makes activities easy or difficult?
❑ Is the child given opportunities to *compare performance* when an activity is completed in a usual way versus when it is completed with special strategic procedures?
❑ Is the child given appropriate informative *feedback* (e.g., peer feedback)?

Planning
❑ Is a *planning guide* available, if needed?
❑ Does the child begin the day by *preparing a plan* on a planning board or in a journal?
❑ Does the child begin each activity by preparing a simple plan?
❑ Do therapeutic activities include attempts to plan meaningful complex events (e.g., snack)?

Organizing: See Figure 14-1.

Self-Initiating
❑ Do everyday people give the child *opportunities to initiate* and wait an appropriate length of time? Are *signals* available to remind the child to initiate activities?
❑ Are all forms of institutional *learned helplessness* avoided?
❑ If initiation cues are necessary, are they provided as much as possible by peers or siblings versus staff or parents? Is nagging avoided?

Figure 14-3. Everyday intervention for preschoolers with executive system impairment: a checklist.

Self-inhibiting

☐ Do everyday people give the child *opportunities to inhibit* (e.g., distractions) that are realistic in their demands?

☐ If inhibition cues are necessary, are they as subtle as possible and provided as much as possible by peers versus staff? Is nagging avoided?

Self-monitoring and self-evaluating

☐ Do everyday people give the child *opportunities to self-monitor and evaluate* performance? If cues are necessary, are they subtle? Is nagging avoided?

☐ Is the child routinely asked to identify what works and what does not work for him or her?

Problem solving and strategic thinking

☐ Is the child maximally involved in *solving everyday problems* as they arise? Are *everyday people* thoroughly oriented to the importance of problem solving?

☐ Is the child maximally engaged in *selecting strategies* to overcome obstacles and achieve important goals?

☐ Is there an appropriate amount of *external support for strategic thinking*?

    ☐ Do everyday people in the environment *expect and cue strategic performance*?

    ☐ Do everyday people in the environment avoid *learned helplessness* (i.e., do they resist solving all of the child's problems)?

☐ Is there *consistency* among staff and family members in how problem-solving tasks are presented and in the kinds of external problem-solving support that are provided?

☐ Is there consistency in *reducing external support* as the child becomes increasingly independent in problem solving?

---

classroom, the day begins with children planning their main activity for the morning. They then engage in active problem solving during the activity and, finally, review what they did and issues that arose. For a 2 year old, planning may be no more than selecting a toy with which he or she will play and listening to the teacher comment on the great plan. However, older children progress in planning so that by age 5, many can select a project, say where they will work or play, identify what they need, and describe the steps they will go through to complete their chosen project for the day. Throughout the "plan-do-review" process, teachers and aides provide the children with the amount of support or scaffolding they need to be successful at these executive dimensions of activity. Furthermore, preschool staff members work intensively with parents to help them to understand their role in facilitating their child's cognitive and social development and, in particular, their child's self-regulation and strategic thinking.

The High/Scope Curriculum has been found to have remarkable long-term effects on the development of high-risk children, measured by appropriate real-world criteria. For example, significantly fewer status offenses and reports of property damage, significantly greater sports participation and appointments to school office, and significantly fewer reports from the children's families that the children were doing poorly were found among the High/Scope graduates, as compared at age 15 with graduates of direction instruction preschools (Schweinhart and Weikart, 1986). At age 27, the High/Scope graduates were compared with a control group who had no preschool intervention (Schweinhart and Weikart, 1993). Among the interesting findings were that significantly more of the High/Scope group had completed high school, more were earning more than $2,000 per month, more owned a home, fewer received welfare as adults, and fewer had been arrested five or more times.

Obviously, between ages 5 and 27, numerous changes occur in every person's life. However, the use of a control group suggests that the executive function focus early in life combined with intensive work with families may have powerful long-term consequences in the life of a child. Application of these findings to children with frank neurologic impairment must be undertaken with great caution. The experimental children in the High/Scope study were at risk for environmental reasons but (presumably) were neurologically intact. Nevertheless, the positive findings should motivate early-childhood professionals to implement a similar executive system focus, combined with intensive family education and support, for other children.

Our goal here is not necessarily to promote this curriculum. Indeed, significant modifications must be made in the High/Scope approach to make it applicable to children with serious organically based organizational and executive system weakness. These children may require smaller groups and more individual attention than neurologically intact children, more concrete support for executive behavior (including modeling, cueing, and visual maps), and recognition of their limitations related to lengthy verbal planning and reviewing. Our points are rather that, with appropriate support, executive functions can and should be a legitimate intervention target for preschoolers, that this intervention can occur in the context of everyday routines, and that parents should be collaborators with professionals in this intervention. Furthermore, children with disability ultimately need to have better-developed executive function skills than do normally developing children: Because children with disability have more obstacles to overcome in life, they must be better at knowing their strengths and weaknesses and at acting strategically than is true of people whose automatic behavior serves them adequately. Finally, children with TBI have a very special need for an executive system focus in their rehabilitation and special education due to the vulnerability of their frontal lobes.

A second explanation for the frequent neglect of executive functions in traditional rehabilitation for preschoolers is the unfortunate tendency in both rehabilitation programs and special education to focus exclusively on short-term goals and objectives. In deciding to target executive functions in preschoolers, family and staff members must assume a very long-term perspective. Consideration must be given to the kind of reflectiveness, self-knowledge, independence, self-control, and strategic skill one would like to see in the individual at age 18 or 21, when leaving school. With this as a guiding vision, family and staff members can patiently facilitate the small steps needed to arrive at the goal 15 or 18 years later. Without this perspective, adults sensitive to the need to focus on executive functions may become frustrated with the child or adopt developmentally inappropriate expectations.

Third, parents and professionals sometimes object to the expectation that a child in need of rehabilitation or special education must achieve a level of self-control and strategic behavior beyond what is expected of normally developing children. Sensitivity to the tragedy that the child with TBI has experienced and the extraordinary effort required of the child to accomplish everyday tasks would seem to justify simple acceptance of the child's dependence or impulsiveness or lack of strategic behavior. Clearly, there is nothing fair about what children with disabilities must do to be successful. Unfortunately, having a disability imposes the burden of needing to behave and think more strategically than do people who have no disability. For this reason, it is critical to begin focusing on these functions as early as possible.

Finally, parents, teachers, and therapists sometimes object that there is simply too much for the child with a disability to accomplish, and they are reluctant to add yet another component to the child's rehabilitation or special education program. Many children receive a variety of therapies that address physical needs; others that address basic cognitive, communicative, and academic needs; and yet others that address social and emotional needs. Some parents and staff argue that there is simply insufficient time and staff to add another curricular content area. However, this objection misses what is most important about executive system intervention. Executive system intervention should not be conceived as another therapy, analogous to physical therapy or speech-language therapy. Rather, all staff and family members can and should target executive functions in the course of all daily routines of and interactions with the children. For example, all therapists and teachers can and should help the children to understand how easy or difficult various tasks are for them, to plan how to accomplish the job, to pay attention to how well they are doing, and to think of clever ways to succeed if they are having a difficult time. In fact, most professionals and parents do attend to this type of stimulation. A rehabilitation or special education program with an appropriate executive system orientation simply organizes and intensifies this focus and keeps careful track of the children's progress.

Appropriate rehabilitation plans and individualized education plans for young children in the area of executive functions might include objectives such as those listed in Table 14-2. Figure 14-4 presents a rating scale that can be used to track progress in children in this area and to remind teachers and others of the areas that need to be integrated into the day's activities.

Using Everyday Activities to Facilitate Development of Executive Functions. Table 14-3 contains suggestions for organizing routine everyday activities for preschoolers so that there is a developmentally appropriate focus on the executive components of the activity. This can be part of group activities (e.g., snack time) or individual activities (e.g., any of the rehabilitation therapies). Children who are very immature may be able to tolerate little of this executive system focus. Certainly, this type of reflection should not become a burden. However, as a child recovers and matures, parents, therapists, and teachers can incrementally add more and more of these components to otherwise engaging daily activities. If a child does not achieve a level of recovery in the hospital at which executive system intervention is relevant, hospital staff must orient family members and community professionals to the importance of this focus and the procedures for adding a developmentally appropriate emphasis on executive functions to all activities.

An attractive visual map can be created that captures the critical components of executive functioning. This map might have at the top a box for the goal, below this four side-by-side boxes for the plan (materials, people, place, steps), below this a box for possible problems and solutions, and below this a box for reviewing the highlights. If such a map is too complicated for a child, it can be omitted. The objective is to create for the child a habit of being thoughtful about activities. Often a clear, visible map, along with daily practice, helps to imprint the desired thought process.

As with organization and memory (discussed earlier), the *vocabulary* of executive functions should be emphasized even before children can be expected truly to grasp the meaning of all terms. For example, adults can begin an activity by asking, "What is our goal?," and, once that has been

Table 14-2. Illustrations of Executive System Objectives for Preschoolers, to Be Used in Rehabilitation Plans or Individualized Education Plans

Self-awareness
1. Given a difficult task, John* will (verbally or nonverbally) indicate that it is difficult.
2. John will accurately identify, with words, tasks that are easy or difficult for him (first physical tasks, then cognitive or academic tasks).
3. John will explain why some tasks are easy or difficult for him.
4. John will request help when tasks are difficult.
5. John will offer help to others when he is more capable than is the other child.

Goal setting
1. John will predict accurately how effectively he will accomplish a task (e.g., pick up all the toys; stay on the balance beam; put all the puzzle pieces in place).

Planning
1. Given a routine (e.g., snack), John will indicate what items are needed (e.g., plates, cups, crackers, juice, napkins) and the order of the events.
2. Given a selection of five activities for a therapeutic or instructional session, John will select three, indicate their order, create a plan on paper (e.g., put photographs in order to represent the plan), and stick to the plan.
3. Given a task that he correctly identifies as difficult for him, John will suggest something special that he can do to accomplish the task.

Organizing
1. John will create a system for organizing personal items in his cubby.
2. To tell an organized story, John will place photographs in order and then narrate the sequence of events.
3. John will assemble all the materials he needs before beginning a project.

Self-initiating
1. When John does not know what to do, he will ask the teacher.
2. With no prompting from the teacher, assistant, or parent, John will begin his assigned tasks and initiate work on his plan.
3. John will initiate interaction with other children.

Self-monitoring and self-evaluating
1. John will state accurately whether he completed what he said he was going to complete.
2. John will indicate whether he did a good job (e.g., cleaning up after snack).
3. John will identify major mistakes in his work without assistance from the teacher.

Problem solving
1. When faced with obstacles to accomplishing an objective (e.g., can't reach the puzzle he wants), John will try at least three alternative solutions.
2. When faced with obstacles to accomplishing an objective, John will offer three suggestions for approaches he could try to overcome each obstacle and will argue for and against each approach.
3. John will offer one or more possible solutions to everyday problems as they arise over the course of the school day.

*The name *John* is selected arbitrarily to represent any preschooler in this context.

identified, can say, "Great, let's make a plan." Comments can be made throughout the process that help children to internalize executive system reflection over time: For example, "How can we organize this?" "Let's think about this." "That's a problem. What can we do?" "That looks like it's hard for you to do. I wonder what would make it easier?"

Psychosocial Aspects of Rehabilitation

Psychosocial Development During Infancy and Early Childhood

A critical developmental achievement of the preschool years is children's ability to coordinate their actions and intentions effectively with those of others. This social coor-

dination is intertwined with and dependent on cognitive development (in particular, the ability to assume another person's perspective), communication development (including the ability to express desires and intentions, to understand others' expression of desires and intentions, and verbally to negotiate solutions to social problems), and development of executive self-regulation (including the ability to inhibit antisocial actions, to initiate social activity, and to plan and organize behavior to achieve social goals).

Children's rates of social development are highly variable. They depend in part on the social experiences and cultural standards that inform the apprentice-child's everyday social routines (Richard and Light, 1986) and, in part, on neurologic maturation. Normal prefrontal lobe development is related to (1) the cognitive transformations that enable children to gradually escape the concreteness and

Child's name: _____ Child's age: _____

Child's hospital/school:_____ Special-ed classification: _____

Person completing this rating: _____

Relationship to the child: _____

How long have you worked with the child? _____

Instructions

In each of the following categories, circle the developmental level that, in your judgment, best fits the student's typical behavior. *Positive behaviors* and *negative behaviors* are listed under each category simply to focus your attention on the types of behaviors that are relevant to your consideration of that category.

Planning and organizing

age 1   age 2   age 3   age 4   age 5   age 6   age 7

Negative impact of behavior in this area on success in rehabilitation or preschool:

1   2   3   4   5   6   7

No negative impact   Major negative impact

Illustrations of problem behaviors in this area: _____

_____

_____

Positive behaviors: integrates several props in representational play; stores school materials and personal articles in an organized manner; formulates a plan before beginning a complex task; completes tasks before moving on; produces organized artwork, craft projects, and the like; speaks in an organized manner; produces well-organized descriptions or stories

Negative behaviors: stores materials in a disorganized way; if given no reminders, begins tasks without a plan or without the needed materials; produces disorganized arts and crafts projects; can express only single thoughts; engages in extended discourse that is disjointed or incoherent

Initiation

age 1   age 2   age 3   age 4   age 5   age 6   age 7

Negative impact of behavior in this area on success in rehabilitation or preschool:

1   2   3   4   5   6   7

No negative impact   Major negative impact

Illustrations of problem behaviors in this area: _____

_____

_____

Positive behaviors: starts tasks with no reminders or cues; when stuck or finished with a task, asks for help or, in some other way, proceeds; initiates interaction with peers and with adults

Negative behaviors: needs cues or reminders to start tasks; when stuck or finished with a task, stops and needs additional reminders to continue; waits for peers or adults to initiate interaction

Inhibition

age 1   age 2   age 3   age 4   age 5   age 6   age 7

Negative impact of behavior in this area on success in rehabilitation or preschool:

1   2   3   4   5   6   7

No negative impact   Major negative impact

Illustrations of problem behaviors in this area: _____

_____

_____

Positive behaviors: stops and thinks before acting; controls emotions; continues play or work in the presence of distractions; perseveres

Negative behaviors: acts impulsively; says or does things without thinking; has frequent tantrums; insults others without intending to; is easily distracted by things going on in the environment; repeats behaviors or actions, even when they are clearly inappropriate

Figure 14-4. Executive function rating scale. The primary purpose of this scale is to highlight for preschool staff the importance of executive function themes in preschool rehabilitation and special education and to facilitate tracking in this important area. The scale does not have psychometric properties necessary for use as a diagnostic tool. Even when used as an aid to program planning, the scale should be completed by more than one person.

Independence (include perseverance, task completion)

age 1   age 2   age 3   age 4   age 5   age 6   age 7

Negative impact of behavior in this area on success in rehabilitation or preschool:

1   2   3   4   5   6   7

No negative impact   Major negative impact

Illustrations of problem behaviors in this area: _____

_____

_____

Positive behaviors: completes work without much help or many cues; sticks to a task even when it is difficult; uses needed resources without much help or reminders; can work alone

Negative behaviors: needs reminders to begin and to continue to work; needs reminders and help to use resources; has difficulty working alone

Orientation to task and flexibility

age 1   age 2   age 3   age 4   age 5   age 6   age 7

Negative impact of behavior in this area on success in rehabilitation or preschool:

1   2   3   4   5   6   7

No negative impact   Major negative impact

Illustrations of problem behaviors in this area: _____

_____

_____

Positive behaviors: easily learns and adapts to new classroom and other routines; with minimal direction, understands how to complete a task; stays oriented to tasks over time; shifts easily from activity to activity and class to class or therapy to therapy

Negative behaviors: has difficulty adjusting to new situations; often does not know what to do; needs frequent reminders to stay on task; has difficulty shifting from class to class and activity to activity

Understanding of task difficulty

age 1   age 2   age 3   age 4   age 5   age 6   age 7

Negative impact of behavior in this area on success in rehabilitation or preschool:

1   2   3   4   5   6   7

No negative impact   Major negative impact

Illustrations of problem behaviors in this area: _____

_____

_____

Positive behaviors: correctly identifies (verbally or in some other way) some tasks as being easy and others as being difficult for him or her; can state what makes a task difficult; sets reasonable goals for concrete tasks; can list or describe own strengths and weaknesses (physical or other)

Negative behaviors: misidentifies difficult tasks easy or easy tasks as difficult; begins difficult tasks, expecting to succeed; cannot list or describe own strengths or weaknesses; sets unrealistic goals

Self-monitoring and self-evaluating

age 1   age 2   age 3   age 4   age 5   age 6   age 7

Negative impact of behavior in this area on success in rehabilitation or preschool:

1   2   3   4   5   6   7

No negative impact   Major negative impact

Illustrations of problem behaviors in this area: _____

_____

_____

Positive behaviors: notices major mistakes; accurately states whether a job has been completed and has been done well; can identify some things that worked and did not work to complete a task; notices the effects of behavior on others

Negative behaviors: does not check work or notice mistakes; inaccurately evaluates the quality of work (overly optimistic or overly pessimistic); having completing a task, cannot identify what worked and what did not work; fails to notice the effects of behavior on others

Strategic behavior

age 1   age 2   age 3   age 4   age 5   age 6   age 7

Negative impact of behavior in this area on success in rehabilitation or preschool:

1   2   3   4   5   6   7

No negative impact   Major negative impact

Illustrations of problem behaviors in this area: _____

_____

_____

Positive behaviors: when a task (physical, academic, communicative, cognitive, social) is difficult, tries a variety of approaches; suggests interesting solutions to practical problems and acts on those suggestions

Negative behaviors: when a task is difficult, either gives up or persists with an ineffective plan; rarely tries varied solutions to problems; rarely suggests meaningful solutions to practical problems; talks about strategic solutions but does not act on that talk

Figure 14-4. *Continued.*

Table 14-3. Executive Function Routine for Preschoolers

Goal
    Preschool children need a concrete goal for their activities. Therefore, activities can begin with identification of the goal of the activity: "Okay, what are we trying to do here?" "Today we are going to make a cake (*or* a wonderful story together about a mouse who lives in a house in a city, *or* a bean plant)." "Today we are going to have a great snack."

Plan
    Once the goal has been identified, a plan is needed: "Great! Now, to get this done we need a plan. Let's make our plan." The plan might include (1) materials, (2) sequence of steps, (3) locations, (4) people, (5) roles (who will do what), and (6) scripts. Ideally, the plan is somehow made visible. For cognitively immature preschoolers, the plan might be very simple (e.g., to choose a toy).

Prediction
    If possible and relevant, the children predict how well they will do: "How many will you get done?" "Will you finish?" "Will it be easy or difficult?"

Problem solving and strategic thinking
    Throughout the activity, opportunities are seized for engaging the children in practical problem solving.

    Planned problem-solving occasions: Snack is a great context for planned problem solving, but any activity will do. At snack, there can be one too few chairs or napkins or glasses or plates. The children must identify the problem and together develop the best solution. This sort of activity may take only 30 seconds. The point is to make it routine so that children know that 10–20 times daily they will be called on to recognize and solve some interesting little meaningful problem.

    Unplanned problem-solving occasions: Every naturally occurring problem can be used to promote strategic thinking: "What exactly is the problem here anyway?" "Can anybody think of a smart thing to do about this?" "Do you think that will work? If so, why?" "Can you think of anything else?" "Who thinks this would be best to try? Did it work?" "Great! That was a smart thing to do, wasn't it? Let's remember to do that again."

Review
    Preschool children generally would rather move on to the next activity than stop to review the last activity. However, if done quickly and in an animated manner, reviews can be part of the activity routine: "We did a great job today. Our job was to make finger paintings, and we all did it. Did we stick to our plan?" "What did we need to get the job done?" "Did it turn out well?" "What was easy and what was difficult?" "What were some really smart things that we learned to do?" "What are some things that didn't work out so we will not do them next time?"

egocentrism of early childhood and to see the world from other perspectives and (2) the development of executive self-regulation of social behavior. The prefrontal part of the brain develops more slowly and variably than do other parts. Therefore, it is not surprising that profound differences are seen among typically developing preschoolers and young school-aged children with respect to their ability to coordinate their actions with those of others.

Earlier, we argued for the usefulness in rehabilitation of Vygotsky's thesis that everyday social-behavioral routines are the crucible within which internal cognitive and executive functions are fashioned. This dependence on social routines, context, and values is even more obviously true of social development. For this reason, the vulnerability of children with brain injury acquired during this critical developmental period is best addressed by effective coaching and support of their everyday communication partners, most notably their parents and siblings.

Social Development During Infancy

Infants have an innate capacity to send social signals that have a markedly arousing effect on others (Lamb, 1989). For example, crying commands comfort and security from caregivers. Smiling commands adults to stay near and maintain social interaction. Reciprocal vocal play is intrinsically reinforcing for both baby and caregiver and creates prolonged social interactions that evolve gradually into predictable, routine "conversations" in the absence of meaningful words.

By the middle of the first year of life, most infants have formed a strong affectional bond with their primary caregivers (Hodapp and Mueller, 1982). Associated with a growing understanding of the world as consisting of independent, persisting things and people who both act and can be acted on, this emotional attachment to important adults is associated also with a growing fear of strangers. Whereas early research in infants' emotional attachment focused on the mother-child bond, more recent investigators have identified contributions to attachment from varied relationships, including those with fathers, grandparents, and siblings (Bratherton, 1992; Richard and Light, 1986). Central to attachment theory is the critical thesis that healthy emotional development requires a committed caregiving relationship with one or a small number of adults. It is within this network of relationships that children develop a sense of emotional security; an understanding of the power of language; a growing perception of the intentions, feelings, and perceptions of others; and, ultimately, the ability to coordinate their actions with those of others, resulting in social acceptance and reciprocal friendships.

Social Development During the Toddler Years

The second year of life embodies a burst of social development most apparent in the child's language. Less obvious is the ability of 2 year olds to recognize distress in others, to offer help, to verbally sympathize and protect the victim, and to attempt to evoke a change in affect in the distressed person (Radde-Yarrow et al., 1983).

Corresponding to this slowly growing appreciation of another's perspective is the progression in peer-related play behavior from socially isolated play with objects, to parallel play (playing in physical proximity and with similar toys), to intersecting play (occasionally sharing objects with a peer but in an unplanned and unsustained manner), to cooperative play (sharing toys and in some way working toward a common goal). By age 2, play objects continue to receive most of a child's attention (vs. social interaction with peers), and a majority of social behaviors directed by one child to another are ignored (Brownell and Brown, 1992). However, children increasingly play in such a way that one child's behavior is contingent on that of another. For example, children at this age might roll a ball back and forth, march together in a circle, or imitate one another's behavior. Mature toddlers might even exchange roles in play. For example, one child might pull the train while the other verbalizes "toot toot," followed by an exchange of these roles.

Social Development During the Preschool Years

Controlled social interaction—including conventional signals to initiate and maintain interaction and the ability to coordinate interaction around a theme, goal, or plan—emerges during the preschool years (Brownell and Brown, 1992). By age 4, a large proportion of preschoolers' play is organized around familiar themes, such as a princess-and-dragon theme, eating out at McDonald's, or other familiar scripts. Organized social play using familiar scripts is made possible by the child's developing language and social knowledge but is also the context within which social uses of language are practiced and social knowledge (e.g., knowledge of social roles) is solidified. Within the context of enjoyable social role playing controlled by familiar scripts, children practice social skills (e.g., initiating interaction, interrupting ongoing interaction, taking turns, sharing, engaging in extended conversations, and using a variety of such pragmatic functions of language as teasing, joking, threatening, promising, warning, complimenting, and criticizing).

Social problem solving is apparent in children's decision making in choosing social games to play, roles to use, and rules to follow and in their repair negotiations as breakdowns in their play emerge. Play scripts offer support to preschoolers who might otherwise yield to their inclination to be egocentric, selfish, and aggressive. For example, it is easier to say, "What do you want? Here, have some french fries" when acting out a McDonald's script than when jealously guarding one's french fries at the lunch table.

Some evidence corroborates persistent patterns of social behavior evident during the preschool years. For example, boys with extreme restlessness and difficulty with impulse control at age 3 tend to show conduct disorders at age 8 (Richman et al., 1982). However, research literature is limited, and some counterevidence is available (e.g., that girls do not show the same behavioral continuity as boys). The possibility that social skill weakness early in life persists or, worse, creates a self-fulfilling dynamic of increasing social isolation combines with the social vulnerability created by early TBI to support an intensive focus on psychosocial development in pre-schoolers with TBI.

Psychosocial Development of Children with Early TBI

Koskiniemi and colleagues (1995) found that adult outcome of children injured as preschoolers was poor (none of the children injured before age 4 was working full-time as an adult). Ominously, outcome was clearly worse than that predicted on the basis of children's early recovery and school performance. Of greatest relevance to the issue of psychosocial development, the best indicator of outcome in this group was a measure of their sense of identity. Other studies of early TBI, particularly prefrontal injury, emphasize the frequency and intensity of long-term behavior problems, which often grow in magnitude over the years after the injury (Eslinger et al., 1992; Grattan and Eslinger, 1991, 1992; Marlowe, 1992; Mateer and Williams, 1991; Price et al., 1990).

With these sobering findings as backdrop, it is critical to highlight social development and behavioral self-regulation in rehabilitation and special education programs for children with early TBI. An injury itself often creates social vulnerability by interfering with the development of social initiation, social inhibition, social perception, and the ability to take the perspective of others. Variability in normal development easily generates in parents and professionals alike a confusion regarding possible consequences of the injury. In our experience, the intensity and duration of emotional and social responses often distinguish developmentally normal phenomena from symptoms of TBI. For example, typically developing children may frequently fail to initiate expected activity but rarely to the degree seen in preschoolers with organically based initiation impairment. Similarly, typically developing preschoolers may occasionally seem emotionally out of control (angry, giddy, or unrelenting in demands for attention) but rarely in response to minimal provocation or for the extended periods seen in many children with TBI.

This organically based vulnerability is exacerbated easily by natural dynamics created within families. For example, it is natural for parents of an injured child to commit themselves to ensuring that the child will never again be hurt physically or emotionally. This admirable protective instinct can lead easily to an overprotective environment in which children are denied social opportunities wherein they might fail but which are nonetheless critical for social maturation.

Similarly, children with acquired disability are often placed in settings where they interact mainly with adults, thereby failing to learn how to negotiate social situations with peers. Many children who have TBI and an organically based difficulty in regulating their emotions and in controlling their anger grow worse in an environment in which well-meaning adults ensure that the child wins

every game, succeeds at every task, and never has to adjust to failure and disappointment. Furthermore, sympathetic adults may translate *understanding* the child's social or behavioral problems (which is a good thing) into *excusing* the child for unacceptable behavior, again blocking normal development of self-regulation. In this case, adults could become enablers of social immaturity and might be contributors to the child's truncated social development.

The importance of psychosocial development in young children with TBI might easily be overlooked in rehabilitation programs understandably focused on medical stability and physical recovery. However, psychosocial development might receive the attention it deserves if staff and family members share a simple creed:

- We want children to think, choose, react, and speak for themselves.
- We want children to be friends and to have friends; to wait, listen, and share.
- We want children to like themselves.

Psychosocial Intervention for Children with Early TBI

In Chapter 13, Ylvisaker and colleagues describe a positive and proactive approach to serving children with social and behavioral needs after TBI. The principles and procedures described in that chapter apply to preschoolers and older children. In particular, preventing the evolution of challenging behavior with creative antecedent control measures and teaching communication alternatives to unwanted behavior (both described in Chapter 13) should be bread-and-butter procedures in all programs for preschoolers with disability.

In addition, growing recognition of the importance of psychosocial development for all children with disability has led to an increased emphasis on social development in general preschool programs for children with disability. This focus extends far beyond simple conversation and basic rules of getting along. In addition, children are taught varied scripts associated not only with school behavior but with a variety of social environments and tasks.

Context of Psychosocial Intervention: Family and Peers

It is not difficult to appreciate the importance of social context in establishing or re-establishing positive, routine social behaviors. Walker and coworkers (1994), long associated with direct instruction approaches to teaching social skills to children (i.e., scripted practice of discrete social behaviors outside the context of real social interaction), outlined 11 cardinal rules of social skills intervention. Interestingly, six of those 11 cardinal rules emphasized the critical importance of natural settings and real social contexts in promoting improved social competence in a meaningful and generalizable way. The emphasis on meaningful contexts in current discussions of social skills intervention is, in part, a consequence of earlier efficacy research, in which a common finding was that social changes created in a training context do not generalize easily to everyday interactions with peers and others in natural settings.

Social Context and Family

Because interaction with parents and siblings is the most natural social context for young children, this is the ideal context for psychosocial rehabilitation. Just as young children serve a *cognitive* apprenticeship at the feet of their parents and other family members (described earlier), they serve a *social* apprenticeship in the same place. Parents who are oriented adequately can play the role of "social consultants" to their children, modeling competent interaction, providing assistance and encouragement, and serving as the authority figures who impose discipline and set limits without inviting battles over control.

Therefore, family members must be welcomed into all aspects of rehabilitation, not just as spectators but as collaborators who both receive information about how to interact most effectively with their child and give insights to staff about the child. In inpatient rehabilitation, it is important to create opportunities for flexible staff hours so that parents who work in the daytime and visit only in the evening can still interact regularly with therapy staff to practice and internalize principles of positive intervention and support. Excellent materials, including training videos and manuals, are available for teaching family members to use their own interaction with young children as the context for instructing children with varying degrees of disability in positive social interaction skills (see Manolson, 1992; MacDonald, 1989; Weitzman, 1992). An important goal of parent education is to demystify therapy, enabling parents to recognize the importance of their role and the simplicity and commonsense nature of good rehabilitation. This goal is achieved more effectively by working elbow-to-elbow with parents than by engaging them exclusively in formal training sessions (see Chapter 20). The effectiveness of early communication intervention—working indirectly through parents—has been demonstrated in several studies (Haney and Klein, 1993; Mahoney and Powell, 1988).

Social Context and Peers

In most small inpatient rehabilitation programs, it is not possible to create meaningful peer groupings for all the children at every age and level of recovery. However, if hospitalization is prolonged, it is important to try to do so. In general, the ideal times to focus on peer interaction are dining and recreation hours, because these settings are natural for varied social interaction. Peer groups can be composed of fellow hospitalized children who are at roughly the same age and level of recovery, siblings and friends who were known before the injury, or contrived groups that might include volunteers (e.g., children of

staff members). With whatever support necessary, the children practice social competencies, including varied pragmatic communication acts and the ability to negotiate social problems or socially awkward situations. Practicing social interactive skills over lunch or during a late-afternoon recreational art project certainly is more natural for children than are contrived therapy interactions and, therefore, less likely to fail the litmus test of generalization and maintenance.

When children return to their homes and to community preschools, play groups with peers and snack and lunch times at school are preferable to contrived professional-child interactions or social skills groups as contexts for coaching children in the competencies that will enable them, over time, to have friends and to mature socially. Within these settings, adults take responsibility for engaging children in play that is instituted at an appropriate level of challenge and that invites social interaction, for redirecting children to peers when they address comments to adults, for coaching children through conflicts, and for anticipating problem behavior and prompting communication alternatives as a means of defusing potential conflict before it escalates.

Family-Centered Services

Philosophy of Family-Centered Intervention

The principles of family-centered care were first articulated in relation to delivery of health care (Public Health Service, 1987) but have subsequently been applied to a variety of fields in a variety of ways. This positive development inevitably has led to some differences in terminology and application of principles. Understood generically, *family centered* refers to "a combination of beliefs and practices that define particular ways of working with families that are consumer driven and competency enhancing" (Dunst et al., 1991, p. 115).

In their landmark text on family-centered care, Shelton and colleagues (1987) identified eight key elements of family-centered care, components that were later refined and expanded by the National Center for Family-Centered Care. Family-centered care includes:

- Recognizing that the family is the constant in a child's life, whereas the service systems and personnel within those systems fluctuate.
- Facilitating parent-professional collaboration in the care of individual children; in program development, implementation, and evaluation; and in the formulation of policy.
- Honoring the racial, ethnic, cultural, and socioeconomic diversity of families.
- Recognizing family strengths and individuality and respecting different methods of coping.

- Sharing with families, on a continuing basis and in a supportive manner, complete and unbiased information.
- Encouraging and facilitating family-to-family support and networking.
- Understanding and incorporating the developmental needs of infants, children, and adolescents and their families into service systems.
- Implementing comprehensive policies and programs that provide emotional and financial support to meet the needs of families.
- Designing accessible service systems that are flexible, culturally competent, and responsible to family-identified needs.

Recent federal legislation has both supported and given direction to family-centered approaches with such laws as the Omnibus Budget Reconciliation Act of 1989 (PL 101-239) and the Individuals with Disabilities Education Act of 1990 (PL 102-119).

Family-centered services must be understood and delivered within a broader philosophical context that includes *community-based services and supports* and *culturally competent services*. A community-based approach includes flexible and easily accessible services, services that are coordinated within a system and that support choice, supports within inclusive settings, and planned use of informal resources and formal services. Culturally competent services recognize and honor diversity (e.g., racial, ethnic, religious, cultural, geographic, socioeconomic, gender), acknowledge the power of culture in shaping the lives of both providers and consumers, and ensure the skills, attitudes, and knowledge that providers require to deliver services effectively across cultures.

Rationale for Family-Centered Care

Earlier in this chapter, we emphasized the importance of context in the cognitive, communication, and psychosocial development of children. In the case of infants, toddlers, and preschoolers, that context is largely the family. In an important sense, young children serve an extended apprenticeship with their parents, grandparents, older siblings, and other important members of the extended family unit. Whereas providers of services come and go in the life of a child, the family is the ongoing caring, teaching, and decision-making unit for the child. Family-centered approaches honor these family roles and facilitate development of family competence so that the roles can be played as effectively as possible.

Besides arising from a compelling philosophical rationale, family-centered services are required by law in serving young children, under the Individuals with Disabilities Education Act. Furthermore, a variety of service providers have found that family-centered practices improve outcomes for children (Als et al., 1994; Johnson, 1995),

increase staff satisfaction in delivering the services, and lower costs (e.g., decreased use of hospital services; Adnopoz and Nagler, 1993; Perrault, 1986; Robinson et al., 1989).

The urgency of a family-centered perspective combined with community-based supports is underscored by draconian funding cuts associated with managed care and by cutbacks in other support programs. As Russell and colleagues point out in Chapter 6, average length of inpatient stay in one pediatric TBI rehabilitation program with which the authors are affiliated decreased by 75% from 1983 to 1993. Countless children who, in the past, were judged to be in need of inpatient rehabilitation are now rehabilitated at home by family members with whatever support they can receive from professional providers. Such an economic environment offers no alternative to empowering families so that they are able to competently play roles thrust on them by economic necessity.

The urgency of a family-centered perspective combined with culturally competent services is underscored by the dramatic social, demographic, and economic changes that have occurred during the last few decades and have transformed the American family (data summarized by Ahlberg and DeVita, 1992, and Hodgkinson, 1992). For example, for most of the 1980s, the "Norman Rockwell" family (working dad, homemaker mom, two school-aged children) accounted for only 6% of all households. Eighty-two percent of children younger than 18 have working mothers. One of every four babies is born to an unmarried parent; 60% of today's children will live with a single parent before they reach 18. The number of children living in multigenerational families (child, parent, and grandparent) doubled to 2.4 million during the 1980s, resulting in part from our sagging economy. In the United States each year, a half million babies are born to teenage mothers. Yearly, more than 1 million babies are born into poverty; in 1991, 25% of children younger than 6 lived in poverty. In that same year, 13.7 million children were being raised by single women with a median annual income of $10,982. More than 8 million children younger than 18 are without health insurance. It is expected that recently legislated changes in the welfare system will make these statistics even gloomier for children.

Many different kinds of families make up our communities: single-parent families, extended families, stepfamilies, foster families, adoptive families, dual-career families, commuting families, widowed families, and gay and lesbian families. Approximately 150 native languages are spoken in U.S. classrooms, with 5% of our nation's children possessing limited proficiency in English. By the year 2010, 12 states will have "minority" youth populations of 40% or higher, making the term *minority* inaccurate and outdated.

The expanded diversity in our communities, combined with the environmental stressors affecting the lives of children in this country, yields the inescapable conclusion that providers must develop new ways to deliver services that are flexible, accessible, and consistent with the need to respect diverse cultures, strengths, and needs of families. Service delivery systems were developed before many of these changes occurred in our social struggle to meet the diverse needs of today's children and families. New issues require new solutions. Cultural diversity combined with frank recognition of the critical importance of family competence in TBI rehabilitation requires a new focus on professional roles, training, and attitudes that will facilitate family competence building within a collaborative and respectful rehabilitation milieu.

Family-Centered Services and TBI

In Chapter 16, Waaland explores a large number of issues in working with families of children with TBI. She emphasizes the importance of a family-professional alliance and methods of achieving this alliance, including ensuring equal family participation in developing rehabilitation plans and discharge plans. In light of shortened lengths of stay in rehabilitation hospitals, this collaborative planning includes parents and professionals working together to anticipate long-term needs, to identify local community supports, to orient community providers (including preschool or school staff) to the potential needs of the child, and to identify those in the local community capable of coordinating services and solving problems associated with service providers. When rehabilitation staff work with family members in developing comprehensive and effective discharge plans, they also provide in vivo modeling and coaching on how to advocate for the child and interact with community professionals.

For family members, Waaland also emphasizes broad circles of support that extend well beyond professional services. Parents may need help organizing the support of relatives, neighbors, churches, civic organizations, recreation programs, employers, respite providers, and others. They may also need emotional support that can be provided by peers who have experienced what they are experiencing and have successfully negotiated the systems and jumped the hurdles with which the current family is struggling. In our experience, support groups in hospitals and local chapters of the Brain Injury Association may not always meet this need. Support groups are intimidating for some families in the early weeks and months after an injury. Brain Injury Association chapters often do not address the needs of parents of young children. Therefore, we have tried to match new families with peer families that, in our judgment, are compatible and are in a position to support and otherwise help the new family. Successful one-to-one family matching can be helpful for families in crisis during the early weeks and months after acquired brain injury in a child.

Respect for cultural diversity may be most problematic for professionals in TBI rehabilitation. For example, it is easy for professionals to become defensive when parents bring faith healers into the hospital or engage in other religious practices that may appear inconsistent with a commitment to scientifically grounded rehabilitation. Child discipline practices that are natural to some families may appear abusive to staff (and, in extreme cases, *may* be abusive, requiring appropriate action). In these and other cases, staff who react judgmentally or who withdraw from the family jeopardize the parent-professional alliance so critical to the child's long-term improvement, including relationships between the parent and subsequent professionals.

Obstacles to Family-Centered Rehabilitation

Despite their solid rationale in philosophy and practice, effective family-centered services are subject to many obstacles. For example, a family-centered approach is based on teamwork, interdependence, and collaboration—values typically not incorporated into professional training programs that tend to highlight the medical-model values of specialization, professional independence, and respect for the expertise associated with technical knowledge. Overcoming this obstacle requires teaching new skills, such as how to work as a collaborator and consultant, how to work on teams, how to facilitate meetings of equals, how to resolve conflicts, and how to solve problems (see Chapter 20). More specifically, many preservice education programs fail to teach students how to collaborate with parents and that it is their job to be competent in this collaborative relationship. Typically, it is the responsibility of rehabilitation programs to equip their professionals with these competencies.

Second, preservice education tends to focus on pathology, impairment, deficits, disability, illness, and weakness. It is only a small jump from this starting point to defining the goals of rehabilitation in terms of curing illness, eliminating pathology, and reducing disability. Applied to families, this perspective directs professionals to look for problems (e.g., dysfunction) and to work to reduce these problems. A family-centered perspective, in contrast, although not blind to problems, seeks capacity and competence first and foremost, and attempts to expand competence so that the family can play its many roles most effectively. This shift in perspective can make all the difference in the world in creating a positive working alliance with family members.

Third, preservice education programs understandably communicate to practitioners the value of their discipline and the importance of the technical competence that their years of education yield. The negative side of professional pride and pursuit of ever-increasing technical expertise is difficulty in releasing to other professionals and family members this expertise and the role with which it is associated. Family-centered and holistic rehabilitation—critical to serving young children with TBI—requires just such a role release and a willingness to play a new role: that of consultant to people who lack specialized training in the field.

Finally, policies and practices in rehabilitation hospitals may be obstacles to family-centered rehabilitation. For example, barring clear conflict with confidentiality rights of other patients or with the possibility of engaging a child in meaningful therapeutic activities, parents should be routinely invited to participate in assessment and intervention sessions. Staff planning conferences should be scheduled at times convenient for parents, or their participation should be facilitated by means of teleconferencing. Pediatric rehabilitation hospitals should have a policy of assisting families with overnight sleeping arrangements and of rendering visits to the hospital positive experiences for siblings, other family members, and friends.

Helping Rehabilitation Professionals to Adopt a Family-Centered Perspective

Creating competence and shaping attitudes necessary for effective family-centered services may require considerable effort on several fronts. Here, we address administrative issues, specific training activities, and ongoing support for this approach.

In the absence of administrative support, the philosophy of rehabilitation in a facility likely will not change appreciably. Administrative support can take many forms. Family-centered care can be tied directly to quality improvement initiatives, marketing, program evaluation, and profits. Policies and procedures may have to be augmented. For example, to staff job descriptions we have added competencies in communicating and collaborating effectively with family members (Ylvisaker et al., 1993; see also Chapter 20). Supervisors may need to be trained in how to supervise family-centered approaches and to evaluate the performance of their staff in this area. Policies and procedures regarding visitation and family participation may have to be rewritten.

Classroom-based learning events can be useful for staff but only as one component of a larger focus on institutional change. Consistent with well-established principles of adult learning, these training sessions should engage the staff members' motivation to learn, connect new practices with past experience, actively involve the learner in critical thinking and in practicing specific competencies, and be conducted in a climate of respect for the learners and for the challenges of their jobs (Moore, 1988; Zemke and Zemke, 1995). Parents should be involved in this training to avoid the contradiction implicit in promoting family involvement without involving families and to make the parents' important insights, observations, and ideas available to staff. Ideally, parents

representing a wide range of experiences should be involved. In recognition of the genuine importance of parental involvement, parents should be paid for their assistance in developing, conducting, reviewing, and evaluating staff training programs (Edelman, 1995; Project Copernicus, 1991). Consistent with the theme of collaboration, staff from diverse professional backgrounds should attend training sessions together.

One-shot in-service programs rarely achieve meaningful and stable change in institutional settings. The process of implementing a family-centered approach in rehabilitation may involve some combination of the following (Jeppson and Thomas, 1994):

- Discussions and planning at team meetings
- Site visits to other programs
- Suggestions from family members acquired by means of surveys, interviews, or focus groups
- Mentoring relationships between veteran family-centered providers and novices
- Curricular changes in preservice programs in local university training programs
- Readings in family-centered services
- Periodic reviews of the program
- Family advisory boards that ensure that families have an opportunity for meaningful participation in the design, delivery, and evaluation of services

Many excellent training programs and materials have been developed for providing family-centered, community-based, and culturally competent services for children and their families. Catlett and Winton's *Resource Guide: Selected Early Intervention Training Materials* (1995) is an excellent reference for products that can be useful in staff training and program development. This guide can be ordered from Camille Catlett, SIFT, Frank Porter Graham Child Development Center, CB No. 8180, University of North Carolina, Chapel Hill, NC 27599-8180, (919) 966-6635.

Summary

In this chapter, we highlighted some of the critical issues for preschool-aged children with TBI, described principles and selected practices related to cognitive and psychosocial disability, and presented a philosophy of family-centered services that is particularly important for this age group. None of the rehabilitation concepts presented in this chapter applies uniquely to TBI. Indeed, we have emphasized intervention strategies that originated in the province of other disability groups. However, we believe that the information presented here may be helpful to rehabilitation professionals who are unfamiliar with this age group or whose practice has not encompassed the cognitive, psychosocial, and familial aspects of rehabilitation.

References

Adnopoz J, Nagler S (1993). Supporting HIV Infected Children in Their Own Families Through Family-Centered Practice. In ES Morton, RK Grigsby (eds), Advancing Family Preservation Practice. Newbury Park, CA: Sage.

Ahlberg DA, DeVita CJ (1992). New realities of the American family. Population Bull 47;2.

Als H, Lawhon G, Duffy FH, et al. (1994). Individualized developmental care for the very low-birthweight preterm infant. JAMA 272;853.

Bratherton I (1992). Attachment and Bonding. In V Van Hasselt, M Hersen (eds), Handbook of Social Development. New York: Plenum.

Brink JD, Garrett AL, Hale WR, et al. (1970). Recovery of motor and intellectual function in children sustaining severe injuries. Dev Med Child Neurol 12;565.

Brownell C, Brown E (1992). Peers and Play in Infants and Toddlers. In V Van Hasselt, M Hersen (eds), Handbook of Social Development. New York: Plenum.

Bruner J (1978). How to Do Things with Words. In J Bruner, A Garton (eds), Human Growth and Development. Oxford, UK: Oxford University.

Catlett C, Winton P (1995). Resource Guide: Selected Early Intervention Training Materials (4th ed). Chapel Hill, NC: Frank Porter Graham Child Development Center, University of North Carolina at Chapel Hill.

Chadwick O, Rutter M, Shaffer D, Shrout PE (1981). A prospective study of children with head injuries: IV. Specific cognitive deficits. J Clin Neuropsychol 3;101.

Diamond A, Goldman-Rakic PS (1989). Comparison of human infants and rhesus monkeys on Piaget's AB task: evidence for dependence on dorsolateral prefrontal cortex. Exp Brain Res 74;24.

Dunst C, Johanson C, Trivette C, Hamby D (1991). Family-oriented early intervention policies and practices: family-centered or not? Except Child 58;115.

Dunst C, Trivette C, Deal A (1988). Enabling and Empowering Families: Principles and Guidelines for Practice. Cambridge, MA: Brookline Books.

Edelman L (ed) (1995). Getting on Board: Training Activities to Promote the Practice of Family-Centered Care. Bethesda, MD: Association for the Care of Children's Health.

Eslinger PJ, Grattan LM, Damasio H, Damasio AR (1992). Developmental consequences of childhood frontal lobe damage. Arch Neurol 49;764.

Evans MA (1987). Discourse characteristics of reticent children. Appl Psycholinguist 8;171.

Ewing-Cobbs L, Levin HS, Eisenberg HM, Fletcher JM (1987). Language functions following closed head injury in children and adolescents. J Clin Exp Neuropsychol 9;575.

Ewing-Cobbs L, Miner M, Fletcher JM, Levin HS (1989). Intellectual, motor, and language sequelae following closed head injury in infants and preschoolers. J Pediatr Psychol 14;531.

Feeney TJ, Ylvisaker M (1995). Choice and routine: antecedent behavioral interventions for adolescents with severe traumatic brain injury. J Head Trauma Rehabil 10(3);67.

Finger S (1991). Brain damage, development, and behavior: early findings. Dev Neuropsychol 7;261.

Fivush R, Fromhoff FA (1988). Style and structure in mother-child conversations about the past. Discourse Proc 11;337.

Goldman PS (1971). Functional development of the prefrontal cortex in early life and the problem of neuronal plasticity. Exp Neurol 32;366.

Grattan LM, Eslinger PJ (1991). Frontal lobe damage in children and adults: a comparative review. Dev Neuropsychol 7;283.

Grattan LM, Eslinger PJ (1992). Long-term psychological consequences of childhood frontal lobe lesion in patient DT. Brain Cogn 20;185.

Haney M, Klein MD (1993). Impact of a program to facilitate mother-infant communication in high-risk families of high-risk infants. J Child Comm Disord 15;15.

Hanft BE (1989). Family-Centered Care: An Early Intervention Resource Manual. Rockville, MD: American Occupational Therapy Association.

Hodapp R, Mueller E (1982). Early Social Development. In B Wolman (ed), Handbook of Developmental Psychology. Englewood Cliffs, NJ: Prentice Hall.

Hodgkinson H (1992). A Demographic Look at Tomorrow. Washington, DC: Institute for Educational Leadership: Center for Demographic Policy.

Hoffmann M, Weikart DP (1995). Educating Young Children. Ypsilanti, MI: High-Scope Education Research Foundation.

Jarrett NLM (1988). The Origins of Detour Problem Solving in Human Infants. Unpublished master's thesis, University of Southampton, Southampton, England.

Jeppson ES, Thomas J (1994). Essential Allies: Families as Advisors. Bethesda, MD: Institute for Family-Centered Care.

Johnson BH (1995). Newborn intensive care units pioneer family-centered change in hospitals across the country. Zero to Three 15;11.

Kennard MA, Fulton JF (1942). Age and reorganization of central nervous system. Mt Sinai J Med 9;594.

Klonoff H, Low MD, Clark C (1977). Head injuries in children: a prospective five year follow-up. J Neurol Neurosurg Psychiatry 40;1211.

Kolb B (1995). Brain Plasticity and Behavior. Hillsdale, NJ: Lawrence Erlbaum.

Koskiniemi M, Kyykka T, Nybo T, Jarho L (1995). Long term outcome after severe brain injury in preschoolers is worse than expected. Arch Pediatr Adolesc Med 149;249.

Lamb M (1989). Social development. Pediatr Ann 18(5);223.

Lange-Cosack H, Wider B, Schlesner HJ, et al. (1979). Prognosis of brain injuries in young children (one until five years of age). Neuropaediatrie 10;105.

Levin HS, Culhane KA, Mendelsohn D, et al. (1993). Cognition in relation to magnetic resonance imaging in head-injured children and adolescents. Arch Neurol 50;897.

Levin HS, Goldstein FC, Williams DH, Eisenberg HM (1991). The Contribution of Frontal Lobe Lesions to the Neurobehavioral Outcome of Closed Head Injury. In HS Levin, HM Eisenberg, AI Benton (eds), Frontal Lobe Function and Dysfunction. New York: Oxford University, 318.

MacDonald J (1989). Becoming Partners with Children: From Play to Conversation. Chicago: Riverside Publishing.

Mahoney G, Powell A (1988). Modifying parent-child interaction: enhancing the development of handicapped children. J Spec Educ 22;82.

Mahoney WJ, D'Souza BJ, Haller JA, et al. (1983). Long-term outcome of children with severe head trauma and prolonged coma. Pediatrics 71;756.

Manolson A (1992). It Takes Two to Talk: A Parent's Guide to Helping Children Communicate. Toronto: Hanen Centre.

Marlowe WB (1992). The impact of a right prefrontal lesion on the developing brain. Brain Cogn 20;205.

Mateer CA, Williams D (1991). Effects of frontal lobe injury in childhood. Dev Neuropsychol 7;359.

McCabe A, Peterson C (1991) Getting the Story: A Longitudinal Study of Parental Styles in Eliciting Narratives and Developing Narrative Skill. In A McCabe, C Peterson (eds), Developing Narrative Structure. Hillsdale, NJ: Lawrence Erlbaum, 217.

McCabe A, Rollins PR (1994). Assessment of preschool narrative skills. Am J Speech Lang Pathol 3;45.

Meichenbaum D (1993). The "potential" contributions of cognitive behavior modification to the rehabilitation of individuals with traumatic brain injury. Semin Speech Lang 14;18.

Moore JR (1988). Guidelines concerning adult learning. J Staff Dev 9(3);2.

Nelson K (1973). Structure and strategy in learning to talk. Monogr Soc Res Child Dev 38; Serial #149.

Paul R, Smith RL (1993). Narrative skills in 4-year-olds with normal, impaired, and late-developing language. J Speech Hear Res 36;592.

Perrault C (1986). Family support system in newborn medicine: does it work? Follow-up study of infants at risk. J Pediatr 108;1025.

Peterson C, McCabe A (1983). Developmental Psycholinguistics: Three Ways of Looking at a Child's Narrative. New York: Plenum.

Piaget J (1974). The Language and Thought of the Child. Translated by M Gabain. New York: The New American Library.

Price B, Doffnre K, Stowe R, Mesulam M (1990). The compartmental learning disabilities of early frontal lobe damage. Brain 113;1383.

Project Copernicus (1991). Parents as Training Partners. In Project Copernicus News. Baltimore: Kennedy Krieger Institute.

Public Health Service (1987). Surgeon General's Report: Children with Special Health Care Needs, Campaign '87. Washington, DC: US Government Printing Office, 184-020/65654.

Radke-Yarrow M, Zahn-Waxler C, Chapman M (1983). Children's Prosocial Dispositions and Behavior. In PH Musson, E Hetherington (eds), Handbook of Child Psychology, vol 4. New York: Wiley.

Raimondi AJ, Hirschauer J (1984). Head injury in the infant and toddler. Child's Brain 11;12.

Reese E, Fivush R (1993). Parental styles of talking about the past. Dev Psychol 29;596.

Reese E, Haden CA, Fivush R (1993). Mother-child conversations about the past: relationships of style and memory over time. Cogn Dev 8;403.

Richard M, Light P (1986). Children of Social Worlds. Cambridge, MA: Polity Press.

Richman N, Stevenson J, Graham P (1982). Preschool to School: A Behavioral Study. London: Academic.

Roberts RJ, Pennington BF (1996). An interactive framework for examining prefrontal cognitive processes. Dev Neuropsychol 12;105.

Robinson JS, Schwartz MM, Magwene KS, et al. (1989). The impact of fever health education on clinic utilization. Am J Dis Child 143;698.

Roth FP (1986). Oral narrative abilities of learning-disabled students. Top Lang Disord 7(1);21.

Schweinhart LJ, Weikart DP (1986). Consequences of three preschool curriculum models through age 15. Early Child Res Q 1;15.

Schweinhart LJ, Weikart DP (1993). Success by empowerment: the High/Scope Perry Preschool study through age 27. Young Child 49;54.

Shelton TL, Jeppson ES, Johnson B (1987). Family-Centered Care for Children with Special Health Care Needs. Bethesda, MD: Association for the Care of Children's Health.

Snow CE, Goldfield BA (1981). Building Stories: The Emergence of Information Structures from Conversation. In D Tannen (ed), Analyzing Discourse: Text and Talk. Washington, DC: Georgetown University, 127.

Vygotsky LS (1978). Mind in Society: The Development of Higher Psychological Processes. Edited and translated by M Cole, V John-Steiner, S Scribner, E Souberman. Cambridge, MA: Harvard University.

Vygotsky LS (1986). Thinking and Speech. In LS Vygotsky (ed), Collected Works: Problems of General Psychology, vol 1. Translated by N Minick. New York: Plenum.

Walker HM, Schwarz IE, Nippold MA, et al. (1994). Social skills in school-age children and youth: issues and best practices in assessment and intervention. Top Lang Disord 14(3);70.

Weitzman E (1992). Learning Language and Loving It: A Guide to Promoting Children's Social and Language Development in Early Childhood Settings. Toronto: Hanen Centre.

Willatts P (1990). Development of Problem-Solving Strategies in Infancy. In DF Bjorklund (ed), Children's Strategies: Contemporary Views of Cognitive Development. Hillsdale, NJ: Lawrence Erlbaum, 23.

Williams D, Mateer CA (1992). Developmental impact of frontal lobe injury in middle childhood. Brain Cogn 20;196.

Yakovlev PI, Lecours AR (1967). The Myelogenetic Cycles of Regional Maturation of the Brain. In A Minkowski (ed), Regional Development of the Brain in Early Life. Oxford: Blackwell.

Ylvisaker M, Feeney T (in press). An Integrated Approach to Brain Injury Rehabilitation: Positive Everyday Routines. San Diego: Singular Publishers.

Ylvisaker M, Urbanczyk B, Feeney T (1993). Developing a Positive Rehabilitation Culture for Communication. In C Durgin, N Schmidt, J Freyer (eds), Brain Injury Rehabilitation: Clinical Intervention and Staff Development Techniques. Baltimore: Aspen Publishers.

Zemke R, Zemke S (1995). Adult learning: what do we know for sure? Training Mag 32;31.

Chapter 15

From Denial to Poster Child: Growing Past the Injury

Elisabeth D. Sherwin and Gregory J. O'Shanick

When young persons experience a brain injury, their worlds, as well as those of their parents, siblings, extended family, peers, and teachers are forever changed. All expectations, dreams, and hopes are set on a course that is not charted in parenting books or delineated in developmental or educational psychology texts, a course in which previous experience with other children becomes null and void. Although much has been written about facilitating family adjustment, maximizing therapies and services, and enhancing medical recovery of a person with a traumatic brain injury (TBI), little attention has been devoted to promoting such an individual's psychological adjustment to the injury. Enhancing adjustment is particularly critical in dealing with a child or adolescent who will live with the repercussions of the brain injury for many years to come.

The purpose of this chapter is to outline the challenges facing professionals committed to facilitating and enhancing psychological adjustment of young persons with TBI. The chapter identifies client and environmental factors that interact with such efforts and recommends ways to address them. Case studies are presented and analyzed to exemplify theoretical issues and practical implications. Our goal, to paraphrase Polonius, is to help children or adolescents be true to their own selves, moving them past denial and even past being a poster child.

The Challenge

Psychological work with a young person with TBI differs unequivocally from work with any other client or patient. The child or adolescent may present with varying degrees of consciousness, ranging from severely confused and poorly oriented to fully oriented and alert. Such children may progress in recovery to resume preinjury activities, or the rehabilitative path may be constrained severely. They may also experience degrees of (obvious and, often,

not so obvious) communication problems in expressing themselves or comprehending others, which may be the result of the injury or simply a reflection of their developmental stage. Memory problems, attentional deficits, and distractibility may become apparent—possible products of the individual's age, injury, or even medication. Behaviorally, impulsivity, emotional lability, and regression to earlier developmental stages are likely to be present and will test the skills and resourcefulness of the therapist, who may feel grossly inadequate or ill prepared for the task.

Developmental Issues Related to TBI

Theoretical Issues

Irrespective of the specific theoretical framework used by a therapist, TBI interferes with children's usual developmental course. Issues and tasks previously mastered may need to be relearned, and stages poorly resolved may need to be revisited before the child can move forward. The young child who previously exhibited age-appropriate autonomy may suddenly become clingy, refuse to part from the mother, exhibit fears previously mastered, and mistrust strangers. Schoolchildren may lose bowel control and experience psychological distress, shame, and self-doubt when they are aware that they have soiled themselves. For adolescents, this regression will certainly be difficult, and they may become extremely sensitive to the invasion of their privacy.

Independence Issues

The Child

After a brain injury, family members may become more protective and constricting, frustrating a child's natural need and desire for independence (Miller, 1993). Field trips, invitations to sleepovers, and the like may be rejected by fearful adults. Sports activities, an essential component in physical and social development, may be ruled out, denying the child an opportunity to resume socialization and bolster self-esteem, even if only through team victories rather than via individual successes. Although concerns over reinjury are valid and must be considered, the child's desire to resume such activities reflects a critical point in the resumption of a normal developmental course.

The Adolescent

The struggle for independence between parents and adolescents who have a brain injury may be expressed in several spheres: substance use (past and future); engagement in specific, potentially high-risk behaviors (such as contact sports and driving); or poor academic effort. If substance use (or abuse) was involved in an adolescent's injury, parents may become even more vigilant and restrictive (Miller, 1993; Sparadeo et al., 1992). Although fear of reinjury is a valid one, sports (particularly contact sports) are a form of social bonding and an opportunity to express personal identity. Young women, however, are less likely (both by virtue of the comparative prevalence of brain injury and by socialization) to express their independence through sports. They are more likely to exhibit their independence through rebellious sexual precociousness and promiscuity.

Parents may assume that sustaining a brain injury precludes future driving, but this is not necessarily the case. Moreover, standard cognitive tests do not adequately predict driving performance, and actual driving skills may have to be assessed (Brooke et al., 1992). Additionally, fear for their children and (perhaps) the cost of insuring their vehicle for adolescent driving may also lead parents either to discourage or to forbid their children from driving. As with sports, the issue of parental fear must be assessed in the context of the adolescent's rehabilitation: the ability to reintegrate socially and possibly to obtain employment.

Identity Issues

The Child

Identity issues emerge as a child moves through puberty. However, identity begins forming in early childhood as children's sense of self is intertwined closely with temporal memory of themselves and their environment (Butler and Satz, 1988). For children with TBI, this process may be derailed as their sense of self is injured by the gaps in their memory and by changes noticed in themselves and in comparison to younger siblings. Such children's position within the family may shift, as younger siblings surpass them in accomplishments. Their sense of self-efficacy and mastery thus becomes vulnerable as a result of the injury and the environment's response to the injury (Leichtman, 1992).

Such damage may result in depression, emergence of fears and anxieties, and failure to attempt tasks that are within the child's abilities (Maddux, 1991).

The Adolescent

As opposed to the children who were dependent on their parents before injury, preinjury adolescents had already begun the struggle to remove themselves from beneath parental wings. Adolescents with TBI tend to perceive themselves as "different" and are "painfully aware of their physical, cognitive, emotional, and behavioral changes, as well as their loss of abilities" (Bergland and Thomas, cited in Miller, 1993, p. 159). This self-awareness is particularly marked as decreased awareness and overestimation of skills and capabilities are sequelae routinely identified with TBI (e.g., Fleming and Strong, 1995; Gasquoine and Gibbons, 1994; Prigatano and Leatham, 1993; Ranseen et al., 1990).

This perception of being a stranger to oneself (Lewington, 1993) may elicit unproductive, constricting belief systems regarding locus of control and efficacy and may result in a learned helplessness and an overgeneralization about the effects that TBI has in an adolescent's life (Moore and Stambrook, 1995). Combined, these belief systems may result in an emotional life limited by "crushed self-esteem, conflict and guilt" (Miller, 1993, p. 159) at failure to meet expectations.

Parental and societal expectations are also intertwined with an adolescent's nascent sexual identity. Issues of homosexuality, if explored or suspected before injury, may be stifled (Mapou, 1990) as the adolescent fears loss of parental support suddenly so necessary for survival. Ability to interact with other homosexual peers may be curtailed by transportation limitations or by fear of censure. Alternatively, difficulties with the opposite gender and inadequate social opportunities or skills may lead the adolescent to same-gender partners, finding in that community the acceptance not found elsewhere. For heterosexual adolescents, impaired social skills, disfigurement, infantilization by parents, and abandonment by peers may restrict their opportunities to test their sexual identity and emerging sexuality.

Social Issues

Often, social difficulties do not emerge until discharge from the hospital and the commencement of attempts to reintegrate children or adolescents into their family and peer groups—even as long as 6 months after the injury (Coster et al., 1994). Even if handled adequately, these problems may continue and influence the young person's ability to return to school (Kaplan, 1988).

The Child

Young children may find, on discharge from the hospital, that their world has changed. The younger the children and the more severe the injury, the less they are able to articulate the awareness that other members of the family have also changed (Jacobs, 1991). As children heal, their natural ebullience returns, and they will make increasing demands on the adults in their life. Concomitantly, a decline in services, therapeutic regimens, and resources occurs as they are judged to have plateaued physically and are weaned from such regimens. In young children, the withdrawal of supports may result in new or re-emerging behavioral problems and a regression from skills that had been recovered since the injury (Jacobs, 1989; Lezak, 1978).

Academic issues per se aside, young persons may find the school environment and its demands frustrating and physically exhausting and may be bewildered by the difficulties they now encounter (Williams, 1994). Acting-out behaviors stemming from frustration or inappropriate behaviors secondary to misprocessing of information may result in an inappropriate placement in "emotionally disturbed, learning disabled or mentally retarded" learning environments (Russell, 1993). The stigma of being labeled a "retard," being thrust among children less socially accepted, and rejection by preinjury peers all raise significant issues of self-esteem, competence, and shame. (See Wright, 1991, for a discussion of the perils of labeling.) For the bright student who regressed to "averagehood," this demotion may be as devastating as the chronic failure experienced by the always-poor student. In either case, both student types may decide to stop trying.

Learned helplessness may be compounded by shame and embarrassment if young persons are experiencing seizures secondary to the brain injury. Fear of having a seizure in front of friends may make young persons with TBI secretive and vigilant, also undermining the social reintegration process (Williams, 1994).

Children and adolescents, anticipating the reunion and resumption of their friendships, may be bitterly disappointed when these do not occur, whether due to their new physical limitations or to their altered personality. Moreover, the "disfigurement paradox" comes most blatantly into play: The greater their disfigurement, the more accepting the environment is of behavioral deficits. Conversely, the more "normal" they appear, the less any deviation from normalcy is tolerated. Furthermore, the greater the disfigurement, the less likely that peers (or their parents) will feel comfortable in their presence. This rejection is experienced by both young persons and their parents, who may feel betrayed by the parents of their child's friends.

The Adolescent

Erikson (1977) notes that in puberty, adolescents are "primarily concerned with what they appear to be in the eyes of others as compared to what they feel they are" (p. 235). Much of their self-worth is derived from their social milieu, their peer group in general, and the opposite gen-

der in particular. Lack of social contact is the most noted complaint of adolescents and adults with TBI (e.g., Davis and Schneider, 1990; Newton and Johnson, 1985; Schmidt et al., 1995; Willer et al., 1990).

As social groups disband, adolescents may have difficulties in establishing new friends. If not privy to the history of such adolescents, these new friends may find social interaction with them aversive and may not pursue the relationship. Although children with TBI may prefer to play with younger children who are more tolerant of their physical and cognitive limitations, such choices can be very disconcerting when exhibited in an adolescent. In the hypervigilant, sexualized world in which we live, concerns about the nature of such a friendship and its appropriateness may arise. Although such concerns may have a basis, they can also severely limit an adolescent's social opportunities. Social interaction at any age is critical because noninjured peers can serve as models for healthy behavior (James and Reynolds, 1994), particularly when they are involved in learning the fine art of establishing intimate relationships.

Sex. If the adolescent is to master successfully the eriksonian stage of identity versus role confusion and advance to that of intimacy versus isolation, sexuality and sex must be addressed. Special attention to an individual's cognitive deficits is merited, so that information is processed and integrated accurately. Information provided in the classroom setting may not transfer, or adolescents may not distinguish when it is appropriate or inappropriate to repeat and share what has been learned about sex and sexuality. Adolescents with cognitive deficits may be inundated with messages about values associated with sex and sexual behavior but unable to identify those values or value systems that they should adopt and emulate. A more insidious problem is that of gender-typing messages, messages about "good girls" and "good boys" and how they behave before, during, and after sex that may be adopted by the adolescent, never to be articulated and perhaps hampering the pursuit and establishment of intimacy and sexual satisfaction (Sigler and Mackelprang, 1993).

Although concerns are expressed about the impulsive expression or exhibition of inappropriate sexual behavior on reentry to school (e.g., Williams, 1994), no mention is made of how to handle appropriate maturation and interest in the opposite sex. Emotional lability, social withdrawal, and inappropriate social behavior (e.g., over-talkativeness, impaired judgment, and concreteness) are often the culprits that mediate poor sexual adjustment as they interfere with the ability to establish relationships that could serve as a basis for sexual intimacy. Furthermore, frontal lobe damage, often associated with aggravated sexual behavior, has been associated more with inappropriate verbalization than with actual sexual behavior (Ducharme et al, 1993).

Substance Use.   For adolescents who are extremely desirous of social interaction (e.g., Schmidt et al., 1995; Willer et al., 1990), alcohol may serve as a means for social engagement and, therefore, be hard to avoid or resist. Even if adolescents are capable of recalling the limitations on substance use that a brain injury has placed on them, they may not circulate or share this information with peers for fear of being ridiculed. Many an individual has thought it "cool" secretly to take out a friend with TBI and to go drinking or to provide a marijuana cigarette, with all concerned feeling particularly pleased with themselves for successfully deceiving the heavy-handed parent.

Assessment

Medical and Psychological Issues

Assessment of children or adolescents with TBI must address both current and premorbid functioning of both the clients and the families within which they function.

Preinjury Child or Adolescent

It appears that some children are more susceptible than are others to TBI; boys are more at risk than girls and are also more vulnerable to both first and second injuries. The child with repeated brain injuries is more likely to be described preinjury as "disobedient, destructive, hyperactive, and prone to fighting with other children" (Miller, 1993, p. 156). Such children often experience a mild brain injury, usually as a result of engaging in forbidden, thrill-seeking behavior.

   Thus, for both the child and adolescent, information should be sought regarding developmental markers that had been attained prior to injury. Extent of independence, initiative, verbal skills, hobbies, relationship with peers, and coping style are relevant. Also relevant is premorbid medical history, particularly possible previous serious or mild brain injuries. In a review of medical records, attention should be given to past use of medications to control mood or behavior. These medications may be required again in the future and may have to be integrated with current injury-related medication. Past behavioral and academic difficulties may also have an impact on recovery. Previous experience with psychotherapy, either premorbidly or since the injury, should also be determined. Therapists should make efforts to review past psychotherapy records to divine those techniques that were successful and those that failed, keeping in mind that such records may not necessarily predict current efficacy. Research has clearly shown a strong relation between premorbid psychological difficulties and postinjury adjustment difficulties (e.g., Cicerone, 1991).

Current Child and Adolescent

Although not often conceptualized thus, both children and adolescents may experience and exhibit symptoms of a posttraumatic stress disorder, particularly if they experienced a mild brain injury (Leichtman, 1992; Miller, 1994a). Furthermore, the presence and extent of a grief response must be assessed: how the trauma of brain injury is being experienced and interpreted (Leichtman, 1992). Children may exhibit magical thinking (DeSpelder and Strickland, 1987), believing that they caused the brain injury and that their parents may be angry or blame them for what has happened. For adolescents, issues surrounding parental expectations and the death of their own dreams may arise. Open acknowledgment or verbalization of these difficulties may not occur, owing to developmental linguistic restrictions, restrictions secondary to the injury, or embarrassment. Furthermore, children or adolescents may have difficulty in recognizing or labeling their emotions. In some instances, efforts to be a "big boy" or "big girl," "macho," or "a strong woman" inhibit them from voicing their feelings.

   Although past medical records are important, current documents are also essential (Butler and Satz, 1988). It is recommended that a therapist obtain copies of any physical, emotional, cognitive, and neuropsychological assessments conducted since the injury. Repeated testing may be necessary as the child or adolescent regains or relearns skills. Retesting may also be necessary as the child or adolescent faces new experiences and challenges (Boyer and Edwards, 1991; Ylvisaker, 1993).

Premorbid and Current Family

Although the family is changed forever when a child experiences a brain injury, its past functioning can suggest how it may respond and cope with this stress and the resources on which it may draw. Cultural norms and values must be identified (DePompei and Williams, 1994; Jacobs, 1989, 1991; Leaf, 1993; Williams and Savage, 1991). Beliefs about discipline, preinjury expectations of the child or adolescent, and beliefs about recovery will affect the family's tolerance for the changed child (Leichtman, 1992). Furthermore, the family's place in its own recovery process from the injury inflicted on it, the members' processing of feelings of guilt and grief for their lost dreams, and their ability to deal with uncertainty associated with recovery from brain trauma will have an impact on familial resiliency (Williams, 1991). Finally, the dawning recognition that their child may depend on them—at some level—for the remainder of his or her life (Kramer, 1991; Leaf, 1993) will affect their ability to respond to their child and to the professionals desirous of helping.

Treatment Issues

Before a therapist develops an extensive and intensive treatment program, basic logistics must be acknowledged. Psychotherapy of any sort may be restricted severely or may not be covered by the parents' health insurance. Although counseling may be reportedly offered by the school system, budgetary restrictions may limit its availability or frequency, the child or adolescent may not bond with the counselor or psychotherapist, or parents may feel that their child is served better by staying in the classroom.

Assumptions about parental appreciation of the need for, and value of, psychotherapy may be fallacious. Families may easily feel overwhelmed as they must incorporate their child's therapies into their schedule and budget. Often, the parents will spare no expense for their child, thereby accruing significant debt (Perlesz et al., 1992). Yet parents may focus on more "obvious" therapies, such as physical therapy, as a focus for their meager fiscal resources (McDowell et al., 1995). The children or adolescents themselves may rebel at any more infringement on their time; may focus on visible, tangible improvements as signs of recovery; or may desire to avoid the pain associated with psychological introspection.

Injury Factors

Obviously, the severity of injury and extent of recovery will play significant roles both in the manner in which psychotherapy is conducted and in its scope. A basic understanding of brain functioning, assessment of severity of damage, and general guidelines for prognosis are critical knowledge for any therapist desirous of helping a young client with TBI. Such books as *Head Injury: The Facts* (Gronwall et al., 1991) may be a good place to start acquiring such knowledge, although more sophisticated knowledge of human neuropsychology will be needed. Such classics as *Fundamentals of Human Neuropsychology* (Kolb and Whishaw, 1996) and Lezak's *Neuropsychological Assessment* (1983) are also recommended.

However, even armed with the latest tome, therapists may find themselves having to cope with the uncertainty associated with TBI and its recovery. Defined sites of injury that "may" result in particular deficits, "best guesses" of prognosis and recovery trajectory that are offered, and the client's defiance of all predictions are a routine and integral aspect of TBI rehabilitation. Moreover, the relationship between severity or extent of damage and subsequent deficits is not linear. Furthermore, subtle deficits may be perceived as severe losses by the individual with a brain injury (Cicerone, 1991). Even mild injury to the frontal lobes can result in difficulties for an individual with TBI in understanding irony and sarcasm or a failure to detect humor in a sentence, creating potentially significant social difficulties to such children or adolescents who otherwise appear to have recovered fully from their injury.

Treatment

Philosophical Issues

Psychotherapy Versus Counseling

The first distinction between psychotherapy for children or adolescents with TBI and that of their noninjured counterparts lies in the nature of the therapeutic interaction. When working with children with TBI, therapists will find themselves taking a more active role within psychotherapy, often acting more as a counselor than as a psychotherapist. Although counseling is often more directive—offering instruction and guidance—psychotherapy is traditionally oriented to a process of self-discovery. Furthermore, although psychotherapy may be focused on maladaptive behavior or specific emotional distress, counseling tends to address "problems of living" (Kaplan and Sadock, 1991, p. 44; Leaf, 1991). Psychotherapists may also find themselves in the role of advocate for young persons with TBI and their families, fighting their cause, representing them to state and federal agencies, and helping them to navigate the rehabilitative maze to access the services to which they are entitled (Miller, 1991; Perlesz et al., 1992; Prigatano, 1991). In response to the unique nature of the therapeutic relationship, it is suggested that psychotherapists (or counselors) begin to think of, and refer to, their young charges as *clients* rather than as *patients*. This perspective is more empowering, much as moving from "victim" to "survivor" (Harrell and O'Hara, 1991) is important for the child and adolescent.

Theoretical Orientation

The deficits associated most commonly with TBI, such as decreased or impaired insight and awareness (Langer and Padrone, 1992; Prigatano and Schacter, 1991), disruption of verbal skills (Coster et al., 1994), emotional and cognitive regression (Levine et al., 1993) interact with developmental factors inherent in working with children and adolescents. The severity of deficits, the client's premorbid skills and developmental achievements, and current developmental issues must effect the theoretical orientation of the psychotherapeutic treatment.

Thus, the younger the client or the more severe the injuries, the more behavioral the perspective and goals. An excellent resource for establishing a behavioral management program is Jacobs's *Behavior Analysis Guidelines and Brain Injury Rehabilitation: People, Principles, and Programs* (1993), which outlines the fundamentals of behavior analysis and goal setting, as well as providing many of the support materials that facilitate the management of such a program.

Psychotherapeutic interpretations may be problematic, as they can confuse clients already experiencing cognitive deficits and may be futile in the face of the rigidity of thought often associated with cognitive sequelae of TBI (Miller, 1991; Prigatano, 1991). However, although traditional insight (in the psychodynamic sense) may not be pursued, existential issues of identity, the meaning of life, and establishment of a hopeful outlook should not be ignored (Cicerone, 1989; Miller, 1994a).

Therapy Issues

Engaging in a psychotherapeutic relationship with a child or adolescent with TBI is riddled with pitfalls, some inherent in any therapeutic relationship, some unique. Countertransference is ever-present, as therapists confront their own mortality (or that of their children) in their client (Miller, 1994a). Issues concerning parenting emotions and skills may seep into the relationship, as therapists may feel inadequate to the task. Feelings of inadequacy can easily arise in therapists (O'Brien and Prigatano, 1991) as the demands of the situation require them (or they believe they should be able) to exhibit expertise in developmental, educational, and rehabilitation psychology and neuropsychology; to be adept in family therapy and sexual counseling; and to be willing to take on the world as advocates for their client.

The bond formed at the bedside of an injured client, developed through many intensive hours of inpatient rehabilitation, may be hard to relinquish (O'Brien and Prigatano, 1991) at discharge. Alternatively, frustration at the lack of, or extremely slow, progress may be transferred to the client, whose neurologic limitations may be interpreted by the therapist as resistance, apathy, or lack of appreciation (Butler and Satz, 1988). Therapists' ability to endure in and to desire a long-term, perhaps lifelong, therapeutic relationship with their clients comes to the fore.

Other Therapies

Therapists working in a hospital or a rehabilitation setting may find themselves sharing clinical time with other therapeutic regimens: physical, occupational, speech, and perhaps cognitive. Moreover, their place on the therapeutic totem pole may be quite low (McDowell et al., 1995), as insurance companies, the family, and even the client may focus on physical improvement. Children or adolescents may be referred to a psychotherapist or counselor only when they become noncompliant or behaviorally inappropriate (Miller, 1993). Therapists working with a child or an adolescent with TBI must be prepared to interface routinely with other therapists and professionals, such as school administrators, coaches, and even lawyers. Territoriality has no place here; only a cooperative, multidisciplinary perspective can maximize outcome (Leichtman, 1992; McDowell, 1995; Miller, 1991; O'Brien and Prigatano, 1991; Prigatano, 1991). Thus, therapists may find themselves engaging in psychotherapy in their office, the physical therapy gymnasium, the speech laboratory, or the ballfield.

The Parents

Although the primary therapeutic bond is established with the client with TBI, it is the parents—particularly when behavioral management is involved—who will implement the treatment program. Sensitivity to the family culture, values, and goals is necessary if such an alliance is to be established and succeed (Bracy, 1994; DePompei and Williams, 1994; Jacobs, 1989, 1991; Leaf, 1993; Williams and Savage, 1991). This sensitivity can be problematic when parental goals differ markedly from those of the adolescent with TBI (Harrell and O'Hara, 1991), such as when the parents insist on postsecondary education and the adolescent is opposed to it. Alternatively, parents who see no harm in engaging in heavy alcohol consumption (or other substance use) may have a difficult time understanding why their adolescent may no longer drink or in restricting such activities (Sparadeo et al., 1992).

Although clients may alternate between overestimation and underestimation of their capabilities (Butler and Satz, 1988; Cicerone, 1991), parents may be invested in overestimating their child's past abilities and unrealistically hoping for a miraculous recovery (Cicerone, 1989, 1991). They may be torn between a belief that devout adherence to the program will result in a cure and the inability to set limits and challenge their child to fulfill (postinjury) potential, instead infantilizing the child and excusing poor behavior and academic performance by labeling the child as *limited* or *disabled*.

The Client

Although client-therapist (e.g., Beutler et al., 1991; Erlich, 1983) and patient-physician (e.g., Kaplan et al., 1989; Wallston, 1989) matching, or fit, and its implications for outcome have long been addressed, such matching is particularly crucial when engaging in psychotherapy with a child or adolescent with TBI. Thus, therapists should avoid statements that are evidently untrue, such as (in trying to appear empathetic) claiming to know how a client feels (Butler and Satz, 1988). Such claims or unrealistic promises of recovery may result in loss of therapeutic authenticity and integrity (Bracy, 1994). Children's or adolescents' premorbid or current attitude to other individuals with brain injury is also important, as it can provide information as to how they view themselves (Butler and Satz, 1988).

Conducting Psychotherapy

Initiation of Psychotherapy

As in traditional psychotherapy and counseling, establishing a bond and a therapeutic alliance is critical. Clients must be able to trust the therapist and believe that the therapist believes in their distress. Such trust is particularly relevant for children and adolescents who have experienced a mild brain injury and whose strengths wax and wane, often in the absence of neurologic findings (Bracy, 1994; Cicerone, 1991). Clients must feel that their therapist believes that every problem they report is valid (Bracy, 1994). Acceptance, empathy, unconditional positive regard, and patience for the client are excellent starting points for any type of therapeutic intervention (Bracy, 1994; Harrell and O'Hara, 1991). Irrespective of clients' cognitive abilities, they will sense true empathy, without necessarily comprehending the details or nuances of the communication.

Establishing Therapeutic Goals

The specific reason for a psychotherapy referral may vary. The presenting problem and its conceptualization should be shared and understood equally by the client and the therapist (Cicerone, 1989). The conceptualization should entail a holistic approach to the client, addressing both the "disordered mind," and the "wounded soul" of the client; both acknowledging the cognitive difficulties that are impeding successful coping and grappling with the existential question of "how can life be worth living after brain damage?" (Prigatano, 1991, pp. 3, 4). Although adolescents must tackle both issues, young children may require focus on the former, the latter appearing as they mature and encounter their limitations.

The Therapeutic Process

Structure

Before progress can be made on goals, therapists must establish a structure within which they and their client will function (Harrell and O'Hara, 1991; Miller, 1994a). Boundaries must be established, particularly as the therapeutic relationship with individuals with TBI is a nontraditional one to begin with. Issues of confidentiality, sharing of personal information, and physical contact are more salient when dealing with an adolescent but may arise over the course of psychotherapy with a child. In an effort to facilitate internalization of control, external limits in the form of behavioral contracts may have to be imposed. As children or adolescents mature and can self-control and better self-regulate, these restrictions gradually may be removed (Harrell and O'Hara, 1991).

Reframing

If a client communicates concerns of a more introspective nature, such concerns must be addressed. The therapist may have to facilitate a transition from what was or could have been to what is and what might be (Bracy, 1994). As they recover some of their skills or attempt to resume past activities, children and adolescents may become very sensitive to the discrepancies between current and expected performance capabilities. For clients with a mild brain injury, any lingering symptoms may be highly distressing as they (and their environment) perceive them to be "cured." This distress may result in psychological magnification of the extent of deficits that they are experiencing. Although validating the distress, therapists may need to facilitate a reinterpretation of the extent of disability that is actually being exhibited (Cicerone, 1991).

Educating

Along with reframing of current difficulties, refocusing must occur. Clients must be provided with information about their injury and current skills and capabilities and must be given conservative estimations for potential recovery (Harrell, and O'Hara, 1991; Miller, 1994a). Information should be tailored carefully to meet both the comprehension abilities and the needs of the client. It is the therapist's responsibility to assess how best to present the information, when to present it and, perhaps most crucially, whether to present it. Children and adolescents may need to hold on to their denial to cope with their reality. As long as that denial is not impeding functional performance and progress, little reason exists to challenge it (Bracy, 1994; Cicerone, 1989; Elliott et al., 1991; Miller, 1991).

Reorienting

After information is provided, clients must be helped to realize that there is a future and that, although restrictions exist, they must be encouraged to find new dreams and challenges. Often two additional issues may have to be addressed: Clients may need to accept that they have experienced a trauma, and they may need to integrate it into their self-schema. This acceptance may be expressed through repeated requests to have others tell them what happened or perseverative recounting of the accident to others. In a piagetian sense, children or adolescents are, in these behaviors, accommodating their self-schema or assimilating their trauma into a new self-schema. Adolescents who were injured in childhood, may minimize, or be encouraged to minimize, the effects of their brain injury. Therapeutic interventions may help the adolescent face these limitations and move past them. These changes are not a uniform process: Clients may express acceptance or awareness of their deficits only to "forget" them and to experience the insight's reappearance at a later stage (Janoff-Bulman and Schwartzberg, 1991). This intermittent forgetfulness and recall can be quite frustrating to both the therapist and the environment (Miller, 1991).

Furthermore, if the trauma occurred through no fault of children or adolescents with TBI, feelings of "why me?" may emerge, as their view of the world as a fair and just place is threatened. Alternatively, if clients were responsible for their trauma, "survivor's guilt" may emerge. Either perspective can undermine rehabilitation efforts, as clients may cease to try or may engage in self-destructive behaviors as a form of self-punishment (Janoff-Bulman and Schwartzberg, 1991; Miller, 1994a).

Reframing of events, realistic appraisal of past events, and ways to avoid future injury may have to be developed to decrease the use of ineffective coping strategies, such as denial, resignation, and escape (Moore and Stambrook, 1994). Woven into the psychotherapeutic fabric must be cognitive-behavioral interventions designed to identify, dispute, and replace dysfunctional or inaccurate beliefs. Such interventions must be combined with, or occur parallel to, neuropsychologically based cognitive rehabilitation skills aimed at reducing black-and-white, concrete ways of thinking (Moore and Stambrook, 1995).

Coping with Failure

As children and adolescents with TBI set out on the course of physical and psychological recovery, setbacks are inevitable. Preparing for them by cautioning the client (Cicerone, 1991) and preparing the family and environment to expect the subsequent distress (Miller, 1993) may both establish the therapist as an expert and contain some of the inevitable disappointment brought on by such setbacks. In cases in which denial or poor self-awareness result in an overestimation of skills, planned failures—occurring in the real world (as opposed to an inpatient setting)—may enable clients to safely learn their limitations (Butler and Satz, 1988). These experiences may have to be repeated before a client, whose limited self-awareness is organically based, internalizes the lesson. As with children who are first learning these skills, these developmental experiences can also serve as opportunities to test newly learned skills (Harrell and O'Hara, 1991) and can become the source of new self-efficacy and a sense of mastery and esteem.

Focal Points of Therapeutic Interventions

Independence

Involving adolescents in consultations during rehabilitation and encouraging them to set the goals they want to accomplish can promote feelings of independence and motivate them to try harder and adhere to the program longer. Goal setting also provides an opportunity to regain a sense of mastery as clients achieve the goals. Further, with appropriate facilitation, goal setting allows adolescents to gradually increase self-awareness of their new limitations (Bergquist and Jacket, 1993; Webb and Glueckauf, 1994). For children who cannot be integrated into traditional sports, organizations such as the Brain Injury Association can often refer parents to recreational programs designed for individuals with more limited capabilities (e.g., Fines and Nichols, 1994).

Education

Although high schools have legal obligations to provide education (Public Law 94-142 and the Education for All Handicapped Children Act, 1975; Savage and Carter, 1991), the legal rights of adolescents with TBI at the college level are different. Both parents and adolescents may need to be encouraged to re-evaluate their expectations and perhaps consider alternatives, such as testing to assess employability (Lam et al., 1991). Vocational training and job coaching may also be alternatives (Brantner, 1992; Kreutzer et al., 1989). When the services of the department of vocational rehabilitation are not needed imminently, contact should be made on behalf of both the child and the adolescent, so that the system will be familiar with their cases and quick to respond should the need arise (Savage and Carter, 1991).

Sex and Sexuality

Parents may have the misguided belief that talking about sex with their adolescent is irrelevant (because of the changed circumstances) or even harmful (i.e., "giving the kid ideas"). Family members must be encouraged to perceive their young adult as able to pursue, and capable of, attachment and, within the limitations set by the injury, competent for and deserving of intimate and sexual relationships. Adolescents may require education in the mechanics of both partnered and self-sex (Miller, 1994b), and in the effects medications may have on performance. The issues of contraception in general and safe sex in particular must also be addressed. If adolescents continuously fail in their efforts to have satisfying sexual experiences, more extreme measures, such as psychological sex therapy in the PLISSIT (Permission, Limited Information, Specific Suggestion, Intensive Therapy [Annon, 1974]) spirit, may be required. Sexual ignorance can be addressed by a sex educator, sexual discomfort can be handled by a sex counselor, sex problems arising from a relationship conflict can be dealt with by a marital therapist, sex problems stemming from a psychological conflict can be addressed by a psychotherapist. When all these problems are intertwined, a client can be referred to a sex therapist (Halvorsen and Metz, 1992). Alternatively, a designated counselor-confidant can be chosen, one who is comfortable in discussing any questions that arise and in providing educated information rather than myth and misinformation.

Therapeutic Techniques

Memory Book

Children or adolescents may use a memory book to document and remind them of past and future events. Cue cards with appropriate responses to certain situations may also be helpful, with a small cue from the environment advising the client to use the card (Bracy, 1994). At the very least, however, clients must be able to remember to have someone read to them from the book or must be able to read it by themselves.

Relaxation Training and Stress Management

Relaxation training can help reduce anxiety in general and social anxiety in particular (Butler and Satz, 1988; Newton and Johnson, 1985). Stress management can be effective in reducing arousal that can precipitate inappropriate expressions of anger (Miller, 1991). Both of these techniques can be adapted to children, using music to facilitate relaxation and computer games to teach biofeedback for tension reduction. An excellent resource is *The Relaxation and Stress Reduction Workbook* (Davis et al., 1995).

Role Playing

Inappropriate processing of social cues and decreased social interaction are particularly common after TBI. Role playing, appropriate for all age groups, can be used to teach social skills (Johnson and Newton, 1987) in general and interpersonal skills in particular (Medlar, 1993). It is also effective in increasing empathy by teaching clients to practice taking another person's perspective.

Checklists and Self-Monitoring Inventories

Asking clients to self-monitor through lists and inventories can be used to increase self-awareness (Cicerone, 1989). In instances when children or adolescents report that they are being treated unfairly or complain of mistreatment, checklists may be effective in gathering concrete data or actual prevalence of these complaints.

Videotaping

Videotaping may be used as a memory aid to allow clients to review psychotherapy sessions or as a basis for feedback after role playing, when they can review their performance (Cicerone, 1989). The use of videotapes also allows clients to objectify their evaluation. It may facilitate increased self-awareness, as clients can learn to self-review and self-critique more accurately, and clients can watch the tapes as many times as needed. Videotaping is also an effective tool to record progress in the mastery of a skill.

Support Groups

Support groups are an excellent opportunity for clients to practice social skills in a real-world setting, increasing social interaction and receiving support from the few people who know what they have gone through (Miller, 1992). Facilitation by a trained group leader is needed to ensure appropriate pragmatics—that is, the give and take of a conversation, maintaining focus, and so forth.

Group Therapy

Much like support groups, group therapy is an opportunity to practice social skills. Because of its professional guidance and therapeutic focus, it can also provide more structured feedback about such performance. Group therapy can facilitate increased self-awareness, as clients receive feedback about their interpersonal style and adroitness (Lynch and Kosciulek, 1995).

Community-Based Activities

Fear of failure and of being embarrassed may inhibit children or adolescents from going into the community. However, a community-based sortie to a place of their choosing may both encourage them to test newly learned skills—from maneuvering a wheelchair to interpersonal activity—and may transfer some control over the rehabilitation process back to them (Cicerone, 1989).

Planning Tasks

Practicing complex processing, or multi-step cognitive exercises, in the office or hospital setting is an artificial way to cognitively retrain children or adolescents. This goal can also be achieved by allowing clients to plan a desired activity, such as going to the movies or making a favorite sandwich or dish, and carefully guiding and cueing the clients to the components of the tasks. After several attempts, clients may be allowed to develop the plans on their own and may also be given the opportunity to fail. The therapist may purposefully not remind them of all the stages of the task. When a difficulty is encountered, clients should be given the opportunity to explore or practice self-correcting tactics (Miller, 1991).

Communication

Variations of traditional psychotherapy and counseling are also effective. However, sessions should be shorter and more frequent to accommodate fatigue, attention span, and the client's limited memory skills. Interruptions such as telephones and other environmental distractions are to be kept to a minimum (Marme and Skord, 1993). Verbal communications should be made in short, simple sentences, repeated and paraphrased if needed. Children or adolescents should be asked to repeat and elaborate on what they have been told, to enhance retention and decrease parroting of the instructions (Bracy, 1994).

During sessions, the use of creative therapeutic techniques and props is encouraged (Jacobs, 1992). Props are helpful in engaging the child and may appeal to the adolescent if appropriately presented. However, both willingness to use and ability to comprehend the metaphor of props is necessary.

Any communication with children or adolescents should be directed to their current strongest sensory modality (Marme and Skord, 1993). Immediately after injury, music may be appropriate, though visual stimulation may be more appropriate later in recovery.

Humor can be an effective form of communication, as long as the client is capable of registering the humor. TBI may limit comprehension of linguistic nuances, curtail affective expression even if the joke was understood, or impede ability to recognize prosodic changes on which the punch line may rely. Before therapists engage in humor, they should test both the strength of their bond with a child (should a misunderstanding occur) and the child's or adolescent's linguistic skills.

Music

Music may be used to stimulate and draw out the comatose patient-client, soothe irritated spirits, and create a sense of familiarity in a depersonalized environment (Claeys et al., 1989). The use of music in this manner may be effective for both a child and an adolescent, for whom music often is a primary mode of expression. It can also be an indirect way to communicate feelings that a client finds difficult to label, admit, or put into words (Prigatano, 1991).

Stories, Myths, and Fables

The telling of stories is a form of communication with which children are familiar. This is no less true of children with TBI, but only if they are not restricted by concrete thinking, which can limit ability to understand the metaphor. Stories and fables are also a safe way for children or adolescents to share of themselves, relating stories about a third person (a variation on "I have a friend with this problem . . .") who may be encountering difficulties (Prigatano, 1991). Using props, such as puppets and stuffed animals, allows clients to neutralize or distance themselves from a painful emotion or a difficult situation. For further suggestions regarding ways to integrate props into therapy, *Creative Counseling Techniques: An Illustrated Guide* (Jacobs, 1992) is recommended. Stories and fairy tales can also offer opportunities to learn how others have mastered a situation and to glean cultural mores and values (Bettelheim, 1975; Prigatano, 1991).

Counseling and Coordination of Services

Bobby was 2 years old when he fell from a second-story window of his mother's apartment. After a protracted neurosurgical and neurorehabilitation inpatient course, he returned to his mother's care. Outpatient rehabilitation efforts were stymied by repeated missed appointments and frustrated attempts to engage social service agencies to intervene. The family eventually relocated out of state so the mother could pursue a new relationship. Therapists in the new town were contacted by the mother on advice of her child's attorney, who was preparing a lawsuit against the former landlord. Evaluation at this point (now approximately 2 years later) revealed a child with precipitous crying outbursts alternating with impaired ability to sustain attention. Initial medication intervention with methylphenidate was unsuccessful. Some question of diversion of this stimulant for recreational purposes arose. The therapist was cast in a surrogate parent role because of the mother's chaotic parenting. A referral to child protective services was made to assess the child's supervision and the overall stability of the household. During a period of intensive supervision, testing revealed the presence of abnormal spike-wave complexes in the left temporal region, and carba-

mazepine therapy was initiated. Improvement in affective lability was noted, and monitoring of drug levels provided a mechanism to supervise and ensure appropriate parenting activities. When Bobby was 8 years old, therapeutic attention was centered on assisting the child to understand the need for medication and to share the responsibility with his mother. Counseling activities also addressed managing the social isolation and chaotic environment of the family and assigning a financial trust officer to oversee the settlement of the legal suit and to ensure that funds were used for treatment for the child.

Self-Esteem and Identity

Throughout his school years, Tom had been an honors student. At the time of his injury at age 14, he was enrolled at a regional high school for the academically gifted. Problems with expressive language and writing cohesion emerged after the injury, which led to significant academic decline. Tom's frustration mounted as he was unable clearly to articulate his distress to his parents and teachers. Lack of TBI education resulted in teacher ignorance of why Tom could remain gifted in certain domains while failing in others. Consequently, the teachers accused Tom of malingering and being lazy. Initial referral for evaluation occurred after a period of progressive social withdrawal, suicidal threats, and suspected alcohol use. Tom endorsed numerous neurovegetative symptoms of depression and focused on how different studying was for him after the injury. Before his injury, he was able to retain information after one reading. He now required several readings to retain information, while still continuing to falter in higher-level linguistic analytic and synthesis skills. Therapeutic interventions included antidepressant medication for his neurovegetative symptoms, neurolinguistic therapy for his language deficits, and counseling for his parents and himself. Counseling with the parents addressed grieving for the lost intellectual capacity of their child and the loss of reflected esteem for their child's accomplishments. Tom's sessions focused on his nonverbal strengths and creativity, including facility with computer hardware installation and auto mechanics. To facilitate the therapeutic bond, treatment sessions as often as not occurred while playing catch in the parking lot of the office. To underscore the strength of the therapist's confidence in Tom, an offer by Tom to detail and accent-stripe the therapist's new car was accepted in lieu of typical copayment. These actions served to acknowledge Tom's emerging independence from his parents and his responsibility to maximize his potential. Assistance with reducing his academic load and supporting his local teachers with technical instructional assistance also decreased his overall distress and improved his sense of self.

Denial, Lack of Awareness, and Substance Abuse

Kelley sustained her brain injury when she was 13 years old, while drinking and driving with older friends. Neurodiagnostic studies demonstrated persistent frontal lobe structural changes and electrophysiologic irritability. As her physical recovery was remarkable, she quickly reentered the social milieu that fostered her injury. Attempts by her mother (the custodial parent) to control her were met with rebellious outbursts. Visits with her father were characterized by an absence of limit setting and a tacit approval of her "resocialization." Clear determination of parental legal responsibility for treatment was defined, and Kelley was engaged in therapy. Treatment issues centered on establishing parental responsibility for limit setting and review of age-appropriate behaviors. Kelley's lack of awareness of her deficits was addressed through an intensive educational program regarding the brain and its function, including review of x-rays and brain scans from her own care. Community-based examples of her irritability were elicited from parents and siblings. Despite these measures, she repeatedly minimized her problems and externalized them. Only when she was attempting to obtain her learners' permit did the therapeutic opportunity of a lifetime arise. Alcohol monitoring and behavioral checklist implementation both at home and in school were used to "grade" her and provide reinforcement with behind-the-wheel driving time. Once the behavioral structure was established, counseling sessions focused on grieving and on injury adaptation issues could begin.

Sex and Impulsivity

Steve sustained TBI at age 12, resulting in significant frontal lobe injury. As he entered puberty, his level of interest in the opposite sex increased; however, due to his impulsive, pragmatically disordered style, few girls of his age would talk with, let alone date, him. The use of carbamazepine to reduce impulsivity during this developmental stage assisted somewhat in reducing his overt intrusiveness. In his late teens, Steve engaged in a series of disastrous encounters, from following women home from work to soliciting phone numbers from every woman he met. Desperate, he sought advice, asking the therapist's beliefs regarding prostitution. In session, the therapist explored the legal nature of such encounters, the potential physical danger associated with the location of such women, and the practical aspects of condom use. Information regarding sexually transmitted diseases and AIDS was also provided. Steve contemplated the level of his estrangement and alienation from the world and initiated a conversation regarding celibacy and monasticism. The therapist indicated that such dichotomous thinking was due to his injury, but that his belief that he was only lovable "when he paid for it" or when he renounced everything suggested lowered self-value.

Steve was encouraged to involve himself at a local animal shelter to foster self-esteem, while interacting with the public in a more controlled and structured context. Practice sessions involving social conversation with office staff and other young adult women were initiated, along with social skills training in a group format, with videotaping of the interactions for group critique.

References

Annon JS (1974). The Behavioral Treatment of Sexual Problems. New York: Harper & Row.

Bergquist TF, Jacket MP (1993). Awareness and goal setting with the traumatically brain injured. Brain Inj 7;275.

Bettelheim B (1975). The Uses of Enchantment: The Meaning and Importance of Fairy Tales. New York: Penguin.

Beutler LE, Clarkin J, Crago M, Bergen J (1991). Client-Therapist Matching. In CR Snyder, DR Forsyth (eds), Handbook of Social and Clinical Psychology. New York: Pergamon, 699.

Boyer MG, Edwards P (1991). Outcome 1 to 3 years after severe traumatic brain injury in children and adolescents. Injury 22;315.

Bracy OL III (1994). Counseling and psychotherapy for those with brain injury. J Cogn Rehabil 12;8.

Brantner CL (1992). Job coaching for persons with traumatic brain injuries employed in professional and technical occupations. J Appl Rehabil Counsel 23;3.

Brooke MM, Questad KA, Patterson DR, Valois TA (1992). Driving evaluation after traumatic brain injury. Am J Phys Med Rehabil 71;177.

Butler RW, Satz P (1988). Individual psychotherapy with head-injured adults: clinical notes for the practitioner. Prof Psychol Res Pract 19;536.

Cicerone KD (1989). Psychotherapeutic interventions with traumatically brain-injured patients. Rehab Psychol 34;105.

Cicerone KD (1991). Psychotherapy after mild traumatic brain injury: relation to the nature and severity of subjective complaints. J Head Trauma Rehabil 6;30.

Claeys MS, Miller AC, Dalloul-Rampersad R, Kollar M (1989). The role of music and music therapy in the rehabilitation of traumatically brain injured clients. Music Ther Perspect 6;71.

Coster WJ, Haley S, Baryza MJ (1994). Functional performance of young children after traumatic brain injury: a 6-month follow-up study. Am J Occup Ther 48;211.

Davis DL, Schneider LK (1990). Ramifications of traumatic brain injury for sexuality. J Head Trauma Rehabil 5;31.

Davis M, Eshelman ER, McKay M (1995). The Relaxation and Stress Reduction Workbook (4th ed). Oakland, CA: New Harbinger Publications.

DePompei R, Williams J (1994). Working with families after TBI: a family-centered approach. Top Lang Dis 15;68.

DeSpelder LA, Strickland AL (1987). The Last Dance: Encountering Death and Dying (2nd ed). Mountain View, CA: Mayfield Publishing.

Ducharme S, Gill KM, Biener-Bergman S, Fertitta LC (1993). Sexual Functioning: Medical and Psychological Aspects. In JA DeLisa (ed), Rehabilitation Medicine: Principles and Practice (2nd ed). Philadelphia: Lippincott, 763.

Elliott TR, Witty TE, Herrick S, Hoffman JT (1991). Negotiating reality after physical loss: hope, depression and disability. J Pers Soc Psychol 61;1.

Erikson E (1977). Childhood and Society. St. Albans, England: Triad/Leaf, Paladin.

Erlich IS (1983). Speaking the same language. J Am Coll Health 31;174.

Fines L, Nichols D (1994). An evaluation of a twelve-week recreational kayak program: effects on self-concept, leisure satisfaction and leisure attitude of adults with traumatic brain injuries. J Cogn Rehabil 12;10.

Fleming J, Strong J (1995). Self-awareness of deficits following acquired brain injury: considerations for rehabilitation. Br J Occup Ther 58;55.

Gasquoine PG, Gibbons TA (1994). Lack of awareness of impairment in institutionalized, severely and chronically disabled survivors of traumatic brain injury: a preliminary investigation. J Head Trauma Rehabil 9;16.

Gronwall D, Wrightson P, Waddell P (1990). Head Injury—The Facts: A Guide for Families and Care-Givers. Oxford: Oxford University.

Halvorsen JG, Metz ME (1992). Sexual dysfunction, part II: diagnosis, management and prognosis. J Am Board Fam Pract 5;177.

Harrell M, O'Hara CO (1991). Meeting the emotional needs of brain injury survivors: an empowerment approach to psychotherapy. Cogn Rehabil 9;12.

Jacobs E (1992). Creative Counseling Techniques: An Illustrated Guide. Odessa, FL: Psychological Assessment Resources.

Jacobs HE (1989). Long-Term Family Intervention. In DW Ellis, AL Christensen (eds), Neuropsychological Treatment After Brain Injury. Boston: Kluwer Academic, 297.

Jacobs HE (1991). Family and Behavioral Issues. In JM Williams, T Kay (eds), Head Injury: A Family Matter. Baltimore: Paul H. Brookes, 239.

Jacobs HE (1993). Behavior Analysis Guidelines and Brain Injury Rehabilitation: People, Principles, and Programs. Gaithersburg, MD: Aspen.

James EM, Reynolds CR (1994). Barriers to Serving Children with Traumatic Brain Injury in the Public Schools: Problems and Solutions. College Station, TX: Texas A&M University. (ERIC Document Reproduction Service No. ED 377 664.)

Janoff-Bulman R, Schwartzberg SS (1991). Toward a General Model of Personal Change. In CR Snyder, DR Forsyth (eds), Handbook of Social and Clinical Psychology. New York: Pergamon, 488.

Johnson DA, Newton A (1987). HIPSIG: a basis for social adjustment after head injury. Br J Occup Ther 50;47.

Kaplan HI, Sadock BJ (1991). Comprehensive Glossary of Psychiatry and Psychology. Baltimore: Williams & Wilkins.

Kaplan SH, Greenfield S, Ware JE (1989). Assessing the effects of physician-patient interactions on the outcomes of chronic disease. Med Care 27(Suppl);110.

Kaplan SP (1988). Adaptation following serious brain injury: an assessment after one year. J Appl Rehabil Counsel 19;3.

Kolb B, Whishaw IQ (1996). Fundamentals of Human Neuropsychology (4th ed). New York: Freeman.

Kramer J (1991). Special Issues for a Parent. In JM Williams, T Kay (eds), Head Injury: A Family Matter. Baltimore: Paul H. Brookes, 9.

Kreutzer J, Conder R, Wehman P, Morrison C (1989). Compensatory strategies for enhancing independent living and vocational outcome following traumatic brain injury. Cogn Rehabil 7;30.

Lam CS, Priddy DA, Johnson P (1991). Neuropsychological indicators of employability following traumatic brain injury. Rehabil Counsel Bull 35;68.

Langer KG, Padrone FJ (1992). Psychotherapeutic treatment of awareness in acute rehabilitation of traumatic brain injury. Neuropsychol Rehabil 2;59.

Leaf LE (1991). Relationship therapy: a psychotherapeutic approach with persons sustaining brain injury. Cogn Rehabil 9;14.

Leaf LE (1993). Traumatic brain injury: affecting family recovery. Brain Inj 7;543.

Leichtman M (1992). Psychotherapeutic interventions with brain-injured children and their families: I. diagnosis and treatment planning. Bull Menninger Clin 56;321.

Levine MJ, Van Horn KR, Curtis AB (1993). Developmental models of social cognition in assessing psychosocial adjustment in head injury. Brain Inj 7;153.

Lewington PJ (1993). Counseling survivors of traumatic brain injury. Can J Counsel 27;274.

Lezak MD (1978). Living with the characterologically altered brain injured patient. J Clin Psychiatr 39;592.

Lezak MD (1983). Neuropsychological Assessment (2nd ed). New York: Oxford University.

Lynch RT, Kosciulek JF (1995). Integrating individuals with traumatic brain injury into the group process. J Spec Group Work 20;108.

Maddux JE (1991). Self-Efficacy. In CR Snyder, DR Forsyth (eds), Handbook of Social and Clinical Psychology. New York: Pergamon, 57.

Mapou RL (1990). Traumatic brain injury rehabilitation with gay and lesbian individuals. J Head Trauma Rehabil 5;67.

Marme M, Skord K (1993). Counseling strategies to enhance

the vocational rehabilitation of persons after traumatic brain injury. J Appl Rehabil Counsel 24;19.

McDowell I, Anderson S, Wilson C, Pentland B (1995). Late rehabilitation for closed head injury: clinical psychologists' interventions. Clin Rehabil 9;150.

Medlar TM (1993). Sexual counseling and traumatic brain injury. Sex Dis 11;57.

Miller L (1991). Psychotherapy of the brain-injured patient: principles and practices. Cogn Rehabil 9;24.

Miller L (1992). When the best help is self-help, or, everything you always wanted to know about brain injury support groups. J Cogn Rehabil 10;14.

Miller L (1993). Psychotherapy of the Brain-Injured Patient: Reclaiming the Shattered Self. New York: Norton.

Miller L (1994a). Civilian post-traumatic stress disorder: clinical syndromes and psychotherapeutic strategies. Psychotherapy 31;655.

Miller L (1994b). Sex and the brain-injured patient: regaining love, pleasure, and intimacy. J Cogn Rehabil 12;12.

Moore AD, Stambrook M (1994). Coping following traumatic brain injury (TBI): derivation and validation of TBI sample ways of coping—revised subscales. Can J Rehabil 7;193.

Moore AD, Stambrook M (1995). Cognitive moderators of outcome following traumatic brain injury: a conceptual model and implications for rehabilitation. Brain Inj 9;109.

Newton A, Johnson DA (1985). Social adjustment and interaction after severe head injury. Br J Clin Psychol 24;225.

O'Brien KP, Prigatano GP (1991). Supportive psychotherapy for a patient exhibiting alexia without agraphia. J Head Trauma Rehabil 6;44.

Perlesz A, Furlong M, McLachlan D (1992). Family work and acquired brain damage. Aust N Z J Fam Ther 13;145.

Prigatano GP (1991). Disordered mind, wounded soul: the emerging role of psychotherapy in rehabilitation after brain injury. J Head Trauma Rehabil 6;1.

Prigatano GP, Leatham JM (1993). Awareness of behavioral limitations after traumatic brain injury: a cross-cultural study of New Zealand Maoris and non-Maoris. Clin Neuropsychol 7;123.

Prigatano GP, Schacter DL (eds) (1991). Awareness of Deficit After Brain Injury: Clinical and Theoretical Issues. New York: Oxford University.

Ranseen JD, Bohaska LA, Schmitt FA (1990). An investigation of anosognosia following traumatic head injury. Int J Clin Neuropsychol 12;29.

Russell NK (1993). Educational considerations in traumatic brain injury: the role of the speech-language pathologist. Lang Speech Hear Serv Schools 24;67.

Savage RC, Carter RR (1991). Family and Return to School. In JM Williams, T Kay (eds), Head Injury: A Family Matter. Baltimore: Paul H Brookes, 203.

Schmidt MF, Garvin LJ, Heinemann AW, Kelly JP (1995). Gender- and age-related role changes following brain injury. J Head Trauma Rehabil 10;14.

Sigler G, Mackelprang RW (1993). Cognitive impairments: psychosocial and sexual implications and strategies for social work intervention. J Soc Work Hum Sex 8;89.

Sparadeo FR, Strauss D, Kapsalis KB (1992). Substance abuse, brain injury, and family adjustment. Neurorehabilitation 2;65.

Wallston KA (1989). Assessment of Control in Health-Care Settings. In A Steptoe, A Appels (eds), Stress, Personal Control and Health. New York: Wiley, 85.

Webb PM, Glueckauf RL (1994). The effects of direct involvement in goal setting on rehabilitation outcome for persons with traumatic brain injuries. Rehabil Psychol 39;179.

Willer B, Allen K, Durnan MC, Ferry A (1990). Problems and coping strategies of mothers, siblings and young adult males with traumatic brain injury. Can J Rehabil 3;167.

Williams D (1994a). Seizures Following Traumatic Brain Injury. (ERIC Document Reproduction Service No. ED 373 476.)

Williams D (1994b). Traumatic Brain Injury: When Children Return to School. (ERIC Document Reproduction Service No. ED 373 475.)

Williams JM (1991). Family Reaction to Head Injury. In JM Williams, T Kay (eds), Head Injury: A Family Matter. Baltimore: Paul H Brookes, 81.

Williams JM, Savage RC (1991). Family, Culture, and Child Development. In JM Williams, T Kay (eds), Head Injury: A Family Matter. Baltimore: Paul H Brookes, 219.

Wright BA (1991). Labeling: The Need for Greater Person-Environment Individuation. In CR Snyder, DR Forsyth (eds), Handbook of Social and Clinical Psychology. New York: Pergamon, 469.

Ylvisaker M (1993). Communication outcome in children and adolescents with traumatic brain injury. Neuropsychol Rehabil 3;367.

Chapter 16
Families of Children with Traumatic Brain Injury

Pamela K. Waaland

The crisis of childhood brain injury challenges the integrity of even the most unified family. Researchers have documented the effects of chronic disabilities on families (Wallander et al., 1989; Wilkins, 1979). Parents of children with chronic disabilities can adapt gradually and do not face the inevitable crisis of brain trauma in a child—one day a whole child, the next a child whose survival is questionable. In contrast, families who face brain trauma in a child must adapt rapidly, not only to expectations and roles but to the multiple needs and uncertain future of their children. Such families are confronted with the medical problems of hearing, visual, and motor impairment. Family members also must adapt to the child's struggle to communicate, solve simple problems, control labile emotions, and regulate aggressive outbursts. These concerns often translate into troubled days, sleepless nights, financial and transportation demands, community embarrassment, and family conflict (Waaland and Raines, 1991).

The 1994 mission for survivors of traumatic brain injury (TBI), as promulgated by the Brain Injury Association (formerly the National Head Injury Foundation), parallels this chapter's mission for its readers: healing, caring, passion, and unity. Its goal is to foster professional understanding, compassion, and services needed to promote family healing. To that end, it provides an overview of common reactions and needs of family survivors of pediatric TBI and offers treatment strategies helpful in addressing family issues.

Effects of Childhood Brain Trauma on Families

"No words are adequate to express the comprehensive sorrow, pain, anger, disappointment, and hope shared by persons and families changed and challenged by the impact of a head injury" (Dell Orto and Power, 1994). In contrast to many illnesses that resolve with resump-

tion of life through cure or with mourning in the event of death, families must adapt to the loss of the "old person" while caring for multiple needs of their new family member (Williams, 1991). The disruption to family equilibrium is even more intense when the injured person is a child.

What happens to families whose child has experienced TBI? Until Lezak (1978, 1986) addressed family issues, TBI was designated as a *medical* rather than a *family* problem. Lezak's seminal work has made professionals increasingly aware that not only survivors but family members experience reactive trauma and a healing process. Polinko and colleagues (1985) modified Lezak's theory to address family reactions to TBI. Both these stage theories link perceptions of the child to injury, tie family expectations to recovery, and connect coping mechanisms to periods of the child's recovery (Waaland, 1990). A summary of Polinko and colleagues' (1985) model and clinical prescriptions paralleling each stage appear in Table 16-1. Understandably, the family's initial shock and disbelief that "this is happening" change to elation and relief on learning their child will live rather than die. However, the family quickly learns that life will not be as it previously was. Their expectations move from believing that they will "get their child back" to depression and mourning when it becomes apparent that deficits are relatively permanent.

These theories recognize that the often delicate balance of family life is destroyed by the tragic injury and threatened life of a loved one. Imagine for a moment that your daughter, Lauren, is injured tragically. You are called to the hospital. You don't remember much of what the caller said—except for such isolated words as "accident," "injured," and "emergency room"—or even driving to the hospital. You see Lauren lying motionless, surrounded by the tubes and machines that sustain her. Passively you hear medical terms, confusing information—but that no, she will not die.

Table 16-1. Common Family Reactions and Prescriptions During Sequential Postinjury Phases

Stage	Reaction	Clinical Role
Injury stabilization	Shock, denial, and panic	Provide simplified, consistent information; lend support; provide reassurance about the quality of care
Return to consciousness	Relief, massive denial	Stabilize family resources and roles; orient slowly to possible realities; attend to siblings' needs
Rehabilitation phase	Variability: continued denial, anxiety, and guilt; anger and depression	Normalize feelings and needs; focus on family communication; address physical, social, and supportive needs of family members
Return to community	Depression, anger, grief	Promote nondefensive attitude; normalize family structure; facilitate transition; work toward acceptance and action

Source: Adapted from PR Polinko, JJ Barin, D Leger, KM Bachman (1985). Working with the Family. In M Ylvisaker (ed), Head Injury Rehabilitation. San Diego: College Hill, 91. Copyright 1997, Butterworth–Heinemann.

And she doesn't. Your family rejoices as she emerges from coma a month later. You celebrate the return of family life. Months later, however, she still speaks little, cannot walk, and seems like a "changed" person—but no, everything will be all right. Your spouse seems to cry all the time. Neither of you sleeps through the night. You have nightmares about the drunken driver who stripped away your child's identity and took away normal family life. You recall how your joyful anticipation of Lauren's return to school turned quickly to anxiety and confusion when the team discussed "special classes" and "retarded functioning—that will get better." You think about that first day, when Lauren threw her video game against the wall and screamed uncontrollably, "I can't do it." She and her sister both refused to go to school the next day. You were late for work, blew up at your secretary, shouted at Lauren's teacher, and went to your office and sobbed, "Why me … Why her?" Mourning for the permanence of Lauren's injuries gradually replaces dreams of recovery promised by her rehabilitation team. Although sadness often returns when you see Lauren's old friends or the soccer field on which she played, over time you come to accept the new little girl and rejoice in her little triumphs.

The foregoing theories and family member's true experiences are validated by our clinical experiences. Thus, writings of Lezak and others have raised awareness of common family reactions after injury. At the same time, the premise that most families follow a predictable course is based on clinical impressions rather than on research. These impressions do not explain the diversity of ways in which families appraise and react to this stressful life event (Rape et al., 1992). Some family members may follow predictable paths. Other family members instead describe a "roller-coaster" ride of emotions. The reader—savvy in rehabilitation terminology, treatment, and expectations—undoubtedly would react to Lauren's injury differently from a high-school dropout with limited resources or life experiences. Thus, the family's life experiences, lifestyle, and perceptions before injury may predict family reactions better than can the severity of, or elapsed time since, the injury (Dell Orto and Powers, 1994; Lezak, 1994; Rivara et al., 1992; Waaland, 1992).

What could possibly change family members' perceptions of such a tragic event? First, *past and present medical experiences* modify family reactions. Lezak (1994) emphasized that "family denial" is not a pathologic response but rather a normal consequence of *expectations, experience,* and *cultural exposure to illness*. In particular, media portrayals of miraculous recoveries rather than realistic outcomes significantly alter family members' expectations for recovery. *Contradictory* or *confusing advice from experts* (e.g., professional statements about recovery rather than improvement) also prolongs the family's healing process. Thus, family confusion about the injured child reflects more than survivor confusion. Practitioners receive and give conflicting information about how, for how long, or to what extent children of different ages are affected by their injuries. Family experience with normal developmental variations, such as children who "grow out of" motor or language disabilities, also kindles beliefs that the former child will be restored.

Second, the *family's resources, values,* and *reaction to past crises* are critical determinants of how members will respond to their current crisis (Dell Orto and Powers, 1994; Rivara et al., 1992; Waaland et al., 1993b). Multivariate theories of crisis help to explain why some children and their families are particularly vulnerable and others are extremely resistant to the strain caused by childhood disability (Billings and Moos, 1982; Wallander et al., 1989). These theories focus not on an injured brain but on a brain that belongs to a child; not on a TBI family but on a group of unique individuals who profoundly influence, and are influenced by, other family members' reactions. On the basis of these models, *vulnerability* (risk) for poor outcome is affected by family developmental stage, extent of child disabilities, and additional adversities and stresses experienced by the family.

Table 16-2. Family and Child Characteristics Affecting Vulnerability, Resilience, and Outcome After Injury

Family resources	Family adjustment affected by family's capacity to:
Cohesion and intactness	Provide support and meet intimacy needs
Flexibility	Respond to change and challenges
Parenting skills	Manage child's behaviors
Parenting knowledge	Understand child's needs
Parent health	Give emotionally and physically
Financial resources	Provide for therapy and educational needs
Geographic community	Receive community support and services
Social support systems	Receive emotional and physical assistance
Limited major stresses	Experience decreased emotional burden and health risks
Child's strengths	**Child's adjustment affected by:**
Psychosocial skills	Receipt of support from friends
Knowledge base	Enhanced relearning ability
Intellect and memory	Enhanced new learning ability
Coping skills	Response to primary and secondary effects of injury
Prior mental health	Enhanced emotional reservoir

Resilience, or positive outcome, is affected by multiple factors. These factors include family access to resources that support rehabilitation (e.g., their financial status, community resources, and family cohesiveness) and personal characteristics that enhance role flexibility, problem-solving, and healthy communication. An adapted summary of these models appears in Table 16-2 (Waaland, 1990).

Finally, theorists recently made the important distinction between the *family's phases in adapting to crisis* and their *reaction to crisis*. All families go through phases of adapting to crisis. However, their reactions and resolution often differ (Weltner, 1985; Zarski and DePompei, 1991). Initially, crisis imposes realignment in family roles, communication, and definition. After the immediate crisis, family members develop unique ways of coping or interacting as a normal response to system disequilibrium. Ultimately, the family develops its unique way of achieving the universal need for intimacy and support. Family characteristics will determine how family members respond during each phase. For example, resilient families are able to mobilize their resources, use support systems, and focus on changing attitudes and circumstances within their control. Less adaptive families become immobilized by their losses and are overwhelmed by uncontrollable events. Family members may maintain old family patterns that do not work in the new family. Out of frustration, spouses or siblings may have needs met through work, affairs, or other unhealthy outlets when needs cannot be fulfilled by overwhelmed family members.

The professional will be unable to answer family questions about the future without understanding not only how families experience injury but how the availability of personal resources affects family members many years after the injury. The course of children who miraculously recover or unexplainably get worse is often charted by understanding the environment from which they came and to which they returned. This enlarged conceptual model forms the basis for the family assessment and intervention sections that follow.

Comprehensive Evaluation

Unquestionably, the professional who begins with an objective evaluation of family strengths, weaknesses, characteristics, and needs sets the stage to document the efficient treatment and outcome sought by payers and family members. Unless these issues are addressed, well-intentioned interventions can be sabotaged. The well-planned assessment provides

- A standardized method to evaluate how family members are adapting and what they need
- A baseline to monitor changes in the family's perceptions, interactions, and behavior
- An understanding of a family's uniqueness, talents, and history and how these unique cultural and personal differences affect their treatment needs
- An understanding of the family's knowledge and perspective of injury
- The family's reason for seeking treatment, priorities, and therapy goals

Thus, by the end of the first several meetings, a professional should understand who the family is, why its members seek assistance, and what they hope to gain. That is, do its members seek education or personal support? Do they seek help in accepting life circumstances or "fixing" the child? Were the parents referred due to physician concerns about family adjustment or by an attorney hoping to strengthen the child's legal case? Even when other issues seem pressing, a clinician can strengthen family commitment to treatment by addressing *its* problems. The clinician first should address the family's major concerns and, second, should reframe therapist concerns in a manner consistent with their world view.

Many standardized instruments are available, with norms that quantify how the family is reacting, interacting, and behaving. Only a select subgroup of these instruments has been normed for families coping with TBI. Also, a variety of techniques can be chosen, including paper and pencil or self-report measures, structured interviews, or direct observation. Family assessment tools are described thoroughly in several reviews (Bishop and Miller, 1988; DePompei and Zarski, 1991; Kay et al., 1995; Schwentor and Brown, 1989; Waaland, 1990) and are not summarized in this chapter. Because many instruments are available, it is important to consider both state-of-the-art practices and the evaluator's informational needs.

Standards for an Effective Assessment Battery

The first standard refers to where and how information is obtained rather than what is measured (i.e., properties rather than content of tests). In particular, the use of a multidimensional battery (getting information from different methods and different sources) assures that conclusions are reliable, generalizable, and interpretable (Schwentor and Brown, 1989). By getting different types of information (e.g., teacher ratings vs. direct observations of school behavior) from important people or perspectives (family members vs. teacher), a clinician is more likely to understand the four *W*s (who, what, where, and why) underlying discrepant reports.

Thus, discrepant ratings of an injured youth's behavior by family members, the youth, and significant others (such as a teacher) should be viewed as grist for family therapy and environmental interventions rather than as invalidation of the ratings of any particular rater. Often, an adolescent client, the parents, and the teacher may seem to be rating different persons on the basis of seemingly irreconcilable differences in their perceptions (Waaland, 1992). These disparities often provide information about their different levels of awareness, experience, and objectivity and can guide therapy hypothesis and interventions. For example, the adolescent may deny any problems to avoid being seen as "different." On the basis of the law of averages, the mother may rate problems as more extreme than would the father—who may attribute behavior to stubbornness, overprotective parenting, or even normal adolescence. Varied ratings from the special and regular education teachers may also be understood by differences in their experiences and expectations of students in their classrooms. Other times, ratings may accurately reflect variations in the youth's behavior, depending on reactions to different people and situations. For example, the youth may control anger successfully during school hours but display uncontrollable outbursts directed at one or more

family members in the more accepting home environment. I often use objective observations (and even videotape) to address disagreement among significant others regarding the cause, extremity, and developmental appropriateness of the youth's behavior.

Siblings—typically left out of the assessment process—are often perceptive observers of family dynamics. Siblings also feel less isolated from family life when given the message that their feelings and views are important. Additionally, parents and counselors are able to address confused feelings, inaccurate beliefs, and special needs of siblings on the basis of their interview (see Table 16-3 for a sample sibling clinical interview). For example, "magical thinking" may cause the preoperational preschooler to accept blame for the accident (e.g., "I didn't kiss him good-bye.") and to develop multiple fears and compulsive behaviors (e.g., "I must kiss everyone good-bye or they will get hurt."). Mixed feelings of guilt (e.g., "Why him?"), anger (e.g., "Why not me? He gets attention!"), and fear (e.g., "What if me?") are common. Often, these feelings are missed by the parent consumed by the injured child's needs but are important to target as family therapy issues.

Another important property of an assessment instrument is its *sensitivity to*, and *ability to quantify*, *change*. Thus, measures should be sensitive not only to family deterioration associated with crises but to improvements due to family healing. After the youth is medically stable, the interviewer should ask family members to compare the preinjury and postinjury skills and behavior of the youth and how changes have altered the family's lifestyle. The degree of change indicated by these ratings is a barometer of the family members' stress level. These measurements can serve as a baseline to assess future family change. Studies of family members of adult (Livingston and Brooks, 1988) and child (Jaffee et al., 1993) survivors have documented that family ratings of behavior management problems and personal burdens often increase rather than decrease over time. Often, the professional can circumvent family "burn out" or crisis through routine monitoring and follow-up assessment of family member's adaptation. Important areas include mental health (e.g., brief symptom checklist), adjustment (e.g., family assessment device), and client behavior (e.g., child behavior checklist) (Achenbach, 1951).

Irrespective of the type of measurement selected, the assessment procedure should ultimately answer the question, "Who is this family?" The checklist presented in Appendix 16-1 (Waaland, 1991) is designed to help the clinician to gain a comprehensive understanding of each family. Kay and colleagues (1995) have developed a comprehensive five-part family interview that addresses both research and clinical needs. Their checklist includes comprehensive demographic and preinjury information, perceptions of the patient and significant others (e.g., peer support, educational progress, and injury-related problems and changes), and explanations of the ways in which

Table 16-3. Sample Sibling Interview

Background information
    Family relations before injury: person to whom child was closest, time spent with each family member, roles
    Leisure time: special talents, activities, interests, church and community involvement
    Antisocial activities (substance abuse, sexual activity, etc.)
    Academic adjustment and progress: grade, history of learning or behavior problems, school marks, strengths and weaknesses, attitude toward school
    Peer relations: popularity, type of peer group, level of support at school and home
    Emotional status: history of anxious, depressed, or agitated mood; problems with attention, concentration, and activity
    Unusual thoughts, experiences, fears, or compulsions
    Sleep and appetite disturbance; headaches, stomachaches, or other physical symptoms
    Sexual and physical abuse history
Injury-related changes and perceptions
    Time spent with sibling before the accident and since return home
    Time spent with parents and friends
    Time family spends together and time parents spend with each other
    Understanding of the sibling's disabilities
    Level of involvement during acute and rehabilitation phases
    Fears and misunderstanding about sibling's disabilities and health
    Fears about safety of self or other family members
    Responsibilities at home before and since accident
    Restrictions in previously enjoyed activities
    Restrictions in future plans due to changes in finances or responsibilities
    Changes in school adjustment, achievement, or relationships
    Supportive persons or systems in extended family, school, and community
    Major concerns and stresses
    Feelings of embarrassment, anger, guilt, or sadness directed toward sibling
    Negative feelings directed toward other family members
    Things liked best and things to change about self and family
    Three wishes

Source: Adapted from B Shapiro (1983). Informational interviews. Sibl Info Network News Lett 2.

these circumstances affect family members. A follow-up interview is also provided to address community needs.

Assessment of Family Characteristics

A thorough assessment includes information about the family's history, roles, and resources before and after injury; ethnicity, religious beliefs, and value system; external stresses; and support systems. These defining characteristics of the family will affect how they appraise stress, their attitudes and beliefs about the child's injury and potential progress, and interpretation of the injury. Figure 16-1 presents a modified version of models of family outcome (Singer and Irvin, 1989). This model illustrates how family members' characteristics and resources (see Table 16-2) affect how they perceive and react to crisis. Following is a discussion of ways in which to assess each of the characteristics included in Figure 16-1.

Life Before Injury

Pianist Scott Ocoutt (1994) coined the terms *before injury* and *after injury* from his own tragic personal experience with TBI. Everyone has heard the tired joke: "Doc, will I be able to play the piano?" "Of course." "Good—I never played the piano." As a renowned pianist, Scott Ocoutt is a stellar example of the need to assess life before injury. The most common cause of communication breakdown is the professional's failure to respect the family's lifestyle and values before injury and the changes they have experienced after injury. *Before injury* may represent an "Ozzie and Harriet" family: A "Let's-talk-out-the-problems" approach to conflict. Children from these families typically have not been exposed to sex, drugs, and alcohol. These children likely enjoy excellent family and peer support, academic achievement, and community involvement. At the other extreme are youths at risk for mild to moderate TBI (Rutter et al., 1983; Waaland, 1992). Often, these families are more disengaged, lacking economic resources, good school systems, and even a dual-parent system or transportation to therapy. The importance of respecting sociocultural differences in family treatment planning is addressed in sections that follow.

The Youth's Former Role in the Family

The response to this question often navigates the therapist's course. Was the youth the "black sheep," "mom's

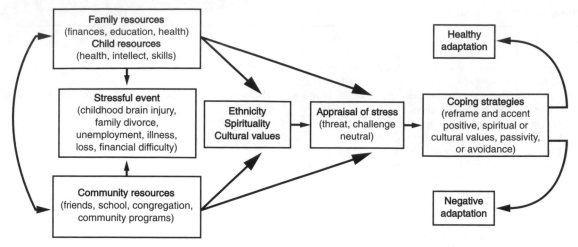

Figure 16-1. Conceptual model of family outcome or adaptation. (Modified from GHS Singer, LK Irvin [1989]. Family Caregiving, Stress, and Support. In GHS Singer, LK Irvin [eds], Support for Caregiving Families: Enabling Positive Adaptation to Disability. Baltimore: Paul H. Brookes.)

favorite," or "marital glue"? What was the youth's birth position and historical importance to the family? Illustrating this point is the Johnson family referred by their physiatrist and guidance counselor for treatment. Professionals were concerned by parents' overindulgence and overprotection of their son, Ronald, following his involvement in a pedestrian accident. Clinical assessment did confirm these parenting behaviors. However, referring professionals did not understand the significance of many years of infertility and multiple miscarriages before Ronald's birth. This information enabled the clinician to defuse defensiveness that previously had been directed toward professionals who "did not understand Ronald" or his significance to the family.

Family Beliefs About the Child's Symptoms, Behavior, and Potential for Recovery

Youths with TBI display many baffling, frustrating behaviors. Some children become withdrawn, anxious, and despondent over many losses and fears about the future. Other children become impulsive, angry, defiant, and even combative. Family members in search of meaning and control develop beliefs about why the child behaves "this way" and how to "fix this problem." Common attributions are that "he was always this way" "she can't help it—it's brain injury," "he got spoiled (fearful) from hospital treatment," or quite often, "Mom just spoils her." Family members often receive contradictory advice from well-meaning friends or relatives. This conflicting advice escalates the family's feelings of confusion, inadequacy, and helplessness. These feelings are particularly pronounced for first-time parents and can cause well-intentioned but unhealthy parenting practices. For example, family members often vacillate between punishing,

rewarding, and ignoring temper outbursts. These inconsistent reactions further confuse the youth with TBI (Waaland and Raines, 1991). Clinical experience suggests that mothers more frequently respond with an attitude of "the flower needs more water and nurturance." In contrast, fathers more often respond with a philosophy of "let nature take its course." Too much or too little sun, water, and nurturance—and particularly inconsistencies in amounts—is harmful to the flower.

Family Members' Interpretation of the Meaning of the Child's Injury

Humans seek not only to maintain security but to explain life events. They naturally seek the cause and meaning of negative events, such as disability (Affleck et al., 1985). Family members may blame the person responsible for the injury, or medical professionals who "did not do things right," or service providers who "didn't tell me that," or even God—"Why me?" When a parent feels personally responsible or blames another family member for injury, these feelings must be assessed and addressed, often repeatedly. Without intervention, the member is likely to develop unhealthy beliefs, parenting patterns, and isolation from family life. Thus, understanding of the family's *world* view or "Mind's Eye" (Lezak, 1994) is critical to understanding the *meaning* of the injury to family life.

Evaluating and Coping with Stress by Family Members

Family perceptions of stressful events and coping mechanisms can show when, where, and how to intervene in ways that will be accepted into family life. A number of measures quantify *environmental stresses* (Holmes and

Rahe, 1967). Common stresses associated with family disability include isolation from the child's friends and other parents, compromised finances, adjustment to the child's disabilities, increased caregiving demands, and coping with future uncertainties (Singer and Irvin, 1989). These constant burdens often increase typical responses to *daily hassles* ranging from a flat tire to a difficult boss.

However, it is the person's appraisal of stress that guides thoughts, attitudes, and behavior. Because individuals in crisis seek stability, family members often rely on comfortable ways of maintaining family integrity (Waaland and Raines, 1991). Before the child's injury, the family may have already displayed unhealthy coping strategies; for example, the mother may have overreacted by striking out, the father may have left passively for work, and the child may have learned to tune out the entire sequence of events. However, the family's prior unhealthy coping strategies will likely escalate to a crisis level after a significant event, such as a child's brain injury. In the face of crisis, the mother is likely to react by escalating her attempts to be heard, the youth by retaliating, and the father by leaving on a business trip. Unable to effectively tune out the problems, siblings may turn to substance abuse or unhealthy peer support for relief. Common coping strategies include passivity or avoidance (minimizing or ignoring problems), reframing or actively solving problems, and relying on the support of religion or significant others (Turnbull and Turnbull, 1991; Waaland, 1990).

Family members' coping mechanisms show where and how to intervene with families. For example, Mr. Lopez always seemed to have emergency trips or late business meetings after Justin's accident. Before the injury, Mr. Lopez enjoyed playing golf, jogging, biking, and camping with his son. Both Justin and Mrs. Lopez felt abandoned when they were in greatest need of his support. His absence also left Mrs. Lopez to provide basic care for Justin and his siblings, to transport them to all appointments, to meet with doctors and teachers, and even to manage complex financial and insurance issues. The reader can see how unhealthy family alliances and interactions and, ultimately, divorce can develop when the coping strategies used by one or both parents interfere with team work and support. These unhealthy relationships must be addressed either directly or indirectly before the family can move forward (see Waaland, 1991).

Finally, often neglected in descriptions of family interactions and reactions is the purpose of assessment: to *address family needs* with respect to the *goal of improved family cohesion, community support, and life satisfaction.* The carefully planned assessment is the vehicle for moving families from crisis intervention to proactive problem solving. After trauma, families must learn quickly about complex medical insurance issues, how to manage finances, and to adapt schedules to meet doctors' appointments and child needs. They must also develop new support networks, negotiate child needs with school systems and other agencies, and cope with emotional strain. Family members understandably differ in the value they place on different services as well as in their perception of how well these needs are being met. The Children's Family Needs Assessment provides the clinician with ratings of family member priorities (ranging from professional, family, and community support to emotional and practical needs) and how well these needs are being met (Kreutzer et al., 1988). These measures help to establish family-directed treatment goals. The therapist who assesses and prioritizes family goals wins the family's confidence needed to help members to look forward rather than dwell on past losses. For example, the mother's highly rated (and unmet) need for respite care should be addressed before the therapist's concern that she caters to the child's every demand.

Meaningful Interventions

Basic to all intervention is respect for changes in treatment paradigms. New prototypes emphasize the movement from patient to person and from therapist to case manager or life skills coach. New models also move from medical- to consumer-based services and, most notably, from crisis management to proactivity and synergy. Within this framework, many helpful tools can enable the family to experience contentment with itself and others.

Respecting Sociocultural Differences

Respect for the values and dignity of each family member—not simply as a family confronted with brain trauma but as unique individuals—is the catalyst to therapeutic progress. From a statistical standpoint, the reader of this chapter most likely is a highly educated Anglo Saxon with values emphasizing independence, self-control, and achievement. The reader also has associated beliefs or "rules" based on family experiences that are reinforced by professional training. These rules offer perceptions of how families should interact, parents should guide children, and individual members should spend productive and leisure time.

In contrast, the recipient of rehabilitative services is represented disproportionately by cultural minority individuals who are poor, undereducated, and underserved. These recipients are often subjected to discrimination and poor treatment by many agencies. Such individuals are more likely to face cultural discrimination on the basis of what they have, believe, and can do (Waaland et al., 1993a). Waaland and colleagues explored the characteristics of families with a child with TBI. Notably, more than two-thirds of high-income caregivers (>$30,000) were married, whereas a majority of the low-income group (<$30,000) were single parents. Over half the former group had a college education, whereas most of the low income caregivers were high-school dropouts. Not surprisingly, these two groups also differed as to the level of their emotional and community support and the presence of other stressful life events or family disability.

Socioeconomic Diversity

Socioeconomic differences also dictate the amount and quality of services families receive. Services received typically stand in stark contrast to service needs. The discrepancy between what the family needs and what it receives typically translates into significant emotional burden on the "have-nots." Such families typically have less money to provide quality rehabilitation or community services and less time to expend on "therapy homework" or even hospital visits. They also have less experience interpreting medical descriptions or negotiating service mazes.

Ms. Miller's experiences with rehabilitative services are not uncommon. Her therapist was recently complaining about Ms. Miller's frequently missed appointments and 8-hour late arrival for her 8-year-old son's discharge. Yet, the same therapist had failed to secure bus tickets for this single parent of three who had no insurance, money, or car. The therapist also had placed Ms. Miller in an educational group with predominantly educated, middle-class parents. Ms. Miller—who attended this group once—concluded that "therapies don't help." This all-too-frequent vignette may help the clinician to understand why persons with limited resources may feel alienated from professionals.

The majority of caregivers with limited resources are more likely to be alienated from not only professionals but from their family members (Waaland et al., 1993a). In contrast, a majority of high-income caregivers react to their child's injury with overinvolvement. Parents without resources often must shut down emotionally to survive. Practical limitations affect parent contact with therapists, educators, and family survivors. These professional and family supports in an ideal world could help caregivers to understand why the patient behaves or thinks differently from before. More importantly, providers could teach family members how to react to these differences and how to get needed services from outside agencies.

Thus, to reach such families with limited resources, the therapist must anticipate (and find solutions for) transportation, job, and respite-care problems. These families need helpful, quality educational services and practical interventions. Therapy assignments, such as charting behavior or carrying out daily reinforcement schedules, often do not fit the routine or lifestyle of many caregivers. Families struggling to survive need

help (and time) to learn how to play, trust, and experience compassion. In contrast, families with bountiful resources often need permission to let go and give greater control to their youngster.

Case Illustration

Illustrating these differences are Shawn and Bobby. Both received moderate injury with prolonged coma and rehabilitation stay. However, Shawn's wealthy family had the resources for extensive private therapeutic regimens, involvement of friends and family, and support from the school where his mother volunteered. Time, parenting skills, and family security also were on his side. Shawn was well-liked by peers and teachers, was very confident in all respects, and was an exceptional student before his injury. Thus, skills learned before the injury helped him to compensate for deficits after his injury. His parents were information seekers who read professional literature, sought second opinions, and adapted a problem-solving orientation toward injury. They made frequent calls to therapists to ensure that they were doing the right thing and to acknowledge their need to "let go." These resources supported successful placement in regular classes and eventually in accelerated courses.

In contrast, Bobby's mother had planned to leave her abusive husband on the night her son was injured in a motor vehicle accident. Bobby—who shared his sister's diagnosis of attention deficit hyperactivity disorder—also shared a bedroom with her in their small one-bedroom apartment. After injury, he received special education services in a preschool classroom but frequently was out of control at school and particularly at home. His knowledge base was limited before the injury. Bobby had great difficulty in self-expression, in learning any types of concepts, and in maintaining any gains after his injury. Mrs. Johnson's history of depression was exacerbated by circumstances surrounding Bobby's injury. Family stress resulted in abusive parenting and referral to child protective services. Understandably, referral for investigation further alienated the family from outsiders. Nevertheless, Mrs. Johnson accepted support from a home-based service team, many community services, and educators. Bobby's therapy team also provided a second family and guided his education program. Supplemental housing, Social Security income benefits, and other forms of governmental support also helped the family to survive financially. Even with these supports, Mrs. Johnson continues to struggle with Bobby's management problems and with personal depression. Bobby and his family have developed a pessimistic, defeatist world view because of their multiple hardships. They have not experienced the successful experiences essential for a healthy image of world and self. These cases are included to help the provider to understand how available resources can direct families encountering trauma in different paths.

Ethnic Background

Ethnicity also affects the types of services appropriate and available to families. Notably, nearly half of all Americans will be nonwhites by the year 2000. Cavallo and Saucedo (1995) have noted that approximately 20 million Hispanics, 1.4 million Native American tribal members, and significantly greater numbers of people of Asian and African descent reside in the United States. Minorities—particularly blacks—are at much higher risk for TBI (Frankowski et al., 1985). Male blacks have a 14.3% rate of disability compared to 9% for male whites; the rate of female black disabilities is nearly double that of female whites (14% vs. 7.8%).

The provider of pediatric services faces many challenges in assisting families from varying cultures. First, *language barriers* can be an obstacle when parents speak limited English and their child's ability to learn even one language is compromised severely. Family members already confused by medical issues and terms need the comfort of communicating with the therapist in their native language; alternatively, a trained interpreter should be provided (American Psychological Association, 1990; Cavallo and Saucedo, 1995).

Second, multicultural families may understand but discard suggestions that conflict with cultural beliefs and values. For example, religious beliefs often affect the family view of injury, professional advice, and different types of treatments (Cavallo and Saucedo, 1995). Many fundamental Christians believe their children were injured because of their sins or "God's will." The church may be a more important support than the nuclear family for many fundamental Baptists, particularly blacks (Baxter and McDuffy, 1993).

Providers often interpret family reliance on God (and belief that prayer, rather than doctors, will cure the child) as reflecting denial and an obstacle to treatment progress. These interpretations are not only judgmental but contrary to the strong emotional and community support that parents often receive from their congregation during crisis. When included in networking efforts, clergy and congregation members can help support practical and emotional needs of family members. At times, family members refuse traditional therapy but accept assistance from their church leader (who in turn may be an important member of the child's rehabilitation team). Youth groups often provide positive experiences and compassionate role models. Otherwise, youths with brain trauma may gravitate

toward antisocial activities and peer groups in their search for a new identity.

Cultural Attitudes

Culture often influences the family's acceptance of professional services and willingness to share personal feelings with outsiders. For example, Asian families typically view physicians as esteemed; they often think that expressing feelings or accepting help is a weakness of character. In other cultures, people may exaggerate problems to ensure that the physician "understands how hard we have it." Many ethnic families have had negative experiences and feel misunderstood or devalued by health care providers. Consequently, the therapist should inquire about the family's health care experiences to address any negative perceptions. For example, the Tellez family's resistance to surgical intervention for their son and their belligerent attitude toward staff led to family therapy intervention. Their resistance and underlying fears were addressed after they were assigned a therapist who shared their ethnic background and native tongue. Because of their comfort level with this therapist, the family was able to disclose their past loss of a family member due to medical malpractice.

The professional will also gain family trust by respecting cultural differences in family structure. Hispanic and Asian families more often have patriarchal structure, whereas matriarchal family control is more common in black families. The family member who attends sessions may not be the person who makes family decisions but is responsible for daily care.

Geographic Diversity

Besides economic and cultural differences, geographical diversity profoundly affects family needs. Rural families who must travel many miles for therapy visits have problems similar to those of low-income families in accessing needed services. Differences in resources available in rural areas in contrast to urban areas are often profound. Rural communities often lack health care specialists, recreational programs, and educational resources that could support the child's recovery. Because of the limited demand, family support groups, respite care programs, or even a YMCA are often unavailable outlets for family members. Consequently, health care providers have the responsibility of developing a treatment team, a supportive community network, and training to community members (see Community Needs).

Matching Therapeutic Interventions to Family Needs

Families need the type, sophistication, and intensity of therapy services fitted to their personal needs. Thus, providers have the responsibility to adapt interactions to family members' intellectual, emotional, and developmental needs rather than fitting family members into traditional paradigms. This approach contrasts with traditions of the "therapy hour," "family group," and "education program." In this spirit, the following discussion is organized by family needs rather than traditional discussion by therapy modalities presented elsewhere (Kreutzer et al., 1990; Waaland and Kreutzer, 1988).

Many different avenues lead to the ultimate destination of helping families to experience satisfaction with their life and control over extremely difficult situations. Irrespective of the type or content of therapy, effective therapy provides for each family member's need for

- *Emotional support*: to help family members deal with anxiety, anger, depression, or grief and to address individual adjustment or psychiatric symptoms affecting family adaptation
- *Family realignment*: to distribute new family and caregiving responsibilities fairly; to strengthen husband-wife, parent-child, and individual-community relationships; and to respect family members' competencies and successes rather than weaknesses and failures
- *Education*: to develop common expectations, goals, and behavioral management strategies and to advocate for service and emotional needs of all family members
- *Stress reduction*: to think in a positive and solution-oriented manner and to communicate in a way that is direct and respectful and to develop healthy ways of managing external and internal stresses

Zarski and DePompei's (1991) matrix model helps families prioritize these goals and helps therapists to match therapy interventions to individual family needs. Their model pairs the family's functional skills, adaptation (realignment, adjustment, or reintegration), and caregiver demands with appropriate strategies and interventions. Families are ranked on a 1–4 level on the basis of the three factors mentioned. Appropriate *strategies and interventions* then are matched to the family's unique needs. The authors defined *interventions* as therapy goals (e.g., providing education, restructuring family roles, or resolving symptoms). In contrast, *strategies* refer to therapy focus (i.e., the family's need for crisis intervention, short-term goals, or long-term change).

On the basis of this model, families who are struggling to survive (defined as level 1 families) are defined by limitations in their emotional, intellectual, and practical resources. These families require basic skill building, including parent education and assigned tasks. In contrast, families with greater resources (level 4 families) are defined by their quick ability to adapt to change and to cope with stress. Therapy goals for these families tend be long-term or proactive and to focus on strengthening family intimacy and problem solving. The reader may recognize the parallel characteristics between level 1 and vulnerable families and level 4 and resilient families (see Figure 16-1). Because of the similarities, these terms are used interchangeably throughout the discussion.

Thus, the family's resources and mental health dictate the type, amount, and focus of therapy goals. In level 1 families with poorly developed coping skills, compromised mental health, or acute crises, individuals typically are so consumed by basic survival and personal needs that they do not have the capacity to address broader family issues. Their participation in a support group is often counterproductive and frustrating to other group members. The needs of these family members must be addressed through intensive individual therapy. Their therapeutic goals help to produce the internal calming in attending to the needs of others. These skills are needed before individuals are ready for effective family or group participation. Individual referral for medication, focus on stress management, and assistance in overwhelming responsibilities are particularly important when family members display prolonged clinical symptoms. The provider should be sensitive to increased rates of psychiatric disorder among primary caregivers. These problems include elevated rates of depression, psychosomatic disorder, and posttraumatic stress disorder, which may be caused or exacerbated by injury of a family member. Without treatment, the needs of these individuals will intensify the burden experienced by other family members and impede efforts to reorganize family roles effectively.

Although emotional support is important for families in crisis, families in later phases (i.e., levels 3 and 4 with focus on long-term goals) need healing through optimism and empowerment. Specific interventions are not as important as helping family members to reframe problems as challenges and to experience mastery in meeting life's challenges. Interventions that work highlight *positive* change rather than negative behaviors and emphasize *family competency* rather than family weakness. Therapy experiences clearly bear out the dictum that people move in the direction in which they think. When a family member dwells on negative feelings or events, mental energy is drained and prophecies are fulfilled. To move families in positive directions, professionals need exceptional interpersonal skills. The effective therapist is insightful and compassionate and has a sense of humor. These skills are used to reframe family perceptions quickly in a way that family members embrace as their own thoughts. The successful therapist focuses on what the family can do rather than reinforcing feelings of helplessness, hopelessness, or anger. Expressions such as "How can I help?" "What goals can we set this week?" or "You managed that well!" will help family members to focus on positive goals. Such statements also deter focus from thoughts of what they would, could, should, or must have done. As noted previously, many types of brief, strategic family therapy approaches—particularly paradoxical interventions—do not address effectively the family's struggle in its search for newly defined roles and identity.

Irrespective of their vulnerability or functional level, family members rank family education regarding TBI as a high priority (Waaland et al., 1993). The authors report that nearly 100% of caregivers in their survey ranked understanding (and understanding by other family members) of their children's injuries and recovery process as most important to them. These needs were also among the most frequently rated *unmet* needs. Family members obviously seek clear, honest explanations of their child's injury, how it affects current thinking and behavior, what they can expect in the future, and how they can help the child now.

Thus, the family *unit* should be provided a *clear, understandable* explanation of how the child has changed. They need to know how to react to these changes and what to expect in the future. Each individual (including siblings) then should be given an uninterrupted opportunity to ask questions and voice concerns. These therapy meetings will ensure that all members receive first-hand information rather than confused or filtered second-hand explanations. Obviously, the technical level and frankness of explanations and advice should be modified on the basis of family level or vulnerability status. Thus, level 1 and 2 (vulnerable) families should be given simplified explanations that are connected to their previous experiences. It is particularly important to provide these families with concrete examples of how their children have changed and with very specific behavioral interventions. They also should be provided with optimistic hope for the future but also frequent follow-up visits to update family needs and intervention plans.

In contrast, the therapist should provide resilient, educated families (levels 3 and 4) with understandable but technical explanations. These families seek both short- and long-term expectations and goals as well as technical information. Therefore, to minimize the effects of horror stories that they might encounter through the Internet or at the library, the therapist should have a well-stocked library of up-to-date reading and video materials.

Creating Effective Teamwork for Challenging Behavior Problems

Similarly, family members should be asked to develop guidelines and intervention strategies *as a team*. Family members especially need to work together in management of such negative behaviors as impulsive risk-taking, anger outbursts, and rebellion. Otherwise, family members individually or collectively may punish, ignore, or reinforce behaviors of a child who can learn only through repeated and consistent guidance. Again, more vulnerable families will need a very easy-to-administer but structured program, whereas more resilient families can be taught general principles and guidelines.

Family feelings of helplessness and impaired decision making often accompany feelings of hopelessness. During initial crisis intervention, most families seek step-by-step instruction. However, family members should be treated as active guides rather than as passive tourists in developing interventions. All families should be in charge of setting target behaviors, formulating behavior plans, and monitoring progress toward goals. Some families (particularly level 1 and 2 families) will require more coaching and direction to help them to feel in control. By taking this approach, the therapist can point to documented gains made when the family predictably expresses concerns that the child is not making progress and even losing ground.

Therapeutic focus on individual strengths and positive reframing is essential for all families. However, family members are at times paralyzed by guilt and confusion. These feelings may prohibit them from providing the consistent, firm consequences for behavior within the youth's control. These families frequently need permission to set limits but often cannot distinguish between behaviors caused by TBI, its secondary emotional trauma, or outright manipulative behavior.

Many family therapy goals for those facing the aforementioned problems can be addressed simply by directing members in the problem-solving task of developing a behavior management plan. Using my approach, family members learn to observe cognitively rather than to react emotionally to problem behaviors. When operating from a cognitive rather than an emotional mode, family members are better able to explore different world views. This altered perspective helps them to understand why their family member is behaving inappropriately. Family members then can explore ways to motivate that changed person. From this experience, family members are often able to reconcile differences in their perceptions not only of cause but of the impact of the child's behavior on family integrity. Most important, family members learn teamwork in setting realistic goals that are within their control: their reaction to persons, places, and things. Therapy efforts often result in both effective behavioral management programs and improved family insight and new family therapy goals. Through this process, the family develops a sense of control, goal-orientation, and cohesion.

For example, one approach to addressing overprotective or guilt-ridden behavior is to emphasize the child's seemingly unhelpful or helpless behavior. This perspective allows the therapist to bypass family-member disputes about why, when, and for whom behavior is a problem. The therapist also avoids taking sides while gaining the family's confidence that the therapist understands that this problem must be addressed.

Finally, the therapist is in a position to test assessment hypotheses about the family's structure, beliefs, cohesion, and problem-solving skills. Using this approach, family members next are taught how to be (1) observers of behavior, (2) recorders of basic information, (3) identifiers of causes and triggers for behavior, and (4) agents for behavior change. Family members' psychological well-being (level of functioning) determines the level of education, guidance, and task difficulty appropriate for family members to accomplish therapy tasks successfully. Family members (especially siblings) first are instructed to stand back and watch carefully what the child does. Then they write information about all the behaviors that are problematic for them (including what triggered what reaction, with whom, where, and when). Parents and siblings next rank-order these problems and negotiate target behaviors. Then (with guidance) they form hypotheses about the reasons for the behavior and ways in which to test these hypotheses. The reader is referred to Chapter 13 for a comprehensive discussion of behavioral intervention strategies.

Problem-solving tasks help not only family members but the therapist to set and reset goals constantly for the family. By assigning tasks and setting measurable goals, the therapist is often able to isolate subtle attempts to sabotage team efforts. The therapist also gains information about family members' knowledge of the effects of injury, beliefs about the causes of behavior, and alliances with other family members. Finally, by assessing daily problem-solving skills directly, the therapist quickly can shift to a more basic approach when families show rigidity or poor problem-solving skills (e.g., shifting to techniques prescribed for level 1 and 2 families). Intervention plans also maintain focus on what the family can change. Families are taught how to modify their environment (e.g., avoiding overstimulating settings), teach the child coping strategies or skills, or change their reaction to behavior.

Therapy outcome with the Ryan family demonstrates the potential success of family task orientation or problem-solving approach. Sherry, a rising middle-school student, was always the vivacious, high-achieving, and agreeable child relative to her 17- and 12-year-old brothers. After a pedestrian injury left Sherry comatose for a day, she became a different person. She received homebound services and eventually was able to maintain average marks in advanced (but not honors) classes. During the next year, however, Sherry became increasingly aggressive, disruptive, and defiant toward family members. She constantly threatened suicide and was failing all subjects.

In the initial family session, family members' descriptions of the cause, context, and intensity of her behavior were as different as their responses to Sherry's behavior. In response to her outbursts, she variously was ignored (by her father and 17-year-old brother), was given sympathy (by her mother), or was subjected to yelling (by her 12-year-old brother, who in turn was reprimanded by the parents). Hypotheses about the cause of outbursts were just as varied: Her father attributed her outbursts to seizures and medication, her mother to adolescent pressures, her 12-year-old brother to anger at her parents, and

her 17-year-old brother had no opinion. In their monitoring of her behavior, their only consistency involved the occasion: Sherry's outbursts typically happened after she had been out with her friends. Sherry apparently gravitated toward a "bad group" of friends after her injury. Parents began to monitor these relations and her social activities more closely. Ultimately, parents' observations (rather than reactions) led to the discovery of Sherry's multiple substance abuse and (unfounded) fear of pregnancy. Her oldest brother was aware of her problems but feared that if he reported her, she would do the same to him. Her youngest brother shared her anger at parents, whose attention to Sherry detracted from his needs. Thus, intervention shifted from behavioral therapy or neurologic intervention to a focus on family issues: Sherry's need for guidance, her parents' guilt that impaired their ability to set limits, and the unmet needs of other family members focused on Sherry's problems. Ultimately, family life (and Sherry's behavior) returned to a more balanced state. Participation in an Outward Bound program and follow-up involvement of the school and therapist helped Sherry to re-establish a positive identity.

Goldfarb and colleagues (1986) provided an excellent family guide with exercises that clarify values, priorities, and needs and promote problem solving, self-advocacy, and stress management. Their approach is similar to my focus on empowering families to better prioritize, manage stress, and focus on positive change. This book provides practical exercises to guide the therapist.

Helping Family Members Through Change

Families also seek continuity in transitions from one setting to another. The assembly-line movement from acute care to rehabilitation to community reentry often leaves family members confused and jettisoned. This discontinuity intensifies family alienation and impedes readaptation (Romano, 1974). Family members seek smooth transitions and providers whom they consider their own. Family needs and convenience rather than professional turf issues and traditions should determine who is involved and how services are delivered.

For example, the child's disorientation and the family's distress caused by rapid moves from the emergency room to intensive-care unit to step-down unit to rehabilitation are reduced when rehabilitation team members guide the family through acute crisis into community reentry. Professional continuity reduces family exposure to contradictory information and selective family member use of information supporting distorted views. Such consistency is vital to the disoriented child and to confused family members. The family needs consistent information, familiar faces, and proactive planning to experience joy in progress rather than to suffer insecurity and fears. The child's return to the community and school typically increases family tensions. Often, previous friends, activities, and classroom placement are gone.

Unless this transition is orchestrated carefully, unhealthy anger, anxiety, guilt, depression, and family conflict can be heightened.

Helping the Family Through Growth

Most parents have experienced the frustration of being unable to soothe an infant's relentless crying, control a toddler's outbursts, or restrain a preschooler's hazardous behaviors. Similarly, many parents do not know how to relieve the middle-school child's fears of bullies, lockers, and classroom changes. The high-school student's anxieties about personal identity often create turbulence in the most smoothly sailing family system. Media, friends, and professionals help most families through these difficult developmental transitions. Parenting magazines, television specials, and advice from experienced others help to guide parents and their children. Parents of youth with TBI do not have these road maps available. Well-meaning advice based on experiences with typical childhood problems often only intensifies the family's confusion.

Consequently, families often rely on professional knowledge about how to modify normal developmental expectations ranging from play and learning to responsibilities and privileges. The background requirements of the clinician working with families of children parallels the clinical guidelines for working with families of ethnic diversity. The clinician who lacks experience with children, knowledge of normal development, and awareness of developmental child and family needs after injury should make an appropriate referral.

For example, the age of children at the time of injury will affect both their ability to acquire new skills and the family's ability to support disrupted emotional growth of their child. In particular, the younger the child, the more profound are expected long-term impairments in cognitive, socioemotional, and physical development. This greater risk reflects the developmental immaturity in neuroanatomy and knowledge base. Illustrating these principles, the infant learns about the world through seeing, touching, and operating on things. The emotional accomplishment of infancy is a sense of security gained by having basic needs met. After injury, the infant's learning process is often disrupted by impaired vision, hearing, and motor skills common to more severe trauma; the trauma of hospitalization and disrupted parent-child bonding further disrupts emotional development.

Each developmental stage presents unique family challenges. How does a parent comfort an infant with severe sensory integration deficits? How does a parent teach a blind or paralyzed infant who has no past experiences on which to rely? Parents express similar confusion in making decisions ranging from selecting an appropriate educational setting to locating appropriate recreational activities. Parents express greatest confusion during the youth's adolescent years. For example, how do parents determine whether their teenager is ready to

Table 16-4. Developmental Tasks and Reactions to Losses

Developmental tasks: 2–5 years
  Learn how to control body and environment.
  Develop rudimentary basics of empathy.
  Develop sense of self and play.
Developmental tasks: 6–12 years
  Develop sense of task mastery in social relations, of school demands, and in cooperation and competition.
Developmental tasks: 13–18 years
  Adjust to growth spurts and hormonal changes.
  Master autonomy and decision making.
  Develop higher-level reasoning skills and insight.
  Develop futuristic thinking (e.g., vocational plans).
  Define *me*.
Childhood reactions to losses
  Experience disrupted sense of self owing to changes in body and skills.
  Develop feelings of "differentness" owing to changes in self and peer reactions.
  Develop generalized acting out or withdrawal as primary emotional reactions (symptoms of depression less likely).
Adolescent reactions to losses
  Incorporate injury into identity via "meaning" of injury.
  Deny effects of injury and engage in risk-taking behavior.
  Blame others and develop rebellious, antisocial behavior.
  Develop self-pity and a pattern of withdrawal and depression.
  Develop self-doubt and anxiety, further compromising abilities.
  Experience underlying loss of identity, independence, rites of passage, and vocational dreams.

drive, date, or even stay home alone? Table 16-4 presents skills of normal development and reaction to the loss of such skills.

For the child with TBI, needs are constantly changing: Needs change from parent-child bonding and appropriate stimulation at the infancy level to behavior management, safety, and environmental stimulation at the preschool level. Intervention focus shifts from family and home to peer and school needs on the child's entry into school. For the child capable of learning strategies, cognitive interventions (e.g., self-monitoring, problem-solving, and social skills programs) should focus on transferring responsibility from the family to the child. This shift helps the family to decrease overprotectiveness. Emphasis on the child also empowers the child, and averts oppositional-defiant patterns that result in the struggle for autonomy. Strengths in athletics, music, art, scouting, or any positive extracurricular activities should be developed in adaptive or regular community programs. These services help youths to develop feelings of worth and identity. (See Waaland, 1990; Waaland and Raines, 1991, for a more thorough discussion of developmental stages and the changing needs based on age at injury and changing developmental stage.)

By far the peak time for TBI to occur—and also the most emotionally traumatic for the recipient—is adolescence. Even under the best circumstances, adolescence is marked by significant turmoil. Adolescents are reacting to social pressures to fit in, to achieve recognition, and (often) to cope with the emotional upheaval of first love. Such questions as Who am I? What should I do for the rest of my life? With whom should I do it? overwhelm a typical adolescent. These anxieties are intensified by peer pressures regarding sexual activity, substance abuse, and many alternative lifestyles available to youths in our society. At this stage, adolescents often experience feelings of immortality, live in a fantasy world, and fight for independence. In contrast, their parents face fears of security, harsh realities of aging, and time pressures to correct all their teen's human failings. This developmental family crisis is disrupted severely—and normal parent-teenager reactions are intensified—by brain trauma. Because of these differences in perspective between parents and children, it is not surprising that adolescents typically show the most diverse range and extremity of reactions in their attempts to reenter their "old world." As a consequence, many teenagers become withdrawn, depressed, anxious, and suicidal, whereas others cope by acting out through sexual promiscuity, substance abuse, aggression, and noncompliance. Often underlying these reactions are the teenager's loss of identity and a growing confusion about growing up.

Thus, the clinician's goal is to guide parents in setting appropriate expectations and boundaries while helping the teenager to learn personal limitations. Vocational issues and, for the teenager who cannot function independently, long-term placement issues should be addressed by the proactive therapist. Otherwise, significant transitional problems (including often lengthy waitlists for supported employment or housing) may add to a family's burden. Because family members still may have unrealistic hopes that the child will complete a 4-year college program, the therapist should present supported living options as long-shot possibilities. Initially, the therapist may even explore options without family involvement when extreme resistance is encountered.

Irrespective of the child's age at injury, both child and family will face new challenges throughout the family life cycle. The proactive therapist will schedule "well checks" on a routine basis to help to avoid crises and to update changing family, school, and community needs. Follow-up visits should include all family members. Additionally, family evaluation forms and updated information from physicians, therapists, and teachers should be reviewed prior to the family's visit. Review of this information will enable the therapist or the entire team to address problem areas and needs. In turn, the family can be provided with updated recommendations about modifications in the youth's responsibilities, privileges, and academic program.

Creating Natural Support Networks and Helping Families to Reenter Community Life

The medical model of the seventies and the interdisciplinary model of the 1980s have been superseded in the 1990s by models of consumer empowerment and community support. Unaffordable services and the fragile state of the health care system in the United States have accelerated a healthy paradigm shift. This shift transfers decision-making control from professionals to the persons who must cope with the aftermath of TBI. Due to the complexity of life and loss of the traditional nuclear family, family members need guidance to experience success in this new role.

Current movement from therapist to case manager and from fixing patient pathology to meeting consumer needs places new demands on professionals. Movement from a medical model to a consumer model requires professionals to know and develop community services. The 1987 principles of the Center on Human Policy, developed to support families of children with disabilities, succinctly describes our current mission. These families need strengthening of existing social networks and natural support systems; availability and control of their choice of services; support in meeting basic family needs; inclusion of their exceptional child into community life; and placement of their child within the nuclear family or an alternative family setting (Center on Human Policy, 1979).

Consistent with this mission is the shifted emphasis from family treatment to family empowerment. The growth of the Brain Injury Association from a small group of families to a commanding force influencing health care providers, community service dollars, and even public policy represents a powerful example of consumer-driven services. Central to this movement are new attitudes toward support groups. Traditional family support programs were based on the premises that (1) the disability should be accepted, cured, or contained; (2) the person with disability should be rehabilitated or removed from community life; and (3) the family should be freed of unrealistic expectations, pathology, or denial. Since the 1980s, many support groups (particularly those under the auspices of the Brain Injury Association) have served an empowerment role in which family members rather than professionals dictate the agenda. Support groups of the 1990s also serve a variety of functions ranging from traditional goals of education and emotional support to a new focus on advocacy and political involvement. Other variations include parent-to-parent programs that provide individuals with support in a natural manner (often via telephone) rather than at infrequent and inconveniently scheduled meetings.

The concept of natural, existing support systems also parallels the movement from physician control over services to community support for family needs. These needs include not only traditional services provided by professionals but creation of a user-friendly environment in which the family lives, learns, works, and plays (O'Brien, 1989). In particular, parents highly value—but struggle to find—quality child and family services in their community (Waaland et al., 1993b). Parents rank school and community recreational services as more important than any other support system (including physicians) but most lacking for children with TBI. Thus, families appear to seek reduced dependency on professional services and increased access to community persons, places, and programs.

The Virginia Department of Rehabilitative Services grant-funded PITON project (Graesser, 1991) is an example of successful building of natural supports. This "train-the-trainer" project targeted individuals who were not successful in traditional supported work, life skills, or housing programs. Eligible individuals also were at risk for hospitalization due to significant behavioral disturbance. Through extensive training sessions, which included the individual with TBI, the family had the benefit of a cohesive network of individuals. The project's goal was to train both family members and other principal players in the family's life in ways to manage dangerous and often aggressive behavior. Family supporters ranged from family, neighbors, and congregation members to school personnel, employers, and community workers. Outcome data highlighted the effectiveness of this program in preventing hospitalization, improving the quality of family life, and providing meaningful community participation for the client. Similar programs have been developed for auxiliary school personnel such as bus drivers and cafeteria workers (Heiden and Goodall, 1992).

Families of children with TBI face immense *practical needs* (Waaland, 1991). These needs range from respite care to technical support and equipment. Again, programs across the country are becoming more creative and flexible in improving family control of services. For example, several states (e.g., Wisconsin and Michigan) use flexible voucher systems or direct cash subsidies to reduce bureaucratic frustrations and allow families to determine service needs. A menu of voucher services provided by the state of Wisconsin is listed in Table 16-5. The reader is challenged to go through this list to determine his or her "service IQ" (i.e., awareness of how to access needs). Scores of 10–15 get the "family supporter" blue ribbon; scores of 5 and below suggest that the reader should stop reading and start calling local agencies to become more familiar with services.

Many creative programs have been developed to deliver services described in Table 16-5. For example, many programs have trained community volunteers or grant-paid workers to provide effective respite-care services for even the most difficult-to-manage child. For many families, failures with typical baby-sitters and guilt over having fun while the child is not interfere with resumption of normal family life and particularly trouble

Table 16-5. Youth and Family Service Needs

Architectural modifications to the home
Child care
Specialized counseling and therapy
Specialized diagnosis and evaluation
Specialty dental and medical care not otherwise covered
Specialized nutrition and clothing
Specialized equipment and supplies
Homemaker services
In-home nursing and attendant care
Home training and parent courses
Recreation and alternative activities
Respite care
Transportation
Specialized utility costs
Vehicle modification

marital relations. Even the most resistant caregiver typically will accept *quality* recreational time rather than traditional baby-sitting services. Avenues for respite services include local social services offices, health departments, and the United Way. Some hospital social services departments, mental health clinics, churches, and local recreation departments maintain listings of respite providers.

In the realm of community services, *recreation and alternative activities* are often rated as lacking but are an important family priority for youths with TBI (Waaland et al., 1993b). Again, many community services ranging from recreational programs to daycare have been modified successfully to include youths with disabilities. These services are most helpful in providing transportation when a family is strained by transporting youths to even essential appointments.

Many individuals whose community life has been restricted by severe physical or communication barriers now profit from the incredible technological growth in our society. Thus, *assistive devices* remove prior obstacles to family inclusion in community life. Accessible buildings and bathrooms are paralleled by computerized devices that help children move, communicate, and play. Again, the provider's unfamiliarity with services rather than a youth's insurmountable disabilities may be the obstacle between family burden and active community participation. Assistive technology teams are developing across the country. Nearly all states have programs through departments of rehabilitative services or other agencies. Recently, many schools have developed similar programs. These specialists are able to evaluate a youngster's need for specialized equipment, can recommend specific software or devices, and may guide families to funding sources to pay for the purchase of adaptive devices.

Supportive services and groups for survivors also have changed in format and focus in many areas of the country. Often, services in medical offices signal to youths with

TBI that they are different. In recognition of both social and recreational needs, support group meetings now often occur in such community settings as parks and restaurants. Traditionally, youths with TBI have been placed in special programs with special providers. Because their poor judgment increases their susceptibility to peer influences, children with TBI need normalized experiences. Thus, many inclusion programs have been developed to meet the need for after-school care, athletic and camp involvement, and even school-related activities.

Clearly, new approaches need to use friends and families and to enlist individuals already involved in family life. The public school system is a unique entity in multiple respects. No other public agencies rival its scope of integration into family life and of commitment to appropriate educational and remedial efforts. Most important, these activities are delivered within the context of family and school life. Public education is a primary vehicle for learning both academics and social and life skills and values.

Many parents view their child's education as a primary yardstick of both the child's success in life and their own. In our society, achievement and competition (particularly the ability to excel over other students) are valued highly. Not surprising, parents of all sociocultural backgrounds cite the quality of school services to be *the* top priority after their child's TBI. Parents also report the greatest dissatisfaction with educational services (Waaland et al., 1993b). Parents often describe their youth's return to school as a peak crisis period for the family. Such youths virtually have lost self. They are struggling with physical changes, emotional confusion, and lost abilities. Family members no longer have the protective net provided by inpatient rehabilitation. Emotional reactions to coping with changes in their loved one's ability and practical realities of integrating the youth's many demands into the family system often cause tension within the family. Family reactions to special education placement or services may be particularly intense for the severely injured student who was gifted academically, artistically, or athletically. Parents of the severely injured student—previously elated that their child has survived—must cope with the changes in their child's lifestyle. Such terms as *TBI* and *special education services* may precipitate disbelief, anger, or grief. Thus, the reader working with families of injured youths should read carefully the chapter on academic reentry to learn how to alleviate family anxieties and stresses associated with negotiating the complex maze of special education services. Successful reentry is discussed also in other writings (Savage and Wolcott, 1994; Waaland, 1992a).

Family support is even more critical as youths make the transition to community shelter workshops, supported employment, specialized college programs, or other-oriented services. Uninformed parents often forfeit extended services for their children (up to age 21 in most states), as they believe that graduating with prior friends and moving on will recommence normal stages of family development. These same families often become embittered when they realize that the young adult is placed on wait lists, that they must pay for many services, and that other needed services do not exist.

Conclusions

The last decade has yielded new perspectives on how to alter the fatalistic outcome charted by early descriptive studies of pediatric TBI. Perspectives have changed from an isolated focus on "the brain-injured child" to a multidimensional understanding of the importance of life before and after injury. The focus on family also has shifted from "the TBI family" that follows a rigid series of reactions to a unique family in crisis. Although all families may go through similar phases in adjustment, their unique experiences and background contribute to differences in reactions to family crisis. The child and family's vulnerability or resiliency appears to depend on myriad factors. Some factors are situational, such as experiences with crises and medical issues. Other factors, such as socioeconomic status, are more pervasive and often dictate family member's available knowledge, time, quality of medical and educational services, and support systems.

In recognition of the importance of individual differences, this chapter has emphasized strongly the objective, multidimensional evaluation that provides a thorough understanding of the family's unique sociocultural background, experiences, and resources. Also critical is an understanding of what family members know about injury and what injury means to their lifestyle and beliefs. Although family economic resources have a tremendous impact on family outcome, emotional resiliency and coping skills of family members are critical and changeable factors. Stress is in the eye—or mind—of the beholder. Thus, assessment must address how family members judge stressful events and the methods they use to manage family burden. Family members' perceptions of having a child with TBI and their historical coping strategies guide them to the place and method of intervention. To understand families, we also have to assess their priorities and how well these needs are being met rather than how they are described by our clinical measures.

The proactive therapist will begin with the end in mind. Family aspirations after trauma are similar to those shared by all: to enjoy financial and job security, leisure activities, a sense of belonging, and particularly the support and well-being of loved ones. The means to this end vary, depending on the family's unique makeup. In particular, not only research but clinical treatment of families has operated from a culturally biased perspective. Families coping with the tragedy of childhood injury need to be understood, not interpreted. Cultural perspectives need to be respected, not changed. Families need to have basic aspirations met, not other-defined goals. Families struggling with pediatric injury need foremost providers who are knowledgeable in childhood injury and its long-term effects on both youths and family members, not generalists who do not understand children and family development. Families struggling to maintain identity in the face of crisis need health care providers who share—or are at least professionally trained to understand—their world view. Thus, hospital administrators should recruit individuals on the basis of area demographic needs and the age of the population they serve.

Based on consumer-guided rather than professionally guided services, therapy interventions are geared to family needs rather than to therapist training. One adaptable intervention approach was presented by this author. Restoration of family balance requires changes both in how family members see their current world and in how the professional actively trains them to change things within their control. Transactional models that recognize that children affect families and vice versa are needed to advance both research and clinical efforts.

Regardless of perspective, therapy models of the 1990s focus on family competency rather than on weakness. The 1990s therapist empowers rather than directs families by helping them to focus on what they can do rather than on uncontrollable events and gains losses. Such families need inspiration to experience joy in their daily triumphs rather than to feel fear about uncontrollable future circumstances. The family's mission should encompass the needs of each family member, including the often forgotten siblings, to restore family normalcy.

Providers are in a challenging, new phase of providing services to families. Now they efficiently must improve the child's outcome and the family's adjustment in measurable terms. Just as the family must readjust to trauma with the child with TBI, so must the health care provider adjust to the new world of "managed care." Many healthcare providers now can empathize better with feelings of anger, frustration, and burn-out experienced by the families they treat. However, managed care also has precipitated a positive and much needed movement in health care. Providers now must scrutinize closely how families are treated, what they need, and how interventions affect their adjustment. Creative, cost-efficient train-the-trainer programs and the development of natural support systems meet these criteria.

Clinicians committed to using the family's natural support systems must be willing also to get outside their offices and participate actively with other agencies to learn about services available to their clients. Although restoration of the "old life" is a goal for adults, children and their families have constantly changing developmental needs. Thus, routine follow-up, newsletters outlining new services or family "tips," creative recreational programs, assistive technology, and educational guidance at all team follow-ups are just a few of many ways in which

professionals can improve services. As limited empirical evidence exists, we also need to evaluate the utility of alternative programs, curricula, and interventions to improve the efficiency of service delivery. Researchers must begin to look at not only what works but at those for whom it is meant to work and at the occasion on which it is most effective in the developmental cycle. Thus, multicenter investigations are needed to evaluate the effects of different types of interventions or programs. Critical variables impacting the type of intervention include family and child characteristics and, most notably, developmental and cultural factors.

This chapter has emphasized the significant contribution of families and of the communities in which children live and to which they return after injury. These natural links emphasize the need to move from describing outcome to linking problems with solutions, the need to create a team atmosphere that moves away from a medical model that leaves families, school, and community members feeling powerless.

References

Achenbach T, Edelbrock C (1983). Manual for the Child Behavior Checklist and Revised Child Behavior Profile. Burlington, VT: University of Vermont Department of Psychiatry.

Affleck G, Tennen H, Gershman (1985). Cognitive adaptation to high risk infants: the search for mastery, meaning, and protection from future harm. Am J Ment Defic 89;653.

American Psychological Association (1990). Guidelines for Assessment and Treatment of Culturally Diverse Populations. Washington, DC: American Psychological Association.

Baxter B, McDuffy T (1993). The Role of the Church in the African-American Community: Partners in the Rehab Process. Presented at the National Head Injury Foundation Symposium, November 7–10, Orlando, FL.

Billings AG, Moos RH (1982). Psychosocial theory and research on depression: an integrative framework and review. Clin Psychol Rev 2;213.

Bishop DS, Miller IW (1988). Traumatic brain injury: empirical family assessment techniques. J Head Trauma Rehabil 3;16.

Cavallo MM, Saucedo C (1995). Traumatic brain injury in families from culturally diverse populations. J Head Trauma Rehabil 10;66.

Center on Human Policy (1979). The community imperative: a refutation of all arguments in support of institutionalizing anybody because of mental retardation. Unpublished paper, Syracuse University, Syracuse, NY.

Dell Orto AE, Power PW (1994). Head Injury and the Family: A Life And Living Perspective. Winter Park, FL: PMD Publishers.

DePompei R, Zarski JJ (1991). Assessment of the Family. In JM Williams, T Kay (eds), Head Injury: A Family Matter. Baltimore: Paul H. Brookes, 101–120.

Frankowski RF, Annegers JF, Whitman S (1988). The Descriptive Epidemiology of Head Trauma in the United States. In DP Becker, JT Povlishock (eds), Central Nervous System Trauma Status Report (GPO:1988-520-149/0028). Washington DC: National Institutes of Health, National Institute of Neurological and Communicative Disorders and Stroke.

Goldfarb L, Brotherson MJ, Summers JA, Turnbull AP (1986). Meeting the Challenge of Disability or Chronic Illness: A Family Guide. Baltimore: Paul H. Brookes.

Graesser R (1991). PITON Networking Project. Richmond, VA: Department of Rehabilitative Services.

Heiden S, Goodall P (1992). PEATC Train-the-Trainer Sensitivity Program for Auxiliary School Personnel Working with Youth Following Traumatic Brain Injury. Richmond, VA: Parent Education and Advocacy Center.

Holmes T, Rahe R (1967). The Social Readjustment Rating Scale. J Psychosom Res 11;212.

Jaffe KM, Fay GC, Polissar NL, et al. (1993). Severity of pediatric traumatic brain injury and neurobehavioral recovery at one year: cohort study. Arch Phys Med Rehabil 74;587.

Kay T, Cavallo MM, Ezrachi O, Vavagiakis P (1995). The head injury family interview: a clinical and research tool. J Head Trauma Res 10;12.

Kreutzer JS, Camplair P, Waaland P (1988). The Family Needs Questionnaire. Richmond, VA: Rehabilitation, Research and Training Center on Severe Traumatic Brain Injury, Medical College of Virginia.

Kreutzer JS, Zasler N, Camplair P, Leininger B (1990). A Practical Guide to Family Intervention Following Adult Traumatic Brain Injury. In J Kreutzer, P Wehman (eds), Community Integration Following Traumatic Brain Injury. Baltimore: Paul H. Brookes.

Lezak MD (1978). Living with the characterologically altered brain injured patient. J Clin Psychiatr 39;592.

Lezak MD (1986). Psychological implications of traumatic brain damage for the patient's family. Rehabil Psychol 31;241.

Lezak MD (1994). Family Perceptions and Family Reactions: A New Look at Denial. Presented at the Thirteenth Annual Symposium of the National Head Injury Foundation, November 6–9, Chicago, IL.

Livingston MG, Brookes DN (1988). The burden on families of the brain injured: a review. J Head Trauma Rehabil 3;6.

O'Brien J (1989). What's Worth Working For? Leadership for Better Quality Human Services. Lithonia, GA: Responsive Systems Associates.

Ocoutt S (1994). Life After Brain Injury. Presented at the Thirteenth Annual Symposium of the National Head Injury Foundation, November 6–9, Chicago, IL.

Polinko PR, Barin JJ, Leger D, Bachman KM (1985). Working with the Family. In M Ylvisaker (ed), Head Injury Rehabilitation. San Diego: College Hill, 91.

Rape RN, Bush JP, Slavin LA (1992). Toward a conceptualization of the family's adaptation to a member's head injury: a critique of developmental stage models. Unpublished manuscript.

Rivara JB, Fay GC, Jaffe JM, et al. (1992). Predictors of family functioning one year following traumatic brain injury in children. Arch Phys Med Rehabil 73;899.

Romano M (1974). Family response to traumatic head injury. Scand J Rehabil Med 6;1.

Rutter M, Chadwick O, Shaffer D (1983). Head Injury. In M Rutter (ed), Developmental Neuropsychiatry. New York: Guilford.

Savage RC, Wolcott GF (eds) (1994). Educational Dimensions of Acquired Brain Injury. Austin, TX: PRO-ED.

Schwentor D, Brown P (1989). Assessment of families with a traumatically brain injured relative. Cogn Rehabil 7(3);8.

Shapiro B (1983). Informational interviews. Sibl Info Network News Lett 2.

Singer GHS, Irvin LK (1989). Family Caregiving, Stress, and Support. In GHS Singer, LK Irvin (eds), Support for Caregiving Families: Enabling Positive Adaptation to Disability. Baltimore: Paul H. Brookes, 3.

Turnbull AP, Turnbull HR (1991). Understanding Families from a Systems Perspective. In JM Williams, T Kay (eds), Head Injury: A Family Matter. Baltimore: Paul H. Brookes, 37.

Waaland P (1991). Pediatric Rehabilitation Research Update. Presented at the Fifteenth Annual Postgraduate Course on Rehabilitation of the Brain-Injured Adult and Child, June 5–9, Williamsburg, VA.

Waaland P (1992). Vulnerability and Resiliency Following TBI: Family and Child Outcome. Presented at the Sixteenth Annual Postgraduate Course on Rehabilitation of the Brain-Injured Adult and Child, June 11–14, Williamsburg, VA.

Waaland P, Burns C, Cockrell C (1993a). Evaluation of needs of high and low income families following pediatric traumatic brain injury. Brain Inj 7(2);135.

Waaland P, Clawson B, Raines S (1993b). Caregivers' Coping Strategies Following Pediatric Brain Injury. Presented at the National Academy for Neuropsychology, November 11–15, Phoenix, AZ.

Waaland P, Kreutzer J (1988). Family response to childhood traumatic brain injury. J Head Trauma Res 3;51.

Waaland P, Raines SR (1991). Families coping with childhood neurological disability: clinical assessment and treatment. Neurorehabilitation 1(2);19.

Waaland PK (1990). Family Response to Childhood Traumatic Brain Injury. In J Kreutzer, P Wehman (eds), Community Integration Following Traumatic Brain Injury. Baltimore: Paul H. Brookes, 225.

Wallander J, Varni J, Babani L (1989). Disability parameters, chronic strain, and adaptation of physically handicapped children and their mothers. J Pediatr Psychol 14;157.

Weltner JS (1985). Matchmaking: Choosing the Appropriate Therapy for Families at Various Levels of Pathology. In MP Mirkin, SL Koman (eds), Handbook of Family and Adolescent Therapy. New York: Gardner Press, 39.

Wilkins D (1979). Caring for the Mentally Handicapped Child. London: Croom Helm.

Williams J (1991). Family Reaction to Head Injury. In JM Williams, T Kay (eds), Head Injury: A Family Matter. Baltimore: Paul H. Brookes, 81.

Zarski JJ, DePompei R (1991). Family Therapy as Applied to Head Injury. In JM Williams, T Kay (eds), Head Injury: A Family Matter. Baltimore: Paul H. Brookes.

Appendix 16-1
Checklist of Intervention Needs

Family Assessment and Intervention Planning

Family Demographics and Resources

Parent education level: Mother _____ Father _____
Parent income level: Mother _____ Father _____
Family psychiatric history: Mother _____
                              Father _____
                              Other family members _____
Number of siblings and ages: _____
Insurance: _____
Litigation: _____
Community size: _____

Family Stressors

(0 = minimal/none; 1 = moderate; 2 = severe)
___ Death of child's parent, sibling, or grandparent
___ Family move
___ Loss of job by primary provider
___ Major illness or disability in child's family
___ Divorce or parental separation
___ Major parent conflict or family abuse history
___ Major financial problems
___ Birth of sibling
___ Parental arrest or hospitalization
___ Parental psychiatric disorder

Support Systems

(0 = need adequately met; 1 = need partially met; 2 = need unmet)
___ Child socializes regularly with several close friends.
___ Spouse generally provides emotional support.
___ Extended family provides emotional support or other help.
___ Family belongs to a church that provides support and help.
___ Community groups and coworkers provide support.
___ Caregiver's close friends provide support.
___ Caregiver's supports provide child care as needed.

Family Needs (based on family needs questionnaire)

(0 = no service needed; 1 = short-term need; 2 = significant need)
Mother   Father
_____   _____ Education (issues: parenting, TBI, other _____)
_____   _____ Counseling: parent-family (issues: _____)
_____   _____ Counseling: individual (issues: _____)
_____   _____ Personal time and support (issues: _____)
_____   _____ Services, patient (issues: _____)
_____   _____ Medical assistance (issues: _____)
_____   _____ Other: _____

Beliefs and Attitudes

Understanding of deficits (0 = good understanding; 1 = some misconceptions; 2 = poor understanding). Provide specific examples of behavior changes.
___ Mother: _____
___ Father: _____
___ Siblings: _____
___ Extended family: _____

History of therapeutic contact and preinjury treatment (0 = none; 1 = outpatient; 2 = inpatient). Specify diagnosis:
___ Mother: _____
___ Father: _____
___ Other family members: _____

Beliefs about who is responsible for injury/personal guilt.
___ Mother: _____
___ Father: _____
___ Siblings: _____
___ Extended family: _____

To whom was the child closest before the injury? _____
What was the child's role in the family? _____
Family pattern of Family Assessment Device: _____
Specific needs and developmental problems of other siblings: _____

Family Intervention Planning

(0 = no need; 1 = referral)
___ Individual therapy. Who: _____ Issues: _____
___ Medication. Monitoring: _____
___ Family therapy. Issues: _____
___ Family education. Issues: _____
___ Parent counseling. Issues: _____
___ Support group. Who: _____
___ Brain Injury Association referral
___ Home intervention. Issues: _____
___ Community needs. Who: _____ Activities: _____
___ Sibling needs. Issues: _____
___ Respite care. Frequency and type: _____
___ Home equipment and modification needs: _____
___ Assistance in placement: _____
___ Insurance and financial issues: _____
___ Transportation needs: _____

___ Coordination of therapies and appointments: _____

___ Long-term follow-up plans: _____

___ Other: _____

_____

Patient Assessment and Planning

Patient History

Current grade: _____

History of failure, retention, or special education services: _____

Type of classroom placement: _____

Academic grades: _____ Strength _____ Weakness _____

Behavior problems: _____

History of inattention, hyperactivity, or impulsivity: _____

Personality style: _____

Type, number, and quality of friendships: _____

Dating and sexual history: _____

Previous dependence in self-care, homework, etc.: _____

Job and driving history: _____

Previous problems with the law: _____

History of drug or alcohol use: _____

Previous athletic and artistic talents or interests: _____

_____

Hobbies, clubs, and community activities: _____

Other: _____

Patient Status

Executive Functions

(0 = no problem; 1 = mild to moderate problem; 2 = severe problems; note problems)

___ Insight and judgment: _____

___ Self-monitoring: _____

___ Attention and concentration: _____

___ Task orientation: _____

___ Initiation and inhibition: _____

___ Process efficiency: _____

___ Endurance and persistence: _____

___ Response to stress: _____

___ Ability to generalize: _____

___ Ability to shift set: _____

___ Ability to abstract: _____

Affect and Mood (specify symptoms)

Changes noted since accident: _____

Self-description: _____

Affect (appropriate, labile, blunted, etc.): _____

___ Depression: _____

___ Agitation: _____

___ Suicide ideation: _____

___ Anxiety: _____

___ Obsessions, compulsions: _____

___ Fears: _____

Primary (neurologic) versus secondary causes: _____

Attitudes and Beliefs

(0 = none; 1 = mild to moderate; 2 = severe)
___ Poor awareness of strengths and deficits: _____
___ Recovery beliefs and attitude: _____
___ Postinjury changes in friends: _____
___ Postinjury changes in family relations: _____
___ Postinjury changes in interests, talents: _____
___ Perceived losses and coping mechanisms: _____
Attitude toward therapy: _____

Sensorimotor Functions

(0 = no problem; 1 = mild to moderate problem; 3 = severe problem; specify problem)
___ Gross motor: _____
___ Fine motor: _____
___ Writing: _____
___ Vision: _____
___ Hearing: _____
___ Tactile: _____
___ Other: _____

Medical Problems and Needs

_____

Intellect

(0 = average or above; 1 = borderline; 2 = retarded or below)
___ Scores and range: _____
Functioning in structured versus unstructured setting: _____

_____
___ Attention capacity: _____
___ Memory capacity: _____
___ Receptive language: _____
___ Expressive language: _____

Academic achievement history
___ Scores and range: _____
___ Oral reading: _____
___ Reading comprehension: _____
___ Math calculations: _____
___ Math reasoning: _____
___ Writing mechanics: _____
___ Written expression: _____

Knowledge base
___ Science: _____
___ Social studies and history: _____
___ Language arts: _____
___ Other: _____
___ Academic issues: _____

Outpatient Needs

(0 = none; 1 = referral)
___ Individual therapy. Issues: _____
___ Cognitive therapy. Issues: _____
___ Group therapy. Issues: _____
___ Computer training. Needs: _____

___ Community needs. Activities: _____

___ Peer counseling. Issues: _____

___ Driver's evaluation. Issues: _____

___ Medication. Monitoring: _____

___ Other: _____

_____

Academic and Community Planning and Interventions

(check if completed)

Predischarge planning

___ Interdisciplinary evaluation and recommendations

___ Audiologic, ophthalmologic, and neurologic evaluations

___ Clear written summary of strengths, weaknesses, and needs

___ Network meeting between school and hospital staff

___ Rehabilitation representative has assessed school resources and layout

___ Predischarge meeting with family and social worker

___ Videotapes and contact persons to demonstrate therapy needs

___ Meeting with peers providing clear explanation and recommendations

___ Classroom teachers provided with in-service and contact persons

___ Parents educated in rights of child and education process

___ Placement (eligibility) and individualized education plan (IEP) development

___ Eligibility meeting and IEP developed before discharge

___ Use of appropriate label (e.g., OHI, TBI)

___ Placement based on services rather than on label

___ Services take into account age, preinjury behavior, and abilities

___ Placement flexible and addresses multifaceted problems

___ Frequent re-evaluation written into educational plan

___ May include transition from home intervention to school

___ May need private placement funded by school

___ Liaison persons between school, family, and therapists

Individual assessment issues

___ Physical layout and environmental needs

___ Transportation and mobility needs

___ Materials, test, and instructional modifications

___ Compensatory strategies and aides

___ Modification in day (e.g., fatigue) and schedule

___ Modified work demands and grading system

___ System for monitoring progress, adjustment, and needs

___ Assistance of friends or "buddy system"

___ Socioemotional needs addressed by guidance or psychology

___ Group therapy to address social training needs

___ Unstructured activities (playground, cafeteria) assessed

___ Behavior or cognitive modification programs established

___ Transitional plans (i.e., preschool to elementary school to middle school to high school to vocational or college level)

___ Feedback system between school, parent, and student

Extended community assessment and interventions

___ Meeting with important support systems (extended family, friends, clergy, etc.) to address patient and family needs

___ System implemented to minimize family need to ask for help

___ Social service and support network expanded as needed

___ Continued information to family regarding appropriate community activities (camps, clubs, adapted aquatics or gymnastics, etc.)

___ Conference and ongoing communication with community service providers (physicians, therapists, coaches, employers, etc.)

___ Other: _____

Chapter 17

School Reentry After Traumatic Brain Injury

Mark Ylvisaker and Timothy J. Feeney

With the passage of the Individuals with Disabilities Education Act of 1990, traumatic brain injury (TBI) became an official educational disability category. TBI is an unusual disability in that knowing that an individual has a history of TBI tells one little about the functional strengths and needs of that individual. Students' needs depend on a variety of factors, including preinjury functioning, the nature and severity of the injuries, time elapsed since injury, quality of rehabilitative and educational services, psychosocial adjustment, family support, and peer support. Some students need no special services or supports to succeed in school, others need a set of services and supports commonly used for children with other disabilities, and yet other students with TBI require a customized, flexible set of services and supports that may have to be adjusted frequently over time.

Students with TBI may share important characteristics with people in other disability groups. For example, those students with TBI who recover generally adequate intellectual functioning but who continue to exhibit learning and other information-processing weaknesses may resemble students with congenital learning disabilities. In contrast to those students, however, students with TBI (1) may change neurologically for months or longer after their return to school; (2) may score at misleadingly high levels on tests of academic achievement because of knowledge and skill preserved from before the injury; (3) may experience particularly acute psychosocial problems because of their need to adjust to a changed profile of abilities and disabilities; and (4) may experience unpredictable difficulty years after the injury because of damage to parts of the brain that are needed for later maturation.

In contrast, when outcome is characterized by seriously impaired general intellectual functioning, children with TBI may appear to resemble closely students with a diagnosis of mental retardation. However, the student with TBI (1) may retain surprising abilities in areas unaffected by the injury; (2) may continue to improve neurologically, thereby potentially growing out of this misleading diagnosis; and (3) may maintain a self-concept based on preinjury abilities. In addition, such a student's family might be hindered in their efforts to assist the child with TBI if they are forced to confront the pessimistic prognosis implied by a diagnosis of mental retardation.

Finally, if children with TBI have serious difficulty with behavioral self-control, they may resemble students in whom behavioral or emotional disability has been diagnosed, but the individuals with TBI might not respond to the management programs commonly used with these other students because of issues associated specifically with TBI (see Chapter 13).

In this chapter, one of our primary goals is to describe a general conceptual framework that supports flexible and creative school programming for the students with TBI. Another primary goal is to highlight three common problematic profiles of such students who are returning to school after injury and the combinations of services and supports worth considering for each of these categories of students. We conclude the chapter with a management plan useful for students with mild TBI.

Premises Underlying the Conceptual Framework

The approach to school reentry described in this chapter is organized around a conceptual framework that has evolved as we have worked with several hundred children and adolescents with TBI. Our goal was to facilitate and maintain these students' successful reintegration into the school system. The 11 premises that follow express themes that, in our experience, have emerged as being most critical for this group.

Premise 1: Variability

Because of extreme variability among students with TBI—the nature and duration of their rehabilitation, the schools they attend (including the school's experience with TBI), their families, and other supports—to seek a single school reentry program or process that is applicable to all students is clearly misguided. At one extreme are those students whose outcome is generally good, whose special needs are few, whose rehabilitation staff are experienced and able to communicate effectively with school professionals, whose school staff are flexible and well oriented to possible needs after TBI, and whose parents are emotionally resilient, well oriented to TBI-related issues, and effective advocates for their child. At the other extreme are students whose needs are many and complex, whose rehabilitation staff are not experienced in pediatric TBI, whose school staff are not well oriented to TBI-related issues and are generally inflexible, and whose families have a troubled history with the school and extreme difficulty adjusting to the child's injury. In these two extreme cases, and in the many possible variations between the two, the school reentry processes will vary, as will the combinations of services and supports needed by the student and family. For these reasons, educational planning for children with TBI must be individualized and flexible. Later in this chapter, we present three common profiles of students with TBI and propose a set of services and supports appropriate to those profiles.

Premise 2: Delayed Consequences

Many children with TBI enjoy rapid recovery and resume their preinjury developmental trajectories. However, the literature on long-term outcome after pediatric TBI increasingly has highlighted the frequency of delayed developmental consequences. Delayed onset of symptoms is often related to frontal lobe injury, a common locus of damage in TBI (Benton, 1991; Eslinger et al., 1992; Feeney and Ylvisaker, 1995; Grattan and Eslinger, 1991, 1992; Marlowe, 1992; Mateer and Williams, 1991; Price et al., 1990; Shallice and Burgess, 1990; Williams and Mateer, 1992; Ylvisaker and Feeney, 1995, 1996). Because this part of the brain continues to mature anatomically during childhood and into the adolescent years and because apparently the possibility is limited that other parts of the brain will assume responsibility for prefrontal functions, early injury may yield its consequences only when the child reaches the age at which the function in question is expected to mature. In this sense, children with prefrontal injury "grow into their disability." The phenomenon of delayed developmental consequences is most apparent in relation to executive functions, including mature self-regulation of social behavior, strategic behavior in relation to difficult tasks such as schoolwork, and the ability to meet demands for increasingly abstract and well-organized thinking as the child advances through the academic curriculum (Diamond, 1991; Goldman-Rakic, 1993; Welsh et al., 1991).

Delayed consequences are easiest to detect in children who are injured as preschoolers (an age normally associated with weak executive functions) and who experience apparently good recovery but in whom cognitive, academic, or behavioral difficulties begin when they enter school. Although most apparent at a very young age, this pattern of delayed consequences might continue throughout adolescence, an observation emphasized by Ylvisaker and Feeney (1995). Delayed onset of symptoms is sufficiently common after TBI in children that educational planners must ensure a long-term monitoring and safety-net system for these students. An unfortunate reality is that many children receive little support when they return to school and begin to have serious academic and behavioral difficulties some years after their injury, which are subsequently attributed entirely to their laziness, oppositional nature, or emotional instability.

Premise 3: Cognitive, Behavioral, and Psychosocial Challenges

Although virtually any function or combination of functions can be spared or impaired after TBI, outcome is more commonly dominated by cognitive, behavioral, and psychosocial disability than by physical disability (Papero et al., 1993; also see Chapter 2). In our experience, unusual profiles of cognitive and behavioral functioning (i.e., so-called personality changes) tend to be more vexing than physical disability for school staff, family, and friends (Feeney and Ylvisaker, 1995, 1997; Lehr, 1990; Perrott et al., 1991; Ylvisaker and Feeney, 1994, 1996, in press). Behavior problems are often a consequence of a school staff's failure to recognize the type and degree of supports that a child needs, which results in a child's academic and, possibly, social failure, which in turn leads to behavioral deterioration. When behavioral reactions are poorly understood and inappropriately managed, an escalating cycle of negative behavior is a natural result (Feeney and Ylvisaker, 1995; see also Chapter 13). The three profiles identified later in this chapter all involve interesting combinations of cognitive and behavioral disability.

Premise 4: Contextualized Assessment

The growing literature on frontal lobe injury in children and adults suggests that standardized, out-of-context assessments often fail to identify an individual's functional disability (Benton, 1991; Bigler, 1988; Dennis, 1991; Eslinger and Damasio, 1985; Grattan and Eslinger, 1991; Mateer and Williams, 1991; Stelling et al., 1986; Stuss and Benson, 1986; Telzrow, 1991; Welsh et al., 1991). This may be associated with what Teuber (1964) referred to as the *riddle of the frontal lobes,* "the curious disassociation between knowing and doing." The important functions associated with prefrontal parts of the brain are infrequently needed to perform adequately on highly structured test tasks. These functions include identifying what needs to be done in a complex or novel situation, planning how to accomplish the task (with consideration of one's ability to perform), organizing behavior around accomplishing the task, initiating goal-directed behavior, inhibiting inappropriate behavior, monitoring and evaluating performance, and finding alternative approaches in the event of failure. In the case of tests, responsibility for most of these activities is assumed by the evaluator. For these reasons, among others, assessment that is functional, collaborative, contextualized, and based on tests of carefully formulated hypotheses is most valuable for individuals with TBI, which frequently includes frontal lobe injury, a point that is developed by Ylvisaker and Gioia in Chapter 10.

Premise 5: Contextualized Intervention

In the chapters of this book devoted to cognitive and behavioral aspects of rehabilitation, we emphasized intervention delivered in the context of meaningful activities and routines in the child's life (including academic life). The literature on transfer of training in both cognitive and behavioral psychology yields a strong rationale for contextualized intervention (Horner et al., 1988; Koegel et al., 1995; Singley and Anderson, 1989). Attention to context (i.e., the setting, people, and activities that compose intervention) is particularly important for people whose thought processes are relatively concrete and inflexible (a common consequence of severe TBI). Appropriately contextualized intervention is also advantageous in that it contributes to the child's orientation and motivation.

A corollary of this principle is that, other things being equal, it is advantageous to return children to their community schools as quickly as possible after an injury and to deliver cognitive, communicative, and behavioral intervention in the context of the children's academic work and daily routines in those settings. Many reasons exist for deviating from this general prescription; however, in every case, intervention should occur within as genuinely meaningful a context as possible. Transitional outpatient or short-term special classroom placements are warranted for some children with TBI (e.g., those children who remain medically fragile or who continue to exhibit behaviors that pose a health or safety hazard in a school environment). If a transitional program is judged to be appropriate, a system for frequent monitoring must be in place because of the natural tendency for transitional programs to extend far beyond their justifiable duration.

Premise 6: Antecedent or Proactive Approaches to Challenging Behavior

The tradition in applied behavior analysis has been to focus heavily on consequences in the antecedent-behavior-consequence formula (Alberto and Troutman, 1996; Martin and Pear, 1996). This tradition has emphasized the elimination of undesirable behavior rather than the teaching of desirable behavior. A traditional approach to undesirable behaviors, such as those associated with aggression or noncompliance, would be to target them for extinction by ignoring them, following them with negative consequences (i.e., punishment), or removing the student from reinforcing interaction (i.e., time out).

For several important reasons, this traditional approach might be inappropriate in the case of students with TBI. First, damage to inhibition centers of the prefrontal lobes, which is common in TBI, might modify a child's ability to inhibit impulsive actions to the level of a young preschooler, in whom behavior is managed poorly by manipulating consequences alone. Second, neuropsychological investigations of prefrontal injury, particularly ventromedial prefrontal injury, have suggested that people with this type of injury do not benefit in the usual way from rewards and, especially, from punishments. Current theory suggests that individuals with ventromedial prefrontal injury fail to attach "somatic markers" to the stored representation of an event, thereby depriving themselves of the component of memory that guides future action in response to past rewards and punishments (Damasio, 1994; Damasio et al., 1990, 1991; Saver and Damasio, 1991). Third, after a life-altering injury in a child, the achievement of consistency in implementing consequence-oriented behavioral programs, which is an important condition of the success of such programs, is difficult.

For these and other reasons, Ylvisaker and colleagues, in Chapter 13, advocate a positive, antecedent-focused, communication-based approach to problem behavior after TBI. Procedures associated with this approach include (1) preventing negative behavior by eliminating the provocation, including unreasonable demands; (2) ensuring orientation to task and providing the student with the supports needed to be successful in completing that task; (3) helping the student to be successful on several nonthreatening tasks before presenting tasks that are difficult; (4) teaching positive alternatives, including communication alternatives, to negative behavior; (5) establishing alternative positive scripts; (6) inducing positive internal setting events (e.g., by giving a student choices and control whenever possible); (7) systematically desensitizing the student to events that cause anxiety; and (8) helping the student to manage his or her own antecedents (e.g., by leaving a situation that is getting out of control). Each of these procedures is explained and illustrated in Chapter 13.

Premise 7: Flexibility in Educational Programming

By definition, all individualized education plans (IEPs) are designed to be flexible to meet the potentially unique and changing needs of the student for whom the plan was developed. Flexible educational programming is notoriously difficult to implement. However, the premium placed on flexibility tends to be particularly high in the case of students with TBI. First, these students may change significantly over the early weeks and months after their return to school—either positively, because of spontaneous neurologic improvement and a return to familiar routines, or negatively, because of emotional responses to failure and frustration or because of delayed onset of consequences (Fletcher et al., 1985). Because these changes are minimally predictable and because the resulting profiles of ability and need might be highly unusual, special education plans must frequently be re-evaluated (possibly monthly or bimonthly in the year after a child with TBI returns to school). In addition, novel combinations of services and supports might have to be considered.

Premise 8: Collaborative Decision Making

Ideally, collaborative educational planning begins long before the child is discharged from the rehabilitation facility and involves respectful negotiation among rehabilitation specialists, representatives from the school, family members and, if possible, the student. Each party brings to the table a unique perspective and area of expertise (O'Brien and Lyle, 1986). Families contribute critical information about the student's preinjury and postinjury abilities and interests as well as a vision of long-term goals. Rehabilitation professionals need to inform others of the nature of the child's injury, current status, projected outcome and needs, and recommendations for ongoing rehabilitation. School professionals help rehabilitation staff understand educational dimensions of rehabilitation, ways in which ongoing rehabilitation can be integrated into school activities, educational priorities for the child, and the possibilities and limitations for the child in the community school. The development of IEPs is discussed later in this chapter.

Premise 9: Systematic Reduction of Supports

Many schools enthusiastically serve students with TBI as effectively as such students can be served. However, educators and school psychologists frequently underestimate a student's need for supports in the early months or years after injury, which in some cases results in significant failure and growing disability for the student. In turn, growing disability may necessitate increasing services over the years that the student is in school.

The opposite pattern is far more desirable: That is, adequate supports should be in place in the early months and years after a child with TBI returns to school, followed by systematic reduction of those supports as the child demonstrates an ability to remain competent with less support. Supports might have to be increased at pre-

dictably critical times (e.g., the transition from grade school to middle school) or when the student has difficulty or becomes vulnerable for unpredictable reasons. However, family and school staff alike should strive to reduce extraordinary supports as quickly as possible, being mindful of the threat of learned helplessness when too much is done for students with potentially greater competence than is attributed to them. To reduce the potential for conflict between family and school staff, a plan and rationale for systematic reduction of supports should be written into the student's IEP. Without such a negotiated plan, family members may perceive a reduction in support as a violation of their rights, and time and resources might be wasted on a conflict that could have been avoided. The special education literature includes several useful planning systems for this purpose.

Premise 10: Resource Specialist

Because the incidence of TBI is relatively low, as compared to other educational disabilities, specialized knowledge in this area is unlikely to be widely distributed among special educators and educational administrators in the foreseeable future. Furthermore, because of the nature of the disability associated with commonly occurring frontal lobe injury, effective educational management of children with TBI often necessitates approaches that deviate from conventional wisdom (e.g., antecedent-focused approaches to challenging behavior) or that are emphasized infrequently in traditional special education programs (e.g., executive function routines). Therefore, school staff often profit from collaborative planning and brainstorming with consultants who have special expertise in the educational integration of students with TBI.

In times of shrinking school budgets, special attention to low-incidence conditions is not a high priority. Iowa, Kansas, and Oregon all have addressed the problem of educational integration of students with TBI in similar ways by designating regional teams of TBI specialists in each of the disciplines and by providing ongoing training opportunities for these teams, organized by a resource coordinator in or supported by the state education department. In each of these states, the resource specialists have developed useful materials for the training of educators. In New York State, a very effective system of regional TBI specialists, originally supported by a grant from the state education department, has been difficult to maintain through local financing. However they are supported, resource specialists with expertise in TBI can play some combination of the important roles outlined in Table 17-1.

Premise 11: Support for Family and Peers

Success in school after TBI is related to the child's recovery of neurologically based abilities to learn and perform and to the school's ability to meet the child's academic

Table 17-1. Educational Resource Specialist or Case Coordinator Functions: School Reentry After TBI

Direct service in schools
- Problem solving; helping school staff test hypotheses about what type of instruction and intervention will be most successful
- Training staff, including providing information about the unique characteristics of students with TBI
- Translating medical information into school language
- Supporting school staff
- Facilitating the development of school-based teams
- Supporting peers

Case management
- Finding needed services, supports, and expertise in the community
- Coordinating school and community providers

Team training
- Training teachers and clinicians to be local resources for one another (e.g., understanding of consequences of TBI; knowledge of where to go for help)

Information dissemination
- Providing general information about TBI
- Developing a library of resources (e.g., books, articles, videos)

Transitioning from hospital to school case management
- Facilitating the transfer of function from hospital case managers to individuals in schools who play the role of case manager (possibly social worker, school counselor, special educator, school psychologist, or other school staff)

Family support
- Helping family members understand medical and educational issues
- Supporting family members through their grieving process
- Providing information about TBI and community resources
- Helping school personnel recognize and understand family issues

Source: Reprinted with permission from M Ylvisaker, T Feeney, N Maher-Maxwell, et al. (1995). School re-entry following severe traumatic brain injury: guidelines for educational planning. J Head Trauma Rehabil 10(6);25.

and other needs. Although perhaps less obvious, success is related equally to the support provided to the student by a resilient and well-adjusted family and by thoughtful and encouraging peers. Because their needs are often intense and their contribution to the child's outcome pivotal, families deserve a central place in the intervention planning of hospital and school teams. Family intervention and support are discussed by Waaland in Chapter 16. Similarly, peers need help to play their role effectively. Support for peers is discussed briefly under Support for School Peers later in this chapter.

School Reentry as a Long-Term Transitional Process

Although it is natural to think of school reentry as a single event or as a short-duration process that begins shortly before a child's discharge from rehabilitation and ends shortly after a child's return to school, a far more effective view is that of a process that begins shortly after a child's admission to rehabilitation and continues throughout the child's school years and transition to adult life. This broad view of school reentry helps to incorporate a healthy educational perspective into rehabilitation and a rehabilitation perspective into ongoing schooling. Integration of services over time and among diverse systems of care is obviously

beneficial to the child, however difficult this may be to implement in a fragmented world of service providers.

An Educational Perspective During Acute Rehabilitation

After severe TBI, children may be hospitalized for several weeks or months, much of that time as inpatients in a rehabilitation facility. Rehabilitation professionals actively pursue many medical and restorative goals for the child. Early in recovery, this medical focus is natural and appropriate and is encouraged by third-party payers as well as organizations that accredit rehabilitation facilities. However, children are poorly served if the focus of their rehabilitation does not gradually shift to functional themes, including preparation for returning to school. For example, physical therapy might begin to focus on the child's need for mobility in busy school corridors, transfers in and out of school desks and chairs, and participation in sports or adapted physical education activities. Occupational therapists might focus increasingly on the child's ability to write or to access a keyboard for academic work, whereas speech-language pathologists might focus on comprehension of schoolbooks and the language of classroom routines. This shift in focus is mandated by the generally accepted need to achieve functional outcomes in rehabilitation and also by the need to simulate the activities, routines, interactions, and demands of school to acquire assessment information necessary for planning a successful school reentry.

Education-Relevant Assessment

A child or adolescent who is hospitalized for an extended period after TBI typically is served by a team of rehabilitation professionals, each of whom conducts an assessment that yields important information about the child's profile of abilities and needs in a specific area of functioning. Assuming that the child's functioning remains fairly stable between the time of these assessments and school reentry, this information, if presented to school staff in a digestible manner, should be helpful in planning the child's school program.

However, the information that is delivered from hospital to school is commonly unhelpful—possibly because the information is delivered exclusively in reports (a notoriously weak mode of communication), because the reports never reach the appropriate school staff, or because they are written in terms that do not appear relevant to educational decision making. More often, however, the unhelpfulness of hospital information is attributable (1) to the child's substantial change between completion of hospital assessments and school reentry (i.e., the assessment results are no longer valid when the child returns to school), (2) to the unpredictable improvement or deterioration in the child's performance in the classroom context versus the hospital assessment context, or (3) to the failure of hospital staff to evaluate classroom-relevant competencies and behaviors in classroom-like settings using realistic academic materials and routines.

The first of these three common threats to the helpfulness of hospital assessments, which is a growing problem as lengths of stay in pediatric rehabilitation programs continue to shorten, requires that hospital staff recognize the limitations of their assessments in relation to educational planning. Rather than using valuable time and other resources to acquire standardized assessment information that will quickly be invalidated by the child's rapid neurologic improvement, hospital staff should explore school-related behaviors as effectively as they can in their setting and should work with school staff to plan ongoing contextualized assessment of the child after his or her return to school. In Chapter 10, Ylvisaker and Gioia discuss this approach to assessment across the hospital-to-school divide and present examples of recommendations for ongoing contextualized assessment that may appear in hospital reports.

The second and third threats to the helpfulness of hospital assessments are partially side-stepped if hospital staff members attempt to create functional assessments designed to meet the needs of educational planners and related service providers in the school. Table 17-2 lists several areas of functioning related to academic performance and variables that affect that performance. Inferences from standardized, out-of-context test performance are notoriously dangerous in the case of people with TBI, especially those with frontal lobe injury (Benton, 1991; Bigler, 1988; Dennis, 1991; Eslinger and Damasio, 1985; Grattan and Eslinger, 1991; Mateer and Williams, 1991; Stelling et al., 1986; Stuss and Benson, 1986; Welsh et al., 1991). (This theme is elaborated in Chapter 10.) Not all factors listed in Table 17-2 need to be explored in every case. However, for many children with prolonged hospitalization, exploration of factors that are directly relevant to school success is critical in providing an assessment that is helpful for educational planners. This exploration requires creative use of hospital settings, activities, schedules, personnel, and materials. An important contribution to functional assessment is the availability of the child's own school materials (e.g., texts, workbooks) and assignments. Even tests from school might be useful for those children who prematurely believe that they are ready to return to school and need a functional demonstration of their lack of readiness.

Transitional videotapes may contribute to the functionality of hospital assessments. (A protocol for developing these videotapes is presented in Chapter 12.) When they organize their discharge assessments around the need to illustrate for school staff, on videotape, important aspects of a child's functioning, intervention, and school-related supports, rehabilitation staff members are forced to think in functional and educationally relevant terms. In addition, if they involve the child and family in development of the transitional videotape, rehabilitation staff members create a practical and motivating context in which to deliver family education and facilitate the student's self-awareness of needs. The list of behaviors and variables in Table 17-2 can serve as a checklist for staff in deciding which aspects of a child's functioning ought to be illustrated on videotape for individual children.

Education-Relevant Intervention

In Table 17-2, we presented education-relevant factors as a guide for exploring a child's functioning with the goal of contributing to the development of an effective school reentry education plan. This same list can be used to guide rehabilitative intervention in an attempt to make that intervention relevant to the child's return to school. Using school-like tasks in school-like settings and systematically varying school-related task parameters to pursue rehabilitation goals and objectives has the distinct advantages of making the activities meaningful to the child and facilitating transfer of training from the rehabilitation context to school. Given the medical focus of inpatient rehabilitation, it is understandable that staff in these settings might overlook the obvious fact that children's school careers are appreciably longer and of

Table 17-2. Variables Related to Educational Performance That May Need to Be Explored as Part of School Reentry Planning

Environmental variables
- Instructional context (e.g., one-to-one versus small-group versus large-group instruction)
- Activity levels in the classroom
- Location in the classroom
- Noise levels
- Consistency in staff
- Physical obstacles

Schedule
- Length of instructional sessions
- Length of day
- Effects of rest periods
- Consistency of schedule
- Effects of unscheduled time

Instructional methods
- Need for task analysis
- Effects of advance organizers; types of advance organizers
- Effects of multiple repetition and direct instruction
- Best input and output modalities
- Incidental versus deliberate learning tasks

Materials and task modifications
- Amount of print on a page
- Size of print
- Visual or auditory presentation
- Rate of instructions and lectures
- Rate of information presented in videotapes or movies, audiotapes, computer programs

Cueing systems
- Assignment book, pager, or other cueing system
- Task cues on desk
- Repeated or written instructions
- Advance organizers
- Maps for navigation
- Buddy system for assignments, navigation
- Behavioral response to cues

Classroom and instructional aids
- Calculator
- Tape recorder
- Positioning equipment
- Writing aids and aides
- Computerized instruction
- Classroom aide

Work expectations
- Length of assignments
- Speed of work
- Use of self-paced materials

Degree of independence
- Independence in navigation
- Independence in completing work
- Independence in recognizing needs and seeking help

Flexibility
- Need for routine
- Need for help in orientation
- Ability to shift among instructional formats
- Ability to shift among testing formats
- Ability to shift from class to class or from social time to class

Test modifications
- Additional time
- Take-home tests
- Test administered by classroom aide
- Format: multiple choice (recognition memory) versus fill-in-the-blanks (cued recall) versus essay (free recall)

Motivational and behavioral variables
- Need for success and reaction to failure
- Need for deliberate preparation for difficult tasks (e.g., positive-setting events, behavioral momentum)
- Need for explicit reinforcement; type and schedule of reinforcement
- Need for choice and control: response to self-selected versus teacher-presented tasks

Social variables
- Ability to interact in social groups
- Ability to read social cues and respond appropriately
- Ability to initiate social interaction and inhibit impulsive responses
- Feelings about disability

Source: Reproduced with permission from M Ylvisaker (1992). Students with TBI: Educational Issues and Challenges. Presented at the conference, Serving Students with Traumatic Brain Injury in Our Schools, sponsored by the University of Florida, May, Tampa, FL.

greater long-term significance than are relatively brief hospital stays.

Education-Relevant Support for Families

Family services and supports are discussed at length in Chapter 16. In addition, Chapter 20 presents procedures for engaging family members and others who interact daily with the child (so-called everyday people) in collaborative alliances with professionals. Our goal here is simply to underscore the importance of family intervention in relation to the child's successful return to school.

There are many ways in which rehabilitation professionals can help family members effectively negotiate the potentially problematic issues involved in school reentry. For example, families need help in understanding education law, school policies and practices, IEPs, and related procedural issues. They may also need training in how to advocate for their child and personal support in their initial interaction with school officials. Most states have procedural guidelines that are written for family members (and are obtainable from the state education department). Several recent publications include information about support for families of children with TBI and the procedural aspects of school reentry (Blosser and DePompei, 1994; DePompei and Williams, 1994; Glang et al., 1997; Savage and Wolcott, 1994; 1995; Singer et al., 1996).

In addition, rehabilitation therapists need to prepare family members for the necessary shift in focus when the child returns to school. Without this support, family members who have grown accustomed to at least an hour a day of each of the specialized therapies in the rehabilitation facility may naturally expect or demand a continuation of this level and type of service in school. In most cases, this both is an unreasonable demand and is generally less than optimal for the child. Ongoing intensive individual therapies in school have several undesirable (and unintended) effects: They deprive the child of necessary academic instructional time, fail to intensify rehabilitative efforts by integrating them into the child's daily schoolwork and routines, create a potentially confusing and exhausting schedule, and potentially interfere with social reintegration. Considerable maturity is required for hospital therapists to tell family members that a substantial reduction in the intensity of individual rehabilitative services may be in the best interest of the child returning to school and that it is not in the best interest of the family to quarrel with school personnel about the frequency of individual therapies unless such a quarrel is demonstrably required by the child's ongoing needs.

It is critical that school staff with whom family members must interact understand the nature of mourning after a life-altering brain injury in a child. Mutually destructive adversarial relationships between staff and families are likely if staff members believe that families should move quickly through the stages of grief, accept the changes in their child, develop "realistic" expectations, and "get on with their lives." As described in Chapter 16, family grieving may not be a stagewise progression, may never result in acceptance of the realities of the child's injury, and may be characterized by ongoing episodic emotional reactions that strain relationships with professionals. These reactions are natural and are best managed by staff who understand the dynamics that underlie them (Maitz, 1991).

Support for School Staff

School staff may benefit from written materials that help orient them to some of the central tendency issues that are critical to understanding TBI in children (e.g., Begali, 1992; DePompei and Blosser, 1995; Glang et al., 1997; Mira et al., 1992; Rosen and Gerring, 1992; Savage and Wolcott, 1994, 1995; Ylvisaker et al., 1991, 1995a). Some state departments of education have developed their own general orientation materials that should be made available to schools receiving a child from a hospital. Excellent videotapes, designed to help school staff understand TBI in children and adolescents, are also available (Pearson et al., 1994; Pearson and Roberts, 1990; Tyler and Williams, 1993). More important, however, is orientation of school staff to the specifics of the student's injury, subsequent disability, projected course of improvement or development of delayed symptoms, and specific accommodations that might be required for the student in various aspects of the school program.

The communication of specific information about a child and his or her needs is often done at a meeting, typically requiring at least 2–3 hours of discussion and held at the school or hospital. This meeting is ideally attended by all school staff scheduled to work with the child, at least one school administrator (e.g., building principal; director of special education), selected representatives of the rehabilitation program, and parents. When possible, selected school staff should visit the rehabilitation center before the child is discharged, observe the child in various therapeutic sessions, and meet with rehabilitation staff. This visit helps to reduce staff members' understandable anxiety associated with serving a student with a novel disability and also facilitates continuity between hospital and school programming. In addition to face-to-face meetings, transitional videotapes (described in Chapter 12) can be very helpful to school staff in understanding the child's experience since the injury and his or her current needs. In the event that a child evidences serious challenging behaviors that are unlikely to be managed effectively by traditional school management practices, typically the rehabilitation center behavior specialist must spend time in the school training teachers and a carefully selected behavior aide in creative management procedures (see Chapter 13).

The staff orientation procedures just described are useful in creating a reentry that is initially as successful as it can be. However, students and their needs change, as do the teachers and other staff who serve the students in subsequent years. Therefore, teachers working with students who are complex may require access to a resource specialist who can help to maintain an effective educational program over time, a program that is sensitive to unpredictable changes in the student and to central themes in outcome after TBI. We do not mean to imply that the general competencies possessed by good teachers and special educators are not applicable to students with TBI. On the contrary, good teaching is good teaching, regardless of the disability group. However, the adjustments that are needed by many students with TBI may not be obvious even to excellent teachers without some guidance from a consultant having a great deal of experience with this special needs group. Ideally, this guidance is provided in the context of everyday school routines and takes the form of support for collaborative, contextualized hypothesis-testing assessment (discussed in Chapter 10).

Support for School Peers

Peers can be supported and supportive in a number of ways. While the student is still in the hospital, peers should receive information about the child's progress and should send greetings and information about school activities to their friend, through cards and class letters and possibly videotapes. Furthermore, students in the school might need counseling similar to that routinely provided to survivors when there is a death in the school: They may need help understanding their own reactions to catastrophic injury and their feelings about disability.

Either shortly before or at the time of school reentry, peers should receive information about the status of the child's injury and his or her potential needs in school. The student with the injury or the family may veto such a presentation, which is their right. However, in the absence of their refusal, this presentation serves many valuable purposes. First, it can eliminate potentially negative myths and fantasies about TBI. Second, the returning child can be presented as a hero who has defied death and has extraordinary knowledge and experience far beyond that of any of his or her peers, rather than as an invalid crawling back to school pleading for mercy and charity from peers. Third, students can be instructed about how to interact with and offer assistance to the injured peer, thereby helping to avoid the withdrawal of friends based on confusion, embarrassment, or uncertainty. Finally, a helpful buddy system can be organized that avoids the potential dangers of unplanned buddy systems (e.g., buddy burnout caused by failure to rotate students in and out of the buddy role; social mismatches caused by helpful students volunteering to help a student with whom they have nothing in common). In most cases, the ideal person to make this initial presentation is a respected and trusted member of the school staff (e.g., the classroom teacher in the case of a grade-school student), supported by rehabilitation staff. In some cases, the student with TBI can contribute powerfully to this presentation.

If it is expected that the returning student will have difficulty re-establishing and maintaining friendships, staff should seriously consider involving the student in extracurricular activities that might be helpful and orienting other students to their role in making the activity positive for the student with TBI. For example, choir may be preferable to speech therapy for students with speech impairment, given its potential to enhance social interaction. Similarly, some type of athletic activity may be a useful context within which a student with TBI can pursue physical therapy objectives as well as social interaction.

Schedules should be carefully examined from a social perspective. Sometimes well-meaning staff, thinking only about a child's disability, create a schedule that eliminates most incidental social interaction that may be central to social life in the school (e.g., by having the child navigate halls when no other students are present or by having the child arrive at school late and leave early to avoid fatigue, thereby causing him or her to miss most social interaction during the school day) (Thousand and Villa, 1990). Procedures for facilitating friendships between students

with and without disability are presented by Cooley and colleagues (1997).

Individualized Education Plans

The IEP is a contract that defines the educational program for students with special education needs. The IEP specifies the student's special education category, placement, services, and supports, as well as general goals and specific objectives in areas of identified need. Most state departments of education have an official booklet that describes the IEP and the process used to create it. Hospital staff should make this booklet available to families of children who will enter the special education system after their hospitalization. In Chapter 18, Szekeres and Meserve describe ongoing development of the IEP for students who have returned to school after TBI. They appropriately emphasize the importance of frequent IEP reviews for those children who may change rapidly during the first several months after their return to school.

In the case of children with prolonged hospitalization, the first IEP is generally written before the child is discharged from the rehabilitation hospital and is designed to address important transitional issues. Generally, two meetings that involve hospital staff, school officials, and parents should be scheduled. The purposes of the first meeting are to exchange information and to come to agreement about the kinds of flexibility generally required in educational planning after TBI. The school-hospital-family team then writes the IEP at a second meeting, which typically occurs shortly before the child's discharge from the rehabilitation facility. Whatever initial educational placement is proposed, the transitional IEP should include a clear statement of guiding principles that direct the flexible development and modification of the student's education. In most cases, the following four principles should be included.

Active Experimentation. *Principle 1 states that active experimentation is required to identify the best educational program.* In Chapter 10, Ylvisaker and Gioia present a rationale for and describe the process of collaborative, contextualized hypothesis-testing assessment. The transitional IEP is an ideal document in which to specify questions that can be answered only by teachers and related service providers as a result of their ongoing experimental instruction and management. Some committees on special education consider this practice a questionable departure from their traditional restriction of assessment to a limited time period and reliance on standardized tests to answer all assessment questions. In our experience, however, clear presentation of the rationale outlined in Chapter 10 generally persuades such committees to modify their approach. The resulting IEP mandates careful hypothesis testing and formulation of goals, objectives, and instructional methodologies based on this flexible experimentation. In some cases, some of the goals, objectives, and methodologies may be confidently written into this transitional IEP on the basis of active experimentation in the rehabilitation center.

Ongoing Review. *Principle 2 holds that the educational program requires ongoing review.* For the reasons given earlier in this chapter, educational plans for students with recent-onset severe TBI require relatively frequent review. The transitional IEP should specify the time frames for at least the first two or three reviews. These reviews do not mandate comprehensive re-evaluation of the student. Rather, the goal is to ensure that the program is modified appropriately to fit the student's changing profile of needs and abilities. For the student who is rapidly changing at the time of discharge from the hospital, the first review should take place within 1 month of school reentry. Subsequent reviews may take place at longer intervals.

Inclusion in Regular Education Classrooms. *Principle 3 states that inclusion of the child with TBI in regular education classrooms and routines is valuable.* An important goal of educational planning is to deliver as much of the program as possible in a regular education classroom. However, many factors legitimately interfere with the ideal of a regular classroom placement and a normal school routine. Chief among these factors for a child leaving a hospital after TBI are the child's health status and endurance, behavior (e.g., possible safety risks to self or others), and need for specialized interventions. In extreme cases, children may be served briefly in their homes by teachers and therapists. Others may begin with an abbreviated school day, possibly with part of that day spent in special settings.

Recognizing inclusion in regular education classrooms as a value should lead the IEP team to specify the criteria on the basis of which the student will be allowed to increase participation in normal school routines. The plan may also specify the supports needed to make this participation successful (e.g., paraprofessional support, a buddy system). In other words, the initial IEP should outline a flexible process of school reintegration that has as its goal as much inclusion in normal school routines as is possible. The general levels of functioning described in Table 17-3 and illustrative collections of supports for frequently observed profiles of ability in children with TBI presented in Appendix 17-1 may contribute to this planning process.

Educational Success and Social Reintegration. *Principle 4 holds that educational success depends heavily on social reintegration.* In recognition of the negative educational impact of alienation from peers and consequent withdrawal or anger and defiance, the transitional IEP should specify the attempts that will be made within the educational program to ensure healthy and active interaction with peers. Some examples of such attempts are listed under Support for School Peers.

A Rehabilitation Perspective After the Child's Return to School

Promoting ongoing rehabilitation after the child with TBI returns to school does not mean attempting to maintain the schedule and type of individualized therapies delivered in the rehabilitation facility. Rather, it means maintaining ongoing assessment necessitated by the unpredictable changes that continue for months or longer in an individual after severe TBI (as discussed in Chapter 10 and in the last section of this chapter). In addition, rehabilitation and education specialists should identify creative ways in which physical, communication, and cognitive goals and objectives established by the rehabilitation team can be targeted within the context of classroom activities and academic tasks.

Integration of Education and Ongoing Rehabilitation

From a cognitive perspective, it is sometimes said that a focus on academic content should be postponed in children with TBI while specialists continue to restore cognitive function with process-oriented cognitive rehabilitation activities. This prescription neglects the important tenet of cognitive science that content and process are not easily separated and that the best approach to improving cognitive processes is to target processing efficiency and strategic processing within the context of academic content: That is, as much as possible, a rehabilitative focus on components of cognition (e.g., attention, perception, organization, memory, problem solving) should occur while students are attempting to master academic knowledge and skills that they either forgot or missed because of the time away from school. Similarly, physical rehabilitation should be integrated as much as possible with school activities, supplemented by specialized services for those aspects of the child's rehabilitation that simply cannot be creatively integrated into school routines.

If individual specialized rehabilitative services continue to be necessary after the child returns to school, those services might best be delivered during nonschool hours, thereby avoiding fragmenting the school day and depriving the child of valuable instructional time. If two service delivery systems are used (i.e., school and outpatient rehabilitation), frequent communication between the professionals is required so that fragmentation and inefficiency of services, as well as confusion for the child and family, are avoided. We often recommend that school staff members inform outpatient therapists about the most critical needs in school. Likewise, we recommend that outpatient therapists send to school staff videotapes that demonstrate their intervention and the types of modifications and interactions that might be most helpful in school.

Table 17-3. Levels of Functioning in Behavioral, Academic, and Cognitive Domains

	Behavioral Domain	Academic Domain	Cognitive and Organizational Domain
Level 1	The student's degree of impulsiveness, impaired judgment, or aggressive behavior creates a danger for self or others (with or without pharmacologic intervention). The student requires maximal external control to be safe in age-appropriate activities.	The student is not capable of processing or benefiting from the grade-level curriculum even with one-to-one paraprofessional support. The student requires a fully adapted curriculum.	Despite possibly adequate psychological test results, the student is dependent on external support to organize and complete tasks (relative to age expectations), even those that are relatively routine and that occur in a structured environment.
Level 2	With the support of a behavioral aide, the student is not a danger to self or others but continues to be disruptive and impulsive even with this support.	The student can process and benefit from aspects of the grade-level curriculum with intensive support, possibly including a one-to-one paraprofessional aide and consulting special educator.	The student needs external cues and reminders to use organizing, planning, and memory supports such as printed schedules, photograph cues, graphic task organizers, log book for assignments, and the like.
Level 3	The student is not a danger to self or others and is at most minimally disruptive and impulsive with paraprofessional support or in a structured or highly routine environment. The student continues to be impulsive and disruptive in novel or unstructured contexts.	The student can process and benefit from substantial aspects of the grade-level curriculum with resource room or consulting special-educator support.	The student requires and is fairly independent in the use of organizing, planning, and memory supports.
Level 4	With no special supports, the student's behavioral self-regulation is within age and grade-level expectations.	With no special supports, the student performs at grade level and acquires new academic knowledge and skill at a rate consistent with age and grade level.	The student's ability to organize, plan, and remember is within normal limits for his or her age and grade level.

Source: Reprinted with permission from M Ylvisaker, T Feeney, N Maher-Maxwell, et al. (1995). School re-entry following severe traumatic brain injury: guidelines for educational planning. J Head Trauma Rehabil 10(6);25.

Educational Planning: Student Levels of Functioning

Several scales are available to describe in a general way levels of functioning after TBI. In rehabilitation hospitals, the Rancho Los Amigos Levels of Cognitive Functioning (Hagen et al., 1981) are commonly used for this purpose. Table 17-3 presents a way to organize descriptions of students after TBI that addresses the three most commonly affected domains and that is written in language familiar to educators. All attempts to divide continuous variables into categories or levels (including this one) should be greeted with healthy skepticism. Within each level there is room for considerable variation and, in some cases, an argument could be made to place a student at more than one level in a single domain. In addition, no scale or system of levels and categories should blind professionals to important individual differences among children and their circumstances, nor should any scale or system relieve educational planners of their responsibility to individualize placement and educational program decisions. Nonetheless, in our experience, this simplified set of domains and categories helps planners think clearly and efficiently about this task.

Educational Planning: Placement, Services, and Supports

The general levels of functioning described in Table 17-3 enable educational planners to organize their planning around very different profiles of ability and disability in students with TBI. In our experience, the most difficult children for whom to plan are those with serious behavior problems at the time of school reentry and those with deceptive profiles, including relatively solid academic performance on testing but serious or perhaps subtle cognitive weakness that interferes with ongoing success in school, perhaps leading to growing behavioral or psychosocial problems over time. We first address students with severe behavior problems at the time of discharge from rehabilitation and then consider options for students with three other problematic profiles of ability and disability.

Students with Severe Behavior Problems

Students at behavioral level 1 (i.e., those who pose a danger to themselves or others, with or without one-to-one behavioral support), whatever their academic and cognitive profiles, typically require services and supports beyond those available in community schools. These students may be served in specialized programs designed especially for students with severe behavior problems. Some are discharged to psychiatric hospitals; others (especially younger children) are discharged to home with substantial support for the family. The focus of the educational program for these students must be behavioral self-regulation and behavior control.

The goal for students who are still in a rapid phase of neurologic improvement is to enable them to recover to higher levels of behavioral self-regulation without injuring themselves or others and without acquiring fixed patterns of negative behavior that will interfere, in the long term, with effective school and social reintegration. Students who are beyond rapid recovery phases and who continue to demonstrate serious negative behavior require intense and appropriately targeted behavior management programs in whatever setting is judged to be most appropriate for them. In Chapter 13, Ylvisaker and coworkers describe a positive, antecedent-focused, communication-based approach to comprehensive behavior management for students with TBI that has been successful with many students we have served (see also Feeney and Ylvisaker, 1995, 1997). The intervention procedures described in that chapter should compose the core of the education program for students at behavioral level 1. Pharmacologic possibilities may also be explored, via consultation with a child psychiatrist or other specialist who has rich experience in treating children with TBI (see Chapter 5).

If students at this level of behavioral self-regulation are served at home, the home-based instructor from the school must be thoroughly trained in positive behavior management and must be aware of the characteristics of many children with TBI with regard to behavior management decisions (see Chapter 13). The primary goal of the home-based instructor should be to educate and train caregivers in the home so that behavior management for the child is consistent and effective 24 hours each day.

Students with severe behavior problems who are served in segregated school settings are typically assigned a behavior aide (a paraeducator or an assistant teacher) who remains with the student throughout the school day. Qualifications for the role of behavior aide include training in crisis intervention for individuals with challenging behavior, experience working with students with cognitive and behavioral needs, training in implementing positive, communication-based approaches to challenging behavior, and a sense of humor and ability to gain perspective in the midst of ongoing crises. A specialist in positive approaches to behavior management should be available to this staff member on an as-needed basis for problem-solving discussions. Because of the student's behavioral and emotional volatility and unpredictability, it is critical that a quiet, safe place in the building be available for the student to return to in the event of a behavioral crisis. This location provides a place in which behavioral strategies can be practiced, and it may be a place where the aide delivers much of the student's academic instruction. The goal of the program, then, is to systematically decrease the amount of time spent in this segregated setting and to increase the amount of time that the individual receives instruction with other students while he or she remains nondisruptive.

Other Profiles That Require Creative Combinations of Services and Supports

In Appendix 17-1, programming options are presented for students who are not severely disruptive or dangerous but who return to school at a generally early level of recovery. In the current era of managed care, with sharply decreasing lengths of stay in inpatient facilities, increasing numbers of students with TBI are discharged at roughly these levels of functioning and need to be served by their local school districts.

Also in Appendix 17-1, programming options are presented for those students whose behavior generally is well controlled in structured environments and whose academic performance, although depressed, is approaching preinjury levels. However, cognitive functioning in these individuals remains severely impaired. These students require more intense cognitive supports than commonly are offered in schools, without which behavior and academic performance predictably deteriorate.

Finally, the third part of Appendix 17-1 presents options for those students who appear to be well recovered and ready to resume their preinjury educational careers but who have cognitive weaknesses that are difficult to detect but that nonetheless must be supported, because failure and negative behavioral reactions are potential consequences if supports are not available.

Students with Mild TBI

Most children and adolescents with concussions or TBI that, shortly after the injury, is judged to be mild enjoy a complete recovery and require few, if any, long-term services, supports, or accommodations to successfully resume their academic and social careers (Bijur et al., 1990; Fay et al., 1994; Jennett, 1972; Rutter et al., 1980; Winogren et al., 1984). However, some clinicians (e.g., Boll, 1983; Marlowe, 1992) and researchers (e.g., Casey et al., 1986, 1987; Gulbrandsen, 1984) have identified persistent cognitive or psychosocial disability after apparently minor injuries in some children. Furthermore, in some cases, children with no identified disability before the injury but major preinjury vulnerability, associated with disadvantageous environmental circumstances or unrecognized cognitive weakness, have experienced serious academic or behavioral challenges after mild TBI (Greenspan and MacKenzie, 1994). Their difficulties after the injury may have more to do with preinjury vulnerabilities than with the injury itself. However, determining the exact proportions of each facet's contribution to the difficulties in school is not germane to discussions about how best to serve the student.

Ylvisaker and coworkers (1995b) described a red-flag or safety-net system designed both to identify those children who, on returning to school after mild TBI, have ongoing cognitive, academic, or behavioral needs and to meet their needs in the simplest way possible. The goal of this management system is to prevent the evolution of serious long-term consequences of the injury that are related more to academic and social failure during the anticipated brief persistence of symptoms than to the injury itself. For instance, if symptoms persist for several days or a few weeks, the student might fail several tests and experience conflicts with peers and teachers during that brief period of recovery. The negative consequences of this academic and social failure may easily outlive full neurologic recovery, with a life and dynamic of their own. Therefore, prevention of this negative dynamic is an important goal of school reentry planning for the student with mild TBI.

Identification

The red flag and safety-net system was designed to serve those students whose injury involves no loss of consciousness or only a brief loss of consciousness, with apparently full recovery of function within a day or two. The process begins with a designated hospital staff person describing the program to parents, assuring them that the expectation is for full and quick recovery but indicating that, in the event of short-lived difficulties, the school would be well advised to make appropriate accommodations so that the student could continue to succeed. With parental approval, the school (ideally the school nurse) is alerted to the child's recent history of mild TBI. The school nurse or other appointed staff person then periodically discusses the student's performance with classroom staff. If red flags emerge in these conversations, the program moves to the accommodations phase. Typical red flags include spotty attendance, cognitive weakness relative to preinjury functioning (e.g., inattentiveness, poor orientation to task, difficulty shifting sets, slowed responses, weak memory, difficulty with organization, generally poor academic performance), and social weakness relative to preinjury functioning (e.g., conflicts with peers, impulsive behavior, little initiation, moodiness, mood swings, defiance, excessive tiredness). Real-world difficulty in school was selected as the identification criterion owing to the notorious weakness of standardized tests in revealing subtle changes in functioning, particularly if such changes are related to prefrontal injury.

Accommodations

If red flags appear in school, the nurse, school psychologist, or other designated staff member discusses with the teacher(s) the minimal accommodations that would be necessary to enable the student to succeed academically and socially during the anticipated brief time that the symptoms persist. Frequently used temporary accommodations include (1) reduced assignments; (2) increased time to complete assignments or tests or to respond in class; (3) an assignment book to keep track of assignments or meetings with the teacher at the end of the day to ensure that the student knows his or her homework assignments; (4) rest periods during the day; (5) clear orientation to task and outlines for large tasks; and (6) explanation to peers of the short-term consequences of mild TBI and counseling of peers to ensure their understanding of impulsive or otherwise socially awkward behavior (Ylvisaker et al., 1995b).

If symptoms persist beyond a month after the injury, the student is referred for psychological or neuropsychological testing and the possibility of initiating the IEP process is entertained. This referral may occur earlier if there are serious persisting symptoms.

Prerequisites for the System to Work

This mild-TBI hospital-to-school protocol was originally developed for a hospital system and school district in a medium-sized city in New York State (Ylvisaker et al., 1995b). After an extended period of development, the protocol was adopted by the city's primary hospital system and was implemented. During the period of its implementation, its usefulness was demonstrated in individual cases. For example, a high-school student with mild TBI had difficulty with mathematics within the first week of his return to school. The teacher in the honors math course noticed his difficulties and recommended that he drop back to the general math track, a move that would have been emotionally devastating for the student. However, with the emergence of this red flag, a TBI consultant was called in to speak to the math teacher, who then agreed to make simple and temporary accommodations that proved successful in keeping the student in his chosen academic track.

Despite its minimal demands on the resources of the hospital and school systems, the mild-TBI hospital-to-school program did not survive the departure of the TBI advocate in the region who had helped shepherd it through the developmental process. This single history suggests that a program such as this, designed to serve a relatively small number of children whose needs appear to be relatively minor, must be supported by an advocate who recognizes its worth, who can promote its benefits in both hospital and school environments, and who can keep the program alive. It should be noted that hospital participation is not necessary. In many cases, school personnel know about the student's injury without a referral from the hospital. In these cases, the school protocol, described by Ylvisaker and colleagues (1995b) and briefly summarized in this chapter, can be implemented without hospital participation. The value of hospital participation is to systematize the referral process.

Summary

In this chapter, we have described a conceptual framework, captured in 11 basic premises, that supports effective school reentry after TBI. Highlighted in this framework are the enormous variability among students with TBI as an educational disability, the need for flexible educational planning, a contextualized approach to assessment and intervention, and a long-term focus in planning. We described four profiles of students who are difficult to serve and have presented recommendations for the educational management of such students. Finally, we presented a discussion of a red-flag and safety-net hospital-to-school protocol for students with mild TBI.

References

Alberto PA, Troutman AC (1996). Applied Behavior Analysis for Teachers (4th ed). New York: Merrill.

Begali V (1992). Head Injury in Children and Adolescents: A Resource and Review for Schools and Allied Professionals (2nd ed). Brandon, VT: Clinical Psychology Publishing.

Benton A (1991). Prefrontal injury and behavior in children. Dev Neuropsychol 7;275.

Bigler ED (1988). Frontal lobe damage and neuropsychological assessment. Arch Clin Neuropsychol 3;279.

Bijur PE, Haslum M, Golding J (1990). Cognitive and behavioral sequelae of mild head injury in children. Pediatrics 86;269.

Blosser JL, DePompei R (1994). Pediatric Traumatic Brain Injury: Proactive Intervention. San Diego: Singular Publishing Group.

Boll TJ (1983). Minor head injury in children—out of sight but not out of mind. J Clin Child Psychol 12;74.

Casey R, Ludwig S, McCormick MC (1986). Morbidity following minor head trauma in children. Pediatrics 78;497.

Casey R, Ludwig S, McCormick MC (1987). Minor head trauma in children: an intervention to decrease functional morbidity. Pediatrics 80;159.

Cooley EA, Glang A, Voss J (1997). Making Connections: Helping Children with Acquired Brain Injury Build Friendships. In A Glang, G Singer, B Todis (eds), Students with Acquired Brain Injury: The School's Response. Baltimore: Paul H. Brookes, 255.

Damasio AR (1994). Descartes' Error. New York: Avon.

Damasio AR, Tranel D, Damasio H (1990). Individuals with sociopathic behavior caused by frontal lobe damage fail to respond automatically to socially charged stimuli. Behav Brain Res 14;81.

Damasio AR, Tranel D, Damasio H (1991). Somatic Markers and the Guidance of Behavior: Theory and Preliminary Testing. In HS Levin, HM Eisenberg, AL Benton (eds), Frontal Lobe Function and Dysfunction. New York: Oxford University, 217.

Dennis M (1991). Frontal lobe function in childhood and adolescence: a heuristic for assessing attention regulation, executive control, and the intentional states important for social discourse. Dev Neuropsychol 7;327.

DePompei R, Williams J (1994). Working with families after TBI: a family-centered approach. Top Lang Disord 15(1);68.

Diamond A (1991). Guidelines for the Study of Brain-Behavior Relationships During Development. In HS Levin, HM Eisenberg, AL Benton (eds), Frontal Lobe Function and Dysfunction. New York: Oxford, 339.

Eslinger PJ, Damasio AR (1985). Severe disturbance of higher cognition following bilateral frontal lobe oblation: patient EVR. Neurology 35;1731.

Eslinger PJ, Grattan LM, Damasio H, Damasio AR (1992). Developmental consequences of childhood frontal lobe damage. Arch Neurol 49;764.

Fay GC, Jaffe KM, Polissar NL, et al. (1994). Outcome of pediatric traumatic brain injury at three years: a cohort study. Arch Phys Med Rehabil 75;733.

Feeney T, Ylvisaker M (1997). A Positive, Communication-Based Approach to Challenging Behavior After TBI. In A Glang, G Singer, B Todis (eds), Students with Acquired Brain Injury: The School's Response. Baltimore: Paul H Brookes.

Feeney TJ, Ylvisaker M (1995). Choice and routine: antecedent behavioral interventions for adolescents with severe traumatic brain injury. J Head Trauma Rehabil 10;67.

Fletcher JM, Ewing-Cobbs L, McLaughlin EJ, Levin HS (1985). Cognitive and psychosocial sequelae of head injury in children: Implications for assessment and management. Austin, TX: University of Texas.

Glang A, Singer G, Coole E, Tish N (1992). Tailoring direct instruction techniques for use with elementary students with brain injury. J Head Trauma Rehabil 7;93.

Glang A, Singer G, Todis B (1997). Students with Acquired Brain Injury: The School's Response. Baltimore: Paul H. Brookes.

Goldman-Rakic P (1993). Specification of higher cortical functions. J Head Trauma Rehabil 8;13.

Grattan LM, Eslinger PJ (1991). Frontal lobe damage in children and adults: a comparative review. Dev Neuropsychol 7;283.

Grattan LM, Eslinger PJ (1992). Long-term psychological consequences of childhood frontal lobe lesion in patient DT. Brain Cogn 20;185.

Greenspan AI, MacKenzie EJ (1994). Functional outcome after pediatric head injury. Pediatrics 94;425.

Gulbrandsen GB (1984). Neuropsychological sequelae of light head injuries in older children 6 months after trauma. J Clin Neuropsychol 6;257.

Hagen C, Malkmus D, Durham P (1981). Rancho Los Amigos: Levels of Cognitive Functioning. Downey, CA: Rancho Los Amigos Medical Center.

Horner RH, Dunlap G, Koegel RL (eds) (1988). Generalization and Maintenance: Lifestyle Changes in Applied Settings. Baltimore: Paul H. Brookes.

Jennett B (1972). Head injuries in children. Dev Med Child Neurol 14;137.

Johnson DW, Johnson F (1991). Joining Together. Group Theory and Group Skills (4th ed). Englewood Cliffs, NJ: Prentice Hall.

Koegel RL, Koegel LK, Rumore Parks D (1995). "Teach the Individual" Model of Generalization. In RL Koegel, LK Koegel (eds), Teaching Children with Autism. Baltimore: Paul H. Brookes, 67.

Lehr E (1990). Psychological Management of Traumatic Brain Injuries in Children and Adolescents. Gaithersburg, MD: Aspen Publishers.

Marlowe WB (1992). The impact of a right prefrontal lesion on the developing brain. Brain Cogn 20;205.

Martin G, Pear J (1996). Behavior Modification: What It Is and How to Do It (5th ed). Upper Saddle River, NJ: Prentice Hall.

Mateer CA, Williams D (1991). Effects of frontal lobe injury in childhood. Dev Neuropsychol 7;359.

Mira M, Tyler J, Tucker B (1992). Traumatic Brain Injury in Children and Adolescents: A Sourcebook for Teachers and Other School Personnel. Austin, TX: PRO-ED.

O'Brien J, Lyle C (1986). Design for Accomplishment. Lithonia, GA: Response System Associates.

Papero PH, Prigatano GP, Snyder HM, Johnson DL (1993). Children's adaptive behavioral competence after head injury. Neuropsychol Rehabil 3;321.

Pearson S, Magel J, Parker S (1994). Families Living with Brain Injury. Videocassette. Available from the Division of Developmental Disabilities, Department of Pediatrics, University Hospital School, 100 Hospital School, Iowa City, IA 52242-1011.

Pearson S, Roberts MA (1990). Traumatic Brain Injury: The Return to School. Videocassette. Available from the Division of Developmental Disabilities, Department of Pediatrics, University Hospital School, 100 Hospital School, Iowa City, IA 52242-1011.

Perrott SB, Taylor HG, Montes JL (1991). Neuropsychological sequelae, familial stress, and environmental adaptation following pediatric head injury. Dev Neuropsychol 7;69.

Price B, Doffnre K, Stowe R, Mesulam M (1990). The compartmental learning disabilities of early frontal lobe damage. Brain 113;1383.

Rosen CD, Gerring JP (1992). Head Trauma: Educational Reintegration (2nd ed). San Diego: Singular Publishing Group.

Rutter M, Chadwick O, Brown G (1980). A prospective study of children with head injuries: I. Design and methods. Psychol Med 10;633.

Savage RC, Wolcott GF (1994). Educational Dimensions of Acquired Brain Injury. Austin, TX: PRO-ED.

Savage RC, Wolcott GF (eds) (1995). An Educator's Manual: What Educators Need to Know About Students with Brain Injury (3rd ed). Washington, DC: Brain Injury Association.

Saver JL, Damasio AR (1991). Preserved access and processing of social knowledge in a patient with acquired sociopathy due to ventromedial frontal damage. Neuropsychologia 29;1241.

Shallice T, Burgess PW (1990). Higher Order Cognitive Impairments and Frontal Lobe Lesions in Man. In H Levin, HM Eisenberg, AL Benton (eds), Frontal Lobe Function and Injury. London: Oxford University.

Singer GHS, Glang A, Williams J (eds) (1996). Families and Children with Acquired Brain Injury: Challenges and Adaptation. Baltimore: Paul H. Brookes.

Singley M, Anderson J (1989). The Transfer of Cognitive Skill. Cambridge, MA: Harvard University.

Stelling MW, McKay SE, Carr WA, et al. (1986). Frontal lobe lesions and cognitive function in craniopharyngioma survivors. Am J Dis Child 140;710.

Stuss DT, Benson DF (1986). The Frontal Lobes. New York: Raven.

Telzrow CF (1991). The school psychologist's perspective on testing students with traumatic head injury. J Head Trauma Rehabil 6(1);23.

Teuber HL (1964). The Riddle of Frontal Lobe Function in Man. In JM Warren, K Ackert (eds), The Frontal Granular Cortex and Behavior. New York: McGraw-Hill.

Thousand J, Villa R (1990). Strategies for educating learners with severe disabilities within their local home schools and communities. Focus Except Child 23;1.

Tyler JS, Williams JW (1993). Perspectives on Traumatic Brain Injuries. Videocassette. Available from the University of Kansas Medical Center, Department of Special Education, (913) 588-5943.

Welsh MC, Pennington BF, Groisser DB (1991). A normative-developmental study of executive function: a window on prefrontal function in children. Dev Neuropsychol 7(2);131.

Williams D, Mateer CA (1992). Developmental impact of frontal lobe injury in middle childhood. Brain Cogn 20;196.

Winogren HW, Knights RM, Bawden HN (1984). Neuropsychological deficits following head injury in children. J Clin Neuropsychol 6;269.

Ylvisaker M, Feeney T (1994). Communication and behavior: collaboration between speech-language pathologists and behavioral psychologists. Top Lang Disord 15(1);37.

Ylvisaker M, Feeney T (1995). Traumatic brain injury in adolescence: assessment and reintegration. Semin Speech Lang 16(1);32.

Ylvisaker M, Feeney T (1996). Executive functions: supported cognition and self-advocacy after traumatic brain injury. Semin Speech Lang 17;217.

Ylvisaker M, Feeney T (in press). An Integrated Approach to Brain Injury: Positive Everyday Routines. San Diego: Singular Publishing Group.

Ylvisaker M, Feeney T, Maher-Maxwell N, et al. (1995a). School re-entry following severe traumatic brain injury: guidelines for educational planning. J Head Trauma Rehabil 10(6);25.

Ylvisaker M, Feeney T, Mullins K (1995b). School re-entry following mild traumatic brain injury: a proposed hospital-to-school protocol. J Head Trauma Rehabil 10(6);42.

Ylvisaker M, Hartwick P, Stevens MB (1991). School re-entry following head injury: managing the transition from hospital to school. J Head Trauma Rehabil 6;10.

Appendix 17-1

Educational Programming: Services and Supports to Consider for Various Behavioral, Academic, and Cognitive Levels

Behavioral Level 2 and Academic and Cognitive Level 1 or 2

With decreasing lengths of stay in children's hospitals and rehabilitation centers, many students with traumatic brain injury (TBI) are discharged when they are at behavioral level 2 and academic and cognitive level 1 or 2 (see Table 17-3). Many schools choose to serve these students with home-based tutoring until the student's behavior can be managed at school without special supports and he or she can profit from the grade-appropriate curriculum. Other schools choose to place these students in special classes for those with emotional or behavioral disturbance. Both of these decisions are potentially dangerous.

In *exclusive home-based services* over extended periods, (1) behavioral problems may escalate because family members are insufficiently trained to manage these issues; (2) the student may fall further behind academically; (3) the student may develop increasing anxiety about returning to school and social life; and (4) home-based instruction might persist beyond the point at which the student could legitimately reenter school. Temporary placement in *a self-contained special education class* is potentially dangerous because (1) transitional placements tend to persist long beyond their apparent usefulness; (2) special education placement may be an emotionally volatile issue for the student and family; and (3) the familiarity of the community school is likely to benefit the student more than a novel environment and new people and routines. For these reasons, it often is best to serve the student in his or her local school, provided the behavioral and cognitive supports necessary for success are made available.

Source: Reprinted with permission from M Ylvisaker, T Feeney, N Maher-Maxwell, et al. (1995). School re-entry following severe traumatic brain injury: guidelines for educational planning. J Head Trauma Rehabil 10(6);25.

Services and Supports to Consider

❑ Consideration of placement in a regular education classroom in a local school, possibly only for partial-day instruction to start. Part of the instructional day might be spent in a specialized area of the school with a special educator or paraprofessional aide and no other students.

❑ Support of a one-to-one paraprofessional aide, trained in behavior management and specialized instruction.

❑ Support of a behavioral consultant (when needed).

❑ A well-designed system of antecedent control behavioral strategies (see Chapter 13).

❑ Support of a special education resource room or consultant teacher who (1) supervises the aide (when used) and develops a plan for fading paraprofessional support; (2) generally oversees the academic program; (3) gathers team members for regular integration and planning meetings (once per week at the outset); and (4) serves as the point of contact for families.

❑ A consistent and clearly displayed daily routine to meet cognitive and behavioral needs:
   ❑ The student has an easy-to-follow checklist or sequence of photographs depicting the daily routine.
   ❑ Before each activity, staff members review the day and orient the student to the next activity.
   ❑ After each activity, staff members mark off the completed activity and briefly review how successful the student was, what worked, and what did not work.

❑ Modified curriculum, at least until the student can realistically be expected to profit from the regular curriculum.

❑ Modifications in testing (e.g., extra time) and possibly also teaching procedures; preferential seating in the classroom.

❑ Possibly a buddy system, peer tutoring, and cooperative learning groups to increase social interaction while at the same time providing unobtrusive behavioral, academic, and cognitive support from peers; possibly a circle-of-friends plan, creating a social connection and organizing peers as members of the collaborative team (Johnson and Johnson, 1991).

❏ Presentation to peers about brain injury, its consequences, procedures for dealing with their own fears and anxieties, and procedures for interacting effectively with the student with TBI.

❏ Focus on the student's strengths and expertise (e.g., use of the student to help teach the brain injury unit in health class).

❏ Generous use of prosthetic procedures for cognitive weakness, including graphic advance organizers, memory aids, and the like. Staff should avoid overuse of verbal cues, because these may be perceived as nagging and might promote long-term dependence.

❏ Use of a TBI specialist to orient and train staff and help with individualized education plan development. The specialist can also train an ongoing program coordinator in the school.

❏ Possible use of direct-instruction procedures for academic content that requires rote learning (Glang et al., 1992). However, for information that must be processed in depth, incidental teaching procedures should be used.

❏ Possible use of simple metacognitive and executive system procedures to begin the process of promoting strategic cognitive behavior (see Chapters 12 and 14):

  ❏ If possible, the entire day and each separate segment or instructional session should begin with the making of a plan, with the student participating as much as possible in the planning.

  ❏ Each activity can end with the completion of a self-monitoring sheet and a review of what the student did, an evaluation of that performance, and an attempt to identify what worked and what did not work.

Behavioral Level 3, Academic Level 3 or 4, and Cognitive Level 1 or 2

In some respects, students who are classified at behavioral level 3, academic level 3 or 4, and cognitive level 1 or 2 are the most vulnerable when they return to school. Because they are not significantly disruptive, appear relatively intact socially and emotionally, and perform adequately on academic measures and, possibly, psychological tests, it is tempting to assume that such students will continue to improve and will be able to succeed in school with minimal to no special services or supports.

Services and Supports to Consider

❏ Placement in a regular education class in a local school.

❏ Paraprofessional support for those aspects of the curriculum that cannot be processed without such support.

❏ Support of a trained special education resource room or consultant teacher who (1) supervises the aide and develops a plan for fading paraprofessional support; (2) generally oversees the academic program; (3) gathers team members for regular integration and planning meetings (biweekly at the outset); and (4) oversees the development of an appropriate set of organization and memory strategies, possibly including:

  ❏ A notebook for assignments, schedules, and the like.

  ❏ Photograph cues or graphic organizers for complex tasks.

  ❏ Maps for navigation.

  ❏ Tape recorder for lecture material.

❏ Daily routine (see above).

❏ Plan for long-term monitoring.

❏ Possibly direct-instruction procedures for academic content that requires rote learning (Glang et al., 1992). However, for information that must be processed in depth, incidental teaching procedures should be considered.

❏ Possibly simple metacognitive and executive system procedures to begin the process of promoting development of strategic behavior (see Chapters 12 and 14):

  ❏ If possible, the entire day and each separate segment or instructional session should begin with the making of a plan, with the student participating as much as possible in the planning.

  ❏ Each activity can end with the completion of a self-monitoring sheet and a review of what the student did, an evaluation of the performance, and an attempt to identify what worked and what did not work.

❏ Use of contextualized hypothesis testing to determine the most effective teaching procedures (see Chapter 10).

❏ Use of a portfolio system to measure progress. At this point, grades might be emotionally explosive. In addition, a well-organized portfolio may offer a demonstration to the student and family of genuine progress.

❏ Use of an integrated, collaborative model of related services. Frequent pull-out therapies may cause fatigue and disorientation and may not yield generalizable outcomes.

❏ In the event of deteriorating social relationships, use of contextualized social skills training procedures and, possibly, organization of a buddy or circle-of-friends system (Johnson and Johnson, 1991).

Behavioral Level 3 or 4, Academic Level 4, and Cognitive Level 3

Students who are classified at behavioral level 3 or 4, academic level 4, and cognitive level 3 appear to be fully recovered and often receive no special supports when they return to school. However, subtle cognitive weaknesses might create more problems than anticipated, problems that can increase over time. Inadequate academic performance may, in turn, generate negative emotional and behavioral reactions, which could set in motion a downward behavioral spiral.

Services and Supports to Consider

❑ Consulting special education teacher to help regular education staff understand the student's mild cognitive weakness and to help him or her compensate (e.g., use organization and memory strategies).

❑ Training for regular education staff so that they do not misinterpret the student's behavior (e.g., misinterpret fatigue or lack of initiation as laziness or oppositional behavior).

❑ Plan for long-term follow-up.

❑ In the case of young children, discussion with peers about impulsive and inappropriate behavior.

❑ Behavioral consultation to develop a behavior management plan that highlights antecedent control procedures.

❑ Refer to mild-TBI hospital-to-school protocol (Ylvisaker et al., 1995b) for possible program modifications.

Chapter 18

Educational Intervention After Traumatic Brain Injury

Shirley F. Szekeres and Nancy F. Meserve

It is important to recognize the fundamental paradigm shift occurring in the field of pediatric traumatic brain injury (TBI)—namely, a recognition that TBI is not merely a medical disability the end point of which is perhaps a year after the child with TBI has received services that were prescribed by rehabilitation professionals for school reentry. Rather, schools and families are coming to an understanding of TBI as an enduring *educational disability* with unpredictable long-term sequelae that are nonetheless responsive to intervention by trained educators (Corbett and Ross-Thomsen, 1996; Lazar and Menaldino, 1995; New York State Education Department, 1995).

Children with TBI exhibit a range of educational needs and return to a variety of educational placements, programs, and services depending on the school district practices and resources, the type and extent of the child's disabilities, and the child's and parents' requests and history with the school (Katsiyannis and Conderman, 1994; Ryndak et al., 1996; Ylvisaker et al., 1995b). Statewide data of New York students with TBI show that more than 80% return to their preinjury school placement, with or without related services (New York State Education Department, 1995). These students may be (1) participating in assessment, receiving instruction, and following the curriculum in a manner similar to other students in the room but using external modifications (e.g., a note taker, word processor, calculator, or scribe); (2) receiving a differentiated curriculum, instruction with a consultant teacher, and other related services; or (3) receiving a modified or parallel curriculum with instruction and assessment in a regular education classroom (Szekeres and Meserve, 1994). Children with severe or multiple cognitive, physical, and management needs may be placed in a self-contained special education class for students with a variety of disabilities that include TBI. In rare cases, children with sustained profound brain damage resulting in complex needs that cannot be managed at home or in a public school setting may be placed in a day-treatment or residential facility.

Variation in educational intervention does not end with the child's placement, program, and services. Teachers' assumptions about the patterns of childhood learning, their knowledge of pedagogic theories, their experience and comfort level with curricular and instructional designs, and their methods of classroom management all lead to classroom procedures that vary significantly, even within the same grade or subject. For example, some teachers may emphasize listening and note taking, independent reading and seat work, and systematic direct instruction of either surface-level rote learning or advanced-level domain-specific content. Others may emphasize student-centered experiential learning that focuses on a student's construction of core concepts from diverse authentic tasks and thinking and problem-solving skills. The child may be asked to work in small cooperative learning groups, in small skill-level groups (e.g., reading groups), or in large groups. Students may be expected to self-monitor and plan their work (e.g., to copy homework assignments accurately from the board and to complete them outside of class, to prepare long-term projects independently outside of class, or to choose learning activities to meet a goal) or they may be expected only to follow very direct short-term instructions. Classroom scripts or rules for operating within the classroom (e.g., when to ask questions or when to speak without permission) may be different from one teacher to another. These scripts have been termed the *cultural* or *hidden curricula of classrooms* (Nelson, 1993, 1994).

Delivery of related services also varies considerably, as does the extent to which the delivery mode is determined by a child's educational needs versus the system's constraints. For example, speech-language pathologists may deliver their service by pull-out individual or small-group therapy, large-group classroom therapy, push-in or pull-over individual or group therapy within the classroom (Christensen and Luckett, 1990; Fujiki and Brinton, 1984; Miller, 1989), or combinations thereof. Collaborative efforts may cover a broad range. Consultation (Butler and Coufal, 1993) may take place between a related service provider and the classroom teacher without direct service delivery. Alternatively, direct service may be provided to the child by a related service provider conferring with the classroom teacher to effect transfer of individual therapy gains into the classroom. Further, joint participation may involve a therapist and teacher in planning and delivery of service or full collaboration of the educational team. Such joint efforts might involve selecting interdisciplinary goals, using consistent intervention across subject domains, and monitoring progress and needs. For some children, related services may be delivered in an outpatient rehabilitation setting during a shortened school day involving limited communication between teacher, therapists, and parents.

Cooley and Singer (1991) distinguish between two general approaches to educational intervention for children with TBI. The service need model generates placements and instructional procedures based on a child's learning needs. The categorical service model generates placements and instructional procedures based on typical characteristics of the child's disability category (e.g., TBI, emotional disturbance, learning disability). Many educators maintain that educational needs of children with disabilities can be met effectively in the regular classroom (Cooley and Singer, 1991; Gersten and Woodward, 1990; Giangreco and Putnam, 1991; Kameenui and Simmons, 1990; Lambie, 1980).

The Case for Collaborative Intervention

The goal of educational intervention after TBI must be to meet the needs of students in the least restrictive environment, which, for the majority of children with TBI, is the regular classroom in the local school (Savage, 1991; Ylvisaker et al., 1991). The needs of most students with TBI can be met effectively in a regular classroom if the child's individualized education plan (IEP) identifies appropriate curriculum outcomes (what the child will know and be able to do), instructional procedures and modifications, ongoing assessment procedures and classroom environment, and whether the staff have the knowledge, skills, motivation, and support to be flexible and responsive (Blosser and DePompei, 1994). The last decade of experience in rehabilitating and educating children with TBI has convinced practitioners in the field that a collaborative, interdisciplinary approach to educational intervention is the best practice and results in cost-effective success on accepted educational measures: achievement tests, state competency tests, dropout and retention rates, referral to self-contained special education, and family satisfaction with school services (New York State Education Department, 1995).

A collaborative approach to educational intervention allows educators to function in ways that benefit children with TBI:

- Targeting specific competencies (knowledge and skills) and consistently addressing them across domains to promote the child's depth of understanding and mastery of a goal (e.g., addressing counting in reading, mathematics, art, physical intervention, science, health, and at home)
- Implementing selected instructional strategies (e.g., use of advance organizers prior to introduction of a new concept) and environmental modifications (e.g., a 5-minute rest period at the end of each subject) throughout the school to promote the child's learning
- Providing planned, consistent mediation through dialogue (e.g., scaffolding or cognitive coaching, described in Chapters 5, 9, 11, and 12) to develop the child's knowledge about tasks, strategies, and self as a learner, thinker, and self-manager (metacognitive knowledge) and to develop self-monitoring, self-evaluation, self-initiation and inhibition, and the use of strategies (i.e., metacognitive skills) (Ylvisaker and Szekeres, 1989)
- Providing practice in using compensatory strategies in a variety of situations to increase the probability of generalization and functional use

By using a collaborative approach, members of the educational team can integrate the acquisition of academic content and the process of learning.

Educators are challenged to develop for children with TBI *collaborative* IEPs that can be implemented effectively. A number of factors can influence the success of collaborative intervention (Szekeres and Meserve, 1994).

- The school administration must establish support for educating staff and allocating resources for needed services to meet the educational needs of the child (Janus, 1994; National Association of State Boards of Education, 1992; Ylvisaker et al., 1991).
- The roles of the members of the educational team must be defined clearly, and any overlap in roles of the service providers must be clarified.
- The educational team must commit to maintaining open communication among its members and with the family and must establish mechanisms (e.g., planning meetings, documentation systems) to do so.
- The team must be flexible and willing to work together to modify traditional or systemic rules and procedures.
- The team must acquire and share a knowledge base about the nature and common sequelae of TBI and must know and appreciate the specific histories of the child's development, TBI, and recovery (Blosser and DePompei, 1994; Corbett and Ross-Thomsen, 1996; New York State Education Department, 1995; Ylvisaker et al., 1991).

Because TBI has been designated an educational disability, it is the responsibility of educators to develop a knowledge base about TBI and to establish a service delivery system that can address the unique needs of these students.

Clarifying and Focusing on the Child's Needs

As the child with TBI returns to school, both school and family typically are focused on immediate reentry concerns, such as the return to a normal school day, relationships with friends and peers, and provision of related services. Schools may be concerned with the logistics of scheduling, health and safety issues, and the decisions around grades and credits for missed work. Often, neither schools nor families perceive the longer-term and more complex issues of determining the rate and degree of new learning, selection and use of appropriate modifications and strategies, and availability of consultation and collaboration for staff working with the student.

Even more obscure to school and family are the child's anticipated educational needs secondary to such cognitive deficits as inefficient information processing, problems in learning and memory, disorganization of thought and behavior, and deficient executive functions (see Chapters 11 and 12). As students mature, expectations for independence and self-management increase, placing a greater demand on organizational skills and executive functions. Follow-up studies have indicated that meeting the educational needs of children with TBI is a long-term commitment and that both immediate and anticipated needs must be addressed in programming (Fletcher et al., 1987; Lehr, 1990; Lazar and Menaldino, 1995; Telzrow, 1990). The federal TBI classification recognized this risk of future problems when it designated children with TBI as eligible for services even if deficits are mild and not reflected in current academic functioning (Public Law 101-476, Individuals with Disability Act of 1990). In Appendix 18-1, we offer four case histories of children who sustained TBI, all of which illustrate the nonstatic nature of these children's performance and the necessity for long-term monitoring and intervention.

The Need for Ongoing Classroom Assessment

Appropriate assessment after TBI is critical in designing an IEP that will promote success in the classroom. In Chapter 10, Ylvisaker and Gioia discuss in detail the targets and procedures of cognitive assessment, with emphasis on a hypothesis-testing process. Of major importance are collaborative, ecologically valid assessment, such as curriculum-based language assessment (Nelson, 1992) and interactional script analysis (Creaghead, 1992), which identify the cognitive, linguistic, socioemotional, physical, and curricular demands of a school or classroom and determine the child's abilities or capacities to meet those demands.

- The speech-language pathologist and teacher might conduct an analysis of the language and communication demands of the classroom (e.g., the type and presentation of directions in the classroom and the student's ability to understand and remember the directions).
- The occupational therapist and teacher might conduct an assessment of fine-motor demands found in the classroom (e.g., the student's ability to write at the required speed for the required duration).
- The physical therapist and teacher might assess gross-motor demands (e.g., the student's ability to ambulate safely around the classroom and school).
- The counselor might observe social interactions in unstructured situations and assess the student's ability to interpret the social or hidden curriculum.
- A consultant teacher might review the unit assessment and determine its congruence with the stated IEP goals, the instructional approaches, and the student's performance modalities.

This type of assessment is productive in planning for transitions to other classrooms or schools or when major changes occur in the student's existing classroom (e.g., placement of a student teacher). The information aids in identifying needs and potentially effective modifications for students and can contribute directly to students' success in classroom activities, their self-confidence, and their sense of control (Ried et al., 1995). For junior-high and senior-high students, cognitive, linguistic, social, and curricular demands likely will vary considerably from subject to subject and teacher to teacher. When students encounter unexpected failure in a class, use of the demands-capacity analysis can prevent blaming and defeatism (e.g., "He isn't trying; he can't pass biology"). It can also identify situations in which staff members have become hypervigilant, subjecting the student with TBI to supports that are inappropriate and inconsistent with the student's capacity or with the supports given to typical students. An example of the relative ease and great importance of such an analysis can be seen in the case of AK, a seventh-grade student extremely gifted in school performance before a motor vehicle accident that left him with significant motor and speech impairments and frequently blurred vision. AK was sent to the principal's office repeatedly for trying to evade the one-to-one aide who was walking him to the bus. The observation that AK was able to find the bus without the help of the aide made the staff members realize that the behavior they viewed as a disciplinary problem actually resulted from a modification that not only was not needed but was in conflict with a 13 year old's drive for independence.

Curriculum-Based Language Assessment

The general purpose of curriculum-based language assessment is to evaluate the student's learning within the context of school, considering the student as a learner

Table 18-1. Six Curricula Students Must Master to Succeed in School

Official curriculum	The outline produced by curriculum committees in many school districts, which may or may not be very influential in a particular classroom. To determine its influence, ask the classroom teacher for a copy.
Cultural curriculum	The unspoken expectation that students will know enough about the mainstream culture to use it as background context in understanding various aspects of the official curriculum.
De facto curriculum	The use of textbook selections rather than an official outline to determine the curriculum. Classrooms in the same district often vary in the degree to which "teacher-manual teaching" occurs.
School-culture curriculum	The set of spoken and unspoken rules about communication and behavior in classroom interactions. Includes expectations for meta-pragmatic awareness of rules about such things as when to talk, when not to talk, and how to request a turn.
Hidden curriculum	The subtle expectations that teachers have for determining who are the "good students" in the classrooms. These expectations vary with the value systems of individual teachers. Even students who are insensitive to the rules of the school-culture curriculum usually know where they fall on a classroom continuum of "good" and "problem" students.
Underground curriculum	The rules for social interaction among peers that determine who will be accepted and who will not. Includes expectations for using the latest slang terms and pragmatic rules of social-interactive discourse as diverse as bragging and peer tutoring.

Source: With permission from NW Nelson (1993). Childhood Language Disorders in Context: Infancy Through Adolescence. Boston: Allyn & Bacon, 416.

who is a part of the "highly interactive school system" (Nelson, 1992, p. 73). Special curriculum expectations are viewed in relation to the student's home experiences and to the culture, values, and interactive strategies learned at home. Teacher, parent, and student interviews and observations of the child as a participant in the classroom are used to explore important relevant aspects of the child's performance.

- The student's academic performance on standardized and classroom tests and in specific classroom learning tasks in different subjects
- The student's interaction and success with various classroom materials
- The teacher's perceptions of the student's strengths, weaknesses, problems, and potential in the classroom
- The family's perception of the child's abilities and school performance and what it considers as priorities and major goals
- The student's perception of personal school performance and specific school events (e.g., what is difficult, easy, fun, frightening)
- The student's goals, plans, and desired changes

Nelson (1992) provides excellent direction and examples of methods by which to conduct an analysis of classroom demands and students' capacities to meet them. Although Nelson focused on language assessment in her discussion, the concept of curriculum-based assessment is extended easily to other subject areas. Table 18-1 shows the scope of the school curriculum and highlights the targets of curriculum-based assessment.

Interactional Script Analysis

Interactional script analysis focuses on assessment of the child's knowledge about "how to act and interact in school," which is "embodied in the script for school" (Creaghead, 1992, p. 66). Creaghead pointed out that students whose learning skills are developing normally learn the scripts of a classroom incidentally from their own and classmates' experiences. Because of inefficient memory, new learning, and poor perception of social cues, children with TBI might need extensive help in identifying classroom scripts and recognizing how the teacher cues students when a particular script is initiated. Table 18-2 lists examples of questions that are relevant to knowledge of classroom scripts. Knowledge of classroom scripts entails three aspects. First is *content* of the classroom scripts: What do children have to know about how to act in this classroom? Second is the *teacher's cues* for defining and activating these scripts: How do children know how to act in this classroom? Third is a *child's knowledge of the script and awareness of the teacher's cues*: What does this child know about the script for this classroom; which cues does the child notice and which ones does he or she miss; and what does he or she know about the significance of these cues?

Information from curriculum-based assessment and script analysis is integrated with other assessment data and used by the educational intervention team to identify and prioritize the needs of the child, to select appropriate goals, and to determine modifications, strategies, and instructional procedures to promote the child's success. Accomplishment of such assessments collaboratively

Table 18-2. Sample Questions That Are Relevant to Knowledge of Classroom Scripts

Questions for determining the behavior script for a specific classroom
  1. How important is being quiet?
  2. When is talking allowed?
  3. When can questions be asked?
  4. Is it permissible to get help from peers?
  5. When is it permissible to talk out without raising one's hand?
  6. What is one supposed to do when help is needed?
  7. When is one supposed to give a specific answer and when is an elaborated answer expected?
  8. How important is it to use correct grammar when speaking and writing?
  9. Does this teacher care if one uses an *X* when the directions say, "Put a check"?
 10. Does this teacher put directions on the board or does one need to write them down if one has difficulty remembering them?
Questions for determining the cues that define the script in a specific classroom
  1. What does the teacher *do* when he or she expects the children to listen attentively?
  2. What is his or her *strategy* for demanding quiet?
  3. What does he or she *do* that lets children know that asking for help is permissible?
  4. How does he or she *indicate* which tasks can be done collectively among peers?
  5. How does he or she *mark* the difference between "hand-raising" interaction and a "speak-out" interaction?
Questions to determine the child's awareness of the teacher's cues for initiating and defining the script
  1. Does he or she know when to be quiet?
  2. Does he or she know when to ask a question?
  3. Does he or she know when to raise his or her hand?
  4. Does he or she notice the teacher standing quietly in front of the room and know that this means it is time to stop talking?
  5. Does he or she notice when the teacher says, "Everyone listen up now," and that this means that the directions will be given only once?
  6. Does he or she notice when the teacher says, "Okay, now back to the lesson," and know that this means that no more questions or comments will be entertained?

Source: With permission from N Creaghead (1992). Interactional Analysis/Script Analysis. In W Secord (ed), Best Practices in School Speech-Language Pathology: Descriptive/Non-Standardized Language Assessment. San Antonio: Psychological Corporation, 65.

---

may prevent misinterpretation of behaviors common after TBI—somatic complaint, yawning, impulsivity, denial of problems, and lack of initiation—by teachers using such common pejorative "psychological" labels as *unmotivated*, *noncompliant*, and *oppositional*.

Dynamic Assessment

Dynamic assessment should be an integral part of curriculum-based assessment. The purpose of dynamic assessment is not to describe a student's static performance (e.g., second-grade reading level). Rather, it is to determine the student's modifiability or potential to change with "guided learning" (Palincsar et al., 1994). Dynamic assessment focuses on the way in which a student achieved a score, the amount and type of assistance that was needed to change performance, and the character of the student's response to assistance (Olswang et al., 1992; Palincsar et al., 1994). Schneider and Watkins (1996) described two formats for dynamic assessment. In a test-intervene-retest format, students first demonstrate their static level of independent functioning (e.g., completing a set of mathematics story problems), then are given a strategy or hierarchy of cues varying from mini-

mal to maximal support to help in solving the problems, and finally are retested on the same or on a similar set of problems. In the intervene-test format, change is assessed during the intervention and test phases. The student's modifiability and the effectiveness of different cues, prompts, strategies, and reinforcement are evaluated.

Dynamic assessment is essential in the selection of modifications and the evaluation of their effectiveness. Further, dynamic assessment is valuable because it can reveal not just errors or failure but the knowledge the child has and the strategies (even those that are ineffective) that the child brings to bear. Ineffective strategies might include rigidly applied sets of rules or scripts for thinking about issues and solving problems (Gardner, 1991). Children with TBI are more likely to be rigid in their application of pretrauma rules or scripts for solving academic and social problems; therefore, it is imperative that educators use assessment procedures that reveal such information.

The first several years after the child with TBI reenters school may be a time for this type of "diagnostic intervention," which involves careful hypothesis testing of the recovery of prior learning and the rate and degree of new learning (Ylvisaker et al., 1995a). This represents a distinct change from traditional views of static assessment of content acquisition and assessment of performance, both of which focus on the child's unaided performance at a particular point (e.g., achievement, IQ, or standardized language tests). The interdisciplinary team, with the teacher occupying a crucial role, will initiate and lead this dynamic assessment, but the child and family should participate actively as well.

Curriculum-based assessment must be ongoing to prepare for new social and academic demands and expectations. It is especially crucial for those students in intermediate and junior high school who have a foundation of early skills but who are faced with demands for rapid acquisition of new concepts, vocabulary and skills, and increasing self-monitoring. Educational demands and expectations change with advancing age and grade level (Nelson, 1994), and the IEPs of children with TBI should be designed to prepare for the anticipated demands (Ylvisaker et al., 1994).

Changes in Educational Demands and Expectations

Nelson (1994) described the changes in school demands that occur from the early elementary level through the secondary level. The following are highlights from her in-depth discussion.

1. In the early elementary years (from first to second grade), children are expected to understand increasingly complex language and deal with decontextualized information (i.e., information not related directly to the immediate natural context, such as a classroom teacher verbally describing the habitats of animals around the world as opposed to students talking about an art project in which they are engaged). To convey decontextualized information, students cannot rely on the variety of signals (e.g., showing or pointing) often used in a natural context; therefore, their verbal communication must be explicit. Children are also expected to use new rules for communicative interaction in the classroom; turn-taking rules in particular are very different from those in a play activity.
2. The middle elementary years (from third to fourth grade) are transitional, with expectations for active learning and independent use of study strategies (e.g., rehearsal) to facilitate learning. Here, students are expected to use language and extended text to learn. The range of content to be learned is expanded, and efficient reading skill is important.
3. During the middle-school years (from fifth through eighth grade), the expectation for independence grows. Also the expectation for self- and task management increases as students must change classes, organize their own study time, and complete assign-

ments outside class. Lectures by teachers often increase during these years, creating greater demands on note taking and organization of information. The linguistic demands continue to increase (e.g., mathematics story problems), and information is more abstract. Changes in the physical, emotional, and social self are occurring and often create stress through these years.

4. During the secondary-school years (from ninth to twelfth grade), the expectation for independent learning and task and self-management is high. In traditional classrooms, students spend the greater part of their school day listening to teachers talk, rendering efficient note taking essential. Disorganized students are at high risk for failure. Students focus intensely on such social matters as dating, driving, and peer friendships at this time, when academic demands are at their highest. During this period, students begin to prepare for postsecondary life (e.g., employment, college).

Understanding these changes in expectations is critical in conducting an effective educational assessment and in planning intervention for children with TBI. Some of the changes, such as those in the physical, emotional, and social selves, may create even greater stress for children with TBI because of the characteristic loss of social status. Even though curriculum-based assessment might indicate that the child can function successfully in a particular classroom without ongoing assessment, the child might begin to experience failures in later years as expectations change and the effects of slower new learning are compounded. On the other hand, the characteristic spurts in recovery in children with TBI might result in a change in readiness over short periods, which renders a child capable of dealing with higher expectations for either content or process learning and social interaction than those confronting him or her in the current classroom.

Educational Intervention

Children returning to school after TBI exhibit complex profiles of academic, cognitive, physical, communicative, and social abilities. They may exhibit any or all of the following:

- Varying degrees of confusion and disorientation to time, place, and person
- Difficulty in remembering recent personal experiences
- A loss of social status and a diminished circle of friends and opportunities for physical and social activities
- A mismatch between what they think they can do and what they actually can do, creating a conflict in self-image
- Cognitive problems in attention, perception, memory and new learning, organization, reasoning, prob-

lem solving, judgment, and self-management, which influence academic performance, communication, and social interaction

- Physical and mental fatigue, leading to reduced tolerance or stamina and inconsistent performance
- Problems meeting behavioral expectations
- Problems in adapting to new situations

Posttrauma problems interact with pretrauma characteristics, creating a unique set of needs. These needs must be addressed by educators immediately after the child reenters school, to promote successful adjustment and re-establishment of old knowledge and to create a learning environment conducive to new learning (Ylvisaker et al., 1991). Educators must recognize that this is a critical time to provide external environmental, social, behavioral and cognitive support rather than expecting the student to use unlearned and unfamiliar compensatory techniques.

Clinical experience and follow-up studies have revealed that children with TBI also "grow into problems" when their development of cognitive and social skills does not keep pace with the demands and expectations of the environment (Ewing-Cobbs and Fletcher, 1990; Fletcher et al., 1987; Klonoff et al., 1977; Telzrow, 1990; Ylvisaker et al., 1994). Telzrow argued that it is important to recognize these *anticipated* needs in educational programming. Ylvisaker and colleagues (1995a) discussed frontal lobe damage resulting in executive-system impairments that can significantly affect self-management and deliberate learning; these authors present the rationale for addressing these impairments early in the education process. The finding that children often grow into problems, the frequency and effects of frontal lobe injury in children with TBI, and the increasing school demands that students be effective self-managers and independent learners all highlight the importance of considering in educational programming the anticipated needs of the student with TBI. In our experience, school staff are most concerned on reentry with the child's physical needs and ability to navigate the stairs, hallways, cafeteria, and classroom. Ironically, physical recovery is often speedy and modifications are relatively easy to engineer. School staff members should concern themselves with the far more common, long-lasting, and insidious difficulty that the child experiences in applying cognitive and social skills so that he or she can function and learn in the complex school environment.

Establishing Intervention Goals

Because of the complex profiles in cognitive, social, emotional, physical, and linguistic needs (immediate and anticipated), determining the focus of educational intervention is often difficult, and educators may differ in their views of which educational goals should be addressed. For this reason, all members of the interdisciplinary team must participate in the goal-setting process. The family and the student also play key roles in determining both short-term goals and desired long-term outcomes. Inclusion of a skill that is not valued by the family and student may lead to miscommunication and futile intervention. Conversely, failure to address a skill that the family or culture sees as central to the child's current role in the family or school or to long-term outcome may lead to the family's sense of alienation from service providers (Cavallo and Saucedo, 1995; Ryndak et al., 1996). Families who have experienced a catastrophic loss of control over their child's very life as the result of severe TBI and who have been encouraged by rehabilitation staff to exercise a sense of control through direct involvement in the rehabilitation process will come to school expecting to continue to be part of the team. Meeting this expectation not only supports the immediate needs of the family but establishes a basis for trust during what may be several years of achieving a new understanding of the child's and the family's long-term goals.

When children return to the schools that they attended before the traumatic injury, both school staff and families might have a strong concern for "catching up" in content. As discussed in Chapter 10, standardized tests may indicate that a student is functioning near the pretrauma level and so expectations may be that the student will resume school at that level, particularly if the injury was classified medically as mild (Ylvisaker et al., 1995b). The content-process dilemma often emerges early in the goal-setting process. Some educators (especially at the secondary level) believe it is essential to focus on learning the specific content that is expected in a particular grade or on making up missed content, whereas others will emphasize that the educational team must be concerned with the process of learning. These educators will likely emphasize instructional and student strategies that will facilitate greater effectiveness and efficiency of learning. In time, both content and process certainly should be addressed because both are essential to a student's success (Wallach and Butler, 1994). A number of educators advise focusing on process over content until the student with TBI is able to function successfully (with modifications) in the school structure (Blosser and DePompei, 1994; Cohen et al., 1985; Mira et al., 1988). After this period of adjustment, the integration of process and content learning is preferred practice (Ylvisaker et al., 1994).

When a child has a complex array of needs, the educational team must set and prioritize both process and content goals with the initial concern of supporting the child in meaningful social and academic contexts. Often this involves a discussion with the child and parents about reducing the academic course load or the schedule of state testing requirements. In establishing priorities, the educational team must consider the following issues (Malkmus, 1989; New York State Education Department, 1995):

- Areas that significantly affect the student's current functioning in school, home, and community
- Areas that can result in immediate increases in school success
- Areas that the student considers major problems
- Areas that the family considers major problems
- Areas that school staff members consider major problems
- Situations or environments that the child will encounter routinely
- The child's readiness to acquire targeted knowledge, skills, and behaviors

Meeting Immediate Needs: Adjustment and Learning

Some modification of the learning goals and context is usually necessary to ensure success in the classroom for the child with TBI. Educators initially focus on the design of learning situations that will promote readjustment, re-establishment of old knowledge, and readiness for new learning. It is important to be aware that although children with TBI may perform at or near their previous achievement levels on tests of old knowledge (e.g., fifth-grade level achievement on a math test by a child who was injured at the end of fifth grade), there may be unpredictable knowledge gaps. Further, the student may be surprised, frustrated, or unaware of these gaps because of expectations for performance based on preinjury functioning or self-image. Background knowledge is very important in comprehension, and the lack of adequate access to background knowledge may account for some comprehension failures (Wallach and Butler, 1994) and inefficient processing (Bjorklund et al., 1990). Because students with TBI may have unique knowledge gaps, attention to re-establishing organized knowledge is essential. Therefore, children with TBI may benefit considerably from an extensive review before exposure to new information in any subject area.

Modification of the learning situation involves establishing compatibility between the student or learner and the content, materials, learning environment, staff expectations, and instructional and assessment procedures. This process of establishing compatibility has been described as "headfitting" (Brown, 1979) or matching of demands and capacities (Lambie, 1980). Students come to tasks with certain functional capacities. For example, a student may be able to solve two-place addition problems correctly (level) if given 5 minutes for each problem (efficiency) with one-to-one supervision in an area with minimal distraction (scope) and cues to maintain place (manner). *Efficiency, scope, level,* and *manner* parameters of learning influence a child's performance not only in functional activities but also in evaluation situations (e.g., tests in subject areas). If a student's capacities are not adequate to meet the curricular or instructional

demands (e.g., 10 minutes allotted for completing some addition problems while sitting at a desk with a group of 20 other students and being offered no cues), the student may fail. The challenge is to modify learning and testing situations so that the child can be successful.

Modifications can be made to materials, instructional methods (including examination procedures and assignments), the learning environment, and expectations for performance. Increasingly, states are identifying approved test modifications that can be included on a student's IEP to allow for accurate assessment of learning in test situations. Many very simple modifications of materials are possible, such as cutting a math worksheet into four parts and presenting the segments one at a time (Lambie, 1980). After the child achieves successful performance, an attempt should be made to fade the modification gradually. For example, after the child can successfully complete one-fourth cut sheets, fading would begin by presenting half sheets and, eventually, whole sheets. If the child demonstrates a continuing need for the modification, an effort should be made to foster independence by moving from a teacher-initiated modification to a student-initiated compensatory strategy.

A number of lists or menus of modifications have been devised for children with special needs (Cohen and Lynch, 1991; Gillet, 1986; Lambie, 1980) and some specific menus have been designed for children with TBI (Blosser and DePompei, 1989; Cohen, 1991). Modification menus reflect typical sequelae and best practices for students with TBI and are useful to educators. They can provide direction for observing behavior, interpreting performance, and identifying needs, and they can suggest options for modification. Modifications, however, should never be based solely on what is "typical" behavior for children with TBI. Rather, they should be determined by a needs-driven process that involves problem solving and headfitting to change the curricular demands so that they match the capacities of the child (Lambie, 1980). Modification must be considered an ongoing, integral part of educational programming for children with TBI, as illustrated in Figure 18-1. Establishing an understanding that instructional modifications can be made by the education team without the cumbersome procedure of an IEP meeting is essential to provide rapid response and to promote staff's flexibility.

After the specific needs of the child are understood, the team selects or creates modifications that can be reasonably implemented by the staff, family, and child and that will promote the child's success. Selection of appropriate modifications should be followed by careful monitoring to confirm the efficiency of such modifications in the domain for which they were designed. It must also be recognized by the team that the time spent formulating, implementing, and evaluating modifications will, of necessity, be required on a recurring basis as the student's capacities and needs change.

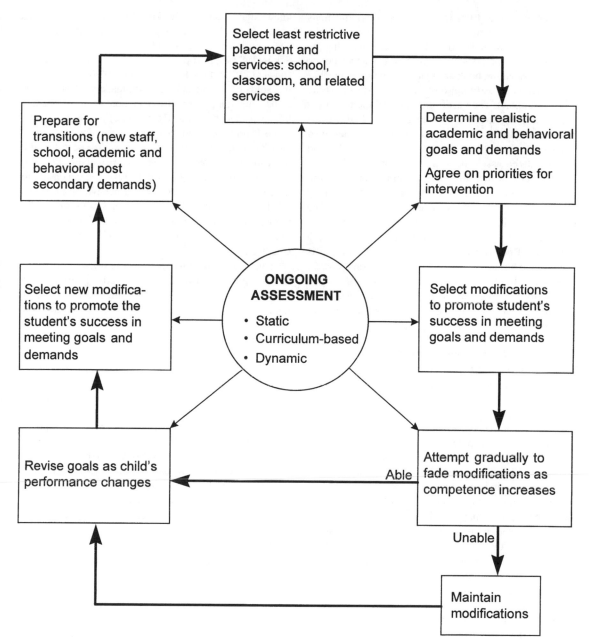

Figure 18-1. Modification as an integral part of educational programming for children with traumatic brain injury.

Lambie (1980) cited three studies of children in regular education (inner-city children and children with "undesirable conduct") that showed that instructional modifications (e.g., altering assignments and feedback, simplifying worksheets) were effective in promoting children's learning. The best practice is that the interdisciplinary team collaboratively identify mismatches in the child's capacity and school demands, make determinations of appropriate modifications, and select those that can be implemented. To be implemented in the classroom and throughout a student's day, a modification must be seen by the team as reasonable and effective in relation to the student's learning (Johnson and Pugach, 1990), as relatively simple, and as ecologically valid (Lambie, 1980). The probability that a modification will be used is increased when it can be used efficiently within the classroom, is effective in the eyes of the teacher and student, and is acceptable for the age, gender, culture, social status, and personality of a student.

Often, school districts ignore low-tech modifications (e.g., affording the student two sets of books, one to be kept in the classroom and the other at home; teaching the student to ask for assistance; providing teacher notes; using a personal log book or organizer notebook) in favor of high-tech or costly options (e.g., a one-to-one aide, pull-out support). The headfitting stage of the modification process is important in helping to avoid such oversights. Individualized modifications should be designed by the educational team from curriculum-embedded and contextualized assessment data and should reflect the unique needs of the child. School staff members who have made modifications for one student with TBI may mistakenly assume that the same modifications will be needed by another student with TBI and might fail to recognize fairly obvious but unique needs. For example, a formerly gifted student who uses a wheelchair and is legally blind has needs that differ markedly from those of an active bilingual student with mild dysarthria and impulsivity, regardless of whether the two students are in the same grade. See Appendix 18-2 for examples of needs-driven modifications.

Anticipated Needs: Helping the Child to Develop as a Learner, Thinker, Self-Manager, and Communicator

Recognition of the long-term effects of frontal lobe injury in children underlies the argument for proactive intervention to address anticipated needs of children with TBI. Educators must collaborate in preparing children with TBI to meet increasing demands (in home, school, and community) for independence in self-management, deliberate learning, thinking, and problem solving. Some educators and families may question teachers' focus on this process-oriented approach for students with TBI when such a focus is minimal or nonexistent for other students in the same grade. Other educators emphasize that a lack of focus on the teaching of thinking skills does not mean that such skills are unimportant. On the contrary, thinking skills are considered a requirement in today's changing and demanding environment, and they should be a focus in educational programming (Nickerson et al., 1985; Resnick, 1987). Students with special needs often have the least access to training in these areas (Means and Knapp, 1991).

Links to Metacognitive Knowledge

Development of self-management, learning, thinking, and problem-solving strategies is closely related to development of metacognitive knowledge. (See Chapter 12 for an in-depth discussion of strategy development and use.) Research results are encouraging for including metacognitive training in instructional programs (Ellis, 1994; Garner, 1990; Nickerson et al., 1985; Rojewski and Schell, 1994). A strong relationship between domain-specific knowledge, metacognitive knowledge and skills, and the acquisition and use of strategies has been noted by a number of researchers (Bjorklund et al., 1990; Borkowski and Schneider, 1987; Clay, 1991; Flavell et al., 1993; Nickerson et al., 1985; Pressley et al., 1987, 1990). For example, in a study of skilled and unskilled readers, metacognitive skills—including comprehension monitoring, error detection, and execution of a "fix-up strategy"—were found to be positively related to the effective use of reading strategies (Garner, 1990). Strategy use has also been found to be positively related to the way one perceives one's ability to perform a task (Garner, 1990). To compensate for neurologically based learning and behavioral problems, children with TBI need to develop and use strategies yet are less likely to develop the prerequisite metacognitive knowledge and skills without specific intervention (see Chapter 12).

Some children with severe diffuse brain injury do not recover to a level at which metacognitive goals are a priority. These children continue to learn best with typically high levels of structure and imposed external modifications compatible with their functional capacities. They are unable to orient to or consistently to act on the abstract goal of learning or remembering (i.e., deliberate memory). For these children, as with normally developing preschoolers, appropriate design of involuntary memory and learning situations is essential to promote learning. In an involuntary learning situation, the teacher's goal (e.g., learning to add two-digit numbers) is embedded in achievement of the child's goal (e.g., selling items in a play-store activity). The child is oriented to meaningful activity rather than to a goal of learning (deliberate learning). See Table 11-6 and Appendix 18-3 for illustrations of involuntary learning situations.

Further, a subset of children with TBI who are at an age and level of recovery at which deliberate strategic learning is expected may not be aware of their needs or might not use deliberate learning strategies (e.g., studying for a spelling test) because of executive-system impairment associated with focal prefrontal lobe injury. This group of children also learns best in involuntary memory and learning situations in which the focus is on meaningful functional activities. Nonetheless, because children with TBI continue to recover for years, it is reasonable to provide ongoing opportunities and stimulation to promote their development as learners, thinkers, and self-managers. As Nickerson and colleagues (1985, p. 62) argued,

> the mere possibility that thinking skills might be taught dictates that efforts to teach them should be made. If we try and discover that it cannot be done, the cost is only a bit of wasted effort. If it can be done, but we choose not to try, the cost in wasted intellectual potential could be enormous.

There should never be a sacrifice of either thinking skills or content. Proponents of teaching thinking skills agree that the optimal context for such teaching in the school setting is during instruction in academic content—for example, during reading, math, or social studies instruction (Meadows, 1993). For students with TBI, teachers must provide the context in which children can acquire knowledge and skills while engaged in the active construction of schemata, scripts, and strategies that can be used in new learning. The youngest child who gains meaning from reading by using memory and visual and semantic cues has discovered that thinking and knowing go hand in hand.

The modification process is also an excellent context for stimulating the development of metacognitive knowledge and skills. Involving the child in this process can promote understanding of task demands (e.g., "A long direction is harder to remember than a short one"), self (e.g., "I have trouble remembering directions"), and strategies (e.g., "Noting a key word in a direction helps me to remember"). The child can be a collaborator at every step of the modification process—identifying a need, selecting a modification, evaluating its effectiveness, and revising the modification if it does not prove to be effective. Through this process, the child is engaged in self-analysis, goal setting, planning, self-monitoring, and self-evaluating, all of which are important to strategy development and use.

Effects of Goal Orientation in the Classroom

Evidence exists that the orientation of the classroom can have a significant effect on whether a child develops metacognitive knowledge and skills (Ames, 1984; Garner, 1990). Ames and Archer (1988) described two types of classrooms: one with a "performance goal orientation," in which there is concern about achieving success and outperforming others, and the other a "mastery goal orientation," in which there is concern about acquiring new skills, improving the process of learning, and using effort. Ames and Archer argued that if strategy-training efforts were to have lasting effects, classrooms must support children's strategy use. Nicholls (1983) contrasted students' attributions in the two types of classrooms. In a competitive, performance-of-goal–oriented classroom, students often attribute their failures to poor ability. When a failure occurs, they respond by asking "Am I dumb?"—an attitude that essentially attributes their performance to an uncontrollable factor. In contrast, students in a mastery-of-goal–oriented classroom, when faced with failure, ask "What must I do differently to master the goal?"—which focuses on increasing effort or revising the strategy.

It has been shown that both high and low achievers' attributions can be affected by the orientation of the classroom (Dweck, 1986). Borkowski and colleagues (1987) showed that through feedback about the relation between strategic behavior and performance, which included discussion of general beliefs about the causes of success and failure and opportunities to perform previously failed items, attributions of failures in a group of hyperactive children were changed permanently. The students learned strategies and still were using them 10 months after the study was completed. The classroom with a mastery-of-goal orientation is well suited to children with TBI and would be particularly beneficial to the child with a mismatch of pretrauma and posttrauma self-image and the child whose learning is highly dependent on the acquisition and functional use of compensatory strategies.

Generalization of Strategy Use Versus Domain-Specific Strategies

Although it is generally agreed that children with TBI can profit from the use of compensatory strategies, generalization of strategy use has been a challenge. Problems in generalization and transfer of strategies in children with TBI provide a strong rationale for teaching domain-specific strategies (e.g., a strategy for borrowing in addition problems) rather than generic strategies (e.g., a general problem-solving procedure that can be applied in a variety of situations) (Ylvisaker et al., 1994). However, generic strategies that can be used across a number of knowledge domains (e.g., use of the self-talk strategy, "stop, think, and ask, Do I understand?" to self-monitor comprehension in reading, math, and history) are powerful. Ellis (1993) found that when strategy training was appropriate and well designed, students with learning disabilities were able to learn general strategies and to use them in a variety of situations. What cannot be expected in students with TBI is that they will generalize a strategy spontaneously across domains without adequate practice and guidance.

One way to provide practice and to promote generalization of strategies is through collaborative intervention throughout the student's school day. See Appendix 18-3 for an example of how the interdisciplinary goal of developing organization knowledge and skills is addressed across disciplines. Developing metacognitive knowledge about organization and its value as a strategy is a primary target in each of the learning contexts presented in the appendix. Because the development of metacognitive knowledge and skills is not content-dependent (i.e., it can be facilitated in the context of any activity, including academic subjects), all staff can contribute to the effort.

Use of Verbal Mediation Techniques to Stimulate Metacognitive Development

The primary means of stimulating metacognitive development in context is through verbal mediation techniques such as scaffolding (Beed et al., 1991; Nelson, 1993; Silliman and Wilkinson, 1994; Wood et al., 1976), coaching (Cognitive Coaching, 1992), reciprocal teaching dialogue (Palincsar et al., 1994), or guided cooperative learning (Brown and Palincsar, 1989). The mediator prompts the student to notice, think, consider options, question, express ideas, see relationships, and the like. A teacher who assumes a role of a cognitive coach guides the child (often through dialogue) to a higher level of performance. A cognitive coach might function in any of the following ways:

- Model the thinking process and mediate children's social and academic experiences to heighten their awareness of themselves as learners, thinkers, and self-managers
- Help children to understand cognitive concepts and terms (e.g., goals, memory, organization, strategies)
- Highlight features and information and keep attention focused on relevant stimuli and prompt children to search for information to enhance processing
- Prompt organization and elaboration of information
- Prompt children to create, discover, and use strategies that aid learning, thinking, and self-management
- Prompt children to identify problems or barriers, generate solutions, and make decisions
- Prompt children to plan, self-monitor, self-evaluate, and reflect
- Give minimal, moderate, or maximal cues to assist the child in successfully completing an activity
- Assist children in clarifying, summarizing, and predicting
- Help children to interpret information
- Provide informative and motivational feedback

See Chapter 14 for a more in-depth discussion of the nature and use of scaffolding in facilitating the development of cognitive and communication skills in young children.

Meadows (1993, p. 30) highlighted a number of points relevant to the use of scaffolding in the classroom:

Students learn best when (1) they are engaged in academic tasks which are clearly introduced to them and which they can proceed through steadily, making consistent progress with few failures (ideally almost none when they have to work independently, and not many when the teacher is there to provide feedback and guidance); (2) the teacher has established a classroom orientation towards conscientious academic work, and supervises and instructs actively within the classroom; and (3) the teacher's behavior supports students' efforts through behavior such as question sequences which establish easy facts which have to be combined to answer a harder problem, allowing an appropriate time for a student to produce an answer, providing regular and extensive feedback, praising specifically rather than generally, and acknowledging achievements in a positive but non-intrusive way.

Meadows pointed out that young students need more scaffolding than do older ones and low achievers need more "active instruction, more feedback, higher success rates and smaller steps in cognitive demands, more practice, more support and more encouragement" (Meadows, 1993, p. 330). Scaffolding, like modifications, must be adjusted to fit the learner.

Palincsar and colleagues (1994) illustrated a scaffolded interaction in a cooperative learning group between a teacher and a child with a language-learning disability. In this interaction, the teacher begins the discussion in the role of leader, with the goal of gradually relinquishing that role to the student (Sara). In the segment, the teacher had just read a short paragraph, and it was Sara's turn to lead the discussion by asking a question (Palincsar et al., 1994, p. 139):

Teacher: "Yes, now Sara think about that section and a question you might ask us." [The teacher then paused; when Sara made no response, the teacher changed the nature of the task.] "Well maybe you could first think of a summary. What did this paragraph tell us about?" Sara: "About whenever that tank is not filled up, he has to come up." Teacher: "Yes. [Building on Sara's idea, the teacher then models generating a question about this information.] Now, we could make a question about that, couldn't we? We might ask, 'Why does the aquanaut have to come up?' Would you like to ask that question?" Sara: "Why does the aquanaut come up? [Calling on another child] Candy?"

Bear and colleagues (1996) described how to use mediation to move from the natural word play of children to playful but deliberate word study, by careful observation and contextual scaffolding of phonics, vocabulary, and spelling instruction to help children master the rules of English orthography.

Leading questions and statements, rhetorical questions, self-talk (thinking aloud), prompting, and cueing are common techniques used in coaching. Although the use of questioning can be a powerful mediator, Gillet (1986) cautioned that educators can become so engaged in prompting a child to think by asking questions that they may deprive the child of needed demonstration, modeling, and practice. This caution is particularly relevant to coaching children with TBI who can become confused if too little structure or guidance is provided. The goal of cognitive coaching is to help children to learn how to think (including problem solving) and to manage their own learning, behavior, and communication. Table 18-3 provides examples of coaching that can be used throughout the child's school day to facilitate the development of metacognitive knowledge and skills.

The Cognitive Apprenticeship Model to Stimulate Metacognitive Development

A more comprehensive approach to facilitating development of metacognitive knowledge and skills in the classroom is illustrated by the cognitive apprenticeship model (Rojewski and Schell, 1994). The model integrates four main elements. The *content* element includes domain-specific knowledge (knowledge of a subject area), heuristics (informal rules of operation, such as when one sees *X*, do *Y*), control strategies (selection of the appropriate strat-

Table 18-3. Collaborative Coaching Throughout the School Day

Cognitive Goals	Target Behaviors	Coaching
Planning and goal setting	Think before acting or speaking.	What do you want to do? What is your goal? What message do you want to send? How do you want this to come out?
Self-monitoring and product monitoring	Think about what is happening at the moment; think about the current status of self and the task.	How are you doing? How does your work look? Are you having any problems? Do you need a strategy? What would be a good strategy? Is the strategy working? Should you try an alternative strategy? Are you making progress toward the goal?
Self-evaluation and product evaluation	Think about the quality and efficiency of performance and the quality of the product.	Did you attend adequately? Was the work accurate? Was the strategy effective? Did you work efficiently? How does it look to you?
Goal accountability	Think about self-management and responsibility.	Did you meet the goal? Was the goal realistic? Should you revise the goal?
Reflection	Think about what was learned from the experience.	What did you do? How did you do it? Would you do it differently next time? What did you learn about yourself? What did you learn about this task? What did you learn about strategies? Were you too demanding of yourself or not demanding enough?
Memory	Think about whether you want or need to remember information from this experience.	Is this going to be difficult to remember? How can you help yourself remember this? Should you do something to help yourself remember?

Source: With permission from S Szekeres, N Meserve (1994). Collaborative intervention in schools after traumatic brain injury. Top Lang Disord 15(1);21.

egy), and learning strategies (procedures used to learn domain-specific knowledge). The *methods* element includes modeling, coaching, scaffolding, fading, exploration, guided practice, articulation, and reflection. The *sequence* element covers what should be taught and when. The *sociology* element includes situated learning (authentic life environments), community of practice (focusing on learning and using a language of learning), and intrinsic motivation (especially through cooperative learning) to make knowledge valuable to the student. Rojewski and Schell (1993) believe that the cognitive apprenticeship model is applicable to education of children with mild disability, including mild intellectual disabilities, learning disabilities, or behavioral disorders. They state that many of these children, though, will need individualized instruction (including modifications) and extensive practice to acquire and maintain the targeted knowledge and skills. Rojewski and Schell (1993) emphasize that the success of the model is related directly to a teacher's knowledge and problem-solving ability, skills in mediation, and willingness to embrace an authentic environment as the context of learning; therefore, staff development and support are essential to successful implementation. They stated that

although budgetary or systemic factors might well preclude full implementation of this model, the cognitive apprenticeship model has important features that can be integrated into traditional classroom instruction (e.g., lectures, worksheets, discussion, unit tests).

The Importance of Automatization in the Learning Process

Implementing appropriate modifications to meet a child's immediate needs for adjustment and learning and creating an environment that promotes metacognitive knowledge and skills to meet anticipated needs are not sufficient to ensure success of educational intervention for children with TBI. In individuals with frontal lobe injury, there is often severe competition for limited resources in attention and working memory (Schmitter-Edgecombe, 1996). Many children with TBI experience great difficulty in managing cognitive resources such as attention and working memory, which results in inefficient information processing, including new learning (see Chapter 9).

Research has shown that one way to decrease the demands on working memory and to make more resources available for processing information or performing tasks is to overlearn or automatize knowledge and skills (both mental and physical) (Case, 1985; Kail, 1990; Schmitter-Edgecombe, 1996). Behaviors become automatic through repetition and practice. A behavior (e.g., a strategy or skill) that becomes automatic requires less working memory space, which in turn increases resources available for more complex tasks or mental operations. For example, when a person is learning to drive a stick-shift car, virtually all that person's mental resources are concentrated on the act of driving, leaving insufficient resources to converse about a complex subject. After the driving becomes automatic, the driver is often no longer aware of the acts being performed and has ample mental resources for other activity. When working memory or attentional capacity is insufficient, overload occurs easily and performance can break down. This condition is likely to occur in children with TBI when they are trying to deal with large amounts of information, learning a new strategy, trying to self-monitor, or working in an unfamiliar or weak knowledge domain.

Repetition and practice, then, are central in educational intervention after TBI for acquisition of academic content (e.g., new vocabulary, new facts about the world, new math concepts), social curriculum (e.g., new scripts, schedules, circle of friends), and metacognitive knowledge and skills (e.g., understanding self, strategies, and tasks; using strategies; self-monitoring; self-evaluation). At times, practice might consist of repetition or drill on a particular task, but more often it can be accomplished through supplemental brief and well-targeted homework assignments incorporating high-interest content, extra instruction time with an older and well-liked student, games that engage the targeted skills, study time with a peer practice partner, or computer work in programs that provide repetition and informative and motivational feedback. A collaborative approach to educational intervention can provide opportunities for practice throughout the student's day, and the increased number of learning trials in a variety of contexts can promote generalization.

Preparing for Transitions

A critical issue in the education of children with TBI is management of transitions (Blosser and DePompei, 1994; Lash and Scarpino, 1993; Mira et al., 1988, 1992; Ylvisaker et al., 1991, 1995). The transition of the child from rehabilitation to school is covered in detail in Chapter 17. In this chapter, we are concerned with the many transitions that lie ahead of the child after returning to school, among which are changing grades, classmates, teachers, and schools. Lash and Scarpino (1993) reported that 17 students in their project on educating students with TBI had gone through multiple transitions and that, at each juncture, documentation and communication of students' previous needs and performance was often

incomplete. The students experienced organizational problems adjusting to new teachers, changing classes, and managing their assignments, all of which were more pronounced at middle- and high-school levels. (See Appendix 18-1 for case studies that describe the range of school districts' planning for transitions and the impact on teacher and student functioning.)

Lash and Wolcott (1992) designed transition worksheets to facilitate the communication of critical information from one setting to another. The following items are components of the worksheets; several additional items are also listed:

- Information on the child's injury
- Information on functional issues (e.g., gross- or fine-motor limitations)
- Information on medical issues (e.g., medications or seizures)
- Dates of IEPs
- Samples of the student's work
- Effective teaching methods
- Behavior management strategies
- Description of assistive technology
- List of compensatory strategies being used
- Descriptions of modifications of learning and test situations that have been effective
- A description of unique behaviors and their typical antecedents

This kind of information can be transferred effectively in a portfolio that would accompany the student to any new situation. The portfolio can be used to communicate information to all individuals involved in the child's education, including school personnel and family.

The student should be involved in determining the kind of information placed in the portfolio (e.g., characteristics or problems that are often difficult to communicate to new teachers or peers). Items could be placed in the portfolio throughout the year and, at the end of the year, the teacher or related service provider could meet with the child to review and update the portfolio before the child moves on to the next grade or teacher. The portfolio should expand and be revised as the child grows, reflecting changes and the child's most recent abilities and needs.

A portfolio review session can be a productive time to introduce and discuss the changes a child will face in the next new situation, including new demands or expectations (e.g., taking more notes, reading longer chapters, sitting for longer periods of time, carrying books from one class to another). Simple maps of a new building supplemented by one or two visits to the school are extremely helpful, especially for a child with spatial-orientation problems. The purpose of the portfolio review is twofold: first, to see that educators in the next setting understand the child's status and needs and can prepare to meet them; and second, to help the child understand new expectations and to prepare for them. The *transition videotape* described by Ylvisaker and coworkers in Chapter 12 is also a valuable tool to facilitate successful transition. The student collaborates with the teacher or therapist in creating the videotape and communicating important information about the student's learning.

Best Practice Instruction

Consultants are often asked for prescriptive advice about curriculum, instruction, and assessment for children with TBI, with the implicit assumption that these aspects of such a child's education will be very different from those offered to other children in the class. Educators must not lose sight of the concept of *best practice* for all children. Children with TBI, like all children (with or without special needs), benefit from quality instruction characterized by features such as

- Clearly defined academic and social outcome goals and selection of learning activities that relate directly to those outcomes (Blosser and DePompei, 1994; New York State Education Department, 1995)
- Well-organized textbooks, lectures, learning activities, and assignments (Scott, 1994)
- Ongoing assessment that is used to identify sources of performance breakdowns and to revise teaching procedures (Lambie, 1980; Palincsar et al., 1994)
- Scaffolded instruction to guide students toward mastery of goals (Silliman and Wilkinson, 1994)
- Teachers' use of multiple modalities in instruction, including visual (e.g., overhead projections, charts, graphic organizers, written directions), auditory (e.g., oral explanations and directions, videotapes), and tactile (e.g., hands-on experience to accommodate different learning styles) (Lazear, 1991)
- Motivating and interesting contexts for learning (Bear et al., 1996)
- Clearly defined rules, expectations, and curricula that are appropriate to students' capacities (Creaghead, 1992; Lambie, 1980)
- Teachers' acceptance of alternate means to demonstrate knowledge and skill (Burke, 1993)
- Teachers' understanding and use of sound behavior management techniques, as discussed in Chapter 13

Conclusions

With the designation of TBI as an educational disability, educators became responsible for identifying students who have experienced TBI, for determining the impact of that injury on the child's functioning, and for developing IEPs that address the student's needs flexibly and responsively. Much has been learned since the 1980s about best practices in educating children with TBI. Common needs have been identified, although the fact that each child has unique needs has also been recognized.

Identification of realistic goals and ways in which the child can achieve them should be the point of departure for all TBI programming and should be derived from not only static assessment but also ecologically valid curriculum-based and dynamic assessment. Some of the child's needs are immediate and must be addressed on school reentry. Others are anticipated because of the likelihood that the child will "grow into problems" as educational demands increase over time and outpace the child's capacity for self-management of learning and behavior. Intervention not only must address the child's immediate needs by promoting adjustment and a readiness for new learning but also must be proactive and prepare the child to meet eventual higher academic and social expectations.

Automatization of new skills and preparation for transitions are important components in the child's educational program. The IEP must be flexible to accommodate the continuing recovery of the child and must include goals that address both the content and process of learning. A collaborative approach to intervention in classrooms that are mastery-of-goal oriented and that promote development of metacognitive knowledge and skills and a positive self-image are particularly well suited to meeting the needs of children with TBI.

The case histories in Appendix 18-1, which illustrate the dynamic nature of performance after TBI, show also that with continuing effort by educators, family, and the children, most children with TBI succeed in advancing to participation in their communities and to achievement of a significant degree of academic success. Modifications to facilitate learning and socialization, family involvement, and a key person who provided staff with a framework in which to conceptualize behavior and skills were important factors in the success of each of the children in these cases. These case studies illustrate the efficacy of well-planned intervention as measured by the students' progress through regular classes, scores on achievement and state competency tests, and social and behavioral competencies.

References

Ames C (1984). Achievement attributions and self-instructions under competitive a individualistic goal structure. J Educ Psychol 76;478.

Ames C, Archer J (1988). Achievement goals in the classroom: students' learning strategies and motivational processes. J Educ Psychol 80;260.

Bear D, Invernizzi M, Templeton S, Johnston F (1996). Words Their Way. Word Study for Phonics, Vocabulary, and Spelling. Upper Saddle, NJ: Prentice Hall.

Beed P, Hawkins EM, Roller CM (1991). Moving learners

toward independence: the power of scaffolded instruction. Read Teach 44;648.

Bjorklund D, Muir-Broaddus E, Schneider W (1990). The Role of Knowledge in the Development of Strategies. In D Bjorklund (ed), Children's Strategies. Hillsdale, NJ: Lawrence Erlbaum, 93.

Blosser J, DePompei R (1994). Pediatric Traumatic Brain Injury: Proactive Intervention. San Diego, CA: Singular Publishing.

Blosser J, DePompei R (1989). The head-injured student returns to school: recognizing and treating deficits. Top Lang Disord 9(2);67.

Borkowski J, Carr M, Pressley M (1987). "Spontaneous" strategy use: perspectives from metacognitive theory. Intelligence 11;61.

Brown A (1979). Theories of Memory and Problems of Development: Activity, Growth and Knowledge. In FIM Craik, L Cermak (eds), Levels of Processing and Memory. Hillsdale, NJ: Lawrence Erlbaum, 104.

Brown A, Palincsar A (1989). Guided Cooperative Learning and Individual Knowledge Acquisition. In L Resnick (ed), Knowing, Learning, and Instruction: Essays in Honor of Robert Glaser. Hillsdale, NJ: Lawrence Erlbaum.

Burke K (1993). The Mindful School: How to Assess Thoughtful Outcomes. Palatine, IL: Skylight.

Butler KG, Coufal KL (eds) (1993). Collaborative consultation: a problem-solving process. Top Lang Disord 14(1);1.

Case R (1985). Intellectual Development: Birth to Adulthood. New York: Academic.

Cavallo M, Saucedo C (1995). Traumatic brain injury in families from culturally diverse populations. J Head Trauma Rehabil 10(2);66.

Christensen S, Luckett C (1990). Getting into the classroom and making it work. Lang Speech Hear Serv Schools 21(2);110.

Clay M (1991). Becoming Literate: The Construction of Inner Control. Portsmouth, NH: Heinemann.

Cognitive Coaching: A Process for Teaching and Learning (1992). Videocassette. Princeton, NJ: Films for the Humanities Sciences.

Cohen S (1991). Adapting educational programs for students with head injuries. J Head Trauma Rehabil 6(1);56.

Cohen S, Joyce C, Rhoades K, Welks D (1985). Educational Programming for Head Injured Students. In M Ylvisaker (ed), Head Injury Rehabilitation: Children and Adolescents. San Diego: College Hill, 383.

Cohen S, Lynch D (1991). An instructional modification process. Teach Except Child 23(4);12.

Cooley E, Singer G (1991). On serving students with head injuries: are we reinventing a wheel that doesn't roll? J Head Trauma Rehabil 6(1);47.

Corbett S, Ross-Thomsen B (1996). Educating Students with Traumatic Brain Injuries: A Resource and Planning Guide. Milwaukee, WI: Wisconsin Department of Public Instruction.

Creaghead N (1992). Classroom Interactional Analysis/Script Analysis. In W Secord (ed), Best Practices in Speech-Language Pathology: Descriptive/Nonstandardized Language Assessment. San Antonio: The Psychological Corporation, 65.

Dweck C (1986). Motivational processes affecting learning. Am Psychol 41;1040.

Ellis E (1993). Teaching strategy sameness using integrated formats. J Learn Disabil 26(7);448.

Ewing-Cobbs L, Fletcher J (1990). Neuropsychological Assessment of Traumatic Brain Injury in Children. In E Bigler (ed), Traumatic Brain Injury. Austin, TX: PRO-ED, 197.

Flavell J, Miller P, Miller S (1993). Cognitive Development. Englewood Cliffs, NJ: Prentice Hall.

Fletcher J, Miner M, Ewing-Cobbs L (1987). Age and Recovery from Head Injury in Children: Developmental Issues. In H Levin, J Grafman, M Eisenberg (eds), Neurobehavioral Recovery from Head Injury. New York: Oxford.

Fujiki M, Brinton B (1984). Supplementary language therapy: working with the classroom teacher. Lang Speech Hear Serv Schools 15(2);98.

Gardner H (1991). The Unschooled Mind: How Children Think and How Schools Should Teach. New York: Basic Books.

Garner R (1990). Childrens' Use of Strategies in Reading. In D Bjorklund (ed), Childrens' Strategies. Hillsdale, NJ: Lawrence Erlbaum, 245.

Gersten R, Woodward J (1990). Rethinking the regular education initiative. Focus on the classroom teacher. Remedial Spec Educ 11(3);7.

Giangreco MF, Putnam JW (1991). Supporting the Education of Students with Severe Disabilities in Regular Education Environments. In LH Meyer, CA Peck, L Brown (eds), Critical Issues in the Lives of People with Severe Disabilities. Baltimore: Paul H Brookes.

Gillet P (1986). Mainstreaming Techniques for LD Students. Acad Ther Pub 21;389.

Janus P (1994). The Role of School Administration. In R Savage, G Wolcott (eds), Educational Dimensions of Acquired Brain Injury. Austin, TX: PRO-ED, 475.

Johnson L, Pugach M (1990). Classroom teachers' views of intervention strategies for learning and behavior problems: which are reasonable and how frequently are they used? J Spec Educ 24(1);69.

Kail R (1990). The Development of Memory in Children (3rd ed). New York: Freeman.

Kameenui E, Simmons D (1990). Designing Instructional Strategies: The Prevention of Academic Learning Problems. Columbus, OH: Merrill.

Katsiyannis A, Conderman G (1994). Serving individuals with traumatic brain injury: a national survey. Remedial Spec Educ 15(3);319.

Klonoff H, Low M, Clark C. (1977). Head injuries in children: a prospective five year follow up. J Neurol Neurosurg Psychiatry 40;1211.

Lambie R (1980). A systematic approach for changing materials, instruction, and assignments to meet individual needs. Focus Except Child 13(1);1.

Lash M, Scarpino C (1993). School reintegration for children with traumatic brain injuries. Neurorehabilitation 3(3);13.

Lash M, Wolcott G (1992). Educating Children with Traumatic Brain Injuries: A Guide on Transitions for Schools and Families. Weston, MA: Wolcott and Associates.

Lazar M, Menaldino S (1995). Cognitive outcome and behavioral adjustment in children following traumatic brain injury: a developmental perspective. J Head Trauma Rehabil 10(5);55.

Lazear D (1991). Seven Ways of Knowing: Teaching for Multiple Intelligences. Palatine, IL: Skylight.

Lehr E (1990). Psychological Management of Traumatic Brain Injury in Children and Adolescents. Gaithersburg, MD: Aspen.

Malkmus D (1989). Community reentry: cognitive-communicative intervention within a social skill context. Top Lang Disord 9(2);50.

Meadows S (1993). The Child As a Thinker: The Development and Acquisition of Cognition in Childhood. London: Routledge.

Means B, Knapp M (1991). Introduction: Rethinking Teaching for Disadvantaged Students. In B Means, C Chelemer, M Knapp (eds), Teaching Advanced Skills to At-Risk Students. San Francisco: Jossey-Bass, 1.

Miller L (1989). Classroom-based language intervention. Lang Speech Hear Serv Schools 20(2);153.

Mira M, Tyler J, Tucker B (1988). Traumatic head injury in children. A guide for schools. Kansas City: Kansas University Medical Center, Children's Rehabilitation Unit..

Mira M, Tyler J, Tucker B (1992). TBI in Children and Adolescents. A Sourcebook for Teachers and Other School Personnel. Austin, TX: PRO-ED.

National Association of State Boards of Education (1992). Winners All: A Call for Inclusive Schools. [The report of the NASBE Study Group on Special Education.] Alexandria, VA: National Association of State Boards of Education.

Nelson NE (1992). Targets of Curriculum-Based Language Assessment. In W Secord (ed), Best Practices in Speech-Language Pathology: Descriptive/Nonstandardized Language Assessment. San Antonio: Psychological Corporation, 73.

Nelson NW (1993). Childhood Language Disorders in Context: Infancy Through Adolescence. New York: Macmillan.

Nelson NW (1994). Curriculum-Based Language Assessment and Intervention Across the Grades. In G Wallach, K Butler (eds), Language Learning Disabilities in School-Age Children and Adolescents. New York: Macmillan, 104.

New York State Education Department (1995). Traumatic Brain Injury Regional Technical Assistance Projects: Annual Report for the 1994–95 Year. Albany, NY: New York State Education Department.

Nicholls J (1983). Conceptions of Ability and Achievement Motivation: A Theory and Its Implications for Education. In SG Paris, GM Olson, HW Stevenson (eds), Learning and Motivation in the Classroom. Hillsdale, NJ: Lawrence Erlbaum, 211.

Nickerson R, Perkins D, Smith E (1985) The Teaching of Thinking. Hillsdale, NJ: Lawrence Erlbaum.

Olswang L, Bain B, Johnson G (1992). Using Dynamic Assessment with Children with Language Disorders. In S Warren, J Reickle (eds), Causes and Effects in Communication and Language Intervention. Baltimore: Paul H Brookes, 187.

Palincsar A, Brown A, Campione J (1994). Models and Practices of Dynamic Assessment. In G Wallace, K Butler (eds), Language Learning Disabilities in School-Age Children and Adolescents. New York: Macmillan, 132.

Pressley M, et al. (1990). Cognitive Strategy Instruction That Really Improves Children's Academic Performance. Cambridge, MA: Brookline.

Pressley M, Borkowski J, Schneider W. (1987). Cognitive strategies: good strategy users coordinate metacognition and knowledge. Ann Child Dev 4;89.

Prigatano G (1995). Sheldon Berrol, M.D. Lectureship: the problem of lost normality. J Head Trauma Rehabil 10(3);87.

Reid S, Strong G, Wood A, et al. (1995). Computers, assistive devices, and augmentative communication aids: technology for social inclusion. J Head Trauma Rehabil 10(5);80.

Resnick L (1987). Education and Learning to Think. Washington, DC: National Academy.

Rojewski J, Schell J (1994). Cognitive apprenticeship for learners with special needs. Remedial Spec Educ 15(4);234.

Ryndak D, Downing J, Morrison A, Williams L (1996). Parents' perceptions of educational settings and services for children with moderate or severe disabilities. Remedial Spec Educ 17(2);105.

Savage R (1991). Identification, classification, and placement issues for students with traumatic brain injuries. J Head Trauma Rehabil 6;1.

Schmitter-Edgecombe M (1996). Effects of traumatic brain injury on cognitive performance: an attentional resource hypothesis in search of data. J Head Trauma Rehabil 11(2);17.

Schneider P, Watkins R (1996). Applying vygotskian developmental theory to language intervention. Lang Speech Hear Serv Schools 27;157.

Scott C (1994). A Discourse Continuum for School-Age Students. In G Wallach, K Butler (eds), Language Learning Disabilities in School-Age Children and Adolescents. New York: Macmillan, 219.

Silliman E, Wilkinson C (1994). Discourse Scaffolds for Classroom Intervention. In G Wallach, K Butler (eds), Language Learning Disabilities in School-Age Children. New York: Macmillan, 27.

Szekeres S, Meserve N (1994). Collaborative intervention in schools. Top Lang Disord 15(1);21.

Telzrow C (1990). Management of Academic and Educational Problems in Traumatic Brain Injury. In E Bigler (ed), Traumatic Brain Injury. Austin, TX: PRO-ED, 251.

Wallach G, Butler K (1994) Creating Communication Literacy, and Academic Success. In G Wallach, K Butler (eds), Language Learning Disabilities in School-Age Children and Adolescents. New York: Macmillan, 2.

Wood D, Bruner J, Ross G (1976). The role of tutoring in problem solving. J Child Psychol Psychiatry 17;89.

Ylvisaker M, Feeney T, Maher-Maxwell N, et al. (1995a).

School re-entry following severe traumatic brain injury: guidelines for educational planning. J Head Trauma Rehabil 10(6);25.

Ylvisaker M, Feeney T, Mullins K (1995b). School re-entry following mild traumatic brain injury: a proposed hospital-to-school protocol. J Head Trauma Rehabil 10(6);42.

Ylvisaker M, Hartwick P, Stevens M (1991). School re-entry following head injury: managing the transition from hospital to school. J Head Trauma Rehabil 6(1);10.

Ylvisaker M, Szekeres S (1989). Metacognitive and executive impairments in head injured children and adults. Top Lang Disord 9(2);34.

Ylvisaker M, Szekeres S, Hartwich P, Tworek P (1994). Cognitive Intervention. In R Savage, G Wolcott (eds), Educational Dimensions of Acquired Brain Injury. Austin, TX: PRO-ED, 121.

Appendix 18-1

Case Studies of Children
with Traumatic Brain Injury

Case 1: The Long Road of Recovery

BJ's case illustrates (1) the ongoing, albeit slow, recovery of function; (2) the importance of a supportive school administration; (3) the need for long-term services to ensure academic success; (4) the importance of teachers' understanding of the effects of TBI and the specific recovery history of the child; and (5) the child's internal struggle for a new self-image.

BJ was injured in a motor vehicle accident in November during his sixth-grade year. He was unconscious for 6 weeks. After 5 months of rehabilitation, he was discharged to home. BJ exhibited severe dysarthria. He used a wheelchair and was ambulatory only with maximum assistance. His handwriting was very slow, and there was evidence of executive system impairments (e.g., lack of initiation, verbal perseveration, insufficient planning for academic demands).

At 10 months after the injury, BJ began a new school year in a self-contained special education class for students with learning and emotional disabilities. He attended for only part of each day and continued outpatient therapy for 2 hours daily. Perceptible gains in cognitive, academic, motor, and self-management skills were made. His family was actively involved with the interdisciplinary school team.

Two years after the injury, at the family's request, BJ returned to a regular seventh-grade class but attended a special education class for English. He used a wheelchair in school for independent mobility and demonstrated continued academic progress and satisfactory grades. However, BJ's teachers reported escalating frustration with BJ, and his family perceived behavioral problems (e.g., perseverative questions, prolonged giggling at a teacher's joke, lack of

initiation to get out his textbooks). Frustration was also created by the IEP "demands" on the classroom teacher for a separate test location, ongoing communication with the parents and special education teacher, and "special treatment" to accommodate BJ's continued outpatient rehabilitation.

The teachers had no training or support for working with a student with TBI and, until March of the school year, school administrators had not firmly voiced their support for meeting BJ's needs in a regular education classroom. By March, family members felt as if they were being held responsible for the fact that BJ was a burden to school staff. BJ's progress was slow, and teachers openly considered whether BJ should be in special education full-time owing to his multiple needs. Several sessions shared by staff and a TBI consultant improved the staff members' level of understanding and acceptance, but the school year still ended on a frustrating note for all. BJ's parents insisted on consultant teacher services for eighth grade and, in ninth grade, BJ was removed from that school and was placed in another school in the same district, which provided a supportive and positive administration.

In the fifth year after his injury, BJ has completed eleventh grade in the same school district. With the assistance of a full-time note-taker and 10 hours per week of support from a consultant teacher, who also acts as case manager among school staff and a liaison between school and family, BJ has passed advanced-level state competency tests in subjects as diverse as English, American history, and chemistry.

BJ now walks with a cane, has improved speech and mild dysarthria, and is well liked by his peers, staff, and administration. He took a noncredit foreign language course at a local college at the age of 16, has traveled alone to see relatives in Europe, and passed the state high school regents examination.

407

BJ attends a monthly support group during the school year. He recently stated, "I have a long road to go. But I think I'm about half-way down the road and I'm still getting better. In my old life I was a good athlete. That's how I think of it—my old life—because everything changed for me after the accident. You have to have goals. It doesn't matter that some people tell you that they are unrealistic. It's trying for those goals that's important, even if you never reach them." BJ's current goal is high-school graduation and admission to a 4-year college. He is optimistic about his success.

Case 2: Growing Into Problems

HM's case illustrates the importance of (1) preparing for the child's anticipated needs and transitions, (2) training staff to develop their knowledge of TBI and interventions, (3) monitoring success and failure, and (4) listening to parents' concerns.

HM was an active 3 year old when he suffered a severe, diffuse brain injury from a fall. He was airlifted to a regional trauma center, where he remained comatose for 1 month and was hospitalized for 3 months before being discharged directly to home. HM's parents, following advice they were given, placed HM in the local special education preschool, where he received speech-language, occupational, and physical therapy several times weekly. HM had double vision for almost 1 year, until eye surgery was performed to correct a damaged muscle. His parents received little prognostic information or direct support from the medical system.

At the age of 4 years, 10 months, HM entered a class for children with TBI. He received collaborative service delivery with a focus on consistent structure for academic and social learning. The staff met weekly to discuss needs and to solve problems. Daily communication was maintained in writing with the family. After 2 years in the TBI class, HM reentered second grade in his regular local school and received resource room support for reading.

He was successful in a regular education classroom with resource center consultation and support provided to the classroom teachers. On the basis of that success and without regard for the complex social and academic demands of the departmentalized fifth grade, school administrators declassified HM and withdrew all services at the end of fourth grade.

In fifth grade, the asymmetric pattern of HM's abilities (eleventh-grade level reading, immature and perseverative outbursts) and the lack of staff knowledge of TBI quickly led to scapegoating of HM by peers, pejorative labeling of HM by teachers, and HM's perception of himself as inadequate. After his

mother insisted that her son be reclassified, that classroom observation by a TBI consultant be instituted, and that staff meet with the TBI consultant, staff attitudes changed, an interdisciplinary educational team (team included teacher, speech-language pathologist, psychologist, and occupational and physical therapists) was identified, collaborative intervention to address behavior problems was initiated, and HM began once again to enjoy success in school.

Case 3: Family and School Collaboration

TD's case illustrates (1) the difficulty of predicting long-term outcome in a young child; (2) the possibility of complicating medical issues; (3) the ways that children "grow into problems" as school demands increase; and (4) the need for intensive partnerships with families to deal with complex decisions.

At the age of 4 years, 11 months, TD sustained a severe TBI in a motor vehicle accident during October of her kindergarten year. She was in acute care for 1 month and a pediatric rehabilitation center for 3 months. Before her discharge, the school met with regional TBI coordinators, family, and rehabilitation staff to identify educational and rehabilitation needs. TD's kindergarten teacher and speech-language pathologist traveled to the rehabilitation center and spent 2 days observing her treatment and developing plans.

TD returned to her same kindergarten class for half-days with push-in speech-language therapy. She spent 1½ hours each day in the special education resource room and collaborative (consultant and teacher) consultation. Team meetings led by a district special education coordinator and counseling by the school psychologist took place weekly. TD received outpatient physical and occupational therapy.

At the outset, TD was nonverbal. With therapy, receptive language improved to age-appropriate levels and expressive language progressed slowly. Because of her young age (November birthday) and the amount of time she had lost from school, the family and school staff jointly decided to keep TD in kindergarten for the next year. She continued to demonstrate new learning, improved peer relationships, and increased speech, language, and motor skills. Monthly meetings were held with school staff, parents, and the regional TBI coordinator to share information and develop consistent interventions.

Almost 2 years after her injury, TD is in a regular first grade with significant educational modifications and related services. The onset of petit mal seizures has complicated her recovery, and the impact of her severe injury on new learning has become more evident with the expectation of emergent literacy and math skills. Because of the support provided and the collaboration between home and school, TD's parents are ready to discuss a possible future need for more intensive support within the district.

Case 4: Value of Case Management

RJ's case illustrates (1) the influence of pretrauma personality; (2) the need for counseling to deal with issues of loss; (3) the importance of assessment and intervention for executive system functions and planning for anticipated needs; (4) the value of planning for transitions between schools; (5) the positive effect of a school principal who allowed staff to forgo grades and other rules in favor of diagnostic teaching; and (6) the value of targeting for intervention independent self-management and use of strategic thinking and behavior (metacognitive functions).

RJ, a highly gifted student, was injured in a car and bicycle collision at the end of her fifth-grade year. She was in a coma for 2 weeks and was in inpatient rehabilitation for 6 weeks prior to beginning sixth grade at her former school.

The school principal and special education coordinator acted as case coordinators for RJ's school reentry. The educational team went to the rehabilitation center for a discharge planning meeting. All professional staff involved with RJ (including the nurse, art and music teacher, school psychologist, physical education teacher, and subject area teachers) attended a planning meeting and in-service training with the regional TBI coordinator before the start of school.

The principal directed that staff members were not to worry about academic grades but were to focus on reintegrating RJ into school and on developing their understanding of how RJ could learn best. Weekly team meetings were facilitated by the special education coordinator. The special education teacher provided both push-in and pull-out support for academic concept and strategy development and worked closely with subject area teachers to analyze academic demands and RJ's capacity to meet them.

RJ's behavior—described before the injury as mature, friendly, and confident—was characterized shortly after reentry by immature giggling and infrequent crying spells. Because of the staff's knowledge base, they responded calmly and minimally to these episodes, which quickly subsided. RJ's ties to her previous studious friends were not re-established, however, and her implicit status as the most gifted child in the class was lost. She demonstrated average achievement during the first 6 months of sixth-grade schooling, which was considered by RJ and her family to be a marked decline and a cause for concern and some denial.

Then the sixth-grade students began independent research projects, and teachers noted that RJ could not handle the demands of such work for planning, organization, synthesis, and self-evaluation. Teachers stated that the effects were subtle but real and unlike anything they had seen in students who were classified as learning disabled. Intervention was initiated to improve RJ's metacognitive skills (e.g., the use of organization strategies). Intensive support was arranged at the end of the sixth grade to prepare for RJ's transition to seventh grade in a much larger middle school in the district.

In the second year after her injury, RJ attended a regular seventh grade. She received counseling by a guidance counselor but no special education support. She developed new peer friendships and was positively supported by teachers as a well-behaved, capable student.

In the fifth year after her injury, RJ completed tenth grade in a regular education setting. She is an independent strategic thinker who requires minimal test modifications. Her achievement is significantly less than would have been expected on the basis of her preinjury level of functioning, but it is still within the high-average to above-average range.

RJ has maintained many of her preinjury characteristics: She is a hard worker, is oriented to achievement, and is quiet and friendly, all of which support her success in high school and beyond. She has fully accepted her new self. Still classified as a student with TBI, she now receives support from a transitional counselor who is helping her to plan for application to 4-year colleges for a career in the health field, though not as a doctor, as she had once hoped. RJ is able to reflect calmly and thoughtfully on her injury and its effects on her school experiences, family life, and career expectations.

Appendix 18-2
Modifying Materials, Instruction, and the Learning Environment to Meet Individual Needs

These options for teacher-initiated modifications are offered only as illustrations of the ways educators can facilitate a child's success in school. No modification should ever be selected because it addresses a "common need of children with TBI." Children with TBI are a heterogeneous group and thorough assessment is necessary to identify individual strengths and needs and the modifications that most effectively enhance performance. To foster independent learning in children, supports should be reduced by gradually fading the modifications. If a modification cannot be faded successfully, an effort is made to shift the responsibility for the initiation of the modification from the teacher to the student. Many modifications can evolve into student-initiated compensatory strategies that promote a sense of control in learning rather than a feeling of helplessness.

Need: Support to maintain orientation to time, place, and person (especially critical if the child changes classes and teachers during the school day)

❑ Designate a person with whom to check in at the beginning of the day and to check out at the end of the day, to reflect on activities and review understanding and organization of assignments and materials to be taken home.

❑ Keep a journal or log book that contains pictures of key staff, maps of the key places in the school, assignment section, schedule, and the like. Complexity of the journal should match the child's capacity for processing information and social appropriateness (e.g., a planning book or day timer for a secondary-level student).

❑ Assign a partner or buddy who will provide support or guidance and who will move close to the student in large congested areas or in times of high activity. Alternatively, allow the student to move before other students.

Need: Support to remember new information, including personal experiences

❑ Keep a journal in which all significant experiences are recorded. (This can be combined with a schedule or plan book.)

❑ Give cues to use the journal book as a memory aid. (For example, if child forgets an event, cue him or her to look in the journal book.)

❑ Provide a special place to keep the journal book so that the child does not misplace it; he or she may need cues to remember where the book is located.

❑ Provide a graphic organizer so that key facts or information is highlighted for review.

❑ Provide graphic organizers that promote elaboration or organization of information to make it more memorable.

❑ Provide targeted homework that is designed to reinforce key skills in meaningful and interesting contexts.

❑ Use review sheets.

❑ Associate information with the child's existing knowledge and past experiences.

❑ Promote experiences that require the child to manipulate, discover, construct, and explain new knowledge and skills in settings that approximate those in which the skill is used authentically.

Need: Support to remember directions, assignments, and upcoming special events

❑ Incorporate a date or assignment book section into the journal book.

❑ Post in the classroom and put in the journal book written or pictorial cues of upcoming major school and personal events.

❑ Give verbal reminders of upcoming significant events.

❑ Repeat or rephrase directions and ask the child to confirm them.

❑ Present oral and written directions with pictorial cues.

❑ Allow the use of a tape recorder for directions and assignments. (The child can use an earphone to listen to the tape during class.)

❑ For secondary students, develop a calendar of long-term assignments with intermediate steps scheduled (e.g., term paper due date with steps: select topic, complete research, write main ideas on cards, organize cards, write rough draft, write final draft).

Need: Help in coping with physical or mental fatigue and stimulus overload

❑ Begin with a shorter school day and gradually increase the course load or time demands.

❑ Designate time and space for rest or time out from stimulation. (This could be a space outside of the classroom, or the child could put his or her head down on the desk.) Alternatively, simply allow the student to gaze out the window as "down time," without viewing the behavior as inappropriate.

❑ Help the child to learn to identify early signs of stress, use signals to inform the teacher of such stress, and establish a plan of action for defusing the stress. (For example, one student who loved astronomy designed his own strategy for dealing with frustration by naming the planets silently; by the time he was finished, he usually was calmer.)

❑ Set shorter work periods separated by brief down times.

❑ Give shorter examinations that require less writing (e.g., a short answer, multiple choice, or true-false).

❑ Give examinations that provide cues and place less burden on free recall of material (e.g., a short answer or multiple choice instead of essay).

Need: Help in maintaining attention or motivation to complete a task

❑ Remove external distractions and background noise.

❑ Ensure that tasks are meaningful to the child and are within the child's readiness range.

❑ Explain the usefulness or importance of the activity.

❑ Use external aids such as a clock marked with tape to show the end of work time.

❑ Set alarm for short time segment.

❑ Keep a graph depicting the child's daily performance in attending to work.

❑ Develop cooperative work groups in which students monitor and help one another.

❑ Seat the child in the front of the classroom near the teacher.

Need: Adaptive equipment or technological aids for eating, writing, speaking, carrying schoolbooks, and the like

❑ Provide computer-access equipment to be used instead of writing, adapted for the child's dexterity and visual acuity.

❑ Provide special eating utensils that are modified for easier management.

❑ Identify the key component of any task and reduce the fine-motor demands when possible. (For example, is the goal of the task cutting out dinosaurs or grasping the attributes of meat eaters versus plant eaters? Cutting is not an essential component of the latter goal.)

❑ Encourage the use of an augmentative communication device or scribe.

❑ Modify pens and pencils for easier grip.

❑ Encourage use of a backpack with pouches for materials and books.

❑ Provide the child with a second set of books to keep at home to prevent balance and fatigue problems.

Need: Support in organizing and structuring behavior (verbal and nonverbal)

❑ Provide checklists or cue card with steps for completing a task; organize the checklists into a small notebook for easy reference.

❑ Provide goal-setting and planning sheets and tell the child the number of steps in a task or the number of items to be completed.

❑ Use graphic organizers as guides (e.g., diagrams showing the proper location of items in one's desk or backpack, the relations of concepts, discourse analysis).

❑ Use color-coded highlighting to show main ideas and supporting details in readings.

❑ Provide a cue sheet to help the child to remember classroom routines or scripts (e.g., a picture of a hand up to remind the child to raise his or her hand and wait for a turn to speak) or to help the child to remember teacher cues for acceptable classroom behavior.

❑ Divide large assignments into a sequence of smaller numbered steps.

❑ Divide complex tasks into a sequences of numbered steps or subgoals.

Need: More time to process spoken language (understanding and formulating utterances)

❑ Repeat and rephrase directions and important information.

❑ Pause more often in lectures.

❑ Use gestural and visual cues.

❑ Provide external aids (e.g., key pictures) for directions that are given frequently.

❑ Promote the use of a tape recorder to tape lectures, directions, or assignments. (The child can use an earphone to replay the tape during class without bothering other children.)

❑ Tape record directions for the home assignment and give the tape to the child. Other reminders also can be put on such tapes.

❑ Use preorganizers to prepare the child for spoken language (e.g., showing a picture that is related to the material to be discussed).

❑ Provide response time when asking the child a question. Directly explain to other students that the student knows the answer and simply needs time to be able to share the knowledge. Students are quickly impressed when they realize this is true.

❑ Provide extra time for the child to formulate utterances to compensate his or her slower word retrieval.

Need: More time to complete written work, including tests

❑ Ask for only written work that is necessary for the student to demonstrate what he or she knows and is able to do. (For example, do not make the student write all the words on the weekly spelling list three times each if some have already been mastered.)

❑ Provide a make-up period at the end of the day.

❑ Allow the use of assistive devices such as a word processor or a scribe.

❑ Allow the child to tape record answers and hand in the tape.

❑ Allow the use of calculators for in-class math computation.

❑ Give examinations that require simple marking rather than extensive writing.

❑ Provide extra time for the child to complete examinations or give examinations in parts.

❑ Request approved test modifications on local and state tests, including college entrance exams.

Need: Support in understanding complex or abstract language

❑ Follow abstract explanations with concrete illustrations. (For example, "He was exasperated, meaning he was ready to give up.")

❑ Follow a long, complex utterance with several simpler sentences that reiterate the main points.

❑ Give information in a series of simple sentences and confirm comprehension periodically.

❑ Give pictorial and written cues.

Need: Support in visual processing

❑ Enlarge the type on worksheets.

❑ Encourage the use of an index card to hold the child's place in reading and math work.

❑ Draw a red line down the sides of pages as cues for scanning.

❑ Use colored lines as cues for organization of written work on a page.

❑ Divide pages into quadrants to facilitate perception.

❑ Encourage the use of notebook paper with well-defined lines.

Need: More feedback and support during independent work

❑ Separate work into segments and provide answer sheets for each segment so that the student can check his or her work immediately after completion.

❑ Have the child work with a partner and periodically have each check in with the other regarding progress and problems.

Need: Guidance in studying and preparing for examinations

❑ Use graphic organizers to guide study of material (e.g., sun diagram to study for a test on a story, main idea and details worksheets for expository text, or Venn diagrams for comparisons).

❑ Prompt the child to make a plan for study and to check off each step of the plan as it is completed.

❑ Give tape recordings with directions for study; involve the family if appropriate.

❑ Assign a partner to engage in study or informal understanding checks.

Need: Guidance in problem solving and judgment

❑ Provide the child with verbal scripts or procedural cues to deal with frequent problems (e.g., teasing, name calling).

❑ Model ways in which decisions to act (judgments) should be made.

❑ Highlight information that is relevant to and necessary for making decisions.

❑ Provide graphic organizers to guide problem solving (see Chapter 11).

Need: Support in re-establishing social interactions and status

❑ Educate other students about brain injuries.

❑ Mediate interactions to promote success and help to identify positive social behaviors.

❑ Give informational feedback about social behaviors (reasons that they were appropriate or inappropriate). (For example, encourage students to follow Grice's conversation rules: be polite, concise, relevant, and truthful.)

❑ Provide information about expectations of peers, staff, and significant others and help the child to re-establish social scripts that guide social behavior.

❑ Provide opportunities to share feelings.

❑ Acknowledge changes in the child and promote acceptance of these changes.

❑ Provide cues to remind the child to use learned social skills.

❑ Provide positive feedback to rebuild the child's self-esteem.

❑ Provide modifications to maintain involvement in sports and other preferred activities (e.g., making a soccer player a student coach or statistician and involving student in practice and games).

   (See Chapters 11, 12, and 17 for additional instructional strategies.)

Need: Support in managing own behavior

❑ Reduce the number of options when choices must be made.

❑ Give prompts or cues to initiate and inhibit behaviors.

❑ Provide charts (e.g., graphs that show the number of times that a goal behavior was achieved) that activate self-monitoring.

❑ Use cue cards (e.g., a stop-and-think cue card to help control impulsivity).

❑ Focus intervention on reducing intensity and duration of behavioral outbursts, rather than initially expecting students to avoid an outburst altogether.

   (See Chapter 13 for behavior management modifications and instructional strategies.)

Need: Help in generalizing skills including strategies

❑ Provide a strategy log so that staff will know which strategies are to be used independently and which are under development; include log in the student's journal.

❑ Note specific skills that have been targeted so that staff can reinforce them in a variety of contexts; record them in the student's journal or log book.

❑ Use consistent terminology across the day for cuing and feedback.

❑ Highlight situations for which a strategy under development is appropriate.

Appendix 18-3
Episodes of Collaboration

The interdisciplinary goal is that the child will demonstrate increased knowledge of organizational schemes and improved ability to impose organization on thoughts, language, and the environment.

Setting and Collaborators	Objectives	Closure and Extended Communication
Art class: SLP, art teacher, and children working in small cooperative learning groups and in a large group.	(A,C) Help the teacher to organize crayons and beads so that children can find them easily. (I) Recognize and appropriately use the perceptual similarity scheme (e.g., grouping by perceptual features such as color or shape).	The class draws conclusions about how and why the scheme helped them to achieve the goals. The class cooperatively writes directions for how to organize the items and then posts the directions in the art room.
Language arts in the regular education classroom: SLP, teacher, and children working in cooperative learning groups, independently, and in a large group.	(A,C) Write or tape record narratives about pictures that depict agents, actions, objects, and locations; present the narratives to the class. (I) Learn story structure (e.g., setting, characters, initiating events) guided by a graphic organizer.	The class discusses features of the narratives and classifies them according to type (e.g., funny, sad, exciting, comic, tragic, adventurous). The children independently write in story journals (or tape record) key ideas from narratives to aid memory; they use their memory aids to tell their stories to friends or family members; children write (or tape record) the listeners' reactions to the stories, and students share those with the class.
Classroom speech-language therapy: SLP, special or regular education teacher, and children working in small cooperative learning groups, in a large group, and independently.	(A,C) As members of a cooperative group, design and set up a grocery store; draw floor plans, and arrange pictures of a variety of grocery store items onto the floor plans to make a store; show, describe, and explain to the class the organizational schemes used for the stores. (I) Appreciate and impose a semantic-similarity (similar features) organizational scheme.	The class discusses similarities and differences in the way groups organized their items and draws conclusions about the best way to organize a grocery store. The children visit one another's stores and engage in buying, selling, and trading communicative interactions.

Setting and Collaborators	Objectives	Closure and Extended Communication
Home: SLP, teacher, family, and children working independently and in a large group.	(A,C) Do surveys of their houses and record how selected areas are organized (e.g., kitchen cupboards, closet, refrigerator). Report the results of the survey.	The class summarizes the different organizational schemes that were identified, discusses them, and draws conclusions about why things were organized in a particular way.
	(I) Distinguish different organizational schemes.	The students write reports of the results of their surveys and take the reports home to their families.
Classroom group speech-language therapy: SLP, teacher, and children working in cooperative learning groups, in a large group, and independently.	(A,C) Play a charades game that involves teams acting out common scripts (e.g., going to the doctor) and others trying to identify the events.	The class summarizes people, objects, events, and language that are typical of the scripts and makes graphic organizers to represent the specific scripts.
	(I) Develop appreciation of a variety of single and embedded scripts and learn how to use a script to guide the organization of verbal descriptions of events.	The children write descriptions of personal experiences using as a guide one of the script graphic organizers.
		The children record their personal experiences in their journals.

SLP = speech-language pathologist; A = activity goal; C = child's goal; I = intervention objective.
Source: S Szekeres, N Meserve (1994). Collaborative intervention in schools after traumatic brain injury. Top Lang Disord 15(1);21.

Chapter 19

Career Development and School-to-Work Transition for Adolescents with Traumatic Brain Injury

Robert T. Fraser

School-to-Work Transition: General Considerations

To discuss the topic of career development and school-to-work transition for youths with traumatic brain injuries (TBI), it is necessary to review the general state of the art of school-to-work transition in our country. This chapter's overview provides a perspective on how much harder those in the school and community must work to improve school-to-work outcome for youths dealing with the residual consequences of a TBI. Glover and Marshall (1993) indicated that the United States has the worst approach to school-to-work transition of any industrialized nation. A 1981 survey by the Educational Testing Service revealed that most high-school students have never talked to a counselor about occupations and that only 6% of high school counselors reported spending more than 30% of their time helping students to find post–high school work (Chapman and Katz, 1981). These authors emphasized that budget cuts during the 1980s eliminated throughout public employment offices those job-counseling services that, at their peak in the mid-1960s, had served 600,000 young people annually.

The United States has undergone a significant change in its economic structure. Formerly, profits were derived from the rapid use of natural resources and the economies of scale that mass production provides. Currently, however, our economic system is fighting for survival in a more competitive global economy in which economic success depends mainly on the quality of output by an employee. For most of the last century, our educational system had provided basic literacy and numeric skills for the majority of the population who were expected to work in mass production in factories or on farms. At that time, school-to-work transition procedures were largely informal, family-related, or promoted through apprenticeship programs in a mass-production, natural resource consumption–oriented occupational context.

In today's more globally competitive environment, companies can compete in two basic ways: focusing on reducing wages or on improving the productivity and quality of the work product. The United States has chosen the easier low-wage strategy, as most other industrialized nations, including Japan and Germany, have focused on the quality of workers as individuals who can adapt and assist in improving technology. These other countries are focused on developing institutions and information systems that truly match workers and jobs, using systematic postsecondary education targeted to the employment market, training opportunities for dropouts, and providing companies with on-the-job training subsidies to support training workers.

The United States simply lacks a well-conceptualized and developed system for bridging the gap from high school (or college for that matter) to stabilization within the employment community. A recent trend in the United States is that of students going on to college or even graduate school due to their lack of awareness about existing job options and perceived lack of relevant skills (Glover and Marshall, 1993). When a high school graduate secures a job with a quality company, it is often a simple function of chance or, at times, survival of the fittest. It is common for students to complete high school, attend a local community college in a nondirected fashion for a year or so, drop out due to lack of direction, and work a number of minimum wage jobs until finally being hired by a company with a reasonable salary schedule and benefits package. This final step is often abetted by a helpful friend or family contact. This is the fortunate young person's scenario. Meanwhile in Japan, the largest industrial firms recruit the better high school graduates with high school outreach programs, a process that rewards students for working hard in school. In the German apprenticeship system, adolescents can spend several days a week in industry-based and nationally approved occupational instructional programs. The Germans also have an impressive counseling and guidance system operated by the employment service for young people. The United States' delay in hiring young people or absorbing them into core manufacturing or technical production jobs gives other countries a significant edge in skill training and also denies the school system immediate feedback relative to the skills of their graduates in the employment sector.

Young people with disabilities have been severely affected by this general lack of transition in the school-to-work process. High school dropout rates for students with disabilities are greater than 25% (MacMillan et al., 1990), and unemployment or underemployment post–high school rates can exceed 75% (Akabas et al., 1992). Approximately 165,000 children and adolescents are hospitalized with TBI each year. A substantial proportion of them encounter the challenge of dealing with an ineffective school-to-work transition system, compounded by their cognitive and associated impairments or lack of relevant school programming and counseling.

Definition of School-To-Work Transition

Transition services are defined in the 1990 amendments of the Individuals with Disabilities Education Act (P.L. 101 476) as

A coordinated set of activities for a student, designed within an outcome-oriented process, which promotes movement from school to post-school activities, including post-secondary education, vocational training, integrated employment (not including supported employment), or continuing adult education, adult services, independent living, or community participation. The coordinated set of activities shall be based upon the individual student's needs, taking into account the student's preferences and interests, and shall include instruction, community experiences, development of employment and other post-school adult living objectives, and when appropriate, acquisition of daily living skills and functional vocational evaluation.

Despite this official definition, a consensus validation conference report (National Institute on Disability and Rehabilitation Research, 1994, p. 4) suggests that some controversy continues regarding the definition of school-to-work transition and interferes with the systematic exploration of the process. However, some successful research trends were noted in this report:

1. Transition appeared to be more successful for students who receive vocational education and early work experience.
2. A series of vocational-education classes was associated with significantly higher wages and rates of employment.
3. The presence of a transition goal for either postsecondary academic or vocational training was related positively to achieving that goal.

In this chapter, I use the term *transition planning* to mean a sequence of planning steps involving all appropriate parties (i.e., the youth, parents, educators, vocational and rehabilitation staff, and other concerned parties) through a sequence of guided activities promoting optimal post–high school economic self-sufficiency in the community.

It should be noted that for individuals with disabilities, particularly neurologic disabilities, moving into a post–high school program, a community college, or even a vocational-technical school does not necessarily assist in later job placement unless the training and transitioning to work are designed specifically to culminate in job placement. Fraser and colleagues (1993) found that only 1 of 20 individuals with epilepsy (and often associated brain impairment), trained in vocational-technical programs by a state rehabilitation agency, actually achieved a job related to that area of training.

Legislation that most directly affects school-to-work transition for students with disabilities includes the IDEA, which requires appropriate education in the least restrictive learning environment and the development of transition plans for students with disabilities at age 16 (or at age 14 or younger if appropriate); the Rehabilitation Act Amendments of 1993, requiring the development of a rehabilitation plan prior to a student's leaving school, and the Americans with Disabilities Act of 1993 that prohibits discrimination in the workplace and guarantees access to the workplace. The challenge facing the schools, rehabilitation service providers, parents, employers, and people with disabilities is to render this legislation genuinely meaningful. This involves not only securing employment or postsecondary education that will result in a job for youngsters with TBI but moving toward independent living and social competence in the community (Wehman, 1990).

Underpinnings of Successful Career Development and School-to-Work Transition: Vocational Assessment

The purpose of vocational evaluation is to set post–high school or employment goals that can actually be tested through work experiences while the student is still in school. This assessment typically includes clarification of vocational interests and work values, review of academic achievement (or actual achievement testing if necessary), assessment of emotional and personality functioning, and testing of cognitive abilities and specific aptitudes. If appropriate, personal and self-care needs may also be assessed. This assessment lays a general framework for the "in vivo" community-based work experience and job tryouts in which a youngster's abilities can be assessed more validly.

Cognitive Assessment

For the purpose of assessing cognitive abilities, a complete neuropsychological evaluation is important, even for individuals with relatively mild brain injuries. Such testing typically includes use of a standard neuropsychological battery, such as the Halstead-Reitan or the Luria-Nebraska battery, or a specifically designed combination of neuropsychological tests. Without careful assessment of a youngster's neuropsychological strengths and weaknesses, vocational planning may not be well grounded, and necessary interventions and compensatory strategies may not be used. The testing should be done before a student returns to school after a significant TBI and again at 1–2 years after injury so as to establish a baseline level of functioning and later to assess potential regain of function.

It must be underscored that traditional school psychology assessments are inadequate for the more sensitive assessment of postinjury cognitive strengths and limitations and are often insufficient for individual education and transition plan development. Telzrow (1991) reviewed these issues and called for assessment using a flexible neuropsychological assessment approach: assessing domains of functioning through the most appropriate psychological and educational tests. She also reviewed the domains of assessment proposed by a variety of authors. The domains proposed by Baxter and colleagues (1985) appear to be most comprehensive: organizational skills, intellectual functioning, sensory and perceptual abilities, language abilities, attention and concentration, problem solving, flexibility of thought, academic functioning, memory and learning, rate of information processing, effects of feedback on performance, sequencing, temporal and spatial abilities, motor functioning, and fatigue. Many of the proposed batteries inadequately assess the domains of cognitive efficiency or rate of information processing and cognitive flexibility. It can be useful to have some core tests administered periodically over the years following a TBI to assess changes in functioning—specifically in relation to initially established areas of deficit.

Neuropsychological testing has some obvious limitations. It can underestimate or overestimate capabilities and does not provide in the assessment process all the environmental cues that are offered through community-based evaluation. It does, however, provide a reasonable framework for beginning to understand areas of asset and deficit plus directions for compensatory efforts by vocational and rehabilitation staff.

Vocational Interest Assessment

Vocational interests are assessed routinely through such inventories as the Career Assessment Inventory (available through NCS Assessments, P.O. Box 1415, Minneapolis, MN 55440), such occupational checklists as the Gordon Occupational Checklist (available through Psychological Corporation, 555 Academic Court, San Antonio, TX 78204-2398), and even slide picture inventories available through Valpar (Valpar International Corporation, P.O.

Box 5767, Tucson, AZ 85703). The Gordon Occupational Checklist can be very helpful in identifying discrete interests at a task level; it also provides a writing sample relative to career aspirations. Some schools have put together specific vocational exploration slide shows based on highly accessible positions available in the local community. Interests can be assessed also as a component activity in a number of computer-assisted career guidance systems (see review by Sampson et al., 1994).

Emotional and Characterological Functioning

If emotional and adjustment concerns are apparent, emotional and personality functioning is assessed by using such inventories as the 16PF (the Millon Adolescent Personality Inventory) and the Minnesota Multiphasic Personality Inventory (MMPI) I–II (all available through NCS Assessments). Depending on the severity of the TBI, paper-and-pencil inventories can become less appropriate. Taped versions can be used if reading or visual concerns are at issue. Use of some of these inventories (e.g., the MMPI) generally is not recommended until the youngster is at least 16 years old. For some youngsters, family input and behavioral rating scales are more appropriate.

Achievement and Aptitude Assessment

Academic achievement can be assessed through the Adult Basic Learning Examination (available through Psychological Corporation), the Apticom System (available through Vocational Research Institute, 128 Walnut Street, Suite 1502, Philadelphia, PA 19102), and other measures. Although the Wide Range Achievement Test (available through Jastak Associates, Inc., P.O. Box 3410, Wilmington, DE 19804-0250) is often used, it is more a quick and easily administered screening tool. The reading comprehension subtest, for example, requires only word recognition and enunciation rather than actual reading comprehension.

The Differential Aptitude Test (Psychological Corporation) assesses not only verbal reasoning and numerical ability but abstract reasoning, clerical speed and accuracy, mechanical reasoning, space relations, spelling, grammar, and general mental ability. It requires only a sixth-grade reading level and takes about 3 hours to administer. The Psychological Corporation also has a number of other specific tests related to mechanical comprehension (Bennett Mechanical Comprehension Test), clerical performance (Minnesota Clerical Test), fine eye-hand coordination (Crawford Small Parts Dexterity, Purdue Pegboard, or the Bennett Hand-Tool Dexterity Test) and other specific aptitudes.

In assessing aptitudes, work-sample evaluation systems are often used (e.g., those developed by Valpar International; the Singer Company, Rochester, NY; or the Vocational Research Institute). These work-sample systems have been reviewed comprehensively by Botterbusch (1985) and can be compared relative to cost and the particular needs of the evaluator's population.

Although often grouped with these work-aptitude batteries, the McCarron-Dial Vocational Evaluation System (McCarron-Dial, P.O. Box 45628, Dallas, TX 75245) is a battery of neurometric and psychological measures that can be very helpful in vocational assessment and, in some states, is used in place of standard neuropsychological batteries—particularly in an area in which neuropsychologists are less available. In addition to measures of neuropsychological functioning, the battery assesses emotional-behavioral functioning and street-survival skills or capacities for daily living. It is one of the few vocationally used batteries that has been cited positively for research because of its capacity to predict the testee's future levels of independent living and vocational functioning. The battery is used better, however, to profile areas of neuropsychological areas of asset and deficit that may require intervention and compensatory strategies. Also, it will draw attention to concerns of independent living and psychosocial adjustment that will benefit from interventions. The battery's predictive utility is compromised today—and rightly so—by the variety of assistive technology interventions that enable an individual to function in the work place despite, for example, substantial motor limitations.

Functional Assessment

Milton and colleagues (1991) advocated for functional assessment of critical thinking skills, skill integration, visual processing, and conversational processing and provided techniques for assessing these functional competencies. These authors presented strategies to assess these abilities or behaviors, overlooked in more traditional assessment. Such behaviors are very critical also to effective school functioning. The reader is invited to review this article and some of the strategies provided, such as the Ennes-Weir Critical Thinking Essay Test or videotaped commercial analysis to assess analytic and abstraction skills. This type of information truly augments and (at times) provides more valid and useful performance data than that secured through more traditional testing.

In making recommendations for school-to-work transition, information is incorporated from vocational evaluators or specialists, educators, and other rehabilitation staff or service providers. Occupational therapists, speech-language pathologists, and physical therapists may be needed to provide information about functioning, speech and language motor capacities, and lifting capacities. Work values are explored in counseling sessions. In conducting job tryouts, it is important to understand the type of work setting that would appeal to youngsters, the type of coworkers they would like, or what they think they might like about work. Because interests are often not defined clearly at high school age, even for youths without disabilities, it is often more important to explore "things about work" that might be interesting to a youngster.

For most adolescents, vocational interests evolve in the context of realistic work experiences. Diverse job tryouts can begin in a school setting and provide a realistic view of potential work competencies. Just as important, they can provide such critical work behaviors as adaptability to work demands, effective communication skills, motivation, the types of work-related supports that are necessary, or capacity for mobility in the community, and the like. Unless work values are explored carefully and the job tryout position actually engages a youth, it can be difficult to have a valid perspective on actual work and interpersonal competencies.

Early Intervention in Transition Planning

Vocational intervention for an adolescent with a severe TBI must begin early. Vocational assessment and incremental involvement in vocational experiences can be critical. Often, such assessment and involvement are difficult because a youngster may not perceive the need or is focused on basic classroom activity and social life. Meanwhile, a number of parents *assume* that the educational experience will be sufficient and that their son or daughter will be able to secure employment through the natural course of events. It must be explained to such parents that their son or daughter might not make the transition into a difficult job market without beginning targeted vocational activity earlier than do schoolmates without a disability. Many adolescents with a TBI need a continuum of vocational programming steps and clarification of barriers to be resolved to reach competitive employment successfully.

Early assessment, planning, and feedback secured from both unpaid and paid job tryouts can facilitate realistic goal setting, maximum use of community resources prior to a youngster's leaving high school, and result in a more seamless continuum of vocational rehabilitation activity. Physicians and members of the allied health team should be encouraged to help parents and others to appreciate the value of targeted vocational activity and household responsibilities.

Parents should be enlisted and engaged in formal individual education transition planning as part of the IEP. Many parents of young survivors refrain from assigning responsibilities around the house and otherwise reduce independent living and household chore responsibilities because such children have a disability. The transition plan should include assigning responsibilities of this nature, because successful transition requires skills learned in household tasks and avocational activities in the home and often depends on the youngsters' ability to maintain themselves in independent living, a group home, or some other type of residential setting. It is critical that parents lay a framework for contributions to home maintenance and independent self-care. The value of self-sufficiency should be conveyed to the youngsters. If these efforts are begun early in the home, the likelihood of vocational progress and successful post–high school outcomes is heightened.

Cross-Disciplinary and Agency Collaboration

Participants at the individual education and transition plan meetings should include the youngster with TBI, the teacher, parents, and any rehabilitation team members still involved. Because human service and allied health professionals have numerous constraints on their time and may not be able to attend meetings, teleconferencing may be useful. Additionally, members of vocational rehabilitation, developmental disability, transitional living, or other community service agencies also should be involved.

As part of the transition planning, the professional or agency representative best suited to carry out a particular function in the plan—despite personal training discipline or agency affiliation—is the person who should carry out this function. In some cases, a physical therapist might be involved, as opposed to a vocational rehabilitation counselor visiting a work site to examine the job's physical demands and to consider a combination of options. Also, a state agency vocational rehabilitation counselor may assume the case manager role, which previously had been the responsibility of a rehabilitation hospital professional. Coordinating and physically getting all concerned parties to a meeting at an assigned time can be difficult, and innovation is encouraged (e.g., use of lunch time, involvement through speakerphone, or breakfast meetings). Johnson and colleagues (1994) reported that academic functioning appears to be better when a rehabilitation professional is involved in the IEP and transition plan development and, in some cases, actually writes the plan, rather than a school system representative performing that function. Provided with a clear and realistic transition plan, a youngster with a disability may be more motivated academically.

In some areas of the country, the local school district has a reintegration team that can educate personnel from a specific school about optimal school integration and school-to-work transition procedures for adolescents with TBI. This situation is ideal, because school personnel may not understand the complexities of cognitive profiles of adolescents with TBI (see Chapters 17 and 18 for further discussion).

Wehman and colleagues (1988) pointed out a number of ways in which agencies can work together. On a basic level, information can be shared. Second, responsibilities can be transferred from one agency to another through a contract or fee-for-service arrangement. Third, several agencies can collaborate and share available funds or in-kind resources for a specific outcome (e.g., a community-based job tryout that effects one's transition to direct job placement activity). In the context of fluctuating or limited funding, this type of shared resources approach is particularly useful and often necessary.

Essential Functions of a School-to-Work Transition Program

Several critical components make up the school-to-work transition process (as summarized in a 1994 report by The National Institute on Disability and Rehabilitation Research).

- A federally mandated individual education plan with identified transition services: Development of this plan includes student and family involvement. For youths with TBI, the maximum number of key individuals from involved state agencies and the treating rehabilitation team should have input into this plan. The identification of transition services often begins at least 2 years before leaving school for many youths with disabilities. For those with TBI, this plan should be developed as early as possible (e.g., at age 14). The plan should be based on vocational assessment data, should describe long-term goals with short-term objectives, should have time lines for integrating services into any cooperative agreements among service providers, and should include strategies for working toward independent living and the other employment-related support activity.

- Plan development using local and state occupational databases: Planning that does not mesh student interests with viable job opportunities available in the proximate community or region simply is not relevant.

- A transition process including active family involvement (as described): This process becomes truly viable if, in the home, the family sets realistic and incrementally more demanding expectations for chore activities, avocational skill development, and steps toward independent living and household management. Family members should be encouraged to use friends and employer contacts in the community to improve the transition experience.

- Skill training for youths that includes marketable vocational skills, job-seeking skills, job-related work habits, and conversational and other interpersonal skills: Appropriate interpersonal behavior is a major reason that individuals secure and maintain jobs. For an individual with TBI and resultant cognitive limitations, the development of social competencies and appropriate work habits can take considerable time and must be initiated early.

- Interagency agreements that combine school and state vocational rehabilitation and other agencies in facilitating activities that range from information sharing to definitive contractual activity of service funding: Writers of these plans can identify the aggregate needs of a youth in transition and assign responsibilities for needed services.

- Critical coordination of services and career activities: The emphasis here is on linking youths and their families with required services and ensuring that appropriate services are accessed as necessary.

- People involved in the transition process who are knowledgeable: They must understand the relevant laws affecting transition (e.g., the Rehabilitation Act Amendments of 1993, and IDEA).
- Career exploration activities and work experiences that are a core element to the transition process: These experiences run the gamut: simply "shadowing" individuals at their jobs to learning about their vocational activities by being coached for a job or other competitive paid work in the community. This activity is an essential component of school-to-work transition and, for a youth with a TBI, it must be initiated as soon as possible.
- Follow-up services: Such services are necessary to ensure that the transition services are effective, that their modifications are based on the needs of the youths and the changing structure of the work economy, and that students requiring additional services are re-referred after leaving school.
- The assurance of expertise relative to the use of specialized procedures or equipment: This expertise will be helpful to the youth in transition. Other vocational mentoring and role models should be available to encourage and further ensure the success of the youth in transition.
- Personnel highly competent in their respective professions: People involved in the transition process should be available to assist youths in developing necessary skills and knowledge and to use available occupational information databases to ensure best practices in a school-to-work transition program.
- Procedures should ensure availability: Such procedures should guarantee to youths in transition that assistive technology, learning aids, and other environmental assists or support (e.g., a job coach) are transferred from school to the post–high school job or training environment.

The Institute report emphasizes that successful transition services encourage the involvement of youths and families in the pursuit of a successful transition, a commitment to eventual employment, and shared responsibilities in reaching that goal, with time lines developed to complete certain tasks and with key players (e.g., parent or community agency representative) being assigned to ensure that these activities occur. The process allows for flexibility, is seamless as regards the progression of events, includes a strong interdisciplinary team whenever possible, and has an established framework for identifying successful outcomes.

A Detailed Look at Work Experience

Work experience is critical in the transition process. Initially, students might be able to visit work places to "shadow" individuals involved in varied jobs. It can be helpful to teach job-seeking skills in the school setting, but it has much more impact if it can be done at company sites, using company applications, with input from company human resource representatives. Sandow and colleagues (1993) recommended use of the Saturday academy model in which businesses and industries provide sites and training for students who are interested in learning more about vocational topics not covered in school. This type of exposure assists in understanding the world of work and creates an appreciation for different work environments. Students can begin work activity also by participating in integrated work experiences in the school as part of a class program (e.g., janitorial work, kitchen work, or operating a sundries store in the school).

Figure 19-1 provides a review of transitional job-placement options for youths with TBI. Despite even a severe TBI, some individuals can be advised from the counselor's office about a job search activity outside the school. Others need some selective brokering of their skills and abilities and accommodation recommendations by vocational, counseling, or rehabilitation staff for part-time or full-time summer jobs. Finally, some youths will need some type of employment support. The support could be a job coach provided by an agency or national support provided by a coworker or supervisor at the job site.

In identifying those individuals best served by a specific type of placement approach, certain variables must be reviewed: the student's and family's vocational goal, neuropsychological strengths and weaknesses, emotional-interpersonal functioning, and work-related awareness and social competence. Under a Department of Labor waiver, a student with TBI can try different jobs in the community for purposes of exploration and assessment for up to 215 hours on an unpaid basis (e.g., 14 weeks at 15 hours per week totals 210 hours and is under limit). A special education representative, a vocational rehabilitation counselor, a school job-placement specialist, or some other designated person then can examine data relating to the student's productivity, flexibility, punctuality, the ability to accept supervision, and other relevant work behaviors. On the basis of data from these experiences, competitive part-time or full-time placement then can be targeted. Some of these "tryouts" transition to paid positions.

Some individuals profit from job coaches who analyze the tasks of the job and use behavioral methods to improve productivity, accuracy, and other work behaviors. A job coach might also supervise a traveling landscaping crew or household cleaning service. Some adolescents may be filtered through work experiences at a small business site in which some members of the work force have a disability, jobs being provided on both a transitional and a long-term basis.

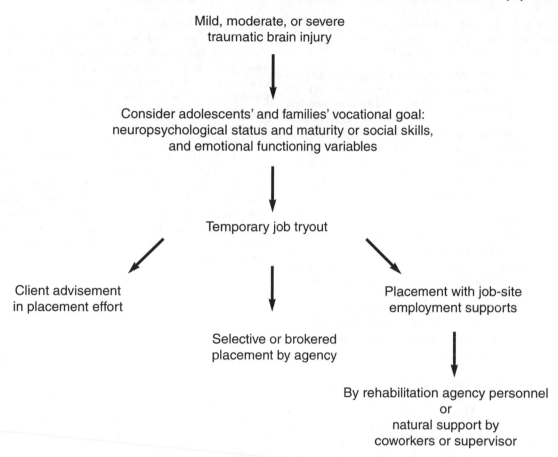

Figure 19-1. Choice of a job placement model in traumatic brain injury rehabilitation. (Adapted from R Fraser, P Wehman, B McMahon [1991]. Traumatic Brain Injury Vocational Rehabilitation: Job Placement Models. Winter Park, FL: St. Lucie Press, 19.)

Curl and Chisholm (1993) demonstrated that coworkers can be taught also to use behavioral training methods (e.g., a tell-show-observe-provide feedback approach) in addition to other behavioral measures. They also provided a stipend for coworkers learning the training methods, with hourly salary increments related to extra time spent on mentoring a youngster on a job site. In other cases, work activity is provided in an enclave located in an industry and supervised by a job coach (e.g., performing a specific type of electronic assembly).

Some students simply will need mentoring by an on-site supervisor or coworker. However, this provision can involve a formal, paid mentoring relationship with a coworker. Many students will be able to be placed on a part- or full-time basis in competitive work, with the benefit of a preliminary job tryout but without the necessity for ongoing coaching. With quality performance feedback, their work performance and behavior often improve appropriately for competitive work access without significant employment support.

Improving School-to-Work Transition Programs with Limited Funding

This chapter has described components of an ideal school-to-work program and has reviewed the types of work experiences that can be sequenced through the high-school years. Funding limitations may have jeopardized the possibility of interagency agreements and cooperative involvement in IEP and transition planning by rehabilitation and community agency representatives outside the family and school. Because of insufficient resources and limited personnel, often the transition process is a piecemeal procedure resulting in limited school-to-work bridging for students with disabilities (particularly those with TBI). However, innovative, helpful activities performed—within a committee planning structure—by parents, by teachers and school counselors, by employers, by relevant state agencies, and by students with the disability can improve the school-to-work transition process despite the lack of ideal funding or collaborative interagency support. One caveat is that an identified person or committee member must ensure the actual occurrence of activities for all key players in the transition process (Wehman, 1990):

- *Parents:* Parents need to be encouraged to start planning for transition at an earlier age, especially for adolescents with TBI. They need to understand their rights and those of their children, to familiarize themselves well in advance of immediate need with agencies that can benefit their youngsters, to encourage around the house a range of responsibilities that will improve the integration of the youngster into the community, to encourage community socialization and participation in activities, to use available social support networks (e.g., friends and other community contacts who can assist a child in having relevant skill-building experiences in the community), to evaluate their youngster's progress in the school-to-work transition program, and to advocate for needed services on an ongoing basis. Many parents believe that school-to-work transition simply will occur in the natural course of events. This process usually is turbulent at best for the youngster with cognitive and other disability following TBI.
- *Educators and school counseling personnel:* These individuals need to forge a closer relationship with business. The recent Oregon education reform effort (Sandow et al., 1993), involved teachers in summer internships with an industry. Both mainstream and special educators learned new technologies being used in the workplace, became aware of company selection criteria and learning curves on the job, began to understand different company cultures, made contacts to develop more meaningful on-the-job tryouts and paid work experiences for their students, and moved into a stronger position to encourage business representatives to become more involved in the school system.
- *Employers:* On a national level, the employment community has engaged only marginally in any linkage to the school system. On a very basic, low-cost level, business representatives can visit schools and create awareness, particularly of the high frequency of jobs in the community. They can serve on advisory committees and provide feedback to special education teachers and other teachers about the relevance of specific vocational-education and job-seeking skills preparation activities. They can assist teachers in revising their curricula to approximate better the activities actually occurring in business and industry.

Oregon has developed workforce quality committees on a regional basis to advise schools on business partnerships (Sandow et al., 1993). These committees are composed of business representatives, educators, and human services professionals and are an excellent source of advice. Employers can be mentors to students who have TBI and are at risk for failure in the community. Mentor activity can be developed through a once-a-week tutoring session, a weekly lunch with a student, or as part of a "lunch bunch" group. Employers can be educated so that they understand better some of the vocational assets and transition concerns experienced by students with TBI and other disabilities.

Sandow and colleagues (1993) encouraged outreaching involvement from businesses that have had no experience in hiring people with disabilities and who for some reason have been out of the transition loop. Employers can be involved in the job-search preparation process for youths who have TBI and are functioning at a reasonable level of independence. Finally, in contrast to the usual practice of administrators and human resource professionals being the only personnel visiting the school or being involved in advisory committees, it is important that master workers be allowed some time off the job to visit schools and provide input on curricula and the general job-preparation activity provided through the high schools. With these individuals engaged early in the process, later student placements should be much more successful, because the students will be better prepared and master or supervising workers' receptivity toward youths will have been increased.

In metropolitan Seattle, the Emerald City Rotary has adopted two middle schools in the central district of the city. This club of 130 members is involved in a number of functions in support of these schools, including one-to-one tutoring, involving students in lunch bunches, and inviting students to the workplace for a day of observing work activities. Some Rotarians individually adopt a classroom teacher and work in support of that teacher's needs. Money has been raised to install computers in each classroom, to buy library books, and to provide post–high school scholarships for the most improved students. (The scholarships are received when they complete high school).

Students completing middle school are sent to a 3-day spring camp. Those who are most at risk due to neurologic and other problems are funded for a 2-week summer camp focused on building self-esteem. Plans are under way to mentor and support these at-risk youths throughout the rest of the summer and the school year. A number of these students are at risk owing to cognitive and behavioral deficits following TBI. This outreach and mentoring effort are examples of the realization by a large group of employers that school-to-work transition is not going to occur without their support and intervention. They have underscored also the belief that, in making the transition to productive work and life activity, this intervention must occur as early as possible to support those students who are disadvantaged or may have diverse disabilities.

Table 19-1. Ideal School-to-Work Transition Program

Level	Student Activity	Activity of Others
Ninth grade	Assessment, including neuropsychological testing, school-site work or business, "shadowing" workers, community service credits, work exploration class, independent living activities	Teacher business internships, parent or advocate support, employer talks, career fairs, employer mentors or tutors, employer lunch bunch, Saturday work academies, teacher internships
Tenth, eleventh grade	Community service credits, school-site work or business, work internships with job-site supervisor (or more intensive support), employment skills class, vocational-education classes, independent living activities	Teacher business internships, parent support, employer talks, career fairs, employer mentors or tutors, employer lunch bunch, Saturday work academies, business advisory council, master worker visits
Twelfth grade	Work internships (continued), paid part- or full-time work (to include employment supports)	Principally same as for tenth and eleventh grade; also interagency agreements
After high school	Paid part- or full-time work (supports), job search, vocational education	Triage or follow-up services, vocational rehabilitation, other service providers' support

- *Youths with TBI:* Generally, most have ignored the issue that many of these youths eventually will have to deal with significant issues in trying to enter the job market. Many youths make the assumption that "return to school" equates with a logical progression into the world of work. Adolescents with TBI should be helped to understand their strengths and weaknesses and to take responsibility for the compensatory behavior needed to succeed despite ongoing disability. In other words: To be successful, youths with TBI must learn to accept their disabilities and the responsibility for teaching others how to accommodate those disabilities in an optimal fashion.

  Despite the Americans with Disabilities Act and other legislation, the responsibility for "fitting in" is often borne in our society by the person with a disability, particularly an invisible disability such as TBI. In addition to accepting cognitive impairments and learning how to work around them, adolescents will do better in the transition to work if they know that they will have to "work a little harder" (and perhaps longer) and often be more organized (e.g., using more structural guides and memory aids) than are their peers. Beginning school-to-work transition steps earlier than their peers may be an important part of "working"; if learning takes longer to reach competency, it simply must begin earlier than for youths without disabilities.

- *State agencies:* Such entities in the school-to-work transition and responsible for vocational rehabilitation, developmental disabilities, mental health, and other services can collaborate on information sharing, assigned transition functions, and funding of needed services (e.g., case management, job development, supported employment, psychotherapy, and community based assessment).

Components of an Ideal School-to-Work Training Program

No specialized school-to-work transition programs have been created specifically for youths with TBI, nor should they have been. Wehman and colleagues (1985) suggested that better employment outcomes result from integrated academic experiences. Similarly, when young people with disability are assimilated into a generic school-to-work transition process, they are more likely to have a broader, more valuable experience. Finally, young adolescents with TBI have varying cognitive profiles, with some requiring no modifications or accommodations in their vocational program and others requiring significant adaptations.

Table 19-1 provides an overview in which are combined the components of an ideal school-to-work transition process for most adolescents and components specific to the needs of a youngster with TBI (i.e., the early ninth-grade start and comprehensive assessment to include neuropsychological testing). The post–high school follow-up and triage services are critical for adolescents with TBI. Siegel and colleagues (1993) indicated that these services, provided for as long as they are needed, are critical to stabilizing youngsters in the world of work and establishing them in a path of upward vocational mobility. Other aspects of the Career Ladders Program as described by Siegel and colleagues (1993) include work internships or 5- to 6-week job tryouts (paid or unpaid, requiring school-paid insurance coverage) and weekly skills classes (e.g., conversational skills) directly related to and in support of the work experiences. Some schools have work activity (e.g., grounds maintenance, janitorial or cafeteria work, or a sundries store) provided for credit before leaving school for the internship experience.

A critical aspect of the transition process for any youngster with TBI or for a student otherwise at risk is having an advocate to ensure that the steps in the transition plan occur; without an advocate, the transition plan likely will fail. In addition to the Career Ladders Program contributions, other aspects of the proposed model are emphasized by Sandow and collaborators (1993) from the University of Oregon and the Emerald City Rotary activities in Seattle. All these activities are used to promote a student's understanding of the work world and its requirements, to improve confidence and competence in making the transition, to ensure relevant curricula and assistance with school resources, and to offer employer input and mentoring in this entire transition process.

Students with TBI can participate in an umbrella-type school-to-work transition program but may benefit from a number of preparatory steps and accommodations:

- An advocate (parent, friend, employer) or nondisabled buddy or sequence of buddies to assist as guides in the process
- Assessment that includes neuropsychological and functional evaluation information to aid in understanding a youngster's cognitive assets and limitations in the program and to improve the experience and better help with goal planning
- Consideration of life skills and community-based skills (including transportation needs)
- Accommodations in the internship and work experiences. These accommodations could include procedural changes in the work, physical modifications to the work stations, or the use of assistive technology (either low cost, such as descriptive charts, checklists, and timers, or higher cost, such as palmtop computers).
- Gradual pacing of work-site exposure. Students with TBI might be prepared for experiences in "shadowing" workers at a work site, using an information-seeking list of questions to ask as they watch a worker perform a job. Employers and master or lead workers might benefit from in-service training on the effects of TBI. They might discuss the times at which to be more animated or active in a presentation and the times at which to proceed more slowly with material, checking with students to ensure that they understand material that they find complex.
- Specialized funding from a state division of vocational rehabilitation, developmental disability, or other services. This funding may include the costs of job coaching, coworkers as trainers, and aides for occasional physical assists; it could include helping in any fashion that can render these experiences more meaningful. It could include extending incentives to employers to convert unpaid into paid work activity and providing on-the-job training funds as an incentive to provide more training and work to a youngster. Adolescents with TBI obviously must meet the eligibility requirements for receiving these different agency services.

All these activities could help to make the school-to-work transition process a reality for adolescents with TBI. Without these considerations and accommodations, such youngsters are likely to be engaged insufficiently in the process; consequently, a solid bridge to stable work will not be constructed.

Summary

School-to-work transition steps and considerations should integrate the needs of youths with TBI into existing programs. This integration requires some obvious tailoring but not distinctly separate programs. Stronger bridging to employment is needed for these youths and must involve refined job goals and schedules for achieving them. This process involves as many relevant parties as possible and true cross-collaboration in reaching goals. Commitments to tasks need to be made though formal and informal agreements. Successful programs acknowledge the need for identified advocates for youths and agreement regarding the definition of success. School-to-work transition programming remains more of a concept in our modern society than a discrete sequence of events. This process demands definition and a significant investment of resources (not simply financial), particularly for adolescents with TBI, or many of them will continue to be outsiders or marginal "hangers-on" in relation to the work force. A good program also includes post–high school follow-up or triage of emerging problem issues to ensure maintenance of positions or reasonable career ladder steps (Siegel et al., 1993). This extra effort will sustain the benefit of all the preceding transition steps.

References

Akabas SH, Gates LB, Galvin DE (1992). Disability Management: A Complete System to Reduce Costs, Increase Productivity, Meet Employee Needs, and Ensure Legal Compliance. New York: AMACOM/American Management Association.

Baxter R, Cohen SB, Ylvisaker M (1985). Comprehensive Cognitive Assessment. In M Ylvisaker (ed), Head Injury Rehabilitation: Children and Adolescents. San Diego: College Hill.

Botterbusch KF (1985). Norms, Reliability, and Validity in Commercial Vocational Evaluation Systems: A Critical Review. In C Smith, R Fry (eds), National Forum on Issues in Vocational Assessment: The Issues Papers. Menomonie, WI: University of Wisconsin-Stout, Stout Vocational Rehabilitation Institute, Materials Development Center, 24.

Chapman W, Katz M (1981). Survey of Career Information Systems in Secondary Schools. Princeton, NJ: Educational Testing Service.

Curl RM, Chisholm LA (1993). Unlocking co-worker in competitive employment: keys to a cooperative approach. J Voc Rehabil 3;72.

Fraser RT, Clemmons D, Trejo W, Temkin NR (1983). Program evaluation in epilepsy rehabilitation. Epilepsia 24;734.

Glover RW, Marshall R (1993). Improving the school-to-work transition of American adolescents. Teach Coll Rec 3;588.

Johnson AO, Chapin B, Buxton JM, Hudson D (1994). Transitioning Students with a Traumatic Brain Injury into Educational Systems: An Exploration of Different Models. Presented at the Thirteenth Annual Symposium of the National Head Injury Foundation, November 9, Chicago, IL.

MacMillan DL, Balow I, Widaman K, et al. (1990). Methodological problems in estimating dropout rates and the implications for studying dropouts from special education. Exceptionality 1;29.

Milton SB, Scalgeone C, Flanagan T, et al. (1991). Functional evaluation of adolescent students with traumatic brain injury. J Head Trauma Rehabil 6;35.

National Institute of Disability and Rehabilitation Research (1994). School to Work Transitions for Youth with Disabilities: Report from Consensus Validation Conference. Arlington, VA: National Institute of Disability and Rehabilitation Research.

Sampson JP, Reardon RC, Wilde CK, et al. (1994). A Comparison of the Assessment Components of Fifteen Computer Assisted Career Guidance Systems. In JT Keyes, M Mastie, E Whitfield (eds), A Counselor's Guide to Career Assessment Instruments. Alexandria, VA: National Career Development Association, 373.

Sandow D, Darling L, Stalick R, et al. (1993). Education reform: opportunities for improving transition from school to work. J Voc Rehabil 3;58.

Siegel S, Robert M, Greener K, et al. (1993). Career Ladders for Challenged Youths in Transition from School to Adult Life. Austin, TX: PRO-ED.

Telzrow CF (1991). The school psychologist's perspective on teaching students with traumatic brain injury. J Head Trauma Rehabil 6;23.

Wehman P (1990). School to work: elements of successful programs. Teach Except Child 3;40.

Wehman P, Kregel J, Barcus M (1985). From school to work: a vocational transition model for handicapped students. Except Child 52;25.

Wehman P, Moon MS, Everson J, et al. (1988). Transition from school to work. Baltimore: Paul H Brookes.

Chapter 20

Everyday People as Supports: Developing Competencies Through Collaboration

Mark Ylvisaker and Timothy J. Feeney

Throughout this book, emphasis has been placed on serving children and adolescents with traumatic brain injury (TBI) in meaningful contexts and working to improve everyday routines in those everyday contexts. Because context includes the people who interact regularly with a child, the places in which they interact, and the activities in those places, rehabilitation professionals face the important task of ensuring that those everyday people in the child's life possess the knowledge and competencies that they need to be successful facilitators of the child's recovery and ongoing development. Many professionals are prepared poorly for this task. The purposes of this chapter are to present a rationale for an approach to intervention that highlights the role of everyday people, to describe some of the competencies needed by those people, and to explain procedures that may be used to teach competencies and otherwise support everyday people. Although we emphasize communicative, behavioral, and cognitive issues, the principles of training and support presented here are also applicable to other areas of rehabilitation and special education.

In this chapter (as elsewhere), we use the term *everyday person* both descriptively (i.e., for people who interact most frequently with the individual with disability) and honorifically (i.e., for people with the potential to have the greatest impact on the person with disability by facilitating that individual's growth, thereby reducing disability and associated handicap).

Intervention Premises

The intervention premises elaborated and illustrated in this chapter underlie a post-TBI rehabilitation approach that highlights the role of everyday people and the associated activities of specialists in helping those everyday people to play their role effectively.

- *Premise I:* For many reasons, it is useful for specialists in TBI rehabilitation to deliver services in part through everyday people in the child's life (including family members, peers, paraprofessional aides, and others). These reasons include respect for everyday people, their insights, and their potential contribution; a likely increase in the intensity, consistency, and duration of intervention; facilitation of generalization and maintenance of learned skills; support for a long-term focus in rehabilitation; and cost-effectiveness of intervention.
- *Premise II:* Many obstacles block the delivery of rehabilitative services through collaboration with everyday people: narrow professional self-perception, territorialism, decreased access to everyday people, some everyday people's reluctance to be active members of the team, and inflexible reimbursement policies. Considerable creativity may be required to overcome these obstacles.
- *Premise III:* Ideally, the life of an individual with disability after TBI is organized around positive everyday routines that involve people who are knowledgeable, skilled in communication and problem solving, optimistic, flexible, creative, and mature. Orientation and training for staff and everyday people must be designed to target all these characteristics.
- *Premise IV:* There are many approaches to staff and family orientation and training, all of which serve a purpose. However, contextualized apprenticeship approaches are most effective in facilitating development of genuine competence.
- *Premise V:* Specialists consult most effectively if they consult as collaborators.
- *Premise VI:* Collaborative rehabilitation, which includes everyday people as collaborators, requires support from administrators whose job is to create a culture that values functional outcomes and real-world collaboration in pursuit of those outcomes.

Rationale for Specialists Working Through Everyday People

Respect

One of the strongest statements of respect that can be issued to parents, direct-care staff, assistants, paraprofessional aides, and others is that they are critical to the rehabilitation and ongoing development of children and adolescents with TBI. Of course, this statement is made not merely by uttering the words but rather by engaging those people as active members of the intervention team and by providing them with the support that they may need to play their roles effectively (Gans, 1987; Giangreco et al., 1993; Hilton and Henderson, 1993). In contrast, when professional staff jealously guard their expertise and their separate roles in assessment and intervention, the message often received by others is one of disrespect, that they are incapable of contributing positively to the individual's rehabilitation.

Use of Insights and Skills of Everyday People

Experienced rehabilitation and educational professionals understand that the people with the greatest insights—into the child's interests and levels of performance and into the supports needed to enhance performance—are often family members and other everyday people (Beardshaw and Towell, 1990; Hilton and Henderson, 1993; Nisbet, 1992; O'Brien and Lyle, 1987). Furthermore, where systematic hypothesis testing is required to identify the precise nature of the disability and the supports and intervention approaches most effective for the child, everyday people are necessary allies (see Chapter 10) (Coggins, 1991).

Intensity, Consistency, and Duration of Services

When everyday people are active allies in the intervention program, it is often possible to increase the intensity of a specific service from a small number of hours per week to several hours per day. With creative and informed use of everyday activities, this intensification of services can be true in the case of interventions focused on behavior, communication, cognition, education, and sensorimotor functioning (Mount and Zwernik, 1988; Timm, 1993). Furthermore, collegial and collaborative relationships with everyday people help to ensure general consistency in intervention (Kasier and McWorther, 1990; Landis and Peeler, 1990; Self et al., 1991). Although complete consistency is impossible and probably not a meaningful goal, it is both possible and desirable to have everybody in the child's life "on the same page," thereby preventing intervention approaches that are at cross-purposes, inefficient, and confusing to the child (Dunst et al., 1988, 1989, 1991, 1992). Finally, if work with family members results in an increase in their competence so that their everyday interactions with the child reach maximum effectiveness, the duration of rehabilitative services might, without additional cost, increase from a few weeks or months to many years.

Transfer or Generalization and Maintenance of Treatment Gains

In most areas of rehabilitation and special education, changing behavior and improving performance might be relatively easy under laboratory conditions or in tightly controlled clinical settings. Historically, however, the Waterloo of treatment programs for many people with chronic disability has been failure of generalization and maintenance (Kasier and McWorther, 1990; Powers et al., 1992; Self et al., 1991; Singley and Anderson, 1989; Stokes and Baer, 1977; Timm, 1993). One response to this classic challenge is to provide services and supports in a variety of settings and with a variety of people throughout the intervention process, thereby encouraging generalization and promoting maintenance, if only because the individuals who will continue to be involved in the child's life understand the skills and behaviors that should be encouraged and the ways in which to do that.

Appropriate Services and Supports Over the Long Term

After severe TBI, a rehabilitation hospital is typically the first in a long series of service providers for the child. Each transition—from inpatient to outpatient services, from hospital to school, from one level of education to another, and from school to adult life—carries with it the potential for breakdowns in continuity and associated regression in performance. However, if family members or others serving as the constants in a child's life are oriented thoroughly to their child's needs and to the role they can play in orienting service providers, breakdowns are less likely (Landis and Peeler, 1990; Smull and Harrison, 1992; Timm, 1993). Playing this role successfully requires a degree of competence and self-confidence that is difficult to acquire without rich experience as an active member of rehabilitation and special education teams (Elkinson and Elkinson, 1989; Stainback and Stainback, 1990; Wetzel and Hoschouer, 1984).

Managed Care and Severe Limitations on Professional Resources

Applying managed care to rehabilitation has reduced (and will continue to reduce) the intensity and duration of services that rehabilitation professionals can provide directly. At the same time, many school districts face shrinking budgets and the need to cut costs. Under these economically challenging circumstances, professionals must make important choices. Those who previously served patients or students in a labor-intensive manner can choose to continue that approach while experiencing the intense frustration associated with failing to accomplish what they were accustomed to accomplishing with ample time and resources. A wise alternative, however, would be to rethink service delivery options and to spend a relatively greater amount of time and energy on training and orienting everyday people. In that way, the child can be served in large part by people who are paid less (e.g., paraprofessional aides) or not at all (e.g., parents) or who are also paid to deliver another service at the same time (e.g., teachers) (Elkinson and Elkinson, 1989; Hagren et al., 1992; Harris, 1990). Our point is not that the goal of rehabilitation planning is to reduce costs as much as possible, nor is it to place an unacceptable burden on family members or others. Rather, given the economic realities of our era, we wish to determine how rehabilitation specialists can have the greatest positive impact on the people they serve.

Obstacles to Professionals Working with and Through Everyday People

Professionals' Self-Perception

Many forces act on young clinicians to shape their understanding of how they should deliver their services and think about themselves as service providers. For example, training programs tend to highlight discipline-specific skills and technical knowledge—a fairly narrowly defined scope of practice—and highly specialized settings in which to deliver the service. This practice combines with the language habitually used to describe the service to create deep-seated and powerful images of how to behave as a professional. For example, routine use of such words as *treatment, treatment room, treatment modalities, treating therapist, diagnosis, prognosis, patient,* and *impairment* inevitably predisposes clinicians-in-training to think of themselves as delivering a service much like that of a surgeon. Routine use of such words as *training, training hierarchy, training program, performance criteria, reinforcement contingencies and schedules,* and *learning trials* inevitably predisposes clinicians-in-training to think of themselves as delivering a service much like that of an animal trainer. Therefore, not surprisingly, many rehabilitation professionals find it difficult to think of themselves (perhaps unconsciously) as anything other than combined surgeon and animal trainer. Under these circumstances, delivering a service through everyday people is perceived as a foreign, possibly threatening, and most certainly dissatisfying professional option.

In their insightful book on the power and pervasiveness of hidden metaphors in everyday language, Lakoff and Johnson (1980) argued that language is thoroughly metaphoric and that people are profoundly influenced in their thinking and acting by the implicit metaphors underlying the language:

> Metaphors may create realities for us, especially social realities. A metaphor may thus be a guide for future action. Such actions will, of course, fit the metaphor. This will, in turn, reinforce the power of the metaphor to make experience coherent. In this sense metaphors can be self-fulfilling prophecies. [p. 156]

These authors offered the word *argument* as an illustration. The way we talk and think about arguments makes it clear that the underlying metaphor is that argument is war. For example, we readily speak about offense and defense in arguments, attack and retreat, winning and losing, strategy and tactics, and the like. More importantly, these associations lead us to want to conquer the opponent when we enter into arguments, to feel defeated when we lose an argument, and to shy away from arguments with intellectual heavyweights.

However, nothing in the nature of arguing mandates a military metaphor. It is conceivable that we just as easily could have selected a dance metaphor: Arguing is dancing. Had we made this choice, utterances such as the following would not seem odd; on the contrary, they would be perfectly natural: "You are a wonderful arguer." "I love arguing with you." "Please save the next argument for me." "Would you like to go out this Saturday, have a nice dinner, and do a little arguing?" However, in our society, we did not choose a dance metaphor; we chose a military metaphor. This has profoundly influenced our feelings and the conduct of our affairs as people who engage in discussions with others about differences of opinion (i.e., as people who argue).

The analogy with clinical conduct should be obvious. Rather than the combined surgeon–animal trainer metaphor that pervades rehabilitation discourse and drives much clinical decision making, rehabilitation professionals could have chosen alternative metaphors, such as consultant, coach, master craftsperson (in relation to an apprentice), counselor, cheerleader, parent, drill sergeant, guardian angel, and mentor. In Appendix 20-1, the meaning implicit in several of these metaphors is analyzed. Our point is not that one metaphor or model best captures the work of rehabilitation professionals; on the contrary, each metaphor—including those of surgeon and animal trainer—is useful for understanding certain aspects of the clinical interaction that is broadly classified as *rehabilitation after brain injury.* Furthermore, most effective interactions include components of two or more of the metaphors. Our point, then, is that rehabilitation professionals must raise to a level of conscious awareness the metaphors that influence their behavior and self-perception as professionals. Having accomplished that difficult task, they must make deliberate decisions about the best approach for serving specific individuals, given that person's needs, context, chronicity of disability, resources, support systems, and so on.

For individuals with chronic disability after TBI, the professional behavior dictated by the coach, consultant, and master-craftsperson metaphors often is preferable to, and more effective in the long run than, that dictated by the surgeon and animal trainer metaphors. Furthermore, the coach, consultant, and master-craftsperson metaphors can be easily applied to interaction between rehabilitation specialists and everyday people in a child's life, enabling the professionals to consider it a natural option to work primarily through those everyday people without feeling their sense of expertise or professionalism threatened.

In preservice training programs, we have found it useful for student clinicians to view a number of varied clinical interactions (on videotape) and to classify them according to the implicit metaphor or metaphors that seem to be driving the interaction and clinical services. Having made and justified their decision, the students are asked to describe how intervention would look if the clinician were to pursue the same goals and objectives for the client but from the perspective of a substantially different metaphor. In our experience, considerable application practice and discussion of this sort are required for student clinicians to achieve clarity regarding alternative metaphors or frameworks, flexibility in designing alternative intervention plans within opposing frameworks, and sensitivity to the extreme importance of the metaphors that dictate professional self-perception.

Territorialism and Lack of Self-Confidence

We have grouped self-confidence and territorialism together because they are frequently connected in the real world: That is, staff who resist interacting with professionals from other disciplines and working intensively with family members and direct-care staff are often people who lack confidence in their own knowledge and abilities. To be sure, territorialism and professional defensiveness may have other roots as well. Whatever their roots, these forces are obstacles to delivering a service with and through everyday people.

In our experience, overcoming this obstacle depends largely on the ability of managers within rehabilitation and school programs to create a culture in which it is a job expectation that staff work collaboratively with a variety of relevant team members, including family members and aides, and that inexperienced staff have available to them the resources to do this effectively. For example, if the staff-staff and staff-family communication competencies (Appendix 20-2) are made part of all staff members' job descriptions, on the basis of which their performance is evaluated, professionals will have a clearer understanding of the importance of this component of their professional lives and will be less likely to dismiss as unnecessary their close collaboration with everyday people.

Access to Everyday People

In many cases, rehabilitation specialists have difficulty finding sufficient time with family members, direct-care staff, professional colleagues, and others to equip those people with the competencies they would need to use everyday activities effectively to facilitate the child's improvement in the professional's area of concern. As we suggest later, an occasional Friday afternoon family conference or 1-hour staff in-service is insufficient time in which to generate competence in otherwise untrained people. Time constraints are an important reality in rehabilitation hospitals and schools alike.

Partial solutions to this problem are available. In rehabilitation hospitals, it is wise (although initially unpopular) to schedule professional therapists so that for 1 day each week they stay into the early evening to interact both with families who visit only in the evening and with the 3:00- to 11:00-PM nursing staff. Creating opportunities for elbow-to-elbow mentoring for families and direct-care staff during those hours can be helpful. Occasional Saturday hours create similar opportunities for working with families and weekend nursing staff.

In addition, alternative forms of communication can be useful. In our work in rehabilitation and other settings, we have made copious use of videotaped communication. In some cases, staff can use videotapes to model, for family members or other staff, therapeutic procedures or important types of interaction with the child. Alternatively, video can be used by family members or direct-care staff to communicate to teachers and professional clinicians important information (e.g., what works in natural settings) (Walther and Beate, 1991; Ylvisaker and Feeney, 1996). In Chapter 12, we described a protocol for transitional or self-advocacy videotapes that help create smooth transitions from one level of care or education to another. We presented the protocol in our chapter on executive functions because one possible purpose for producing the videotape is to help individuals with disability to understand better their strengths and needs. Another purpose is to engage family members, direct-care staff, and others in the production of the videotape in an effort to increase their understanding of the disability and appropriate intervention approaches. The collaborative activity of producing a transitional video can be a powerful training procedure for people who need to acquire understanding and competence in order to serve the individual with disability.

In some cases, parents resist entering into a therapeutic alliance with professionals because they simply lack the time and energy to play a role beyond that which comes naturally to them as family members and for which they have time in their busy days. Professionals must be sensitive to the limits on family resources (including time) and must not apply pressure on families to do more for their child than the families believe themselves capable of doing. A broad understanding of the term *everyday person* will encourage professionals to create alliances with people who might not initially emerge as obvious collaborators (e.g., extended family members, baby sitters, neighbors, siblings).

In other cases, parents might resist a role in rehabilitation suggested to them by professionals because the cultural or family values to which they are committed are (or appear to be) inconsistent with that new role. In this case, professionals must work with family members from within the family's cultural perspective and help them to play the most positive role possible that is consistent with their values (Van Kleek, 1994).

Characteristics of an Effective Everyday Coach, Facilitator, or Partner

If an important goal of rehabilitation is to help everyday people in the child's life effectively use everyday activities and interaction to facilitate improvement in a variety of areas of functioning, identification of the characteristics and competencies of effective everyday coaches is important. In some ways, desirable characteristics vary with the characteristics of the child. For example, some children profit from having active, enthusiastic initiators and cheerleaders as everyday coaches, whereas other children profit from being with coaches who do their work quietly in the background and who make their presence felt only when absolutely necessary.

Ideally, children with disability after TBI are surrounded by adults who are knowledgeable, effective communicators; who are optimistic, flexible, creative, and mature; and who are effective and enthusiastic problem solvers. We propose this list of characteristics, skills, and competencies as relevant in hiring paraprofessionals and direct-care staff and also in setting goals for orientation, training, and support programs for family members and staff.

Knowledge

Everyday people, including family members, direct-care staff, and others, should understand the consequences of TBI, including both general consequences and consequences particular to the child in question. Furthermore, they should understand the principles and intervention procedures associated with all relevant domains of rehabilitation (e.g., cognitive rehabilitation, physical rehabilitation, behavior management, psychosocial rehabilitation, communication intervention, academic intervention). The most frequently used training procedures—namely informational in-services, reading materials, and training

videotapes—are designed to achieve this goal and have an important place in a comprehensive orientation and training program. However, everyday people who are given the opportunity to work elbow-to-elbow with specialists in an apprenticeship role may be best served by the teaching of relevant information along with competencies, routines, and values in this setting.

The potential danger of placing knowledge first on our list of training goals is that knowledge (i.e., possession of information) might be last in a ranking of those goals in order of importance. For example, if one were forced to choose between a knowledgeable person who interacted badly and was pessimistic, inflexible, unimaginative, unenthusiastic, and immature and a person who lacked knowledge but possessed all the other attributes in abundance, the choice would be clear. We make this point not to discourage programs that offer informational in-services but rather to underscore the fact that information is only a small first step. Far more important is competency-based training and ongoing support for everyday people so that their routines of interaction with individuals with disability are as positive and effective as they can be.

Interactive Competence

Individuals with disability, particularly those with cognitive, behavioral, and communication disabilities, must have a good relationship with the people who help them achieve independence and advance in all the skill areas related to their disability. Everyday coaches are required to challenge the children, give them honest feedback, model target behaviors, and set increasingly high expectations. Therefore, it is critical that the children respect those coaches, which in turn requires that the coaches respect the children and know how to communicate effectively with them.

Elsewhere, we have described a comprehensive training program designed to facilitate development of a positive communication culture in rehabilitation programs and other settings in which individuals with TBI are served (Ylvisaker et al., 1993). That program highlights (1) a general philosophy of social-environmental intervention; (2) communication competencies in everyday communication partners that facilitate improved communication, cognitive functioning, and behavior in individuals with TBI through positive everyday interaction; (3) the importance of integrating communication, cognition, and behavior in training staff and family members; and (4) procedures that can be used to orient and train everyday people.

Appendix 20-2 presents organized lists of communication and behavioral competencies that should be included in the job descriptions of all rehabilitation staff and that should be reviewed with family members and other everyday people. We include staff-staff and staff-family communication, in addition to staff-client communication, because of the importance of positive and effective communication to establishing collaborative relationships among staff members and between staff and family. Each list is divided into five subcategories: (1) the *content* of communication (e.g., choice of topics, levels of concreteness); (2) the *form* of communication (e.g., length and complexity of utterances, word choice, manner of speaking); (3) *encouragement* offered by the communication partner (e.g., inviting and prompting the individual to communicate, prompting use of the easiest communication modality); (4) the *environment* in which communication occurs; and, most important, (5) techniques for communicating *respect* (e.g., giving clients choices, including family members in assessment and rehabilitation planning).

The behavioral competencies listed in Appendix 20-2 may appear to identify professional activity that is exclusively in the province of behavioral specialists. To be sure, staff with expertise in behavior play the leading role in functional analysis of behavior and in formulation of a comprehensive intervention plan. However, behavioral intervention is certain to fail if everyday people in the child's life are not competent in the areas outlined by that list. This list of behavioral competencies is placed with communication competencies to highlight the intimate connections between communication and behavior, which are explored in Chapter 13.

Appendix 20-3 includes a proposed outline for a competency-based training session focused on communication and related cognitive and behavioral competencies. The goals of a general training session of this sort are (1) to create a common conceptual framework for communication, cognition, and behavior; (2) to ensure that staff and family members recognize the many connections among communication, behavior, and cognition; (3) to improve the ability of staff and family members to interpret communication-in-context, particularly in cases in which communication impairment interacts with cognitive and behavioral disability; (4) to begin the process of equipping staff and family members with important communication and behavioral competencies; (5) to create enthusiasm for a positive communication culture; and (6) to motivate all staff and family members to work collaboratively toward creating such a culture. In our experience, training sessions focused on communication and related behavioral and cognitive competencies must be at least 3–4 hours long if participants are to begin to achieve these goals.

Later in this chapter, we emphasize the limitations of decontextualized in-service training (i.e., "out-service" training), particularly for staff or family members whose learning needs in the area of interactive competence and "people skills" are substantial. In those cases, in-service training must be followed by some combination of in vivo modeling and coaching, video instruction, and apprenticeship procedures (discussed later). Furthermore, for staff members, performance in this area must be part of the ongoing supervisory process, including employee performance evaluations. We emphasize these points because of the frequency with which programs discontinue training in the area of interactive competence after in-service training has been completed. In our experience, little enduring change in staff communication and behavior management competencies can be expected from in-service training alone.

Appendix 20-4 includes sample vignettes that could be used as part of competency-based training for staff, family members, and other everyday people. These vignettes are merely illustrations of what trainers in a specific program might wish to use—either on videotape or acted out live—to stimulate discussion and role-playing practice of positive alternatives. We use negative models for this purpose for several reasons. When they are exaggerated, negative models are humorous, serve as icebreakers, and can readily encourage participants to become actively engaged in the training session, by identifying the obvious mistakes made in the negative model and by proposing a variety of positive alternatives. Exaggerated negative models also hold the potential to illustrate vividly the dangers of certain common types of communication or behavior management errors by demonstrating the undesirable consequences of those errors. Finally, using funny, exaggerated negative models followed by brainstorming about a variety of positive alternatives communicates the important point that there are many ways to communicate positively and effectively. In other words, it is not necessary for all staff and family members to try to emulate the model exactly, which is the potential message when trainers use videotaped or live *positive* demonstrations of how to interact.

Optimism

It is critical that people who work with a child or adolescent with TBI have a positive vision of where the affected individual can be 1, 5, 10, and 20 years from now and that they be inspired by small steps the individual makes toward that vision (Mount and Zwernik, 1988; O'Brien and Lyle, 1987; Provencal, 1987). Because progress sometimes is frustratingly slow, people involved in the child's life can easily become discouraged, but individuals with disability need to see optimism in the people around them.

Many people are, by nature, optimistic and need no special support to maintain this orientation in their work with individuals with disability. Others are less optimistic and easily become discouraged. Staff and family members who fall into the latter group benefit from support and encouragement from people whose opinions they respect (Condeluci, 1991). Family members might find comfort and encouragement in a formal support group, such as those sponsored by the local chapter of the Brain

Injury Association or other organization that serves families of people with disability. In many cases, encouragement and support are more effectively delivered by individuals who bear a special relationship to the individual in need of such assistance. Professionals can help by ensuring that families have thoroughly explored their world of family, friends, and others (e.g., religious leaders, selected peer families) for needed support.

Staff similarly need support when their patients' or students' progress is slow and frustration levels are high. If adequate peer support systems have not evolved naturally in a workplace, managers should create regular opportunities for staff members to express their concerns and to receive the encouragement they need to see the big picture and to gain confidence that their work is bearing fruit.

In addition, both staff and family members may need to be encouraged to engage in regular "positive scanning," as opposed to the negative scanning that is more natural for many people. *Positive scanning* is simply surveying the realities surrounding work with the individual and identifying everything in that world that is positive. In contrast, negative scanning is looking for everything that is negative. When tired, discouraged, or depressed, most people slip into a negative scanning mode, which only darkens their mood. Routine positive scanning at team conferences and at other times may be a useful antidote and might contribute to the goal of providing for the individual with disability a circle of optimistic people. Team leaders may need to insist that time be devoted to responding to the question, "What are the good things that are happening in this child's life and what are the positive resources?"

Flexibility, Creativity, and Problem Solving

In the next three subsections of this chapter—devoted to flexibility, creativity, and problem solving—we recommend routines that are open ended. Although there is a script, the outcome is unknown, which can generate a sense of anxiety and vulnerability in many people. A sense of vulnerability increases when staff or family members are expected to say things such as, "I'm not sure what's best; let's think about it." People who are uncomfortable with ambiguity and vulnerability will probably always be so. However, if these people understand their own needs, have a script to follow, and observe extremely competent people professing the same uncertainty and the need to think aloud about the issue in question, they are in a better position to facilitate flexibility, creativity, and problem-solving skills in the child.

Flexibility

Hospital, school, and home life with a child or adolescent with TBI is filled with unpredictable events, unexpected deviations from routine, unwelcome changes in behavior, and alterations in plans. The emotional roller coaster that the child or adolescent often rides for some time after the injury may carry with it resistance to apparently useful intervention activities and well-conceived plans. Under these circumstances, it is easy for staff, parents, and others to become frustrated or confused and, as a consequence, to insist on sticking to their own plan, with the unfortunate outcome that they lose effectiveness as a helper for the child.

Many people are, by nature, flexible and adapt easily and effectively to the unpredictable twists and turns in the life of the child; others are inflexible. Flexibility is not easily taught. However, relatively inflexible people can learn that this is a weak area for them and can practice *routines of flexibility* that might help them and most certainly will help the person with TBI. The following example of a script could be rehearsed by an inflexible person until it is routine:

Adult: *(presents activity or plan)* How about if we do ... now?
Child: *(resists)* No, I don't want to do that!
Adult: *(routine response)* Okay, maybe you're right; maybe it's not a good idea. Let's think of some other way to get this job done. Any ideas? *(pauses to give the child time to respond)* How about ...? Or maybe ...?

We have worked with rigid staff and family members who remained relatively rigid but who used a script such as this to create flexibility routines that gave them the comfort they needed and, at the same time, significantly reduced their negative interaction with children with disability.

Creativity

An effective coach is one who can turn any activity or interaction into an occasion to teach something critical or to facilitate some important type of reflection. Effective coaches will be able to follow the child's lead but always find a way to use real-world, everyday activities to facilitate development in an important area.

As is true of flexibility, some adults are very creative and others are not. Teaching people to be creative is very difficult. However, well-rehearsed *creativity routines* are a step in the right direction. For example, let's assume that an issue arises and the child becomes upset.

Adult: *(attempting to create thinking time)* We need to think about this.
Child: Okay. *(Alternatively, the child may not respond.)*
Adult: *(attempting to focus on the goal)* What are you trying to accomplish here?
Child: I want to finish this and I can't. I'm angry.

Adult:	*(attempting to focus on the big picture and the availability of support)* You've done some good work here. That's great, and I know we can figure out some way to get this done.
Child:	*(grumbles)*
Adult:	*(communicating helpfulness and openness to alternatives)* How can I help you? Let's think about it together.
Child:	*(grumbles)*
Adult:	Are you ready to try? I'm not sure I will come up with anything good, but let's brainstorm. I know we can get this done. *(if in a group)* Let's all think about this. *(if no good ideas emerge)* Is there somebody we can talk to who might have a good idea?

The adult may or may not have an alternative idea or be able to generate a creative idea. However, routines of this sort are preferable to an adult's (mistaken) belief that it is his or her responsibility at any given moment to know what is best to do next, to tell the child to do it, and to insist on cooperation at the first sign of resistance. Adults who are not particularly creative or good at thinking on their feet tend to become anxious without a script and therefore slip into the trap of assuming total control and giving *some* instruction, however ill-considered it may be. A script such as the one presented here provides comfort to adults who need to know concretely what to do next, but such a script also creates opportunities for creative reflection that adults might otherwise avoid.

Problem-Solving Ability and Enthusiasm

An effective coach is not only a good problem solver but also a person who *welcomes* difficulties because *real* problems are the best context in which to engage individuals in problem-solving activity. Good coaches are not discouraged when dilemmas inevitably arise. Rather, they react with the thought, "How can I work with people to solve problems and at the same time help them to become better problem solvers?"

Some people are naturally good and enthusiastic problem solvers and others are not. Those who are *not* typically look immediately for *the* answer or *the* solution, thereby avoiding the problem-solving process. As a consequence, children with TBI lose yet another opportunity to practice solving their own problems. People who are not good problem solvers or who do not welcome problems may need to practice and internalize problem-solving interaction routines such as the following:

Child:	*(having a difficult time doing something)*
Adult:	Boy, Fred, that looks like a hard thing to do.

Child:	*(persists unsuccessfully in his attempts to do what he wants to do)*
Adult:	I wonder what would make that go easier.
Child:	I don't know.
Adult:	Let's see. Maybe you could do *(A)* or *(B)* or *(C)*.
Child:	I'll try *(A)*.
Adult:	Okay, you could do that. But hold on; let's think about this for a minute. If you do *(A)*, will it solve the problem? Will it take a lot of time? If you do *(B)*, will it solve the problem and will it take a lot of time? How about if you do *(C)*?
Child:	Don't know.
Adult:	Let's think. *(A)* would take all day. *(B)* might not get the job done because.... *(C)* is easy and quick and probably would be successful. What do you think?
Child:	I'll do *(C)*.
Adult:	Good choice. This was hard to figure out, but we thought of several possibilities and I think you chose the smartest one. Good thinking!

We have worked with professionals, paraprofessionals, and family members who were not natural or enthusiastic problem solvers but who practiced a script of this sort until it became routine. They then were able to facilitate problem-solving development in the person with TBI as effectively as were adults who are natural and enthusiastic problem solvers.

Maturity

People who work with individuals with disability must be sufficiently emotionally mature that they do not take those individuals' mood swings or occasional expressions of anger personally. Furthermore, rather than needing to take credit for solutions, they must be sufficiently mature to help children or adolescents with TBI to create their own solutions to problems. Finally, they must be sufficiently mature to know that their ultimate goal is to work themselves out of a job, to do everything possible to turn over to the person with disability the self-coaching function so that the helpers are no longer needed. People with disability do not benefit from the assistance of aides who feed their own ego by creating dependence.

Assisting staff people to deal effectively with apparently personal attacks—from the child or the child's family members—might require organizing support systems among staff members so that they can remind one another that they are doing good work, that they are good people, and that there are probably understandable reasons for attacks that have nothing to do with the staff members per se. Helping staff and family members turn over their coaching role to the child may require an explicit focus on independence and self-regulation as a primary long-term goal and a focus on small steps toward that goal as an immediate goal. Specifically, executive function objectives should be written into the rehabilitation plan or the individualized education plan so that staff can receive some feedback on how effectively they have helped the child acquire executive or self-coaching behaviors (see Chapter 12). When staff members are clear that it is their job to let the child attempt to solve problems and initiate useful behavior—and when staff members are explicitly rewarded for doing so—the pernicious evolution of learned helplessness can be avoided.

Training Options

Several methods are available to help everyday people, including family members and staff, acquire the knowledge and competencies that put them in the best position to help the child with disability. Selection of teaching and support procedures varies with the goal of the teaching, the learner's background and competence, the setting, available time and resources, and other factors.

Informational In-Services, Family Conferences, and Written Instructions

We have grouped informational in-services, family conferences, and written instructions because they are all appreciably limited in relation to the goal of generating enduring competence in staff and family members. Issues related to TBI are typically far too complicated to be explained in 1 hour or less. Furthermore, just as professionals in their training programs need help translating textbook and lecture material into clinical competencies—that is, they need practical clinical training with coaching from experienced clinicians—so too do everyday people need coached practice to develop their competence, whether it is related to medical, physical, cognitive, communicative, or behavioral aspects of rehabilitation. Therefore, the realistic goal of brief in-services or family conferences should be restricted to introducing themes that can be developed later or to dealing in a problem-solving way with issues that have arisen after the trained staff or family members have attempted to apply their learned competencies.

Rehabilitation facilities and schools that overestimate the potential of in-service training combined with written instructions tend to generate frustration that easily leads to conflict among staff. For example, commonly, therapists, psychologists, and others provide brief in-service training for staff or family members, which is followed by patient-specific instructions regarding management of some aspect of physical or behavioral disability. The predictable result is that many direct-care staff members fail

to follow the instructions as required. This, in turn, might be followed by laments that nursing staff members are uncooperative, oppositional, or even unprofessional. Most often, the problem has nothing to do with cooperation, opposition, or professionalism. Often, the problem is that insufficient attention was paid to teaching competencies in the context in which they must be applied, to giving opportunities for feedback about how realistic the instructions are in that context, and to ensuring that the people who receive the instructions fully understand the purpose of the instructions as well as the procedures used to follow them.

Family conferences, informational in-services, and written instructions all have their place in a comprehensive program of training and support for family and staff. Furthermore, videotaped education and training programs are increasingly available in a variety of rehabilitation domains. However, in the absence of some combination of the training options discussed next, one must maintain appropriately low expectations for outcome after training that does not focus on competencies.

Decontextualized Competency-Based Training

Unlike informational in-services, competency-based training sessions include coached practice of the skill to be learned. The communication and behavior training session outlined in Appendix 20-3 is an example of such training. Although more time-consuming than informational in-services (typically a minimum of 3–4 hours), competency-based training is superior to informational in-services, in which skills are not practiced. At the very least, such training can serve as the basis for legitimately including a skill in staff job descriptions. However, it is unrealistic to expect that staff who are in need of considerable improvement in a specific area will be transformed from incompetent to fully competent over the course of 3 or 4 hours of lecture, discussion, and coached practice of the skill. Again, some combination of the training options discussed next is almost always required for staff members with weak skills.

Apprenticeship

Like long-standing apprenticeship programs in the trades and crafts, apprenticeship as a training option for family members and staff is characterized by (1) working together with the mentor (the master craftsperson) in the context in which the knowledge and competencies to be learned will be used; (2) starting with few responsibilities and gradually increasing involvement as competence increases; and (3) routinely reviewing performance, competencies, and needs in relation to the actual job in the actual context.

Apprenticeship is the most effective training context in which to acquire functional competencies. It is also the ideal context in which to acquire self-confidence and important attitudes about rehabilitation and about people with disability. For example, working with a specialist in cognition can give everyday people the insight that promoting cognitive development often means *not* having the answer. Working with a master teacher can give everyday people the insight that teaching does not necessarily require demanding performance from the child. Working with a master behaviorist can give everyday people the insight that managing behavior does not necessarily entail explicitly controlling the child's behavior.

Training in Vivo

Guided Observation.   The first stage of in vivo training is guided observation, in which the trainee observes the competencies to be learned as they are demonstrated by a clinician or other competent person (live or on videotape). The coach points out specific behaviors, the child's as well as the clinician's. In the case of communication and behavior, the coach and trainee discuss the possible communicative intent of observed behaviors, brainstorm about how to identify the real intent, and identify precursors and consequences of the behavior. They consider alternative ways to communicate messages and to prompt and respond to communication. Throughout this observation, the emphasis is on communication as a two-way interaction. The trainee's competence is demonstrated by adequate identification of communication behaviors, interpretation of communicative intent, identification of the effects of communication behaviors, and flexible consideration of alternative ways to prompt and respond to communication.

Coached Interaction.   The coach then prepares the trainee, with role-playing practice if necessary, for interaction with the child who requires the competencies to be learned. The interaction can be three-way, with the coach only gradually turning over to the trainee responsibility for maintaining the interaction. Alternatively, the trainee can interact with the child, with the coach intervening only if the trainee signals the need for help. This interaction is followed by discussion (possibly including videotape review) of the interaction. This discussion highlights those aspects of the interaction that worked (in relation to the goals of the interaction), those that did not work, and alternatives to the aspects that did not work.

Follow-Along Coaching.   As the trainee demonstrates increasing competence in coached interaction, the coach increasingly assumes the role of resource person, problem solver, and intermittent observer. Initially, there may be planned review and problem-solving sessions with the trainee. As the trainee's competence increases, he or she can begin to play a coaching role for peers (e.g., family members helping other family members; staff members helping other staff members at their job level). The high-

est level of mastery of a competence is the ability to teach it to someone else. Even if the trainee does not desire to become a coach, this level of competence (i.e., consultant's competence) should be a goal.

Self-Observation on Videotape

Increasingly, self-observation has been recognized as an effective training procedure in a wide range of fields. The procedure is clinically less obtrusive than is live observation and creates the possibility of repeated viewings and microanalysis of behavior. Many people fail to become aware of some of their interactive habits without self-observation, even when an excellent verbal feedback system is available. The interaction to be viewed can be contrived or can occur naturally. The first self-viewing can be guided by a trainer (cheerleader and coach), whose job is both to encourage the individual and to identify areas in need of improvement. The coach identifies specific aspects of the interaction that are positive and also discusses the general tenor of the interaction (e.g., respectful, encouraging). The coach then helps the individual focus on specific areas for ongoing improvement. Usually, it is better for the trainee to watch the first videotape alone, as considerable embarrassment is often associated with the first self-viewing. Coached self-observation will be more effective once the trainee has moved beyond this natural reaction. Furthermore, coaches must understand that self-observation on videotape creates a powerful sense of vulnerability that must be respected in coaching interactions.

Coached self-observation includes highlighting the positive aspects of an interaction, giving the trainees ample opportunity to explain their reasons for acting as they did, exploring in a nonthreatening way the aspects of the interaction that did not go well, and practicing positive alternatives to any aspect of the interaction that was unsuccessful. The effectiveness of video feedback has been demonstrated in the training of individuals with disabilities and their peers (Booth and Fairbank, 1984; Kern et al., 1992; Walther and Beate, 1991).

Community Meetings

Particularly when one's work involves a difficult child or adolescent, staff meetings should be understood as community meetings—that is, as opportunities for staff at all levels to support, to encourage, and to learn from one another. Often, staff meetings are focused on the latest crisis or apparently unsolvable problem. As *community meetings*, in contrast, the focus is on collaborative problem solving, on sharing information about the interventions that may be working, and on ensuring that all staff have the script that, at least for the time being, is considered most effective in working with the child or adolescent. The focus of a community meeting is not today's potentially discouraging news but rather the overall story, what is positive about that story (in historical perspective), and how to make the story better. Sharing folklore and brainstorming in a positive way during such meetings are powerful training tools for inexperienced staff.

Peer Training

Staff and Family Training Chains

The creation of high levels of competence in all staff and all family members connected with the child with disability is difficult and time-consuming. However, with appropriate encouragement from trainers and administrators, competence can be passed from person to person much as one communicates by means of a chain letter. For example, parents can pass knowledge and skill on to siblings, grandparents, baby-sitters, and others. Similarly, direct-care staff can support one another, showing untrained staff how to interact with a child or how to use a specific physical, cognitive, or behavioral intervention.

In our experience, training chains of this sort can be effective only in a setting in which peer competence is respected and managers explicitly support this procedure. In unhealthy settings, staff who take responsibility for orienting peers may be disregarded or even ridiculed. Managers may need to ensure that staff members understand that peer support is a job expectation. They may also need to identify some area of expertise for each staff member, so that everyone in the culture has the experience of helping others as well as being helped. Peer training of this sort is one mechanism for promoting ownership of the culture generally and ownership of individual intervention plans specifically (Bernstein, 1982; Bogdan et al., 1974; Wetzel and Hoschouer, 1984).

Child Peers

Thus far, we have restricted the scope of everyday people to adults. However, a child's world is also filled with other children, whose knowledge, skill, attitudes, and sensitivity play a large role in the injured child's recovery and creation of a positive sense of self. Thus, peers in the hospital, at school, and in the neighborhood play an important role in rehabilitation. To play this role well, they may require specialized orientation and support (Christopher et al., 1991; Thousand and Villa, 1990).

In hospitals, it is wise to provide information to visiting friends, particularly if physical or behavioral issues exist that might alarm peers or that peers might misinterpret. Generally, very little time is required for therapists, social workers, or others to show peers how to interact and play with their injured friend. Ideally, enjoyable activities are available in the hospital for children at varied developmental levels. Peers may need help understanding their own feelings and reactions to the injury and to the observable disability.

In schools, teachers can keep peers apprised of their classmate's progress during the rehabilitation phase, orga-

nize letter writing, and possibly send a get-well videotape from school to the hospital. At the time of the child's transition back to school, a presentation to peers about the child's experiences and possible needs when he or she returns to school can be valuable. We have worked with children with a disability who, with coaching, made this presentation themselves. Others were not able to make the presentation or refused to do so. If the child with disability is unable to make this presentation, the best alternative is a respected and well-liked member of the school staff, possibly the teacher in the case of grade-school children. The primary goals of the presentation are to characterize the child as a hero for having survived an extraordinary injury and to help peers to understand the child's ongoing disability and the ways in which they might help. In the absence of such a presentation, peers may withdraw because they feel anxiety associated with ignorance; they may create bizarre fantasies about the reasons for the child's behavior; they may even tease the child who returns to school with physical, cognitive, or behavioral challenges. School staff may need to assist peers in dealing with their own feelings, just as they do when a classmate dies.

Several school supports are designed to facilitate positive social interaction. Buddy systems can be effective, particularly if teachers are sensitive to and do all they can to prevent "buddy burn-out" (i.e., through implementation of a rotational system). Teachers must recognize also that buddies must be people who are compatible with the injured child. Carefully selected extracurricular activities can help the injured child and also provide support for peers, giving all a natural context for interaction.

Self-Advocacy or Transition Videotapes and Staff and Family Training

In Chapter 12, we described a protocol for developing videotapes designed to introduce the child to staff at the next level of service or in the next year's classroom. We included this discussion in a chapter devoted to executive functions because one of the primary reasons for the videotape is to heighten children's awareness of their strengths and needs and to underscore their role in charting their own course. Transition videotapes can also play a useful role in developing staff and family competence. If staff members at all levels work with family members to identify a child's strengths and needs and to devise intervention services, procedures, and supports that are effective in meeting these needs, a great deal of cross-training occurs incidentally. The process of brainstorming about a script for the videotape and determining which important illustrations to include often results in effective sharing of insights and competencies among staff and between staff and family. Furthermore, if staff and family develop a sequence of these videotapes over time, they will have a meaningful historical record that can provide encouragement and a sense of direction during periods of minimal progress.

Working with Reluctant Families

Most families do their best, under extraordinarily stressful circumstances, to support the injured child and to contribute in the most positive way to the child's rehabilitation. For a variety of reasons, relationships between family members and staff sometimes are rocky. Because of the acknowledged importance of the family's contribution and the benefits of staff working with family members, every effort should be made to establish effective working relationships.

Respecting Diversity

Some parents fit easily into the culture of rehabilitation hospitals and schools, confidently establishing effective working relationships with staff members and enthusiastically accepting an active role in their child's ongoing rehabilitation. Others are less comfortable, appear withdrawn, uninvolved, or inaccessible, and do not respond readily to staff members' overtures. In some cases, staff must communicate directly to family members that what needs to be done for the child can be done within the scope of that family's values and routines.

Seeking Capacity and Respecting Family Expertise

Sometimes the professional is tempted to find fault with families and to dismiss them as dysfunctional and unable to contribute positively to a child's rehabilitation. In extreme cases (e.g., families guilty of serious abuse and neglect), this assessment may be a correct. However, in most cases, professionals who look beyond surface conflicts and apparent family disorganization can find capacity and expertise that can be mobilized in the child's interest. Furthermore, barriers between family and staff often crumble when staff members communicate respect for family expertise (e.g., by finding ways for family members to be active contributors in the child's ongoing assessment and program planning) and find a way to integrate that expertise into the child's program.

Understanding Family Grief and Victimization

In Chapter 16, Waaland explores issues surrounding family grieving after severe TBI in a child or adolescent. Because these issues are complex, specialists in family counseling might be engaged to help staff to understand family grief. The point we wish to stress in this chapter is that many families appear to staff to be difficult because staff members have failed to appreciate the family's ongo-

ing grieving process and the intensity of emotions that can emerge and re-emerge for years after TBI.

In addition, it is helpful for staff to remember that families move through many groups of professionals over the years after such an injury. If some of these relationships are negative, as inevitably some are, the likelihood increases that families will be defensive and suspicious of the next set of professionals. Creating a working alliance under such circumstances requires that staff thoroughly understand family reactions and effectively communicate respect and empathy.

Identifying an Effective Communicator

Families with whom staff generally consider it difficult to work often have positive relationships with one or two staff members. The person in the best position to communicate effectively with the family may be a counselor or other professional; alternatively, it may be an aide or any other staff person. Occasionally, nobody in the program communicates effectively with the family, but a priest, family friend, or other person outside the program can be identified as a communication bridge. Having identified this person, staff can funnel their communication in part through this trusted individual, thereby increasing the likelihood of successful communication and the establishment of a working alliance.

Ensuring that Families Are Supported

Families cannot be expected to play their role well if they are without their own support system. Often, family counselors help them to mobilize their network of support, including extended family, friends, and church members, so that they can maintain sufficient emotional and physical energy to support the child. Some families in which a loved one has had a serious brain injury have acquired a helpful perspective and can share this perspective with families that are at an earlier stage of the process, which might be beneficial to all. This one-to-one pairing of families often is more useful, particularly in the early months after the injury, than is a formal support group, such as those sponsored by the local chapter of the Brain Injury Association. In many parts of the country, the regional Brain Injury Association chapter takes responsibility for pairing families that can provide support for one another.

Specialists as Consultants and Collaborators

In this chapter and throughout the book, we have promoted the idea of specialists working (in part) with and through everyday people. This model of intervention is not new, having a long history in programs for infants with disability and a growing history in special education, mental health, and rehabilitation. Increasingly, special educators and therapists are serving children with special needs largely through staff in regular education classrooms. At least two critical themes have emerged from these histories: First, specialists working as consultants must be sensitive to the routines and culture of the setting in which they are consulting. Second, specialists working as consultants must approach the people whom they wish to help more as servants than as experts who intend to impose their will.

The Specialist as Houseguest

The first tasks that must be undertaken by specialists entering classrooms, homes, or other settings is to decipher important features of the culture, so that recommendations will be compatible with values and interpersonal relationships in that setting, and to identify established routines and resources, so that recommendations will be realistic and efficient within the routines of that setting. Just as a houseguest would not play a radio loudly at 3:00 AM, invite additional unwelcome guests, and demand time from the hosts beyond what is reasonable, so too effective consultants would not make recommendations without understanding the practices that will fit the setting. For example, it is unreasonable to ask a single mother, who works two shifts in order to put bread on the table, to devote 1–2 hours per day to physical therapy activities and homework with the child. As in so many similar situations, respectful negotiation and collaborative brainstorming are the keys to success, within constraints imposed by the critical reminder, "I am a guest in your home."

The Specialist as a Support Person

The interactive posture of effective consultants is not "I know what is best for this child and I'm telling you; you have to do it this way." Rather, it is "Here is my background; how might I be able to help you?" To be sure, at times consultants must persist in their offer and find effective ways to promote their usefulness. Occasionally, potential recipients of consulting help are defensive or hostile, and some effort is required to break down their resistance. However, family members and professionals alike generally will act on the recommendations of specialists if they respect those specialists and if the recommendations from the specialists are both respectful and effective.

In the face of resistance, an experimental attitude may be the best. The flavor of the specialist's recommendation might be to concede that his or her services are not needed if indeed things are going as well as possible. If, however, the situation is not ideal, the specialist might suggest that the family work with him or her to identify successful approaches through experimentation. If the experiments fail, then the two parties can collaborate again to try to find another option that might be effective.

Administrative Support for Cross-Training and General Competencies

If managers in rehabilitation hospitals express interest only in billable one-to-one therapy hours, and if their counterparts in schools indicate satisfaction with their staff members working in isolation from colleagues and family members, then the vision of everyday intervention and support described in this chapter will remain just that—a vision. Highly motivated staff in such settings might be best advised to deliver collaborative services in a countercultural manner, but in such situations systems will not be created for the efficient operation of an everyday approach to rehabilitation. Clinicians and managers must work together to identify procedures that will have a maximal effect on the well-being of the consumers of their services. We believe that these procedures will include (1) the promotion of a blurring of boundaries among professionals and between professionals and everyday people, while retaining respect for the expertise of specialists (2) a focus on the skills of collaboration and consultation in hiring and promoting staff, (3) the creation of time for staff training in competencies outside of their traditional sphere of competence, and (4) the creation of time and occasions for staff to facilitate development of genuine competence in everyday people.

Case Illustration: TBI Specialists Collaborating with School Staff

When our involvement began, JK was a 13-year-old boy with bilateral frontal lobe injury and severe behavior problems (including frequent aggression directed at people and objects). Eight years after his injury, a behavioral specialist began working with his family and the staff in his school. JK's educational services were delivered in his community middle school, largely as a result of family insistence that he be educated in an inclusive setting. There was a history of negative interaction between the family and the school, as well as an ongoing threat of litigation.

Like many children with prefrontal injury, JK's behavior had deteriorated steadily over the years since his injury (Feeney and Ylvisaker, 1995; Ylvisaker and Feeney, 1994). The original request from the school was for a behavioral evaluation and behavior plan. Because it was clear that stop-gap measures would be insufficient in this case, the goal shifted to development of a functional long-term plan for JK's future, coupled with identification of concrete means to achieve the long-term goal.

Previous behavior plans for JK had focused on external control and consequence management (reinforcement, ignoring, time out, punishment). For reasons discussed in Chapter 13, this approach had not been successful. A new antecedent-focused approach, involving an executive system plan-do-review routine (see Chapter 12) was proposed. Because the approach was novel for staff and family alike, training was provided in the context of JK's daily routines. Each new element of JK's routine was added experimentally: That is, each element was tried, its effectiveness was carefully documented, and the possible need for revision was assessed. Furthermore, the behavioral consultant was flexible in exploring variations in implementation of the routine at home and in school, consistent with the constraints of those settings. Experimentation was carried out while the consultant was present so that review of the experiments could be guided and possible variations could be explored with the consultant's help. Ongoing contextualized experimentation and review were designed in part to instill in staff and family members a sense of confidence that they could creatively and flexibly design and fine-tune effective interventions for JK. This collaborative experimentation also began to generate understanding on the part of both staff and family members of the others' perspective, which allowed them to retreat from what had been an ongoing threat of litigation.

To help determine long-range goals and short-term objectives, to maintain a functional focus, and to communicate respect for the family's perspective, the COACH functional educational planning system was used (Giangreco et al., 1993). This process helped staff members to understand why the family had made what originally appeared to them to be the unreasonable demand that JK be educated in an inclusive setting. It also helped to clarify overlapping roles of staff and family members.

Furthermore, planning functional intervention throughout the day resulted in the recognition that many members of the team, including family members, could make unique contributions. For example, JK's mother was the expert at getting him out of bed; his father was able to identify many creative teaching opportunities involving electronics, one of JK's interests; the teacher was expert in developing positive behavioral momentum before requesting that JK perform a nonpreferred activity; the aide was very good at encouraging peers to help JK. Meetings became an opportunity for team members to share their expertise with one another.

After several side-by-side experimentation sessions involving school staff and the behavioral specialist, a videotape-and-analysis protocol was implemented. At least once per week, staff members videotaped themselves working with JK in a variety of settings. This videotape then was reviewed with the behavioral consultant in a nonjudgmental manner, and the staff was largely responsible for identifying what approaches did and did not work. This process resulted in a substantial increase in staff insight, in their ability to solve problems, and in their sense of optimism that they could help JK and that they could manage what had previously appeared to be unmanageable behavior. In particular, videotape viewing allowed staff to see clearly how JK's behavior escalated when staff members allowed themselves to be drawn into control battles, which in turn helped them to recognize the importance of choosing their battles wisely, giving JK as much choice and control as possible, distinguishing between structure (a good thing) and overt external control (a provocation for JK), and teaching JK the distinction between choice and no-choice situations. To facilitate this increase in staff competence, the consultant gradually decreased his involvement in these videotape analysis sessions.

After several weeks, the consultant's role was reduced to that of coach and cheerleader at periodic problem-solving and brainstorming sessions with school staff. Staff had acquired a routine of nonjudgmentally identifying problems in the implementation of their intervention, brainstorming about and selecting a potential solution, carefully experimenting with the proposed solution, and patting each other on the back when they experienced success. Although JK's injury was of such a magnitude that he will always be vulnerable and in need of careful, antecedent-focused behavioral intervention, staff at his school had acquired the competence to manage the intervention creatively and flexibly, working cooperatively with JK's family. Two years after the consultant began his work with JK and his family and school staff, JK remained in an inclusive educational setting, the family had not brought legal action against the school district, and episodes of serious behavioral outbursts on JK's part were infrequent.

Case Illustration: TBI Specialists Collaborating with Families

DF was injured at age 2 in an automobile accident. His brain injury included widespread diffuse damage, with focal damage to the visual system and evidence of prefrontal injury. After inpatient rehabilitation, DF received services for 2 years as a day student in a developmental disabilities setting and then was placed in a self-contained special education classroom in a community school. His physical and cognitive functions continued to improve during the first 4 years after he was injured, presumably as a partial consequence of excellent therapeutic intervention and instruction. Throughout this period, services were largely delivered to DF directly rather than through his parents.

When DF was 6 years old, a TBI specialist became available to the family through a state education department TBI project. DF's parents generally were pleased with the services their son had received and with his progress but had two major concerns: first, that DF was so dependent on routine and predictability that the family was virtually held hostage by this inflexibility, and second, that although his speech and grammar were fine, DF never connected his thoughts in language and typically rejected invitations to talk about his experience or any other topic. These two issues became the themes for problem-solving discussions with the TBI consultant, who met with the parents in their home.

The most critical issue, DF's inflexibility and need for routine, was addressed in a 45-minute brainstorming session involving both parents and the consultant. The parents described DF's tantrums when a routine was violated (e.g., a new bus driver appeared in the morning) or an expectation could not be met (e.g., an expected visit from his cousin had to be canceled). The parents said that they had found nothing that worked for DF other than maintaining consistent routines and ensuring that his expectations were met.

The consultant introduced the important concept of a routine to deal with changes in routine, and a brainstorming session ensued that resulted in the parents' decision to experiment with a new routine in their home. Each time DF's routine had to be violated or an expectation could not be met, DF's parents would take him to a choice board (a small chalkboard on which his favorite activities were listed) and present the news while encouraging him to select an enjoyable alternative activity. Within 4 months, this metaroutine (i.e., a routine to deal with changes in routine) was sufficiently well established in the home that deviations from routine or expectation were no longer a major family issue. DF's family used this metaroutine for approximately 1 year, with decreasing frequency toward the end of that year. Four months later, DF spontaneously commented about the chalkboard, "I used to use that when I didn't know what to do; but now I know, so I don't need it anymore."

DF's inability to organize his thoughts and his language were addressed similarly by working through the parents. Like many parents and professionals, DF's parents had come to believe that one way to help DF remember information more effectively was to quiz him regularly about the past. Because of his difficulty in remembering, organizing his thoughts, and organizing his language, DF had developed the habit of resisting all attempts to

have him talk about the past or about complex issues; for example, he routinely replied, "You say it!" Despite ongoing progress in specific cognitive and preacademic domains in school, he similarly resisted organizing his language in that setting.

The consultant introduced the parents to the competencies associated with a collaborative and elaborative style in socially coconstructing narratives about the past. (These competencies are listed and discussed in Chapter 14.) After viewing a training videotape designed to model the competencies, the parents were invited to interact with their son about everyday topics, shifting from the pedagogical and interrogational style to which they had become accustomed to a positive elaborative and collaborative style, designed to help DF organize his thoughts, remember more information, and express himself in an easy manner. The parents audiotaped or videotaped some of these interactions for monthly review with the consultant. After 5 months of daily practice, with monthly coaching and cheerleading from the consultant, the parents had developed a style of interacting that included all the elaboration and collaboration competencies listed in Table 14-1. Meanwhile, DF had begun to volunteer to describe past events and to explain complex issues both at home and in school. Five months after this intervention was initiated through the parents, the consultant observed DF in school and witnessed him organizing eight units of information while providing the teacher with an explanation of what the students had done in art class that day.

It is possible that a comparable outcome could have been achieved through direct professional services for DF. However, in an era of tight budgets, it is highly unlikely that labor-intensive professional work of this sort can be provided. Furthermore, the 6 hours of reimbursed professional consulting time contributed to improvement in DF's cognitive and verbal competence (which was the result of approximately 100 hours of deliberately focused interaction with his parents during that time), to the parents' satisfaction in interacting with their son, and to their growing confidence that they were capable of dealing with a wide variety of challenges that would inevitably arise as their son progressed through the developmental years. In effect, 6 hours of professional time generated several hundred hours of high-quality intervention and ongoing problem solving for DF during his years at home with his parents.

Summary

The goal of rehabilitation is to help people with disability to re-establish competence so that they can achieve the goals that they have set for themselves. An important means to that end is to ensure competence in everyday people so that they can readily use everyday interactions to facilitate development of generalizable skills and competence in the individual with disability.

Rehabilitation professionals who work with children and adolescents with TBI are well advised to create and maintain a vision of a world in which the child with disability is surrounded by people who are informed, competent, optimistic, flexible, and creative, who communicate effectively, and who are enthusiastic and effective problem solvers. This vision will be realized only if specialists in rehabilitation enthusiastically embrace the role of collaborative consultant, a role that may not be traditionally associated with their discipline. In this chapter, we have highlighted themes and practices that are critical if professionals are to play this role effectively.

References

Beardshaw V, Towell D (1990). Assessment and Case Management: Implications for the Implementation of "Caring People." London: King's Fund Institute.

Bernstein GS (1982). Training behavior change agents: a conceptual review. Behav Ther 13;1.

Bogdan R, Taylor S, DeGrande B, Haynes S (1974). Let them eat programs: attendants' perspectives and programming. J Health Soc Behav 15;142.

Booth SR, Fairbank DW (1984). Videotape feedback as a behavior management technique. Behav Disord 9;55.

Christopher JJ, Hansen DJ, MacMillan VM (1991). Effectiveness of a peer-helper intervention to increase children's social interaction: generalization, maintenance, and social validity. Behav Modif 15;22.

Coggins TE (1991). Putting the context back into assessment. Top Lang Disord 11;43.

Condeluci A (1991). Interdependence: The Route to Community. Orlando, FL: Deutsch.

Dunst C, Trivette C, Deal A (1988). Enabling and Empowering Families. Cambridge, MA: Brookline Books.

Dunst CJ, Deal AG (1992). Early intervention practitioners to work effectively with families. Fam Involve 5;25.

Dunst CJ, Johanson XX, Trivette CM, Hamby D (1991). Family oriented early interventions policies and practices: family centered or not? Except Child 58;115.

Dunst CJ, Trivette CM, Gordon NJ, Pletcher LL (1989). Building and Mobilizing Informal Family Support Networks. In GHS Singer, LK Irvin (eds), Support for Caregiving Families: Enabling Positive Adaptation to Disability. Baltimore: Paul H. Brookes, 121.

Elkinson LL, Elkinson N (1989). Collaborative consulting: improving parent-teacher communication. Acad Ther January;261.

Feeney TJ, Ylvisaker M (1995). Choice and routine: antecedent behavioral interventions for adolescents with severe traumatic brain injury. J Head Trauma Rehabil 10(3);67.

Gans JS (1987). Facilitating Staff/Patient Interaction in Rehabilitation. In B Caplan (ed), Rehabilitation Psychology Desk Reference. Gaithersburg, MD: Aspen, 185.

Giangreco MF, Cloninger CJ, Iverson VS (1993). Choosing Options and Accommodations for Children (COACH): A Guide to Planning Inclusive Education. Baltimore: Paul H. Brookes.

Hagren D, Rogan D, Murphy S (1992). Facilitating natural supports in the workplace: strategies for support consultants. J Rehabil 58;29.

Harris K (1990). Meeting Diverse Needs Through Collaborative Consultation. In W Stainback, S Stainback (eds), Support Networks for Inclusive Schooling. Baltimore: Paul H. Brookes, 139.

Hilton A, Henderson CJ (1993). Parent involvement: a best practice or forgotten practice? Educ Train Ment Retard 28;199.

Kasier A, McWorther C (eds) (1990). Preparing Personnel to Work with Persons with Severe Disabilities. Baltimore: Paul H. Brookes.

Kern L, Dunlap G, Clarke S, et al. (1992). Effects of a videotape feedback package on the peer interactions of children with serious behavioral and emotional challenges. J Appl Behav Anal 25;355.

Lakoff G, Johnson M (1980). Metaphors We Live By. Chicago: University of Chicago Press.

Landis S, Peeler J (1990). What Have We Noticed as We've Tried to Assist People One Person at a Time? Chillicothe, OH: Ohio Safeguards.

Mount B, Zwernik K (1988). It's Never Too Early, It's Never Too Late (pub. no. 421-88-109). St. Paul, MN: Metropolitan Council.

Nisbet J (ed) (1992). Natural Supports in School, at Work, and in the Community for People with Severe Disabilities. Baltimore: Paul H. Brookes.

O'Brien J, Lyle C (1987). Framework for Accomplishment. Lithonia, GA: Responsive Systems Associates.

Powers LE, Singer GHS, Stevens T, Sowers J (1992). Behavioral parent training in home and community generalization settings. Educ Train Ment Retard 27;13.

Provencal G (1987). Culturing Commitment. In S Taylor, D Biklen, J Kroll (eds), Community Integration for People with Severe Disabilities. New York: Teachers College, 67.

Self H, Benning T, Marston D, Magnusson D (1991). Cooperative teaching project: a model for students at risk. Except Child 58;26.

Singley M, Anderson J (1989). The Transfer of Cognitive Skill. Cambridge, MA: Harvard University.

Smull MW, Harrison S (1992). Supporting People with Severe Reputations in the Community. Alexandria, VA: National Association of State Mental Retardation Program Directors.

Stainback S, Stainback W (1990). Facilitating Support Networks. In W Stainback, S Stainback (eds), Support Networks for Inclusive Schooling. Baltimore: Paul H. Brookes, 25.

Stokes TF, Baer DM (1977). An implicit technology of generalization. J Appl Behav Anal 10;349.

Thousand J, Villa R (1990). Strategies for educating learners with severe disabilities within their local home schools and communities. Focus Except Child 23;1.

Timm MA (1993). The regional intervention program: family treatment by family members. Behav Disord 19;34.

Van Kleek A (1994). Potential cultural bias in training parents as conversational partners with their children who have delays in language development. Am J Speech Lang Pathol 3;67.

Walther M, Beate D (1991). The effect of videotape feedback on the on-task behavior of a student with emotional/behavioral disorders. Educ Treat Child 14;53.

Wetzel RJ, Hoschouer RL (1984). Residential Teaching Communities. Dallas: Scott, Foresman.

Ylvisaker M, Feeney T (1994). Communication and behavior: collaboration between speech-language pathologists and behavioral psychologists. Top Lang Disord 15(1);37.

Ylvisaker M, Feeney T (1996). Executive functions after traumatic brain injury: supported cognition and self-advocacy. Semin Speech Lang 17;217.

Ylvisaker M, Feeney TJ, Urbanczyk B (1993). Developing a Positive Communication Culture for Rehabilitation: Communication Training for Staff and Family Members. In CJ Durgin, ND Schmidt, LJ Fryer (eds), Staff Development and Clinical Intervention in Brain Injury Rehabilitation. Gaithersburg, MD: Aspen, 57.

Appendix 20-1

Alternative Ways of Understanding the Relationship Between Rehabilitation Professionals and the Individuals They Serve

Physician-Patient Model (Medical Model)

In the medical model, the rehabilitation specialist functions like a surgeon (Figure 20A-1).

Goals: The basic goals are to diagnose and cure a disease or disorder that is *in* the patient. The focus is on illness or deficits.

Power, authority, decision making: All are assumed by the professional. This is an *expert* model. The professional is the expert, sets the goals, and makes the decisions. The patient's job is to comply and get well.

Process: The professional diagnoses the disease or disorder and prescribes a cure or remedial program. The patient's job is to comply with the curative process.

Values: The technical expertise of the professional is positively valued. Illness and disability are negatively valued.

Relationship: The relationship is 100% asymmetric and paternalistic. The patient plays the sick role and is not expected to play a positive or active role in the process of cure. The patient accepts little responsibility for the outcome and is excused from fault or blame while sick.

Setting: Services (versus supports) are generally delivered in highly specialized medical or rehabilitative treatment settings. However, the setting is not the critical feature of this model. Medical-model services can be delivered in any setting.

Stereotypic utterance: "This battery of tests not only yields a diagnosis and a prognosis but also contributes to the development of a treatment plan."

Trainer-Trainee Model (Behavioral Model)

In the behavioral model, the rehabilitation specialist functions like an animal trainer (Figure 20A-2).

Goal: The basic goal is to equip the trainee with a set of behaviors selected by the trainer and that will enable the trainee to accomplish specific tasks successfully. This also tends to be a *deficit* model, the goal being remediation of deficits or extinction of undesirable behaviors. As with the medical model, the problem is *in* the trainee: The individual lacks necessary behaviors or skills.

Power, authority, decision making: All are assumed by the trainer. Like the medical model, this is an *expert* model. The trainer is the expert, and the trainee is expected to comply.

Process: The trainer identifies present and absent behaviors in relevant contexts, identifies relevant goals and objectives, prescribes a regimen of exercises, and engages the trainee in this practice. The trainee imitates and practices.

Values: The technical expertise of the trainer is positively valued. The lack of skill in the trainee is negatively valued.

Relationship: The relationship is 100% asymmetric and paternalistic.

Setting: Traditionally, training has been delivered in specialized training settings, such as treatment rooms and behavior units. Increasingly, behaviorally oriented clinicians have come to realize that training must occur in settings in which the behavior or skill is needed. The setting is not the most critical feature of the model.

Other: In the developmental disabilities model (which includes much of the trainer-trainee model), families are increasingly seen as possessing power and decision-making authority; the focus is increasingly on community supports versus remedial services; and supports are increasingly provided in natural community settings versus institutional settings.

Stereotypic utterance: "When the client achieves 90% mastery on 3 consecutive days, we will move on to the next step in the training hierarchy at the acquisition phase."

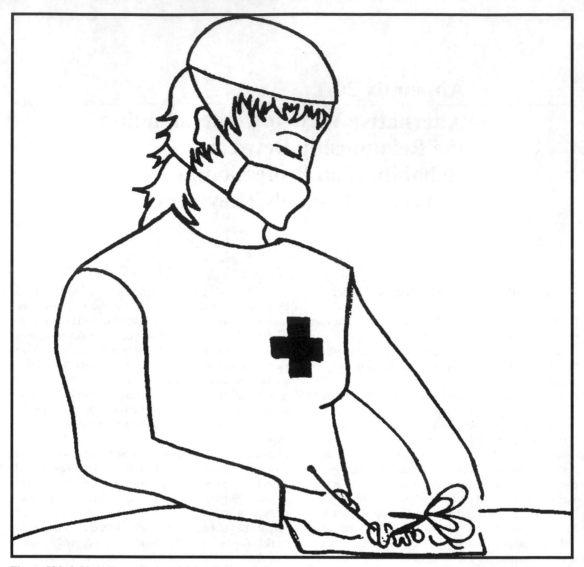

Figure 20A-1. Physician-patient model (medical model).

Teacher-Student Model (Educational Model)

In the educational model, the rehabilitation specialist functions like a teacher (Figure 20A-3).

Goal: The basic goal is to equip the student with new knowledge and skills. It can be a *deficit* model (the goal being to eliminate ignorance) or a *strength* model (the goal being to increase and expand existing knowledge and skill).

Power, authority, decision making: Power, authority, and decision making are generally assumed by the teacher, making this another *expert* model. The teacher sets the goals, determines the curriculum, identifies the learning tasks, and monitors and evaluates performance.

Process: The teacher identifies the student's level of knowledge and skill, selects a curriculum (goals, sequenced objectives, and learning tasks), and provides instruction. The student's role is to comply and thereby learn.

Values: The knowledge and expertise of the teacher are positively valued. The ignorance of the student is negatively valued. However, students are valued for their intelligence, potential, effort, initiative, compliance, achievement, and the like.

Relationship: The relationship has traditionally been asymmetric and paternalistic.

Setting: The service is generally delivered in a specialized educational setting.

Stereotypic utterance: "I will explain this concept today in class; I expect you to do the workbook exercises as a homework assignment."

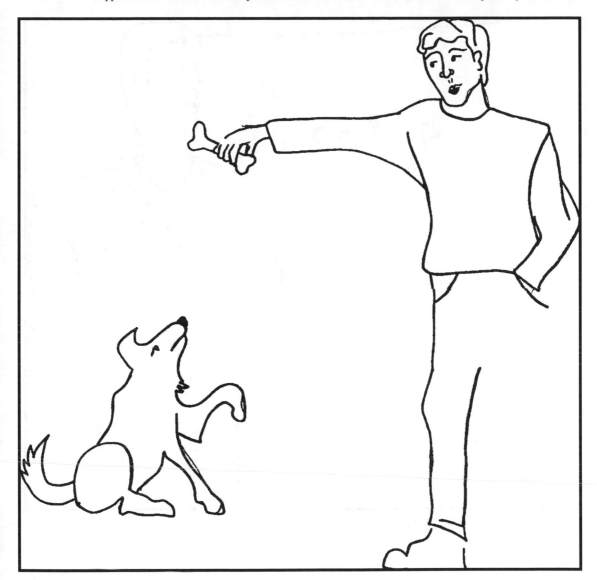

Figure 20A-2. Trainer-trainee model (behavioral model).

Mentor-Student Model

In the mentor model, the rehabilitation specialist functions like a mentor (Figure 20A-4).

Goals: The broad goal is to equip the student (or "disciple") with more than knowledge and skills. In addition, the mentor seeks to promote the student's development of wisdom, self-confidence, autonomy, and other personal characteristics. It is a *strength* model, in which the mentor helps the student to capitalize maximally on strengths.

Power, authority, decision making: Power, authority, and decision making are initially assumed by the mentor but quickly are passed on to the student. Given

resources for learning, the student must accept responsibility for growth and take the initiative in learning from the mentor.

Process: In addition to standard instruction, the mentor models expert performance and the student attempts to be like the model (mentor) in every way possible. Often the student does things that the mentor does without (initially) understanding why.

Values: The knowledge, skill, and wisdom of the mentor are highly prized by the student. The student is valued as a developing expert.

Relationship: The relationship is evolving and dynamic, with the mentor encouraging rapid development of independence and autonomy. Mentors are not only teachers

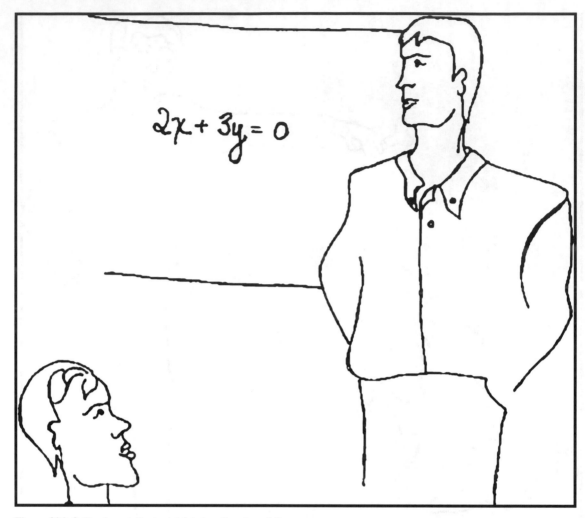

$$2x + 3y = 0$$

Figure 20A-3. Teacher-student model (educational model).

but also heroes to and sometimes friends of the student. This relationship is the key to this model.

Setting: The process generally occurs in settings that are natural in relation to the mentor's expert activity. However, the setting is not the critical feature of this model.

Stereotypic utterance: "You have the tools; do it!"

Master Craftsperson–Apprentice Model

In the master craftsperson–apprentice model, the rehabilitation specialist functions like a master cabinetmaker (Figure 20A-5).

Goals: The goal is to equip the apprentice with the skills and values necessary to produce a product well.

Power, authority, decision making: Initially, power and decision making are assumed by the master, with the exception of the apprentice's long-term goal, which is set

by himself or herself. However, as quickly as possible, autonomy is fostered in the apprentice.

Process: The master takes on an apprentice who has set for himself or herself a goal of being like the master. The master models the skills of the trade and encourages and coaches the apprentice to perform similarly. Teaching occurs within the context of the functional, productive activity at which the apprentice wishes to become skilled.

Values: The skill of the master craftsperson is valued. The evolving skill of the apprentice is also valued.

Relationship: As in the case of mentors and students, the relationship is evolving and dynamic. The master craftsperson encourages rapid development of independence and autonomy. The apprentice often tries to be like the master in ways that extend far beyond the specific skills needed to produce the product.

Setting: The process typically occurs in a setting that is natural in relation to the activity of the craftsperson.

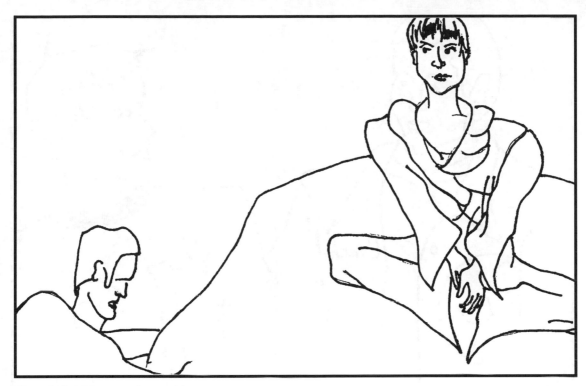

Figure 20A-4. Mentor-student model.

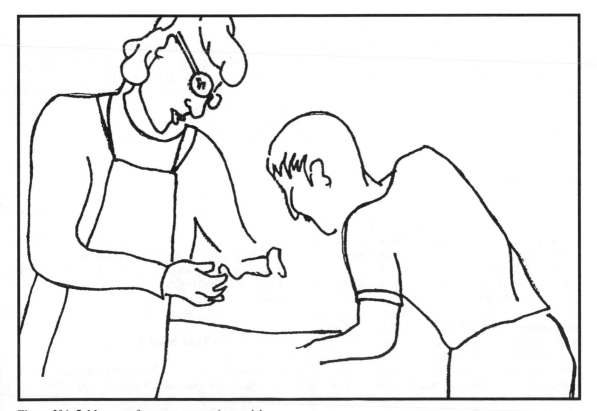

Figure 20A-5. Master craftsperson–apprentice model.

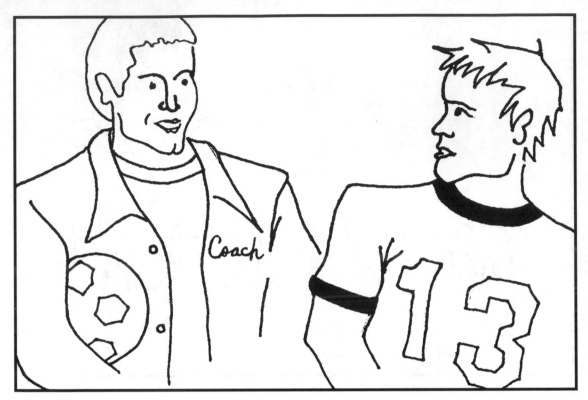

Figure 20A-6. Coach-athlete model.

Stereotypic utterance: "I think we've done a good job with the outline. Why don't you go ahead and work on the introduction section by yourself? Let me know if you have problems; we can work on those together."

Coach-Athlete Model

In the coach-athlete model, the rehabilitation specialist functions like a coach (Figure 20A-6).

Goals: The athlete's goal is to improve skills and achieve personal success and, if relevant, team success.

Power, authority, decision making: The athlete decides which sport to pursue. Within the context of a team, the relationship is asymmetric, as the coach reserves most decision-making functions.

Process: The coach teaches skills (e.g., batting practice) and develops the athlete's capacities (e.g., weight lifting) in specialized teaching or training sessions. Practice activities become increasingly gamelike, with the coach offering verbal instruction, modeling, feedback, and encouragement as the athlete performs, and creating opportunities for the athlete to practice in real competition. (These activities, interactions, and opportunities are the critical features of this model.) The coach also takes responsibility for motivating the athlete, if that is necessary.

Values: The knowledge, skill and athletic history of the coach are valued. The skill, capacity, hard work, and sportsmanship of the athlete are also valued. This is a *capacity* model in that the focus is on an individual's capabilities, not deficits.

Relationship: The relationship is largely asymmetric and paternalistic, without, however, embodying the negative attributions of the medical and training models.

Setting: The coach might initially teach skills in a practice setting. However, the most critical aspects of coaching occur under gamelike conditions.

Stereotypic utterance: "You did a great job of talking on the phone! There were just a couple of times you forgot your targets and stuttered. Listen to this tape . . . Okay, how about a couple of quick trial runs, paying close attention to the targets? Then I know you'll be ready to make the big call about which you've been so anxious."

Consultant-Client Model

In the consultant-client model, the rehabilitation specialist functions like a business consultant (Figure 20A-7).

Goals: Clients engage professional consultants to help them achieve whatever goals they set for themselves.

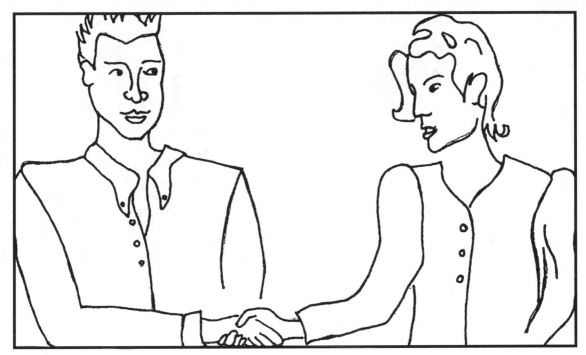

Figure 20A-7. Consultant-client model.

Power, authority, decision making: Power and authority for making decisions reside with the client. The consultant simply provides technical assistance or decision-making support, which is the critical feature of this model. In this respect, this model is distinct from all others. It is a *strength* model, embodying a symmetric relationship.

Process: The client recognizes a need and contracts with a consultant to help him or her address the need. The consultant uses special expertise to help the client achieve the targeted goal. This may involve working directly with the client or with other significant people (e.g., the client's employers, family, teachers). If the consultant is unsuccessful, the client disengages that consultant and finds another.

Values: Individuals with disability are valued in the same way that one would value anybody else. Professionals are valued to the extent that they can play a competent consulting role. Institutional services and the medical model of services are perceived with skepticism and restricted to a narrow domain of issues that necessitate institutional medical management.

Relationship: Interdependence is highlighted as the critical relationship between people with disability and others, including professionals. Thus, this is a symmetric and nonpaternalistic relationship.

Setting: Services are delivered wherever the client wants them delivered, generally in the setting in which the client needs help. However, the setting is not necessarily a critical feature of this model.

Other: The consultant-client model of professional supports is advocated in the independent living movement. The client (e.g., individual with physical disability) sets goals and makes decisions, hires and supervises professionals or paraprofessionals who may be able to help the individual achieve self-determined goals, and decides when the service or support should end.

Stereotypic utterance: "Our first meeting will include a conversation about your goals and the obstacles as you perceive them. We can then make a decision about a role that I might play in helping you achieve those goals."

Counselor-Client Model

In the counselor-client model, the rehabilitation specialist functions like a counselor (Figure 20A-8).

Goals: There are many possible counseling relationships. For our purposes, assume that the basic goal is to help clients achieve sufficient self-understanding and adjustment needed to pursue effectively their primary and realistic goals.

Power, authority, decision making: Power and authority reside with the client. The counselor does not assume the right to tell clients what their goals should be or specifically what they should do.

Process: Counseling processes vary. However, generally the counselor attempts to engage the client in discussion or expose the client to experiences that lead to insight and personal growth.

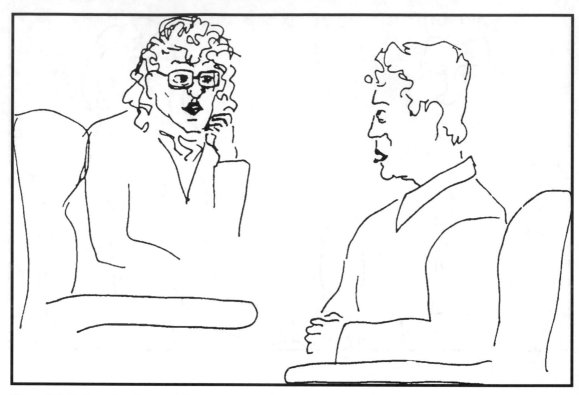

Figure 20A-8. Counselor-client model.

Values: The wisdom and insight of the counselor are valued. The potential strength of the client is also valued. This is a *strength* model.

Relationship: The relationship initially is asymmetric. However, the goal is to create a symmetric relationship.

Setting: Traditionally, counseling occurs in a specialized counseling place. The setting is not a critical feature of the model.

Stereotypic utterance: "What I think I hear you saying is . . ."

Parent-Child Model

In the parent-child model, the rehabilitation specialist functions like a parent (Figure 20A-9).

Goals: The goal is to nurture and protect the child.

Power, authority, decision making: Power and authority reside with the parent. Parents reserve the right to set goals for their children, direct children to do what is necessary to achieve the goals, and restrict their activities to protect them from physical, emotional, or cultural harm.

Process: Parents make judgments about what is best for their child, serve as the child's advocate, encourage growth and development, and protect the child against all real and perceived threats.

Values: When children are young, parents value the child's health, safety, and happiness as well as the child's achievement of important developmental milestones.

Relationship: The relationship is asymmetric and paternalistic or maternalistic.

Setting: Parenting occurs in homes and other natural settings.

Stereotypic utterance: "Honey, I'll never let anything or anybody hurt you; I just want you to be happy."

Figure 20A-9. Parent-child model.

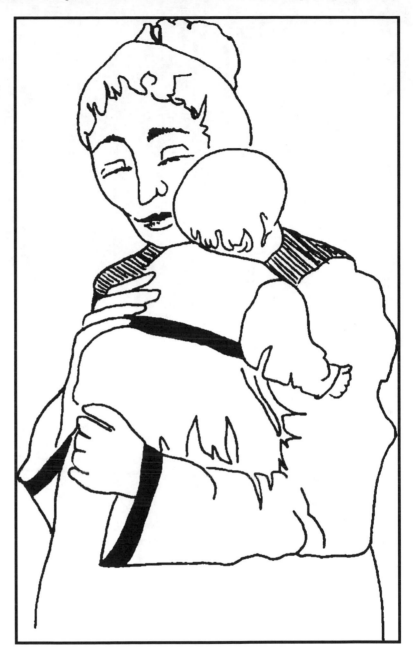

Appendix 20-2

Rehabilitation Staff: Communication and Behavioral Competencies

Communication Competencies

Communicating with Patients or Clients

Content: The staff member will:
- ❑ Talk comfortably with patients about topics that are of interest to them
- ❑ Use a vocabulary that is meaningful
- ❑ Use vocabulary that is adequately concrete yet respectful of each patient's age
- ❑ Use language that is culturally sensitive
- ❑ Give information needed to keep patients oriented

Form: The staff member will:
- ❑ Use gestures, writing, and physical prompts if necessary
- ❑ Use a natural tone of voice and inflection
- ❑ Repeat information if necessary
- ❑ Use short sentences if necessary to ensure understanding
- ❑ Give adequate processing time between messages
- ❑ Use simple grammar if necessary
- ❑ Talk clearly

Partner encouragement: The staff member will:
- ❑ Initiate topics that are of interest to patients
- ❑ Use appropriate prompts to encourage communication
- ❑ Give patients time to respond
- ❑ Give patients words if they are struggling
- ❑ Respond to patients' verbal and nonverbal communication
- ❑ Encourage nonverbal communication
- ❑ Offer choices whenever possible
- ❑ Seek confirmation of patients' understanding

Source: Adapted with permission from M Ylvisaker, T Feeney, B Urbanczyk (1992). Developing a Positive Communication Culture for Rehabilitation. In C Durgin, J Fryer, N Schmidt (eds), Brain Injury Rehabilitation: Clinical Intervention and Staff Development Techniques. Gaithersburg, MD: Aspen.

- ❑ Reinforce (e.g., through additional conversation time, praise) successful communication attempts
- ❑ Avoid ridiculing, teasing, or punishing inappropriate or unsuccessful communication

Communication environment: The staff member will:
- ❑ Minimize distractions
- ❑ Maintain a patient's attention when communicating (e.g., redirect as necessary; use the patient's name; touch the patient to gain attention if appropriate)
- ❑ Interact in a familiar setting
- ❑ Control the number of people present

Communicating respect: The staff member will:
- ❑ Actively encourage patients' participation in treatment planning at the level at which they are capable of such participation
- ❑ Avoid talking about patients in their presence
- ❑ Avoid a condescending style (e.g., baby talk) and condescending words (e.g., "sweetie," "honey")
- ❑ Communicate respect directly (e.g., "I am sure that it is difficult for an intelligent person like yourself to accept some of our rules.")
- ❑ Use polite requests rather than abrupt commands
- ❑ Choose an appropriate time and place to discuss personal issues
- ❑ Pay attention to patients' emotional states and communicate to them that their feelings are understood and are appropriate
- ❑ Communicate in a culturally sensitive manner
- ❑ Never punish, ridicule, or demean patients' atypical behavior
- ❑ Use humor that is appropriate and meaningful to the individual

Communicating with Family Members

Content: The staff member will:
- ❑ Actively invite family members to identify their own concerns and interests and avoid making assumptions about the family members' concerns and interests

❏ Actively seek from family members information about the patient that will be useful for the treatment team
❏ Provide information to families that will help them to stay informed about their family member's care
❏ Clearly explain facility programs, treatment regimens, staff roles, family roles in rehabilitation, and other related matters

Form: The staff member will:
❏ Use meaningful vocabulary and avoid jargon
❏ Speak clearly and use natural inflection
❏ Use illustrations and repetition as needed to ensure comprehension
❏ Communicate openness, warmth, flexibility, and humor (if appropriate)
❏ Use culturally sensitive language
❏ Use techniques of active listening
❏ Use effective and encouraging coaching techniques during family training

Encouraging family participation and communication: The staff member will:
❏ Actively invite family members' participation in assessment, goal setting, and intervention
❏ Actively invite expressions of concern and family problem solving around treatment issues
❏ Act on family recommendations unless these are harmful to the patient
❏ Be available to family members to discuss their concerns

Communication environment: The staff member will:
❏ Minimize distractions and interruptions during interaction with family members
❏ Use a private setting to discuss confidential or personal issues

Communicating respect: The staff member will:
❏ Take family members' questions and recommendations seriously and act on them unless contraindicated by the patient's needs
❏ Avoid a condescending or self-righteous manner in communicating with families
❏ Communicate genuine interest in and concern for family members' issues
❏ Respond promptly to family letters or calls
❏ Avoid ridiculing or devaluing a family member's behavior
❏ Respect racial, cultural, ethnic, and religious differences
❏ Respect the family's right to self-determination (freedom of choice)

Communicating with Other Staff

Content: The staff member will:
❏ Provide other staff with information that is relevant, useful, reliable, and accurate

❏ Ask relevant questions of other staff (including supervisors) regarding patients, policies, treatment, and other issues
❏ Describe minor concerns to supervisors before they become major concerns

Form: The staff member will:
❏ Speak clearly and concisely, avoiding professional jargon
❏ Use natural inflection and tone of voice
❏ Avoid defensive responses, particularly in connection with professional "turf" issues
❏ Demonstrate initiative in interdisciplinary discussions and, at the same time, patience, flexibility, and a cooperative attitude
❏ Be supportive of colleagues
❏ Maintain perspective and a sense of humor, particularly during times of stress
❏ Give instructions to subordinates in a respectful manner

Partner encouragement: The staff member will:
❏ Initiate interaction with other staff
❏ Initiate problem-solving discussions, actively seeking others' opinions
❏ Actively seek out whatever guidance is necessary
❏ Use techniques of active listening
❏ Make time for communication with other staff
❏ Make expectations of others clear
❏ Maintain active communication during stressful times
❏ Freely admit mistakes

Communication environment: The staff member will:
❏ Choose the correct time and place to discuss issues, particularly confidential issues
❏ Be respectful of other staff members' needs for work time and quiet in a busy workplace

Communicating respect: The staff member will:
❏ Treat all staff with respect, fairness, and courtesy, regardless of academic degrees, professional training, or level of employment
❏ Assume that all staff members' time with patients is important
❏ Take others' opinions seriously

Behavioral Competencies

The staff member will:
❏ Facilitate positive behavioral routines for the individual with TBI:
   ❏ Create a concrete, meaningful daily routine (events, sequences, people, places, activities)
   ❏ Create positive setting events (external and internal) before requesting difficult tasks
   ❏ Create positive behavioral momentum before requesting difficult tasks

❏ Create as many opportunities for choice as possible; teach choice making if necessary
❏ Create positive scripts and roles for the individual
❏ Eliminate chronic behavioral provocations
❏ Ensure that the patient is capable of performing all requested activities

❏ Model, prompt, and reward positive communication alternatives to challenging behavior:
   ❏ Collaboratively identify the communication intent underlying challenging behavior (e.g., *escape* task, person, place; *access* activity, person, place, object)
   ❏ Operationally define the communication behavior(s) selected to replace the challenging behaviors
   ❏ Collaboratively decide when it is acceptable to respond affirmatively to the new positive communication acts for escape or access
   ❏ In appropriate contexts, prompt the positive communication alternative and reward that alternative with escape or access as appropriate. Ensure that a large number of successful learning trials occur daily
   ❏ Fade cues and prompts or increase the variety of contexts and tasks in which the child is willing to use positive communication alternatives

❏ If necessary, teach relevant social knowledge (rules, roles, routines, and scripts), including specific pragmatic communication acts
❏ If necessary, teach social perception and social decision making
❏ Prevent behavioral crises:
   ❏ Eliminate known provocation for behavioral crises

❏ Eliminate known environmental stressors (e.g., noise, activity levels)
❏ Separate incompatible individuals
❏ Avoid threats
❏ Avoid power conflicts
❏ Avoid demands that cannot be met
❏ Distract or redirect individuals to neutral activities in the earliest stages of behavioral outbursts
❏ In the case of a mild behavioral episode, remain focused on the task, thereby directing the individual back to task

❏ Manage behavioral crises:
   ❏ Stay calm
   ❏ Appear confident
   ❏ Help the person identify feelings
   ❏ Be a helper, not an antagonist
   ❏ Seek help
   ❏ Keep others safe
   ❏ Avoid suggesting negative behavior (e.g., "Don't hit")
   ❏ Avoid threatening with consequences
   ❏ Avoid presenting commands as questions or pleas
   ❏ Avoid having more than one person talk simultaneously
   ❏ Avoid escalating the individual's behavior by increasing demands
   ❏ Avoid physical interaction or confrontation
   ❏ Avoid attempting to "teach lessons" during a crisis
   ❏ Avoid rehashing the crisis or re-escalating the individual's behavior

❏ Self-management: If possible, teach the individual to manage his or her own antecedents

Appendix 20-3

Outline of a General Communication Training Session

I. Introduction: motivation

A. *Social-environmental approach:* The trainer explains the importance of a social-environmental approach to rehabilitation from brain injury and the role of communication in that approach.

B. *Roles:* The trainer explains everybody's role in this approach and highlights the importance of family members and direct-care staff—that is, those individuals who interact most frequently with the patients or clients. The trainer makes clear that everybody's role is the same with respect to establishing a communication environment.

C. *Payoff:* The trainer highlights the payoffs that flow from a positive communication environment:
   1. Fewer problematic behavioral issues
   2. Better outcome for clients
   3. More satisfying interaction among staff, family members, and clients

II. Introduction: content

A. *Communication*
   1. Communication is pervasive; it is not limited to speech and language. Every behavior or absence of behavior is potentially communicative.
   2. *Exercises*
      a. Given one simple message (e.g., "I am hungry"), the group lists 15 or more distinct behaviors that could communicate

that message. The point: Any behavior—or absence of behavior—can communicate in the correct context.

      b. Given a single behavior (e.g., persistent screaming), the group lists 15 or more messages that this behavior might communicate and the contextual evidence that might help decipher the message. The point: A given behavior might have many possible meanings. If we are committed to a positive communication culture, we will work hard to interpret correctly the communicative intent of the behavior we observe.

   3. Communication is powerful. The trainer highlights the many functions or purposes served by communicative behavior (with or without language) and the extraordinary frustration associated with communication deficits.

   4. Communication is important. A positive communication culture contributes in many ways to recovery and to everybody's quality of life. The trainer highlights the components of a positive communication culture.

   5. Communication problems after TBI are common. The trainer briefly highlights the variety of communication challenges that individuals are likely to experience at various stages of recovery after TBI.

B. *Relation between cognition and communication*
   1. Brainstorm: How would severe confusion and disorientation manifest themselves in communication in this environment?
   2. Brainstorm: How would cognitive disorganization manifest itself in communication in this environment?

Source: Reprinted with permission from M Ylvisaker, T Feeney, B Urbanczyk (1992). Developing a Positive Communication Culture for Rehabilitation. In C Durgin, J Fryer, N Schmidt (eds), Brain Injury Rehabilitation: Clinical Intervention and Staff Development Techniques. Gaithersburg, MD: Aspen.

3. Brainstorm: How would weak attention and memory manifest themselves in communication in this environment?

C. *Relation between behavior and communication*

1. Brainstorm: How would severe disinhibition manifest itself in communication in this environment?

2. Brainstorm: How would impaired initiation manifest itself in communication in this environment?

3. Brainstorm: How can miscommunication or inappropriate staff communication create behavioral problems? Staff-family interaction problems?

4. Brainstorm: How can effective communication prevent behavioral problems? Staff-family interaction problems?

III. **Initial competency training**

A. *Communicative competencies*

1. The trainer introduces the five categories of communicative competence: form of communication; content of communication; environment for communication; techniques for encouraging communication; techniques for communicating respect.

2. The trainer discusses the implications of these general areas of competence for interaction between staff and patient or client, staff and family, and staff and staff.

B. *General outline of competency training*

1. Identifying positive and negative aspects of communication; explaining communication breakdowns

a. Select an important communication competency and context.

b. Provide an exaggerated negative model— that is, one in which the communicative competency is not present, with clearly negative consequences. This can be done using videotaped or role-played models. An exaggerated negative model is used for two reasons:

(1) It can be funny and attention grabbing.

(2) Starting with positive models often communicates that there is only one way to negotiate a given communication task but, in fact, there are many, depending on one's communication style.

c. Practice interpreting the communication in the model. Practice explaining the communication breakdown from cognitive and behavioral perspectives and from the perspective of failures at both the giving and receiving end of the communication.

d. Continue this practice in identifying positive and negative aspects of communication and explaining communication breakdowns until all the group members have had an opportunity to contribute and feel comfortable with the process.

2. Practicing positive alternatives

a. After viewing and discussing a negative model of interaction, list a variety of positive alternatives to the unsuccessful interaction.

b. Practice: The larger group must be divided into dyads or small groups for this practice. The trainers should move among the groups, providing suggestions, encouragement, and other coaching assistance. The trainer's goal is the trainee's acquisition of the targeted competencies, within the context of the individual's preexisting communication style. The training will be resisted and ultimately unsuccessful if the implicit demand is that staff and family members fundamentally revise their manner of relating to other people.

c. Dyads who are particularly good at illustrating a particular competency can be asked to role-play the competency for the entire group.

d. Dyads or small groups can also be asked to create their own negative model of a new competency and, subsequently, a positive alternative. Facility with both types of role play indicates clear mastery of the competency in question.

e. This supervised practice should continue for the duration of the training session.

IV. **Summary.** The trainer should close by highlighting the forest in the trees: A vision of a positive communication culture and its benefits for clients, family members, and staff.

Appendix 20-4
Sample Vignettes for Role Playing in Staff Communication Training

Notes to the trainer:

1. During competency-based communication training, vignettes such as these can be shown on videotape or role-played live. They are designed to present exaggerated negative models of communication. The rationale for using negative models is presented in the text. When the vignette is completed, trainees (a) identify as many communication and behavior management errors as possible, (b) explain why the staff's communication is inappropriate, (c) describe the cognitive and communicative characteristics of the patient that make the staff's communication inappropriate, (d) brainstorm about positive alternatives to these negative models, and (e) practice positive alternatives with trainer coaching.

2. The three vignettes that follow are merely illustrations. After two or three vignettes have been presented by the trainer, the trainees can create and act out their own negative model scripts, given a small set of communicative competencies that they are to violate in the vignette.

Vignette 1: The Know-It-All Therapist

Main points: One should include alert patients in problem solving. One should avoid talking about patients in their presence, at least without permission to do so. One should avoid blaming patients. One should speak respectfully to other staff. One should avoid jargon.

Script: A nursing assistant (NA) pushes an alert but physically impaired patient in a wheelchair into a physical therapist's (PT's) office.

Source: Reprinted with permission from M Ylvisaker, T Feeney, B Urbanczyk (1992). Developing a Positive Communication Culture for Rehabilitation. In C Durgin, J Fryer, N Schmidt (eds), Brain Injury Rehabilitation: Clinical Intervention and Staff Development Techniques. Gaithersburg, MD: Aspen.

NA: Excuse me, but Jane's got a problem with the footrest of her wheelchair. Her foot constantly comes off and then she complains. It's driving us crazy.

PT: (*checking the footrest and not greeting or paying attention to Jane*) Well, Jane can't seem to follow simple rules, can she? I've told her a hundred times to keep her foot on the footrest. She doesn't know what's good for her. But, you know—you probably won't understand this—but she does have significant hypertonus in her lowers and dorsiflexion contractures that interfere with optimal positioning.

Jane: (*trying to interrupt*) Excuse me, but it's very uncomfortable.

PT: (*to Jane*) Don't interrupt! We don't have all day!" (*to the NA*) I think I'll have to just Velcro this foot down. It might hurt, but she has it coming to her for all the fuss that she has caused. It's not as though I was looking for more things to do today. This place is a zoo." (*PT walks off, muttering.*)

Positive alternative: NA invites Jane to explain the problem. PT invites Jane to give any information that she thinks is relevant. PT invites Jane to join in the problem solving. If NA and PT need to discuss Jane, they ask her in advance for her permission to discuss her situation.

Vignette 2: Orientation Group

Main points: One should give disoriented patients personally meaningful information that promotes orientation. One should avoid quizzing patients. One should respect-

463

fully help patients who have difficulty expressing themselves. One should communicate understanding of emotions. One should encourage nonverbal communication strategies.

Script: A therapist is conducting a morning orientation session for three to four disoriented patients.

Therapist:	All right, guys. Let's try to get you ready for the day. Here we go. What's the date? *(pause)* C'mon, what's the date today?
Patient 1:	*(struggling)* Wed … Wednesday
Therapist:	I didn't ask for the day, I asked for the date. John, you tell me.
John:	I think, March...
Therapist:	No, you're way off. I can't believe you guys don't know this simple stuff. Get with the program here! Don't you read the newspaper? You better find this stuff out. Okay, who's the assistant foreign minister of Iraq? Mary, do you know?
Mary:	I want to go home.
Therapist:	Enough already with this "I want to go home" stuff *(mimicking Mary's speech)*. I get sick of hearing you guys talking about home all the time. You're not going to get out of here at this rate. Besides, you should be grateful for all the help we give you. Bill, who is your occupational therapist?
Bill:	I don't know.
Therapist:	I can't believe you don't know your OT. You see her every day.
Bill:	She's . . . ah, ah, got . . . *(gestures long hair)*.
Therapist:	Bill, I asked for her name. How can you be oriented without names?
Bill:	*(getting up to leave)* Go to hell.

Positive alternative: The therapist gives meaningful, person-specific orientation information to the patients; reminds them of ways in which they can find the information (e.g., from their log books); encourages gestured answers; encourages them to help one another; and indicates understanding of the strong desire to get home.

Vignette 3: The Outburst

Main points: The way staff approach and interact with patients can either trigger or prevent behavioral outbursts; patients who lack cognitive and behavioral flexibility must be dealt with flexibly by staff.

Script: A nurse enters the room of an easily agitated patient to draw blood. The patient had not anticipated this interruption. The patient is lying in bed watching TV.

Nurse:	Jim, I need blood. Give me your arm.
Jim:	Wait till this show is done.
Nurse:	I can't wait. I'm busy. I have to do it now *(turning off the TV)*.
Jim:	*(becoming very upset)* Turn that on! Get out of my face! Nobody told me about blood. Leave me alone! Leave me alone! I'm getting out of this damn place! *(throws a magazine at the nurse)*

Positive alternative: The nurse knocks on the door, apologizes for the intrusion, and explains the unexpected need for blood. The nurse explains that it will take only a minute and then might wait for a commercial or offer options (e.g., draw blood during a commercial or after the show). The nurse might, for a few minutes, make pleasant conversation about the show. The nurse does not physically approach the patient without permission.

Index

Note: Page numbers followed by f indicate figures; page numbers followed by t indicate tables.

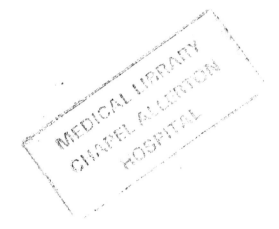